MEDICAL RADIOLOGY

Diagnostic Imaging

Springer
Berlin
Heidelberg
New York
Barcelona
Hong Kong
London
Milan
Paris
Singapore
Tokyo

C. Schiepers (Ed.)

Diagnostic Nuclear Medicine

With Contributions by

W. Becker · R. Campisi · J. J. Frost · S. S. Gambhir · D. A. Hillier · C. Hoh · F. Jamar
C. L. Johnson · F. Y. J. Keng · G. Lucignani · G. D. Luker · K. E. Luker · H. R. Nadel
J. Nuyts · D. Piwnica-Worms · V. V. Rao · H. D. Royal · H. R. Schelbert · C. Schiepers
V. Sharma · M. E. Stilwell · J. L. C. Urbain M.-C. Vekemans · K. Verbeke · A. Verbruggen
I. Virgolini · S. I. Ziegler

Series Editor's Foreword by

A. L. Baert

With 123 Figures in 159 Separate Illustrations and 36 Tables

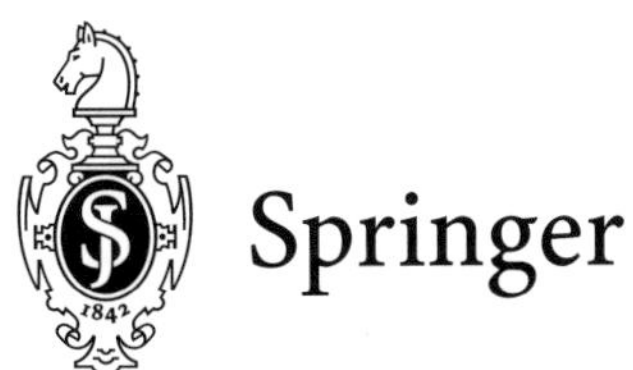

Springer

Christiaan Schiepers, MD, PhD
Associate Professor
Department of Molecular and Medical Pharmacology
UCLA School of Medicine
10833 Le Conte Avenue, AR-144 CHS
Los Angeles, CA 90095-6942
USA

MEDICAL RADIOLOGY · Diagnostic Imaging and Radiation Oncology

Continuation of
Handbuch der medizinischen Radiologie
Encyclopedia of Medical Radiology

ISBN 3-540-63467-3 Springer-Verlag Berlin Heidelberg New York

Library of Congress Cataloging-in-Publication Data.
Diagnostic nuclear medicine / C. Schiepers (ed.); with contributions by W. Becker ... [et al.] p. cm. -- (Medical radiology) Includes bibliographical references and index. ISBN 3-540-63467-3 (alk. paper) 1. Radioisotope scanning. I. Schiepers, C. (Christiaan), 1947- . II. Becker, W. W. (Wolfgang) III. Series. [DNLM: 1. Nuclear Medicine. 2. Diagnostic Imaging. 3. Radionuclide Imaging. WN 440 D536 1999] RC78.7.R4D467 1999 616.07'579--dc21 DNLM/DLC for Library of Congress 99-33012 CIP

Springer-Verlag is a company in the specialist publishing group BertelsmannSpringer

Printed in Germany

Typesetting: Verlagsservice Teichmann, Mauer

SPIN: 106 431 85 21/3135 – 5 4 3 2 1 0 – Printed on acid-free paper

Foreword

Clinical diagnosis of pathological conditions has benefited enormously during the past decade from the impressive progress achieved in diagnostic radiology and in diagnostic nuclear medicine. While diagnostic radiology is now able to provide astonishingly detailed morphological information on living human beings, nuclear medicine can reveal specific information about the function of organs and their physiopathological disturbances.

In nuclear medicine revolutionary new techniques such as PET scanning have now reached maturity. PET scanning techniques now play a major role in the detection of metastatic spread and the staging of malignant neoplasms, in the study of heart function and in many other conditions in various parts of the human body.

This volume includes the up-to-date information that nuclear medicine specialists, radiologists and other clinicians are looking for in order to allow them to provide the best possible care to their patients and to maintain their high standards of good clinical practice. It is my pleasure to congratulate the editor and all the contributing authors for their excellent contributions to this outstanding book.

The editor, Christiaan Schiepers, is a leading expert in the field of nuclear medicine. He has to be congratulated for achieving the collaboration of so many internationally known specialists on the different topics dealt with in this book.

I sincerely hope that this volume will meet the expectations of all those interested in updating their knowledge about modern nuclear medicine techniques and their potential contribution to the good practice of clinical medicine. I wish this book the same success as the previous volumes published in our series *Medical Radiology*. I would appreciate any constructive criticism that might be offered.

Leuven ALBERT L. BAERT

Preface

Imaging studies using nuclear medicine techniques have kept increasing in the past decade. Certain fields such as nuclear cardiology have diversified and stimulated development of new equipment and imaging protocols. The ever-increasing speed of computers has led to improved image quality, faster and more sophisticated software, and highly automated acquisition and processing protocols, resulting in higher patient throughput. In addition, database management, automated reporting, and tele-radiology have made higher workloads possible even with the ever-decreasing amount of money available for health care.

In this volume, current contributions in the nuclear medicine field are presented and put in perspective. The influence of molecular biology is readily appreciable and a shift from functional to biological imaging has emerged. Promising results of gene imaging and therapy are visible on the horizon and are touched upon herein.

Some have predicted the demise of nuclear medicine as a separate and independent imaging specialty. While this may be true from a certain viewpoint, such as managed care, the future of nuclear imaging physicians appears bright, if they see themselves as part of a team of specialists caring for patients. Pharmacological interventions and new radiopharmaceuticals have broadened the number of applications and increased the accuracy of available tests.

This book documents many of the advances that have been realized or are taking place at the turn of the century, and provides an update of this challenging field. It consists of three parts: clinical applications, basics and future prospects. The publishers and I are grateful to the many participants who devoted their valuable time to the contributions, granting the readers, students and professionals, an overview and taste of the field at the end of the decade of the brain. Radiologists, nuclear medicine specialists and technologists, and interested physicians should find this book useful.

Los Angeles, California — Christiaan Schiepers

Contents

1 Introduction
CHRISTIAAN SCHIEPERS 1

Clinical Applications 5

2 Neurochemical Imaging with Emission Tomography: Clinical Applications
GIOVANNI LUCIGNANI and JAMES J. FROST 7

3 Assessment of Myocardial Viability by Radionuclide Techniques
ROXANA CAMPISI, FELIX Y. J. KENG and HEINRICH R. SCHELBERT 37

4 Thromboembolism Imaging
HENRY D. ROYAL and DAVID A. HILLIER 57

5 Renal Imaging
FRANÇOIS JAMAR 79

6 Skeletal Scintigraphy
CHRISTIAAN SCHIEPERS 95

7 Imaging Infection and Inflammation
WOLFGANG BECKER 103

8 Gastrointestinal Nuclear Medicine
JEAN-LUC C. URBAIN, CYNTHIA L. JOHNSON, and MARIE-CHRISTINE M. VEKEMANS 123

9 Peptide Imaging
IRENE VIRGOLINI 135

10 Clinical Positron Imaging in Oncology
CHRISTIAAN SCHIEPERS and CARL K. HOH 159

11 Pediatric Nuclear Medicine – A Coming of Age
HELEN NADEL and MOIRA E. STILWELL 177

Basics of Scintigraphic Imaging 195

12 Radiopharmaceuticals: Recent Developments and Trends
KRISTIN VERBEKE and ALFONS VERBRUGGEN 197

13 Instrumentation and Data Acquisition
Sibylle I. Ziegler 221

14 Image Formation and Data Processing
Johan Nuyts 237

Outlook 251

15 Imaging Gene Expression: Concepts and Future Outlook
Sanjiv S. Gambhir 253

16 Imaging Gene Expression in Cancer: Functional Identification of Multidrug Resistance (MDR1) P-glycoprotein In Vivo
David Piwnica-Worms, Gary D. Luker, Kathryn E. Luker, Vallabhaneni V. Rao, and Vijay Sharma 273

17 Quo Vadis?
Christiaan Schiepers 285

Glossary 287

Subject Index 291

List of Contributors 293

1 Introduction

C. Schiepers

Contents

1.1 Introduction 1
1.2 Perspective 1
1.3 Objectives 2
1.4 Clinical Overview 2
1.5 Basics and Future of NM Imaging 3

1.1 Introduction

In the present volume of the "Medical Radiology" series the advancements in the field of nuclear medicine (NM) are presented with an emphasis on progress in the 1990s. The various contributions in this challenging imaging field, such as new tracers and equipment, modifications of existing tests, diagnostic algorithms for specific organ systems, and general applications for whole-body imaging, are discussed. Major achievements during the last decade of the 20th century were the contribution of 2-^{18}F-fluoro-2-deoxy-D-glucose (FDG) in positron imaging, receptor and peptide imaging, pharmacological augmentation to enhance the accuracy of neuro-, cardiac, renal, and hepato-biliary imaging. This progress has broadened the field and strengthened NM as a functional imaging modality.

Given these advancements and the refocusing of NM on imaging of biological processes, the question as to how we will enter the new millennium comes rapidly to mind. In order to address this question, topics were selected which are considered to be representative of the mainstream events. Our selection is aimed at elucidating key processes in cellular mechanisms of the human body, under normal conditions as well as in disease.

C. Schiepers
Department of Molecular and Medical Pharmacology, UCLA School of Medicine, 10833 Le Conte Avenue, AR-144 CHS, Los Angeles, CA 90095-6942, USA

1.2 Perspective

Nuclear medicine started as a field in which radioactive products were put to use for the benefit of mankind, e.g., thyroid scintigraphy and therapy. The performed studies in the field have fluctuated tremendously since the early years. Flow imaging of the brain was a frequent procedure in the NM clinic until CT was introduced. Later, sophisticated triggering techniques were developed and true functional imaging of cardiac function became a reality. At present, we take the results of these pioneering efforts for granted.

The next major step was the distribution of tomography over all NM facilities. Introduction of faster computers made reconstruction possible within minutes, and allowed for standardization of imaging protocols for acquisition, processing, and review. Image interpretation and reporting, as well as database management, became easy tasks with the help of computers.

The well-known techniques of whole-body scanning were reintroduced (although they never truly disappeared from the older NM clinics) and the equipment became tuned to Tc-99m as the radionuclide of choice. Radiochemistry was geared toward the Tc-99m pharmaceuticals, and kits that could easily be labeled in the lab at room temperature replaced more and more of the older products.

The main achievement, in this editor's view, is the shift of the attention, which occurred in the late 1980s and early 1990s, when NM changed from functional to biological imaging, with a major change of focus to the cellular and molecular level. The enormous strides in molecular biology (e.g., genome project), and awareness that defective genes cause disease, have revived mechanistic models of studying nature, a trend similar to the one that propelled modern physics at the turn of the past century. Two factors played an important part in this refocusing of NM: the advancements in immunology and receptor imaging, and the glucose analog FDG as a tracer of metabolic imaging.

In the present volume the interdisciplinary nature of NM imaging is emphasized: the view of clinicians, radiologists, nuclear medicine specialists, and, where appropriate, scientists and molecular biologists, is put forward to highlight their thought on development and implementation of tests to study organ function in vivo.

1.3 Objectives

This volume is meant for the general NM practitioner who wants to keep abreast of the latest clinical developments as well as the interested student and professional. This volume was not meant as a textbook, but as an addition to these readily available texts. There are three sections, the first of which deals with clinical applications. Contrary to other volumes, the clinical point of view is central and comes first, and the state of the art in the major fields is presented. In the second section, the principles upon which these scintigraphic imaging techniques are based is discussed and new trends are outlined. The progress in the past decade of this century is the main subject of this second section about basics. In the final section, the horizon of genetic imaging is explored and some of the early results useful in the clinical arena are presented.

Selection of topics in the preparation of this volume is one of the prerogatives of an editor. The emphasis has been put on clinical progress in the field as well as on new modalities that are likely to stay. The typical radiological format was chosen, i.e., review by topology, and mixed with the classic internal medicine approach of organ-system description.

In the clinical section, standard tests in neurological, cardiac, pulmonary, gastrointestinal, renal, and skeletal scintigraphy are discussed. In addition, typical multiorgan fields, such as oncology, infection, and inflammation, are subjects of detailed review.

As in any volume, choices have to be made. In this volume monoclonal antibodies are not presented in a separate chapter. Over 15 years of research have resulted in only a few applications such as granulocyte imaging, some tumor imaging applications, and thrombosis detection. The hopes were high but did not materialize as widely applicable routine clinical tests. The switch to smaller molecules, such as peptides, looks far more promising (see Chap. 9).

Positron and single photon emission imaging are dealt with both from the instrumentation point of view and the clinical applications in oncology, and, where appropriate, protocols for metabolic imaging are discussed (Chaps. 10, 12).

1.4 Clinical Overview

In the first chapters the main organ systems are presented. In Chap. 2 brain imaging is reviewed for clinical entities such as stroke, epilepsy, and degenerative disorders. Neuroreceptors and their potential in neurodegenerative disease, as well as applications in psychiatric illness, are discussed. Currently, the use of emission tomography allows assessment of cerebral blood flow, glucose utilization, oxygen metabolism, rate of incorporation of amino acids into proteins, and rate of transport of substrates into the brain. Measurement of the rate of neurotransmitter storage, release, and binding to specific receptors is possible but is not used in clinical practice yet. This possibility has raised high expectations among clinical neurologists and psychiatrists for future developments.

Dysfunctional myocardium in patients with poor left ventricular function can be caused be several mechanisms. The concepts of "hibernation" and "stunning" which both represent viable myocardium are discussed in Chap. 3. Distinction of viable myocardium from scar tissue is crucial to determine whether revascularization is a therapeutic option or not. The available clinical evidence to assess myocardial viability prior to coronary revascularization is presented. Various techniques are highlighted indicating that viability assessment will lead to the correct use of resources, with the potential of decreasing health care costs.

Pulmonary embolism is a common clinical entity, and the imaging diagnosis remains a topic of fierce debate. The emphasis on evidence-based medicine and outcome significantly affects our thinking about diagnosis and treatment. "Do we need to treat all pulmonary emboli?" and "How do we identify the patient in whom the risk of treatment is less than the risk of no treatment?" are questions posed in Chap. 4. It is the authors' firm belief that only new reasoning will allow us to make progress with diagnosis and management of pulmonary embolism.

Bone scintigraphy has been around for a long time and no new developments occurred in the 1990s. It remains an exclusively sensitive procedure for evaluating a variety of skeletal disorders. Main referrals are screening of patients with malignancy, trauma, and orthopedic problems. Sports injuries also appear to be a major indication for performing bone scans. Long ago ^{18}F-fluoride was introduced as a bone-imaging agent, which has been revived since positron emission tomography (PET) is more available. The

PET technique now allows for true regional quantification of bone blood flow.

Studies of the urinary tract are directed to quantification of renal flow and function. New tracers are discussed and compared with the older generation, and a detailed analysis is given as to how they affect the measured parameters. The addition of pharmacological augmentation became popular for several existing tests of the gastrointestinal and the GU tract. These topics are dealt with in Chaps. 5 and 8. Specific applications for pediatric NM are given in Chap. 11.

In order to localize an infectious process, we need procedures with high sensitivity in all areas of the body. The studies available and their clinical effectiveness are discussed in Chap. 7. A typical diagnostic dilemma, posed daily, is the differential diagnosis of inflammation versus infection, e.g., after a surgical procedure. A wide variety of tracers, clinical conditions, and correct way to read, interpret, and report the images, are presented.

The field of receptor imaging became popular again in the 1990s with the introduction of new peptides. Receptors are proteins which bind specific ligands and subsequently respond with a well-defined event. Historically, these radioligands have evolved from monoclonal antibodies, which are large proteins, via "molecular recognition units" to small peptides. Recognition of tumor-specific properties can be used to detect cancers, and peptide receptors appear highly expressed on tumor cells. Chapter 9 illustrates that peptides have been proven effective in clinical practice.

In the field of oncology, the 1990s showed an emerging role for the glucose analog FDG, which is the most frequently used PET radiopharmaceutical. High rates of glycolysis are found in many malignant tumor cells with increased membrane transporters and upregulated hexokinase enzymes. The uptake of FDG varies greatly for different tumor types. High uptake is usually associated with a high number of viable tumor cells and/or rapidly proliferating cells. Increased FDG uptake is not specific for neoplasms and many inflammatory processes have also increased uptake. An overview for the common cancers in the Western world is given in Chap. 10.

1.5 Basics and Future of NM Imaging

The second section of the book deals with the basics in radiopharmaceuticals, instrumentation, and image processing. The potential variety of radiopharmaceuticals which can be developed is unlimited which will keep nuclear medicine in the forefront of clinical imaging. Some NM applications will become obsolete in the future, but new tracers with different biological characteristics will be developed and will adapt the clinical diagnostic imaging possibilities.

The technological improvements of the standard gamma camera include higher spatial resolution, better uniformity, higher rate-count performance, and multidetector geometry. New hybrid devices have been manufactured for both single-photon and coincidence imaging, bringing the advantages of PET to the general NM clinic. At present, there is insufficient evidence on the routine clinical effectiveness of these devices, and the references in the clinical chapters are limited to oncology (Chap. 10). The option of combining both imaging modalities appears promising.

Computer speed tends to double per year, an exponential growth curve that will continue up to the limit set by physics. New reconstruction techniques, leading to improved image quality, are discussed and compared. The effects on quantification of tracer distribution are also discussed. In addition, simple and handy techniques for image enhancement are presented.

The third section of the volume gives an introduction to gene imaging and another chapter covers a specific example of multidrug resistance. The advances in molecular biology are making it possible to image specific molecular processes, and by inference the expression of gene(s) controlling these processes can be visualized. Conventional nuclear imaging techniques can be used by manufacturing a radiolabeled substrate which interacts with the protein of the gene of interest. More general methods are emerging to image gene expression, which is the subject of Chap. 15. Many phenomena in disease leading to altered cellular functions, which can be imaged with molecular biology assays in living animals and humans, is also a subject of Chap. 15.

Chapter 16 deals with a specific multidrug resistance characterized by the failure to respond to diverse drugs despite initial treatment with only a single drug. This refractory behavior to multiple chemotherapeutic agents has been observed in recurring tumors. Clinical data have indicated that tumors can exhibit a multidrug resistance phenotype. The molecular mechanisms of these observations and the role in the clinic is discussed. The presented evidence supports the use of ^{99m}Tc-Sestamibi and ^{99m}Tc-Tetrofosmin to image function and modulation of the multidrug resistance P-glycoprotein in vivo.

Clinical Applications

2 Neurochemical Imaging with Emission Tomography: Clinical Applications

G. Lucignani, J. J. Frost

Contents

2.1 Introduction 7
2.2 Physiologic and Biochemical Basis of Radionuclide Brain Imaging 8
2.2.1 Cerebral Blood Flow and Energy Metabolism 8
2.2.2 Neurotransmission 9
2.3 Methodology 9
2.3.1 Detection Instruments 9
2.3.2 Dynamic and Static Acquisition Procedures 9
2.3.3 Data Analysis 10
2.4 Tracers for Brain Imaging 12
2.4.1 Cerebral Blood Flow and Metabolism Tracers 12
2.4.2 Neurotransmission Function Tracers 12
2.5 Clinical Applications 13
2.6 Dementias 15
2.6.1 Cerebral Blood Flow and Metabolism in Patients with Degenerative Dementias 15
2.6.2 Neurotransmission Function in Degenerative Dementias 16
2.7 Movement Disorders 17
2.7.1 Cerebral Blood Flow and Metabolism in Movement Disorders 17
2.7.2 Neurotransmitter Function in Movement Disorders 17
2.8 Cerebrovascular Diseases 19
2.8.1 Cerebral Blood Flow and Metabolism in CVD Patients 19
2.8.2 Imaging of Neuronal Viability by Central Benzodiazepine Receptors 21
2.9 Epilepsy 21
2.9.1 Cerebral Blood Flow and Metabolism in Seizure Disorders 22
2.9.2 Neurotransmission Function in Seizure Disorders 24
2.10 Brain Tumors 25
2.10.1 Imaging of Tumor Metabolic Processes 26
2.10.2 Imaging of Cerebral Tumors by Antibodies and Receptor-Bound Tracers 27
2.10.3 Differential Diagnosis of Lymphoma and Infectious Diseases in AIDS 27
2.11 Outlook for the Future 28

G. Lucignani
Department of Nuclear Medicine, University of Milan, H.S. Raffaele, Via Olgettina 60, I-20132 Milan, Italy
J. J. Frost
Johns Hopkins Hospital, 600 N. Wolfe Street, Nelson Tower Bl-130, Baltimore, MD 21205, USA

2.1 Introduction

The assessment of neurochemical and neurophysiologic variables by emission tomography can be based on two strategies in relation to the goal to be achieved. A first approach is aimed at the assessment of basic variables related to brain functional activity and energy metabolism, such as blood flow, rates of glucose and oxygen metabolism, and incorporation of amino acids into proteins. A second approach is based on the measurement of neurotransmitter synthesis and reuptake, receptor density, and enzyme activity, variables related to the function of the chemically heterogeneous neuronal populations that compose the central nervous system. The two approaches are complementary and can be used for the assessment of regional derangements of cerebral energy metabolism and chemical transmission. As most CNS disorders entail neurochemical alterations involving the synthesis of neurotransmitters and the disruption of synaptic function, imaging of neurotransmitters and neuroreceptors has become crucial in helping to understand the intrinsic neurochemical basis of neurologic and psychiatric diseases.

The first studies aimed at the in vivo assessment of cerebral function by using radioactive tracers and external monitoring by gamma-ray detectors were focused on measuring cerebral hemodynamics and energy metabolism (Ingvar and Lassen 1961; Hoedt-Rasmussen et al. 1966; Obrist et al. 1975; Phelps et al. 1979; Reivich et al. 1979; Frackowiak et al. 1980; Herscovitch et al. 1983). Following these milestones of radionuclide brain imaging in humans, there has been further development of methods and tracers over the past two decades that permit the assessment of other neurochemical variables, in particular neurotransmission. The first images of brain receptors were those of dopamine (D_2) receptors (Wagner et al. 1983) with positron emission tomography (PET), and those of muscarinic cholinergic receptors (Eckelman et al. 1984) with single photon emission computed tomography (SPECT). Following this seminal work many tracers have been developed (Stocklin 1992) and are currently used. Basic neuroscientists and clinical neuropsychiatrists use these methods for the assessment of regional cerebral functional activity and of neurochemical transmission under physiologic or pharmacologic conditions. Currently, the use of emission tomography allows assessment of cerebral blood flow, glucose utilization, oxygen metabolism, oxygen extraction ratio, rate of incorporation of amino acids into proteins and rate of transport of substrates across the brain capillaries into the brain, as well as of the rate of neurotransmitter storage, release, and binding to specific receptors. The assessment of neurotransmission by emission tomography has attracted the interest of neuroscientists with an expertise in nuclear medicine and has raised high expectations among clinical neurologists and psychiatrists, many of which have been realized.

2.2 Physiologic and Biochemical Basis of Radionuclide Brain Imaging

The CNS is a heterogeneous entity composed of numerous neuronal systems for transferring signals along their own body surface and, by secreting highly selective chemical substances, transfer this information to down-stream neurons. This function requires a continuous supply of nutrients through the cerebral circulation. As nutrients are delivered to brain structures for their energy metabolism, the rate of delivery, and their consumption is indicative of neuronal functional activity, and also of functional derangements when they occur. Since the function of the nervous system is based on the communication among its components, the characterization of the neuronal circuits and of neurotransmission constitute a primary goal of neuroscientists and neuropsychiatrists. A description of the fundamental body of knowledge is reported elsewhere (Feldman et al. 1997; Siegel et al. 1999).

Neuronal communication represents the ultimate function of the nervous system. It requires the integrated function of ion channels, classified according to the mechanism controlling their gating as either voltage sensitive or receptor operated, and neurotransmitters, defined by their presence and release at the presynaptic sites and by the capability to evoke a response at the postsynaptic site. The sequence of events characterizing neurotransmission can be schematically summarized as follows: the propagation of an action potential in the presynaptic neuron activates voltage-sensitive channels at the nerve ending, which turn on the fusion and release of synaptic vesicles, containing the neurotransmitter, into the synaptic cleft; the neurotransmitter then binds to postsynaptic neuroreceptors and initiates a cascade of events by modifying the ionic permeability of the postsynaptic neuron. This event in turn may result in the excitation or inhibition of the postsynaptic neuron, by either depolarization or hyperpolarization states produced by changes in neuronal membranes' permeability to ions such as calcium, sodium, potassium, and chloride. The depolarization results in an excitatory postsynaptic potential (EPSP), whereas the hyperpolarization results in an inhibitory postsynaptic potential (IPSP). Both EPSP and IPSP have a short duration, of the order of milliseconds; therefore, they represent temporary states during which the threshold for neuronal response is either decreased (depolarization) or increased (hyperpolarization). The electrical impulses and the chemical messengers act sequentially and synergistically, the former for intraneuronal conduction, the latter for interneuronal communication.

2.2.1 Cerebral Blood Flow and Energy Metabolism

The normal energy metabolism of the nervous system is dependent on the obligatory consumption of oxygen and glucose. Due to the lack of significant storage of glycogen, brain functions are sustained by a continuous supply of nutrients via blood. The rate of glucose and oxygen utilization throughout the brain is very heterogeneous and is tightly coupled to the rate of blood flow. Thus, the assessment of any of the three variables, i.e., blood flow, oxygen or glucose utilization, provides a measure of the degree of cerebral functional activity (Sokoloff 1960). Normal values of regional cerebral blood flow and metabolism and other neurophysiologic variables are listed in Table 2.1. Because of the close relation between blood flow, metabolism, and brain function, the as-

Table 2.1. Normal values per 100 g brain tissue in a healthy resting young adult man. (Modified from Sokoloff 1960)

Cerebral blood flow	57 ml/min
Cerebral O_2 consumption	3.5 ml/min
Cerebral glucose utilization	5.5 mg/min
Cerebral blood volume	4.8 ml
Mean RBC volume	1.5 ml
Mean plasma volume	3.3 ml

sessment of blood flow is currently performed not only with the aim of detecting cerebrovascular disorders, i.e., pathologic states originated by alterations of cerebral circulation, but also to assess other diseases of the nervous system that, due to neuronal death or to neuronal loss of function, require less blood supply compared with normal regions. In the latter case the reduction of blood flow is secondary to a reduced metabolic demand.

2.2.2 Neurotransmission

The function of the different neuronal systems of the brain hinges on the synthesis and release of several neurotransmitters, each acting selectively on specific neuroreceptor types and subtypes. Thus, neurons, receptors, and entire neuronal networks can be classified according to the neurotransmitter utilized. Neurotransmitters can range in size from small molecules, such as amino acids and amines, to peptides. They are contained in small intracellular vesicles and are released in the synaptic cleft by exocitosis. Neurotransmitters act by influencing the excitability of target receptors, located either on postsynaptic neurons or effector organs. The mechanism of action of neurotransmitters depends on the features of the two types of receptor subfamilies. Ligand-gated receptors contain an intrinsic channel that is rapidly opened in response to transmitter binding, whereas G protein-coupled receptors activate G proteins in the membrane which then stimulate various membrane effector proteins. Membrane proteins act on the synthesis of second messengers (e.g., cAMP, cGMP, and Ca ions) which in turn act on intracellular protein kinases. The action of neurotransmitters may produce rapid and short-term changes, or initiate long-term processes by modifying gene expression. The neurotransmitter action is terminated after metabolic degradation or cellular reuptake. Many neurons possess autoreceptors at their surface, which by responding to the cell's own transmitter initiate feedback mechanisms that reduce transmitter synthesis and release.

2.3 Methodology

The development and use of methods for brain radionuclide studies must take into account cerebral morphologic heterogeneity, neuronal circuitry complexity, neurotransmitter specificity, nonuniform blood flow and metabolism, and presence of the blood-brain barrier (BBB). Each experimental and diagnostic procedure must be tailored to examine the physiologic and biochemical process of interest.

The methodologic research has been aimed at constructing instruments to detect and reconstruct the temporal distribution of tracer substances in three dimensions and at developing methods of data analysis for the transformation of the radioactivity distribution data into relevant neurophysiologic and neurochemical parameters.

2.3.1 Detection Instruments

The process of detecting photons emitted, either as singles or in pairs, constitutes the basis of SPECT and PET, respectively (see Chap. 13). In order to appreciate the potentials and limitations of SPECT and PET with respect to their applications in brain studies, it is worth pinpointing some features of both techniques. Image quality in emission tomography results from a compromise between spatial resolution, which affects the ability to discriminate small structures, and count density, which depends on the system detection efficiency and determines the level of noise in the image. The temporal resolution of emission tomography, defined as the minimum time needed for acquisition of counts, even with recent increases in detection efficiency, remains of the order of seconds/minutes to obtain acceptable, i.e., low noise levels in the image. It is noteworthy that detection efficiency in PET is approximately 10–15 times higher than in SPECT. Whereas PET remains for the brain an instrument primarily devoted to research with many opportunities for clinical applications still unexplored, SPECT is presently widely used for clinical purposes, and will mature as a research tool in time. The features of state-of-the-art PET and SPECT scanners are defined according to their physical performances, including field of view, spatial resolution, system sensitivity, and count rate (see Chap. 13).

2.3.2 Dynamic and Static Acquisition Procedures

Two main approaches can be used for SPECT and PET brain data acquisition. One approach is based on the acquisition at one fixed time interval after tracer administration. The second approach is based on the measurement of changes in time of the brain radioactivity distribution. The two approaches are sometimes referred to as autoradiographic and dynamic imaging, respectively. Both methods may require sequential sampling of peripheral arterial or venous blood to determine the time course of radioactivity in blood. Blood sampling is usually necessary for quantitative assessment of physiologic or biochemical processes, whereas it is not required for assessing uptake ratios of radioactivity distribution between cerebral structures, also referred to as semiquantitative indices of function.

2.3.3 Data Analysis

Data analysis presents a major intellectual and practical challenge in SPECT and PET. Quantification is, in general, a requisite of research studies and is often a complex procedure that may require the assessment of the fractions of radioactive metabolites in blood by chromatography and scintillation counting, as well as scanning times in the order of hours. Data acquired for quantification must be analyzed by kinetic models; these are in general schematic representations of the behavior of tracers in the body spaces, i.e., compartments (GJEDDE and WONG 1990). Kinetic models represent the basis by which to calculate the variables of interest, e.g., tracer rate of transfer across compartment boundaries or rate of tracer accumulation in a compartment. The application of these models requires measurement of radioactivity concentrations in blood and brain after tracer injection. These models may require the a priori knowledge of parameters that are applicable to any subject; two such kinetic models are shown in Fig. 2.1.

Models representing biologic events never can fully account for all relevant factors and conditions that occur in vivo and consequently are imperfect. The experimental procedures must therefore be designed to minimize the possible errors arising from limitations and imperfections of the method. Semiquantitative

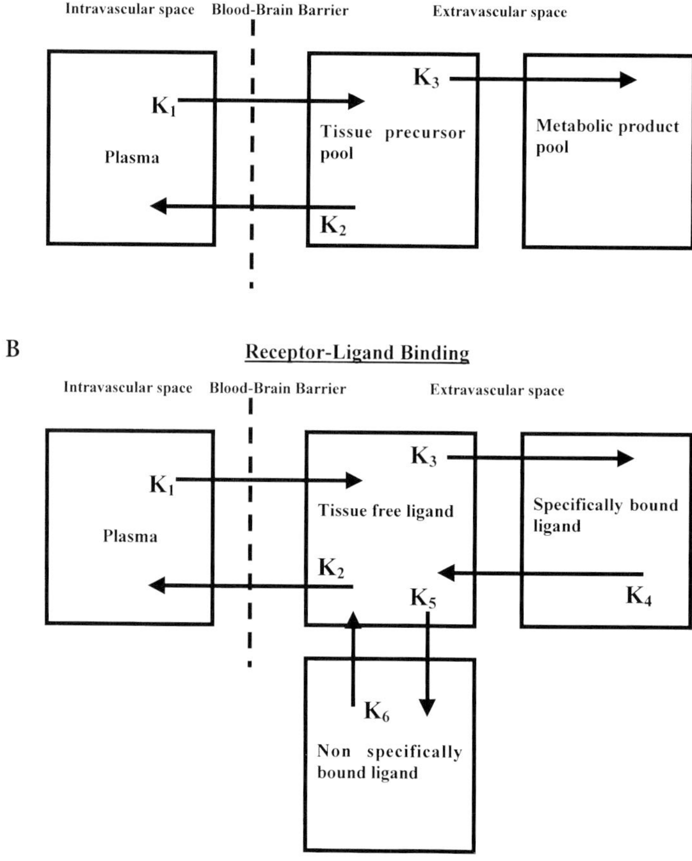

Fig. 2.1. Compartmental models used to calculate physiologic and biochemical parameters. **A** Cerebral glucose utilization; **B** receptor-ligand binding. *K1–K6* are the rate constants or diffusion rates between compartments

assessment is considered adequate in most clinical studies with emission tomography, when only localization of phenomena is sought. Quantification may also not be required in activation studies, i.e., performed under baseline conditions (unstimulated) and then repeated under physiologic or pharmacologic stimuli, where localization of neuronal function is sought. For many studies that address clinical and research questions, location may be only a part of the information sought; assessment of the magnitude of the alterations is also important. Furthermore, it is often impossible without quantification to make comparisons between individuals, e.g., patients, groups, and normal control subjects. Relative changes, as assessed by semiquantitative methods, may be inadequate because the reference region may be affected by the same process as the area under investigation. Nevertheless, semiquantitative assessments are generally preferred because they are less cumbersome for patients, physicians, and technical staff, since blood sampling can generally be avoided and data acquisition can be performed in a shorter time span, with an acceptable tradeoff in accuracy.

Regional cerebral radioactivity is usually measured by drawing regions of interest (ROIs) of either regular or irregular shape on the images. This procedure is time consuming and can be biased because it is based on arbitrary subdivision of cerebral structures into small discrete volumes. To overcome these problems noninteractive voxel-by-voxel-based techniques have been developed. One such method that was developed by Friston et al. (1995) for activation studies with PET and ^{15}O-labeled water has become very popular and is known as statistical parametric mapping (SPM). The use of this method has been extended to other tracers. It offers a series of noninteractive techniques that permit: (a) spatial normalization of brain images into a stereotactic space; (b) normalization for differences in global cerebral radioactivity distribution depending on intersubject variability; and (c) higher spatial resolution than that achieved with subjective ROI-based analysis.

Methods have been developed specifically for estimating in vivo regional variables of blood flow, metabolism, neurotransmitter synthesis, and receptor binding. A selection of these methods is reported in Table 2.2.

Whereas numerous procedures for quantitative measurement of hemodynamic and metabolic variables have been established and fully validated, semiquantitative assessments are performed for clinical use. Methods developed for the assessment of neuro-

Table 2.2. Major neurotransmitters and receptors

Neurotransmitter	Receptors	Clinical application
Glutamic acid	NMDA, AMPA, kainate, quisqualate	Epilepsy Movement disorders Ischemia
Gamma-amino-butyric-acid linked to benzodiazepine receptors: GABÂ/BZD	GABAÂ and GABAB̂	Movement disorders Mood disorders
Acetylcholine	Nicotinic (peripheral) Nicotinic (central), some abnormal in AD Muscarinic (central), five subtypes	Movement disorders Dementia Epilepsy
Dopamine	Five subtypes	Movement disorders Drug addiction Schizophrenia
Noradrenaline	Five subtypes	Vascular tone Movement control Mood control
Serotonin	Seven subtypes	Sleep Depression Food intake Pain
Opioid	Mu, delta, kappa	Drug addiction Pain syndromes Epilepsy Eating disorders

For details see: Feldman et al. 1997; Siegel et al. 1999

transmission function have been most often semiquantitative, although fairly simple quantitative methods exist for assessing the maximum concentration of binding sites (B_{max}) and the affinity of the ligand for the receptor (K_D). A frequently adopted measure of the functional status of brain receptors is based on the assessment of the binding potential (BP), which is equal to the ratio of receptor density (B_{max}) to receptor affinity (K_D).

Analytical methods have also been developed which allow the assessment of the rate of uptake and storage of neurotransmitters precursor into neurons. One such method, which has interesting applications for the analysis of the behavior of any tracer and permits the assessment of volumes of distribution, as well as rate of trapping, has largely been applied for the assessment of dopamine storage in nigrostriatal neurons (Patlak et al. 1985). However, there is a widespread use of semiquantitative methods based on the assessment of ratios of radioactivity concentration in target regions, i.e., known to contain specific receptors and in which there is specific tracer binding, to that of regions devoid of receptors, in which tracer uptake is nonspecific.

2.4 Tracers for Brain Imaging

Numerous tracers have been developed for studying the chemical processes in the brain (Stocklin 1992). The availability of radiotracers for the in vivo assessment of biochemical variables, as well as the physiologic and pharmacologic processes, is a major advantage of PET over SPECT, but the short half-life of the positron emitters makes the presence of a cyclotron mandatory in the proximity of the PET scanner, thus increasing the cost and limiting the diffusion of PET compared with SPECT. It is noteworthy that for some neurochemical studies, tracers labeled with single photon emitting radionuclides may be more suitable because they decay slowly and allow the assessment of tracer kinetics over several hours. This feature is particularly relevant for tracers with high affinity for receptors.

2.4.1 Cerebral Blood Flow and Metabolism Tracers

Cerebral blood flow can be measured both with SPECT or PET by using either diffusible or nondiffusible tracers. To the group of diffusible tracers belongs ^{133}Xe, a gas which decays by single photon emission and employed with SPECT (Kanno and Lassen 1979), as well as ^{15}O labeled water and ^{15}O labeled carbon dioxide (which is converted to ^{15}O-water in vivo), both decaying by positron emission and employed with PET. The use of molecular ^{15}O-oxygen, along with ^{15}O-water, permits the assessment of oxygen extraction fraction, cerebral blood flow and oxygen metabolism (Herscovitch et al. 1983; Frackowiak et al. 1980). To the group of the nondiffusible tracers belong the so-called chemical microspheres, i.e., tracers that cross the BBB after venous administration, and which are retained in the brain in proportion to blood-flow-dependent delivery; chemical microspheres are labeled with ^{99m}Tc and employed with SPECT (Leveille et al. 1992). The assessment of cerebral metabolism can be achieved by PET only, as for this purpose glucose, or its analogs, and oxygen itself can be used, which cannot be labeled with single-photon-emitting radionuclides. The measurement of glucose utilization is performed with ^{18}F labeled 2-fluoro-2-deoxy-D-glucose (^{18}F-FDG; Phelps et al. 1979; Reivich et al. 1979), since glucose itself, labeled with ^{11}C, undergoes a rapid metabolic degradation to water and carbon dioxide, which are partially lost during the measurement of the radioactivity concentration. ^{18}F-FDG instead remains trapped as ^{18}F-labeled fluorodeoxyglucose-6-phosphate, and accumulation is a function of the glucose metabolic rate.

2.4.2 Neurotransmission Function Tracers

The dopaminergic system has been extensively investigated in terms of both presynaptic and postsynaptic processes by means of selective positron emitting radiotracers. The large number of studies performed has also facilitated the development of methods and procedures for studying other neurotransmitter systems. ^{18}F-Fluoro-DOPA has been extensively used as a probe of the presynaptic dopaminergic system, and is transported across the BBB and incorporated into the sequence of processes for dopamine synthesis and subsequent conversion of dopamine to homovanillic acid and 3,4-dihydroxyphenylacetic acid (DOPAC; Cumming and Gjedde 1998). Although this tracer does not permit the measurement of endogenous dopamine synthesis, turnover, and storage, it has been used as a probe of amino acid decarboxylase activity (the rate-limiting enzyme in the synthesis of dopamine) and thus of nigrostriatal neuron density and presynaptic function.

The dopaminergic system has also been studied with tracers binding to the presynaptic dopamine reuptake system, such as ^{11}C-nomifensine, ^{18}F-GBR 13,119, ^{11}C-cocaine, ^{11}C-CFT, ^{11}C-WIN 35,428 and ^{123}I-β-CIT. WIN 35,428 (DANNALS et al. 1993) and ^{123}I-β-CIT (NEUMEYER et al. 1991) are the tracers that are being used currently. The first agent for assessing dopamine reuptake labeled with ^{99m}Tc, TRODAT-1, has been synthesized and tested in human subjects (KUNG et al. 1997).

The activity of the mitochondrial enzyme monoamine oxidase B (MAO-B) can be investigated by using ^{11}C-L-deprenyl, a so-called suicide inactivator, since it covalently binds to the MAO-B flavoprotein group, which results in the labeling of the enzyme itself. Following intravenous administration of this tracer, there is significant uptake and retention of radioactivity in the striatum and thalamus. This tracer can be used to measure the effect of therapy in patients under treatment with MAO-B inhibitors as well as the rate of turnover of MAO-B (ARNETT et al. 1987; FOWLER et al. 1987, 1993).

Dopamine receptors can be grouped into two major families: one including D_1 and D_5 receptors, and the other including the D_2, D_3, and D_4 receptors. PET tracers to measure D_2 and D_1 receptors have been developed; however, there are currently no specific PET ligands to differentially evaluate D_3, D_4, and D_5 receptors.

The first visualization of dopamine receptors in live human subjects with PET was reported by WAGNER et al. (1983) using ^{11}C-N-methyl-spiperone, a D_2 receptor antagonist. Subsequently, several other D_2-receptor tracers have been synthesized including ^{11}C-raclopride and ^{18}F-fluoro-ethyl-spiperone (COENEN et al. 1987). For SPECT studies of the D_2 receptors ^{123}I-Iodobenzamide has been used (KUNG 1990). The specific D_1 ligands SCH 23,390 and SCH 39,166 labeled with ^{11}C have allowed investigation of D_1-receptor subtypes in human subjects with PET (HALLDIN et al. 1986, 1990).

Tracers have been developed for the assessment of cholinergic presynaptic function including acetylcholinesterase activity, by ^{11}C-N-methyl-piperydinil-proprionate (KUHL et al. 1996), and vesicular acetylcholine transporter, by vesamicol and benzovesamicol labeled with either ^{11}C or ^{18}F or ^{123}I (KILBOURN et al. 1990). Nicotinic receptor function assessment has been pursued with ^{11}C labeled nicotine, whereas muscarinic receptor function assessment has been evaluated with ^{123}I-quinuclinidylbenzilate (QNB; ECKELMAN et al. 1984), ^{11}C-scopolamine, ^{11}C-tropanylbenzilate, and ^{11}C-N-methyl-piperydil-benzilate (MULHOLLAND et al. 1992, 1995; KOEPPE et al. 1994). The pharmacokinetics of ^{11}C-scopolamine are not optimal in human subjects because its interaction with the receptor system is limited by poor blood-brain barrier permeability and rapid receptor binding of the extracted activity. ^{11}C labeled derivatives of tropanyl benzylate and N-methylpiperidyl benzylate have the same pattern of distribution as scopolamine, but their extraction by the brain is not limited as it is for scopolamine. From the clinical point of view, a major problem with muscarinic receptors is still the lack of radiolabeled tracers for differentiating the cerebral M_1 postsynaptic receptors from the presynaptic M_2 subtype.

Opiate receptors have been studied with two ligands: ^{11}C-carfentanil, a potent opiate agonist that is highly selective for mu receptors, and ^{11}C-diprenorphine, a partial agonist of the same system but with no specificity for the opiate receptor subtypes: mu, delta, and kappa (FROST et al. 1986, 1990; JONES et al. 1988). This lack of specificity limits the use of diprenorphine due to its widespread uptake in the cortex, whereas the uptake of carfentanil is more selective to the areas that contain mu receptors. Delta receptors can be imaged using and ^{11}C-methyl-naltrindole (MADAR et al. 1996).

Tracers for central-type benzodiazepine (BZD) binding sites, which are postsynaptic membrane receptor ionophore complexes with a $GABA_A$ receptor ($BZD/GABA_A$), have been developed for studies in humans: ^{11}C-flumazenil (SAMSON et al. 1985; SHINOTOH et al. 1986) and ^{123}I-iomazenil (PERSSON et al. 1985; BEER et al. 1990; DEY et al. 1994).

For the assessment of the serotoninergic system only a few tracers are available, including ^{11}C-ketanserin, ^{18}F-setoperone, and ^{18}F-altanserin (BERRIDGE et al. 1983; CROUZEL et al. 1988). Some of these tracers are mixed and bind to dopamine as well as serotonin receptors such as ^{11}C and ^{18}F labeled spiperone analogs.

2.5 Clinical Applications

Progressive increase in life expectancy is leading to an increase in the number of subjects with degenerative and cerebrovascular diseases. At the same time, there is an increasing demand for diagnosis and treatment of all neuropsychiatric diseases, due in part to increasing public health awareness. The investigations carried out over two decades by emission tomography have permitted the in vivo assessment of physiologic and neurochemical processes in several clinically relevant conditions. The PET and SPECT studies have been aimed at clarifying the natural history of cerebrovascular diseases, characterizing the metabolic features of neuronal degeneration in dementia syndromes, assessing the neurochemical impairment in movement disorders, establishing the neurochemical correlates of the clinical and electrical alterations in epilepsy, as well as a variety of syndromes and pathologic states (Table 2.3). The PET and SPECT brain studies have also contributed significantly to a new vision in the area of mental illnesses. Methods originally developed for research are slowly entering the clinical domain.

The use of emission tomography for assessing brain function under clinical circumstances is somewhat overshadowed by its use in research investigations. This is in sharp contrast with the trend in other organs and systems, namely in cardiology, oncology, and endocrinology. On the one hand, this is due to the large number of unanswered questions in neuroscience stimulating research activities, and on the other hand, to the limited therapeutic resources for the treatment of many CNS diseases. In particular,

Table 2.3. Synopsis of clinically relevant tracers

Physiologic variable	Method	Tracers
Blood flow (CBF)	PET	^{15}O-carbon dioxide; ^{15}O-water; ^{11}C-butanol; ^{18}F-fluoro-methyl-fluoride; ^{13}N-ammonia
	SPECT	^{133}Xe; ^{99m}Tc-hydroxy-methyl-propileneamine oxime (HMPAO); ^{99m}Tc-ethyl-cisteinate-dimer (ECD)
Oxygen extraction fraction (OEF) and metabolism ($CMRO_2$)	PET	Molecular oxygen ($^{15}O_2$) (CMRO is calculated by multiplying CBF by OEF)
Glucose metabolism	PET	^{18}F-fluoro-deoxy-glucose
Blood volume	PET	^{15}O-carbon monoxide-labeled RBC
	SPECT	^{99m}Tc-RBC
Protein synthesis and amino acid transport	PET	^{11}C-methionine, ^{18}F-fluoro-L-tyrosine
Tumor viability and proliferation	PET	^{18}F-fluoro-deoxy-glucose; ^{11}C-thymidine; ^{11}C-methionine; ^{18}F-fluoro-L-tyrosine
	SPECT	^{201}Thallium; ^{99m}Tc-methoxy-isobutyl-isonitrile (MIBI); ^{123}I-methyl-tyrosine
Gamma-amino-butyric-acid (GABA)	PET	^{11}C-flumazenil; ^{18}F-fluoro-ethyl-flumazenil
	SPECT	^{123}I-iomazenil
Acetylcholine	PET	Acetylcholine-esterase activity: ^{11}C-methyl-phenyl-piperidine Nicotinic receptors: ^{11}C-nicotine Muscarinic receptors: ^{18}F-fluoro-dexetimide; ^{11}C-N-methyl-piperidil-benzilate; ^{11}C-Tropanyl benzilate; ^{11}C-scopolamine
	SPECT	Acetylcholine transport: ^{123}I-iodo-benzovesamicol Muscarinic receptors: 123I-iododexetimide; 123I-QNB;
Dopamine	PET	MAO-B: ^{11}C-deprenyl Presynaptic function: ^{18}F-fluoro-L-DOPA; ^{18}F-fluoro-L-m-tyrosine Dopamine reuptake: ^{11}C-nomifensine; ^{11}C-cocaine; ^{11}C-WIN 35,428 D_2-receptors: ^{11}C-raclopride; ^{18}F-fluoro-ethyl-spiperone; ^{18}F-N-methyl-spiperone; ^{18}F-fluoro-alkyl-benzamides D_1-receptors: ^{11}C-SCH 23,390
	SPECT	Dopamine reuptake: ^{123}I-beta-CIT D_2-receptors: ^{123}I-Iodobenzamide (IBZM)
Noradrenaline		^{18}F-Fluoro-norepinephrine
Serotonin		5HT reuptake: ^{11}C-McN5652 5HT receptors: ^{18}F-fluoro-ethyl-ketanserin; ^{18}F-setoperone; ^{18}F-altanserin
Opioid	PET	^{11}C carfentanil (mu selective); ^{11}C methylnaltrindole (delta selective); ^{11}C diprenorphine (mu, delta, and kappa selective); ^{18}F cyclofoxy (mu and delta selective).

lack of effective neurologic therapies makes the in-depth characterization of patients for whom there are only limited therapeutic resources of limited utility for many specialists, especially after a diagnosis has been established. Unfortunately, morphologic imaging and electrophysiology are also of little help in understanding the nature of the CNS diseases and remain largely descriptive techniques. Morphologic imaging can only depict advanced disease states, often characterized by gross neuronal loss and irreversible changes in the primary site of the lesion. Electrophysiologic studies can provide us with information having very high temporal resolution, but barely acceptable spatial resolution, unless based on invasive intracranial exploration; both provide limited insight into the neurochemical basis of functional mechanisms in the CNS. Thus, the goal for the future is the characterization of biochemical abnormalities of the CNS at as early a stage as possible during the disease, and to treat each patient with the most appropriate and tailored treatment. In this respect, emission tomography is a unique tool.

2.6 Dementias

The term „neurodegenerative dementia" comprises various diseases, including Alzheimer's disease (AD), Pick's disease (frontotemporal lobar atrophy), diffuse or cortical Lewy body disease (DLBD), and multiple system atrophies. The disease with the highest prevalence is AD. Degenerative dementias are classified on the basis of postmortem neuropathologic assessment. Thus, the in vivo diagnosis of AD by clinical and instrumental assessment is only a probabilistic statement based on evidence of progressive cognitive decline, and lack of an alternative diagnosis of intoxications, systemic metabolic disturbances, infection, cerebrovascular ischemic disease, cerebral mass lesions, and normal pressure hydrocephalus. Several imaging strategies have been applied to the study of dementias. From the perspective of clinical diagnosis, glucose metabolism and blood flow are key variables. The assessment of other neurochemical variables is crucial for testing pathophysiologic hypotheses of the etiology of AD and to assess the efficacy of new drugs as they are developed and introduced into clinical practice (Frey et al. 1998).

2.6.1 Cerebral Blood Flow and Metabolism in Patients with Degenerative Dementias

Glucose metabolism imaging with ^{18}F-FDG is the most sensitive and specific imaging modality available presently for the diagnosis of AD. Automatic analysis of PET images yields a sensitivity as high as 95%–97% and a specificity of 100%, in discriminating patients with probable Alzheimer's disease from normal subjects (Minoshima et al. 1995). Probable AD patients have reduced glucose utilization in the posterior parietal and temporal lobe association cortex and posterior cingulate cortex (Benson et al. 1983; Friedland et al. 1983; Cutler et al. 1985). In moderate-to-severely affected individuals, the reductions of metabolism are bilateral, yet there is often an asymmetry of the severity or the extent of hypometabolism. Patients with more advanced clinical symptoms have reduced metabolism in the dorsal prefrontal association cortex as well, although the typical AD pattern is characterized by more severe parietotemporal than frontal involvement. In AD patients, metabolism is relatively spared in cortical regions other than the above, including the primary somatomotor, auditory, and visual cortices and the anterior cingulate cortex (Fig. 2.2). Subcortical structures, including the basal ganglia, thalamus, brain stem, and cerebellum are also relatively preserved in typical AD. The metabolism in the involved regions decreases with disease severity as shown by longitudinal studies that reveal an overall reduction in glucose metabolism throughout the brain in AD, with progressively decreasing metabolism in the association cortex. The region least affected by AD is the pons, whereas the posterior cingulate cortex is the area in which the hypometabolism occurs in the earliest stage of the disease.

Several lines of evidence suggest the high sensitivity of ^{18}F-FDG PET in the early detection of AD. Many subjects with AD have already an abnormal PET on the initial examination performed for mild memory loss. These studies suggest that hypometabolism actually precedes both symptoms and the clinical diagnosis of AD. Thus, the ^{18}F-FDG PET scan appears to have excellent sensitivity in mildly symptomatic patients and performs well in the diagnostic setting. Patients with frontal or frontotemporal dementia have also typical metabolic patterns. In instances of autopsy-proven Pick's disease, and in patients with a neuropsychometric suggestion of frontal dementia, ^{18}F-FDG PET reveals the greatest reduction in the frontal and anterior temporal association cortical regions,

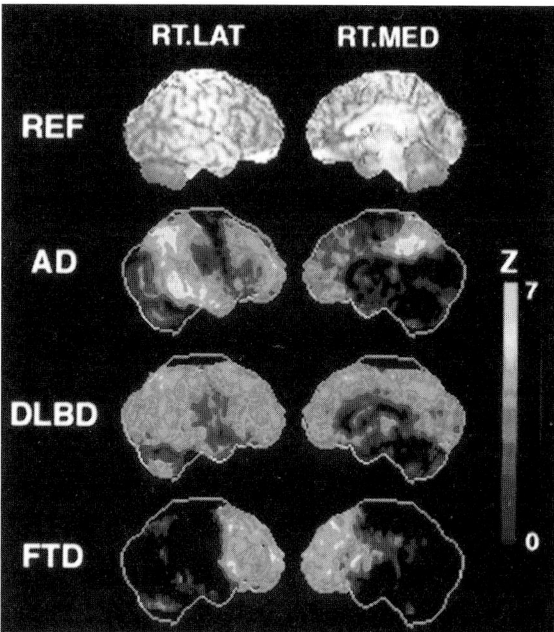

Fig. 2.2. Stereotaxic surface projection maps of glucose metabolism deficits in patients with dementia. Two columns of images are presented, representing the lateral (*left*) and medial (*right*) surface projections of the right cerebral hemisphere. The *top row* demonstrates surface-rendered MRI of a normal subject for anatomic reference (*REF*). The other rows of images depict stereotaxic surface projections of cerebral glucose metabolic decreases in individual demented patients, displayed in Z-score scale in comparison with an elderly normal database. The *second row* depicts a typical AD patient with prominent temporo-parietal and prefrontal hypometabolism on the lateral projection, and posterior cingulate hypometabolism on the medial projection. The *third row* depicts deficits in an autopsy-proven case of diffuse Lewy body disease (*DLBD*) with reductions in the association cortical areas as in AD, but with additional involvement of the occipital cortex on both medial and lateral projections. The *bottom row* depicts deficits in a patient with isolated frontal lobe hypometabolism (frontal lobe dementia, *FTD*). The metabolic decreases are depicted in Z-scores (standard deviations from normal) according to the *gray scale on the right*, extending from 0 to 7. (From Frey et al. 1998)

with the least reduction in the parietal association cortices (Kamo et al. 1987). Patients with pure AD and those with pure DLBD or mixed AD and DLBD, the so-called LB variant AD, can be distinguished (Fig. 2.2). In this latter group, the typical AD pattern of reduced temporoparietal and prefrontal hypometabolism is seen in association with additional hypometabolism of the primary visual cortices, whereas the metabolic patterns of DLBD and LB variant AD do not, at this time, appear separable on the basis of cerebral glucose metabolism (Albin et al. 1996). The pattern assessed with PET ^{18}F-FDG in AD patients may also be detectable using SPECT and blood flow tracers. However, comparative studies of metabolism and flow have shown that SPECT may be a slightly less accurate methodology for the assessment of demented patients in the earliest stages of the disease (Messa et al. 1994).

2.6.2 Neurotransmission Function in Degenerative Dementias

Studies of the presynaptic function have been carried out by ^{123}I-iodobenzovesamicol (^{123}I-IBVM), which is a marker of the vesicular acetyl choline transporter (VAChT; Kuhl et al. 1994, 1996; Hicks et al. 1991). Studies in normal subjects revealed modest reductions with advancing age, approximately 3%–4% per decade. Application of the ^{123}I-IBVM SPECT method for studying AD revealed further losses of cholinergic cortical innervation. The average reductions are distinctly greater in AD patients with symptom onset before age 65 years (30%) than in those with later age at onset (15%). These neocortical reductions were, however, less than the expected 50%–80% losses reported for choline acetyl transferase (CAT) enzyme activity in autopsy series. Whereas CAT activity was reduced over 50% in the neocortex of AD, a parallel 15% reduction in VAChT was not statistically significant. Thus, there is the possibility that these two presynaptic cholinergic markers may be differentially regulated or differentially lost in AD. There may be upregulation of VAChT expression to compensate for cholinergic terminal losses, or alternatively, CAT expression may be reduced within otherwise intact presynaptic nerve terminals. Further studies are underway to explore each of these hypotheses. ^{11}C-N-methyl-piperidinil propionate (PMP) is a substrate for hydrolysis by acetyl choline esterase (AChE; Kilbourn et al. 1996); thus, PET measurements of PMP hydrolysis, accomplished by measuring regional radiolabeled product retention in the brain, provide an index of AChE activity. Preliminary studies of patients with probable AD reveal approximately 20% reductions throughout the cerebral cortex (Kuhl et al. 1996b; Iyo et al. 1997).

Postsynaptic cholinergic studies have also been carried out. Studies of muscarinic cholinergic receptors with ^{11}C-tropanyl benzilate (TRB; Koeppe et al. 1994; Lee et al. 1996) and ^{11}C-N-methylpiperidyl benzilate (NMPB; Mulholland et al. 1995; Zubieta et al. 1994) indicate minor losses of cholinergic receptors function with advancing age. In probable AD patients there is no evidence of significant neocortical losses of muscarinic receptors, whereas significant ligand delivery reduction is found in the association cortical areas, paralleling reductions in glucose. PET studies of the central benzodiazepine binding site on the $GABA_A$ receptor with the antagonist ligand ^{11}C-flumazenil are amenable for the assessment of neuronal viability. In patients with probable AD, a modest reduction of benzodiazepine binding sites has been observed in the association cortex only in the most clinically advanced cases, thus indicating the presence of viable neurons in the early phases of the disease. As this reduction is of a lesser degree than glucose hypometabolism, it is conceivable that the reductions in glucose metabolism seen in the early stages of AD are not just a reflection of synapse and neuron losses, but a correlate of a synaptic dysfunction that precedes the structural losses (Meyer et al. 1995).

2.7 Movement Disorders

The balance between cholinergic and dopaminergic neuronal activity in the basal ganglia is required for normal motor function. Damage to dopaminergic nigrostriatal neurons is found in various forms of parkinsonism. In patients with Parkinson's disease (PD) clinical symptoms occur when dopaminergic nigral neurons have undergone a loss of 40%–50%. The neurons projecting to the putamen have been estimated to decline most, as compared with those innervating the caudate and those projecting to the nucleus accumbens. A reduction in dopamine metabolites 3,4-dihydroxyphenylacetic acid (DOPAC) and homovalinic acid (HVA), and the number of dopamine reuptake sites is also observed. The reduction in dopamine content occurs also in the mesocortical and mesolimbic projections of the ventral tegmental area (VTA) possibly as a consequence of the destruction of dopaminergic neurons in the VTA. Other neurotransmitter systems have been shown to be damaged in parkinsonism, including noradrenergic, cholinergic, opioidergic, and serotonergic circuits (Dubois et al. 1983; Hornykiewicz and Kish 1984, 1986; Dubois et al. 1987; Uhl et al. 1985; Baronti et al. 1991). Such alterations may explain the occurrence of depression, dementia, and other symptoms in patients with PD.

2.7.1 Cerebral Blood Flow and Metabolism in Movement Disorders

In the early studies various patterns of flow and metabolism have been observed in movement disorders, related to the duration and degree of the disease. In the early phase of hemiparkinsonism an increased metabolism was found in the putamen and globus pallidus (Wolfson et al. 1985; Miletich et al. 1988), along with a decrease of metabolism in the frontal cortex, contralateral to the affected limbs (Perlmutter and Raichle 1985; Wolfson et al. 1985). In bilaterally affected patients the cortical alteration is more widespread; however, this effect could be due to concurrent degenerative processes (Kuhl et al. 1984). The significance of the cortical hypometabolism remains unclear. All studies have shown inconsistent and minor changes that have led to abandoning the use of ^{18}F-FDG and flow tracers to measure functional activity in the basal ganglia and cortex of patients with movement disorders. Overall, the assessment of flow and metabolism does not appear to be a useful approach in studying patients with movement disorders.

2.7.2 Neurotransmitter Function in Movement Disorders

The assessment of the dopaminergic presynaptic function has been pursued by two strategies: one aimed at assessing the incorporation of a metabolic substrate of dopamine synthesis in the nigrostriatal neuronal terminals, and another aimed at assessing the density of the presynaptic dopamine reuptake sites.

For the first goal the most used tracer is ^{18}F-6-fluoroDOPA (^{18}F-DOPA) which is metabolized to ^{18}F-fluoro-dopamine by amino-acid decarboxylase (AADC) and subsequently stored in vesicles in the presynaptic nerve endings. Following ^{18}F-DOPA administration in patients with early PD and hemiparkinsonism, a reduced accumulation of tracer is observed, reflecting reduced-AADC activity in the putamen contralateral to the affected limbs, with relative sparing of the caudate (Nahmias et al. 1985). Significant correlations between ^{18}F-DOPA uptake and motor symptoms have been reported (Leenders et al. 1988; Brooks et al. 1990; Martin et al. 1988, 1989). These results are sustained by a lack of AADC activity due to a selective destruction of the ventrolateral nigrostriatal neurons projecting to the putamen in PD. However, the rate of ^{18}F-DOPA uptake is the expression of both the neuronal density as well as of the AADC activity. Whereas ^{18}F-DOPA has shown potential for the early and preclinical detection of PD, it must be noted that ^{18}F-DOPA uptake in the basal ganglia is not proportional to the degree of degeneration of the ventrolateral substantia nigra, due to adaptational increases in AADC function in the surviving cells. This is made evident by the observation that at the onset of symptoms, ^{18}F-DOPA uptake in the affected putamen is reduced by approximately 35%, with no significant reductions detected in the caudate. On the other hand, at symptom onset, putamen dopamine content is already decreased by 80% and at least 50% of pigmented nigra cells are lost. From these observations it can be concluded that the activity of DOPA decarboxylase, as assessed with ^{18}F-DOPA is a sensitive but inaccurate measure of dopaminergic neuronal loss. In fully symptomatic patients, reductions of ^{18}F-DOPA uptake range from 40%–60% in the posterior putamen, and 15%–40% in caudate and anterior putamen, respectively (Otsuka et al. 1991; Brooks et al. 1990).

Functional imaging of the presynaptic sites, aimed at assessing neuronal density by methods independent of dopamine synthesis, offers a more accurate alternative to ^{18}F-DOPA studies. This goal has been achieved by several cocaine analogs that bind to the presynaptic dopamine transporter (DAT) sites (Scheffel et al. 1992; Dannals et al. 1993; Lever et al. 1996). Among various tracers, ^{11}C-WIN 35,428 seems to be the most sensitive tracer for DAT imaging in PD, and PET studies have revealed markedly reduced DAT levels in early PD (Frost et al. 1993). In patients with stage-2 PD, specific binding of ^{11}C-WIN 35,428 in the posterior putamen is reduced more than in the anterior putamen and the caudate nucleus (Fig. 2.3). SPECT imaging with ^{123}I-β-CIT also shows severe loss of striatal DA transporters in idiopathic PD compared with healthy human subjects, with markedly abnormal striatal uptake, more pronounced in the putamen than in the caudate nucleus. ^{123}I-β-CIT uptake is related to clinical findings including degree of akinesia, rigidity, axial symptoms, and activities of daily living. The striatal uptake is reduced by 35% in Hoehn-Yahr stage 1 to over 72% in stage 5 and is correlated to disease severity. In general, abnormalities of dopamine transporter binding are more pronounced than ^{18}F-DOPA abnormalities (Brucke et al. 1993; Seibyl et al. 1994; Marek et al.

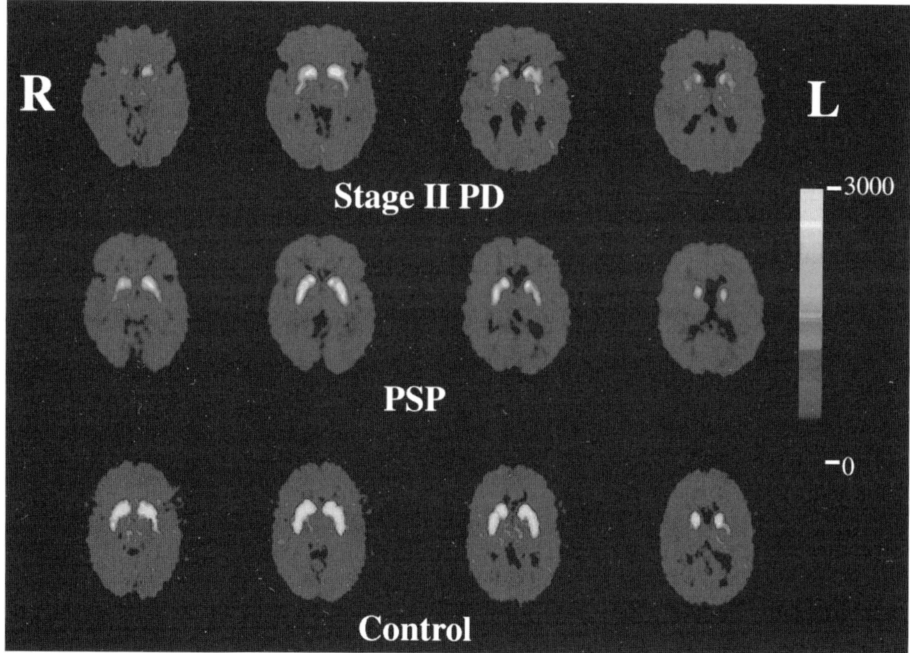

Fig. 2.3. Images of ^{11}C-WIN 35,428 binding at four different levels throughout the striatum of a healthy control, a stage-2 PD and a PSP patient. The images are obtained after averaging the data acquired from 35 to 82 min following administration of the tracer and are normalized for the administered activity. Higher binding in the basal ganglia is seen in the healthy age-matched control subject compared with patients diagnosed with PD and PSP. In PD, reduced ^{11}C-WIN 35,428 binding is seen predominantly in the posterior putamen while there is more uniform reduction throughout the entire striatum in PSP

1996). The assessment of presynaptic function may permit both the early detection of PD and a differential diagnosis between PD and progressive supranuclear palsy (PSP) in a single study since PSP is associated with a more uniform loss of DAT compared with PD which shows more specific loss in the posterior putamen (Fig. 2.2; ILGIN et al. 1995). This goal can conveniently be achieved with SPECT tracers that selectively bind to the presynaptic dopamine transporters such as ^{123}I-β-CIT (MESSA et al. 1998).

Ligands available for studying D_2 receptors with PET are raclopride and spiperone derivatives labeled with ^{11}C and ^{18}F. D_2 receptors can also be assessed with SPECT and ^{123}I-IBZM (GIOBBE et al. 1993; NADEAU et al. 1995). ^{123}I-IBZM SPECT and ^{11}C-raclopride PET findings in patients with PD are significantly correlated (SCHWARZ et al. 1994). In patients not treated with DOPA, either small increases or no changes in basal ganglia D_2 receptor density are observed (RINNE et al. 1990). In patients treated with L-dopa, D_2 receptor density is reduced or unchanged (HAGGLUND et al. 1987). Longitudinal studies have shown that ^{11}C-raclopride uptake is increased in the putamen in the early stage of PD, compared with controls, whereas after 3–5 years ^{11}C-raclopride binding is significantly reduced in the putamen and caudate nucleus in these patients compared with baseline (BROOKS et al. 1992a; ANTONINI et al. 1997). These results indicate long-term downregulation of striatal dopamine D_2 receptor binding in PD. Besides idiopathic Parkinson's disease, there are other distinct diseases, such as progressive supranuclear palsy (PSP) and multiple system atrophy (MSA), which can start with tremor, akinesia, or rigidity. As the diagnosis may be difficult in some cases, hampering the adoption of a proper therapeutic strategy, tools for the early differential diagnosis are of relevant and of clinical interest. PSP and MSA are characterized by a decrease of striatal D_2 dopamine receptor activity, as demonstrated by ^{123}I-IBZM uptake, compared with control subjects (VAN ROYEN et al. 1993). D_2 receptor density is less markedly reduced in the basal ganglia of patients with PSP, with frequent overlap with controls. The decrease in D_2 dopamine receptor activity in the early phase of PSP and MSA, contrary to the initial phases of PD, allows us differentiation between idiopathic PD and parkinsonian syndromes (BUCK et al. 1995). The differential diagnosis between essential tremor (ET) and PD is also crucial to implement an appropriate therapeutic strategy. This is a relevant issue as up to one third of the patients presenting with tremor will eventually develop PD (GERAGHTY et al. 1985). Thus, the demonstration of reduced dopaminergic marker binding in the putamen of individual patients presenting with isolated postural tremor may provide the diagnosis and a targeted therapy. Familial essential tremor is characterized by putamen and caudate ^{18}F-DOPA uptake within the normal range, whereas ^{18}F-DOPA uptake in the basal ganglia appears reduced in patients with essential tremor that eventually develop typical PD (BROOKS et al. 1992a,b).

2.8 Cerebrovascular Diseases

Patients with cerebrovascular disease (CVD) are conventionally studied after the onset of symptoms, by morphologic imaging techniques, such as CT and MRI. Morphologic imaging, although crucial for distinguishing between ischemia and hemorrhage, is not sufficient for the complete assessment of these patients. In particular, within the first 6 h after the onset of symptoms, CT and MRI T2-weighted sequences may be normal, as only MRI diffusion techniques (available only at a few sites) can indeed show the signs of early ischemia. Therefore, assessment of cerebral hemodynamics with emission tomography can be crucial for patient management in cases of transient ischemia and cerebral infarction, and for monitoring cerebrovascular reserve and reperfusion. The same methods can be used in patients with cerebral or subarachnoid hemorrhage. Local cerebral blood flow can conveniently be assessed with SPECT, whereas other key variables, such as glucose utilization, blood volume, oxygen extraction, and oxygen metabolism, can be assessed with PET. Although PET has permitted a detailed description of the natural history of CVD from a hemodynamic and metabolic standpoint, it is not easily amenable to individual patient assessment and management, due to the complexity of such studies.

We present a brief summary of the pathophysiology of stroke, with emphasis on CVD patient evaluation in clinical practice by SPECT with perfusion and viability tracers.

2.8.1 Cerebral Blood Flow and Metabolism in CVD Patients

Perfusion is determined by hemodynamic variables, including vessel patency, arterial blood pressure, cardiac output, as well as functional activity, i.e., the tissue metabolic demand. Thus, blood flow measurements represent the result of the balance between these two concurrent variables, i.e., delivery and demand.

With PET it has been shown that the regional cerebral metabolic rate of oxygen ($rCMRO_2$) is maintained by continuous oxygen delivery, adjusted to the metabolic demand by variations of regional blood flow (rCBF), regional oxygen extraction rate (rOER), and regional blood volume (rCBV). Reductions of perfusion pressure can be compensated by increases in rOER and rCBV. These compensatory mechanisms may leave the patient asymptomatic. Further reduction of perfusion pressure causes cerebral infarction (Frackowiak et al. 1980). The acute phase is followed by reperfusion and 1–3 weeks after the stroke by a marked increase of rCBF in the infarct area (Lassen 1966) without increase in $rCMRO_2$ (Wise et al. 1983). Such changes in rCBF, uncoupled to the metabolic demand, are attributed to loss of vascular autoregulation mechanisms, capillary hyperplasia, and tissue reperfusion, and has been termed „luxury perfusion" by Lassen (1966). The assessment of perfusion in the postischemic phase may be relevant for prognostic evaluation as reperfusion within 1 week of stroke is suggestive of neurologic recovery, whereas delayed reperfusion, beyond 1 week, is indicative of poor outcome (Jorgensen et al. 1994).

Another phenomenon that is observed in stroke patients, in the subacute and chronic phase, is the presence of reduced perfusion and metabolism in areas distant from the site of ischemia. Such reduction in neuronal function is attributed to deafferentation and is termed diaschisis. This phenomenon has been the object of several PET studies (Baron et al. 1981; Lenzi et al. 1982; Serrati et al. 1994). With respect to the location of the infarct region, the areas of diaschisis may be localized in the cerebellum contralateral and in the thalamus ipsilateral to a cortical lesion, in the cortex ipsilateral to a subcortical lesion and in the homotopic cortex contralateral to a cortical lesion.

With SPECT, one can study perfusion and assess the local hemodynamics in the ischemic territories, and the degree of focal neuronal dysfunction due to deafferentation and diaschisis in areas distant from the ischemic zone. In transient ischemic attacks (TIA), i.e., reversible episodes of temporary focal neuronal dysfunction caused by a transient cerebral hypoperfusion, SPECT perfusion studies within hours of the event demonstrate a persistent perfusion reduction, which in some cases may last for up to several days following the clinical recovery. This condition, i.e., persisting hypoperfusion with normal CT and complete clinical recovery termed „incomplete infarction," may be due to reduced vascular reserve, i.e., the capacity of the cerebral circulation to comply to increases in metabolic demand with vasodilatation. When this occurs, vascular reserve, an important predictor of stroke, can be measured in individual patients by assessing perfusion before and after pharmacologic challenge. Acetazolamide, 5% CO_2, or adenosine administration cause vasodilatation and increase blood volume and perfusion only in areas supplied by normal vessels (Vorstrup et al. 1986; Choksey et al. 1989). Lack of an increase of perfusion after challenge indicates a condition termed misery perfusion and is predictive of high risk of cerebral infarction. An alternative to pharmacologic challenge is the assessment of the rCBF/rCBV ratio. Due to the rapid modifications of the two variables, they should be measured concurrently by using two tracers labeled with different radionuclides, i.e., either ^{133}Xe or ^{123}I-iodo-amphetamine for the assessment of rCBF and ^{99m}Tc-RBC for the assessment of rCBV (Sabatini et al. 1991).

The flow pattern at the time of cerebral infarction and thereafter is characterized by a high degree of spatial and temporal heterogeneity due to the imbalance of hemodynamic status and functional demand. In the acute phase of a stroke reduced uptake of the perfusion tracer is seen in an area corresponding to a vascular territory. The CT lesion that eventually develops is usually smaller than the area of the initial hypoperfusion, and at the same time areas of diaschisis are identifiable in cerebral and cerebellar territories. In the subacute phase of infarction, SPECT and CT studies show consistent volumes of ischemic tissue. As shown by SPECT, the core of the lesion is characterized by more severe tissue hypoperfusion than its periphery. Moreover, areas of hypoperfusion due to diaschisis can be observed in areas that are morphologically normal. The area of hypoperfusion surrounding the core lesion may show a response to the acetazolamide test and may reveal luxury perfusion. The chronic phase is characterized by an area of absent perfusion in the infarcted territory.

The clinical applications in cerebral ischemia are limited to SPECT both for diagnosis and prognosis due to the logistic difficulties. The use of SPECT for the early diagnosis of complete ischemic stroke is currently not considered necessary, in view of the fact that there is no substantial difference in the therapeutic approach, even though SPECT may provide information on the severity of hypoperfusion prior to the occurrence of morphologic alterations (Fieschi et al. 1989). On the other hand, the assessment of perfusion with SPECT is the only procedure that shows circulatory derangements underlying the occurrence of completely reversible symptoms in patients with

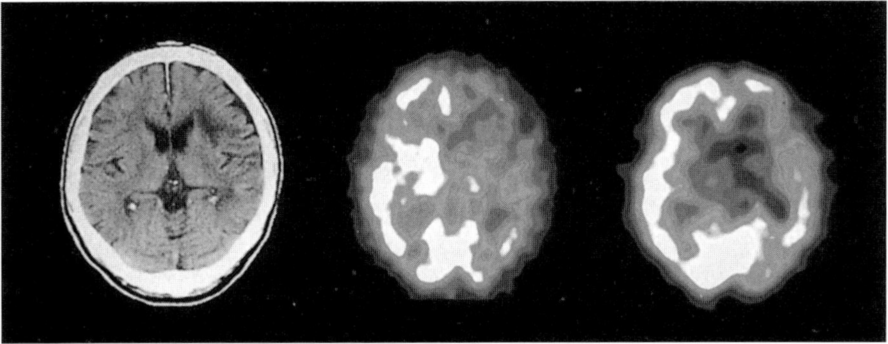

Fig. 2.4. ^{123}I-iomazenil SPECT study (*right*) in a 61-year-old patient with purely subcortical infarction 46 days after onset. A CT scan (*left*) shows hypodensity in the frontal deep white matter with no involvement of the cortical area. Blood flow measured with ^{123}I-IMP (*center*) was reduced in the frontal and temporal cortices, basal ganglia, and thalamus. ^{123}I-iomazenil image demonstrated reduced uptake in the Broca area and milder reduction in the frontal and temporal lobes that were normal on the CT images. The patient presented with global aphasia. (From Hatazawa and Shimosegawa 1998)

TIA. The assessment of TIA by using a pharmacologic challenge can provide useful information prior to EC–IC bypass surgery (Vorstrup et al. 1986).

As for the prognostic use of SPECT in stroke patients, it has been shown that the greater the perfusion deficit, the worse the outcome. This seems to hold particularly when the assessment is performed within 6 h of the onset of symptoms, but also up to 24 h post onset of symptoms (Giubilei et al. 1990; Limburg et al. 1991). The occurrence of diaschisis has been related to outcome, as permanent diaschisis 15–56 days after stroke is correlated with poor outcome (Serrati et al. 1994). Although some hypotheses have been raised about the possibility of using this approach to select patients for thrombolysis with recombinant tissue plasminogen activator in acute stroke, many perplexities still remain and prospective studies are needed (Alexandrov et al. 1997).

Another frequent application of SPECT is the assessment of vasospasm in subarachnoid hemorrhage (SAH), an event that occurs 4–12 days after a SAH. SPECT can detect early the occurrence of ischemia, the worst complication of SAH in a non-invasive and reproducible manner (Davis et al. 1990; Soucy et al. 1990).

2.8.2
Imaging of Neuronal Viability by Central Benzodiazepine Receptors

One limitation of SPECT perfusion studies is the inability to distinguish whether hypoperfusion is due to ischemia or to diaschisis, or to distinguish between glial and neuronal damage. The assessment of neuron-specific damage in CVD has become possible using ^{11}C-flumazenil and ^{123}I-iomazenil, two selective high affinity antagonists of the BZD/GABA$_A$ receptors. Biousse et al. (1993) and Minoshima et al. (1993) have demonstrated reduced glucose metabolism with preserved distribution volume of flumazenil as a result of diaschisis, laying the groundwork for benzodiazepine GABA$_A$ (BZD/GABA$_A$) receptor studies in ischemia. In stroke patients, BZD/GABA$_A$ receptor imaging with ^{123}I-iomazenil and SPECT has been pursued. Hatazawa et al. (1995) have studied the relationship between iomazenil uptake, CBF, CMRO$_2$, morphologic and clinical findings (Fig. 2.4); they reported a decrease in iomazenil uptake beyond the CT hypodense area. This finding is suggestive of either a CT-negative ischemic damage in the area surrounding a complete infarction, or an inhibition of iomazenil binding due to the release of endogenous substances specifically binding to BZD receptors following ischemia. Perfusion reductions with a normal ^{123}I-iomazenil distribution indicate diaschisis, i.e., abnormalities in areas distant from the stroke region, due to deafferentation.

2.9
Epilepsy

Epilepsy is a heterogeneous group of neurologic disorders characterized by recurrent seizures. Seizures may manifest as focal or generalized motor jerks, sensory or visual phenomena, or more complex alterations in behavior, awareness, and consciousness, and are influenced by the age of the patient, the degree of

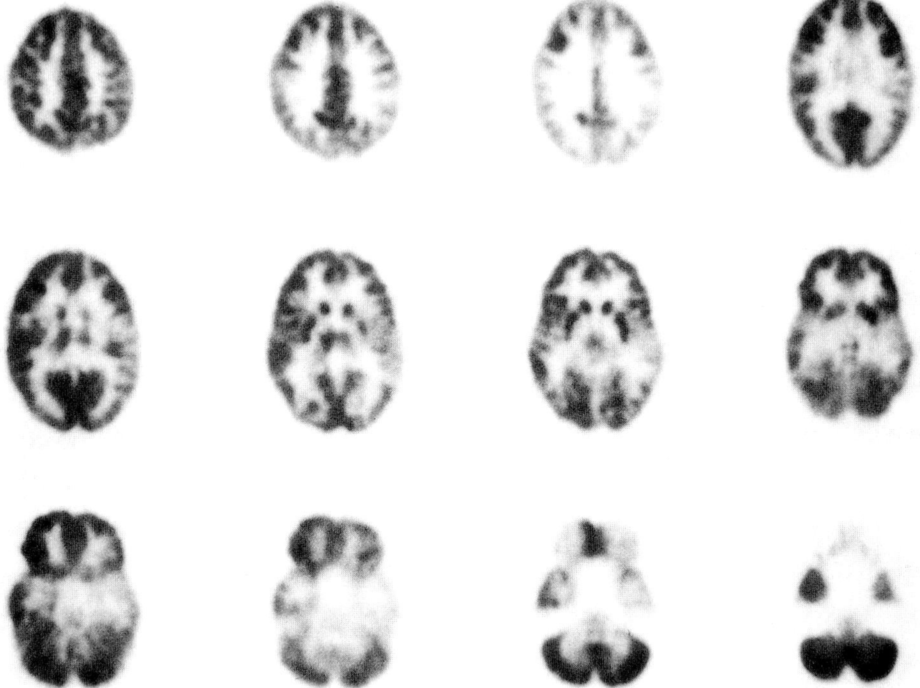

Fig. 2.5. ^{18}F-FDG-PET images of a patient with partial complex epilepsy. There is left temporal lobe interictal hypometabolism corresponding to the left temporal lobe seizure focus. In addition, the area of hypometabolism extends into the left frontoparietal region and ipsilateral thalamus, even though these areas were normal on the electroencephalogram

brain maturation, underlying focal lesions, and the electroencephalographic (EEG) correlates present at the time of seizures. Epilepsy is common, affecting 1% of the population with approximately 50 new cases per year per 100,000 people. Ten to 20% of these new cases will go on to have „medically intractable seizures“ and therefore become candidates for surgical treatment if they can be shown to have a localized seizure focus. Noninvasive localization of seizure foci can be achieved in many patients with PET and SPECT imaging, and these methods have a solid clinical role in management of epilepsy. Nevertheless, it is important to keep in mind that the diagnosis of epilepsy is made largely on clinical and electrophysiologic grounds and accordingly, it is important to carefully integrate functional brain imaging studies into the diagnostic process in patients who have been determined to be candidates for seizure surgery.

2.9.1 Cerebral Blood Flow and Metabolism in Seizure Disorders

The cerebral metabolic consequences of epilepsy were first investigated using ^{18}F- FDG and PET (Kuhl et al. 1980; Engel et al. 1982a–c; Yamamoto et al. 1983; Theodore et al. 1984; Franck et al. 1986; Abou-Khalil et al. 1989). Following the development of blood flow tracers for SPECT imaging, many reports of blood flow abnormalities in epilepsy have appeared (Bonte et al. 1983; Sanabria et al. 1983; Lee et al. 1988; Stefan et al. 1987a; Lang et al. 1988). In recent years there has been a parallel recognition of the usefulness of PET and SPECT in evaluating patients for seizure surgery, but few systematic studies have been performed comparing these two modalities.

Most interictal PET studies demonstrate that approximately 70% of patients with severe partial seizures have reduced regional glucose utilization. Interictal hypometabolism is more common in patients with mesial temporal lesions such as hippocampal sclerosis, small tumors and hamartomas, but is less frequently seen in patients without radiographically visible lesions (Engel 1982a; Henry 1990). Whereas the region of interictal hypometabolism corresponds grossly to the location of interictal EEG abnormalities, its size is consistently larger than the area of the EEG abnormality, as demonstrated in Fig. 2.5 (Engel 1982a; Theodore et al. 1988; Henry 1990). For example, in patients with seizure foci well localized in the temporal lobe, reduced metabolism is seen in the mesial and lateral temporal cortex and at times in the ipsilateral frontal and parietal cortex, basal ganglia, and thalamus (Fig. 2.5; ENGEL 1982c; HENRY 1990; SACKELLERAS 1990). However, subsequent studies indicated that within the temporal lobe the metabolic pattern may differ according to whether the patient has temporal lobe epilepsy of lateral neocortical or mesial basal origin (HAJEK 1993). Patients with temporal lobe epilepsy due to mesial gliosis display a generalized mesial and lateral hypometabolism, whereas patients with a lateral neocortical gliosis have relatively little mesial basal hypometabolism. Accordingly, PET may provide noninvasive information that helps stratify patients for mesial basal vs lateral neocortical selective temporal lobe surgery. Patients with bilateral hypometabolism have a worse surgical prognosis that those with unilateral hypometabolism (BLUM et al. 1998). Interestingly, no quantitative relations have been observed between the presence and magnitude of regional hypometabolism and interictal or ictal electrical parameters (ENGEL 1988b). Accordingly, ^{18}F-FDG metabolic studies appear to be measuring processes different from those reflected by regional electrical activity.

False-positive identification of the side of a seizure focus by ^{18}F-FDG PET has been observed in only a few individuals and was attributed to artifacts resulting from depth electrode placement (ENGEL 1982c; ENGEL 1984). Conversely, erroneous lateralization using scalp and sphenoidal EEG is observed in 10%–15% of patients (Engel 1988; RISINGER 1989). Accordingly, for clinical management of patients with intractable seizures ^{18}F-FDG PET is commonly used together with scalp EEG studies. Close correspondence of scalp EEG and ^{18}F-FDG PET results provides strong evidence for lateralization of epileptogenic tissue and in many instances patients undergo focal resections without invasive electrical monitoring. If ^{18}F-FDG PET and EEG data do not correspond then invasive electrical monitoring is needed (ENGEL et al. 1990). Although ^{18}F-FDG PET is clearly useful in noninvasive localization of epileptogenic tissue, there is no general correlation between the presence and degree of hypometabolism and the surgical outcome (ENGEL 1988). However, SWARTZ et al. (1992a) has demonstrated that patients with widespread areas of hypometabolism tend to have a worse postoperative prognosis. The lack of a clear relation between hypometabolism and outcome undoubtedly relates to the fact that ^{18}F-FDG PET overestimates the extent of epileptogenic tissue, and conversely, extratemporal seizure foci may cause temporal lobe hypometabolism. Clearly new and more specific tracers are needed in order to identify epileptogenic tissue more precisely.

The site of interictal hypometabolism corresponds to sites of ictal onset as shown by EEG, but ictal PET studies are difficult to perform since the tracer may not be available due to its short half-life. Nevertheless, the fortuitous occurrence of seizures at the time of ^{18}F-FDG administration has provided ictal ^{18}F-FDG PET scans (ENGEL et al. 1982b, 1983; THEODORE et al. 1984; ABOU-KHALIL et al. 1989). Due to the propagation of seizure activity beyond the focus and the problems in timing of the injection of ^{18}F-FDG, ictal PET scanning has received relatively little attention, particularly in the context of the clinical management of patients with intractable epilepsy. Additionally, images reflect average metabolic activity over an approximate 30-min time interval after injection. Accordingly, images reflect an admixture of interictal, ictal, and postictal metabolism, which may be difficult to interpret. For example, some ^{18}F-FDG PET studies acquired during an ictus have shown global hypometabolism. In these instances it is thought that the ^{18}F-FDG PET image reflects predominantly postictal depression of metabolism when the actual seizure activity occurs during a small portion of the uptake period. Since some seizures may be subclinical, it is important to monitor the EEG during the uptake period (BARRINGTON et al. 1998). Ictal and postictal blood flow changes in epilepsy have been more extensively investigated with SPECT.

Although most ^{18}F-FDG PET studies have been performed in patients with complex partial seizures originating in the temporal lobe, the same methods can be used to localize frontal lobe lesions (SWARTZ et al. 1989, 1992b; FRANCK et al. 1992; HENRY et al. 1992; ROBITAILLE et al. 1992). Interictal hypometabolism is observed in the region of frontal lobe seizure foci and, as in temporal lobe epilepsy, may extend beyond the areas of electrical abnormality (HENRY et al. 1992; SWARTZ et al. 1989, 1992b). The relation of PET to other imaging modalities in epilepsy has been recently reviewed (DUNCAN 1997).

SPECT imaging in epilepsy has employed ^{123}I-IMP and ^{123}I-HIPDM (MAGISTRETTI and UREN 1983; LEE et al. 1986, 1987, 1988) and subsequently ^{99m}Tc-HMPAO and related tracers (STEFAN et al. 1987b; ANDERSEN et al. 1988; RYDING et al. 1988; DEVOUS and LEROY 1989; ROWE et al. 1989, 1991a; GRÜNWALD et al. 1991; KRAUSZ et al. 1991; NEWTON 1992; THOMAS et al. 1992). Overall, these results demonstrate the high sensitivity in localizing seizure foci comparable to that of ^{18}F-FDG PET (70%), but some studies have shown a lower sensitivity, stimulating the use of ictal SPECT scanning.

Due to the longer half-life of SPECT blood flow radiopharmaceuticals, the use of ictal and postictal scanning in patients with epilepsy has been explored in recent years (Magistretti and Uren 1983; Lee et al. 1987, 1988; Devous et al. 1989; Rowe et al. 1989; Marks et al. 1992; Newton et al. 1992; Ramsey et al. 1992). Numerous studies have suggested that ictal imaging is more sensitive than interictal scanning in temporal lobe epilepsy (Rowe et al. 1989). In these studies a simultaneous EEG recording is obtained and the radiopharmaceutical injected within 1 or 2 min of the onset of seizure. Areas of interictal hypoperfusion convert to areas of hyperperfusion during the ictus. Ictal SPECT imaging has the potential to identify multiple and bilateral seizure foci, but carries with it the possibility of identifying areas of secondary seizure activity depending on the timing of the radiopharmaceutical injection and the rapidity of seizure spread. In addition, one study has provided evidence for an increase in regional blood flow prior to the initiation of seizure activity, implying that the blood flow changes may not directly reflect regional seizure activity (Baumgartner et al. 1998). However, studies of localized simple partial seizures using ^{99m}Tc-HMPAO demonstrate well localized areas of hyperperfusion that correlate with the electrical and clinical localization. Ictal SPECT has also been applied to frontal lobe epilepsy, demonstrating a 91% sensitivity of correctly localizing lateralized seizure foci. Peri-ictal scanning in pediatric patients has been specifically evaluated and found to be beneficial (O'Brien et al. 1998; Shulkin 1997).

Post-ictal SPECT imaging (i.e., imaging within minutes after a seizure) has also been employed and the results demonstrate an improvement in sensitivity compared with interictal scanning (Rowe et al. 1989, 1991b; Duncan et al. 1993). The largest of these studies reported a sensitivity of 69% for post-ictal imaging compared with 38% for true interictal scans. The reasons for the low interictal sensitivity in this study are unclear. Within approximately 10 min after the completion of a seizure, the pattern of hyperperfusion in the anterio-mesial temporal lobe and hypoperfusion in the remaining temporal lobe is often observed. After approximately 15 min, the mesial hyperperfusion disappears and the hypoperfusion becomes less pronounced. Accordingly, the time from ictus is important in interpreting post-ictal SPECT images. It is important not to misinterpret severe post-ictal hypoperfusion ipsilateral to the seizure focus and hyperperfusion on the contralateral side. As with ^{18}F-FDG-PET imaging, SPECT perfusion imaging is more sensitive than MRI (Cordes et al. 1990). The presence of interictal hypoperfusion is similarly more common in patients with T2-weighted MRI abnormalities, as compared with patients with normal MRI scans (Ryvlin et al. 1992).

Another application of ^{99m}Tc-HMPAO is to map the distribution of amobarbital in the intracarotid Wada test (Hietala et al. 1990; Jeffery et al. 1991; Hart et al. 1993). Administration of intracarotid amobarbital was first used to indicate hemispheric dominance for language in patients who were to undergo surgery for intractable epilepsy and is currently also used to identify patients at risk for amnesia following temporal lobe surgery. Subsequently, the Wada test has been used to aid in the lateralization of epileptogenic regions. A good correlation exists between interictal PET and intracarotid amobarbital administration in the lateralization of seizure foci (Salanova et al. 1998). Intracarotid amobarbital administration is used not only to localize language function, but also to predict memory disturbance following temporal lobectomy. In this regard, delivery of amobarbital to ipsilateral mesial lobe structures is the key. In 90% of individuals the posterior two thirds of the hippocampus is supplied by the vertebrobasilar system via the posterior cerebral artery. Accordingly, administration of amobarbital via the intracarotid artery probably does not result in anesthesia of the entire hippocampus in many patients (Jeffery et al. 1991). If the amobarbital is not delivered to the hippocampus, false-negative memory lateralization may occur. Co-administration of ^{99m}Tc-HMPAO and amobarbital via the internal carotid artery can be used to assess areas of perfusion during the Wada test. If present, contralateral hemispheric perfusion via the circle of Willis during the Wada test can also be identified.

Recent studies support the added value of PET over interictal SPECT studies (Lamusuo et al. 1997) and comparable accuracy with ictal SPECT and interictal PET (Markand et al. 1997). However, the final conclusions regarding the relative merits of PET and SPECT will have to await studies using state-of-the-art instrumentation for both modalities.

2.9.2 Neurotransmission Function in Seizure Disorders

Although scalp and invasive electroencephalography is the mainstay of diagnosis, classification, and lesion identification in epilepsy, PET and SPECT have advanced our understanding of the basic ictal and interictal blood flow and metabolic events that correlate with the electrical abnormalities. Flow-metabolism imaging alone is limited in its potential to elucidate the neurochemical mechanisms responsible for initiation and termination of seizures. More specific tracers are needed to further improve localization of the epileptogenic foci, predict prognosis following seizure surgery, and stratify patients for various drug therapies. New methods to image and quantitate neuroreceptors have provided the first approach to realizing these goals.

Studies using PET and SPECT have been conducted with tracers for opioid receptors: ^{11}C-carfentanil, ^{11}C-diprenorphine, ^{18}F-cyclo-foxy, and ^{11}C-methylnaltrindole (Fig. 2.6; Frost et al. 1988; Mayberg et al. 1991; Madar et al. 1997); benzodiazepine receptors: ^{11}C-flumazenil and ^{123}I-iomazenil (Savic et al. 1988; Innis et al. 1991); muscarinic cholinergic receptors: ^{123}I-iododexetimide (Mueller-Gaertner et al. 1993); and histamine receptors: ^{11}C-doxepin (Iinuma et al. 1993). Increased levels of mu and delta opioid receptors (Fig. 2.6) and reduced benzodiazepine and muscarinic cholinergic receptors have been observed. In some, but not all, cases receptor imaging has provided additional localization information over flow/metabolism imaging alone. Comparison of ^{11}C-flumazenil and ^{18}F-FDG in patients with partial complex seizures has shown that ^{11}C-flumazenil may provide improved localization of seizure foci (Koepp et al. 1997a,b; Richardson et al. 1997, 1998). However, another study showed that ^{11}C-flumazenil was less accurate (Debets et al. 1997). Changes in benzodiazepine receptors may vary as a function of seizure activity (Savic et al. 1998).

Some studies have begun to examine the effect of seizure activity on ^{11}C-diprenorphine binding in patients with primary generalized absence seizures (Bartenstein et al. 1993) and seizures induced by reading (Koepp et al. 1998). These studies demonstrate that active seizure activity alters opioid receptor binding, probably due to release of endogenous opioid peptides. This demonstration of a functional change in opiate receptor binding following seizures introduces a new paradigm for investigation of the role of the opiate system in epilepsy.

2.10 Brain Tumors

For the past two decades the diagnostic work-up of brain tumors has been based on morphologic imaging, first with CT and more recently with MRI (Atlas 1991; Fishbein 1988; Goldberg 1991). Contrast-enhanced CT is, in general, the first examination performed in patients with suspected brain tumor. It is possible with CT to make a differential diagnosis with other cerebral lesions and, to a limited extent, also among different types of intracranial tumors. Investigations with CT and MRI, however, may yield partial answers, and must be complemented by biochemical imaging. Biochemical imaging of brain tumors may indeed be crucial for the early differential diagnosis, for a prognostic assessment and for differentiating between edema and gliosis, as well as between recurrence and radionecrosis, and is best achieved by emission tomography. The mechanisms of uptake and retention of each tracer in normal tis-

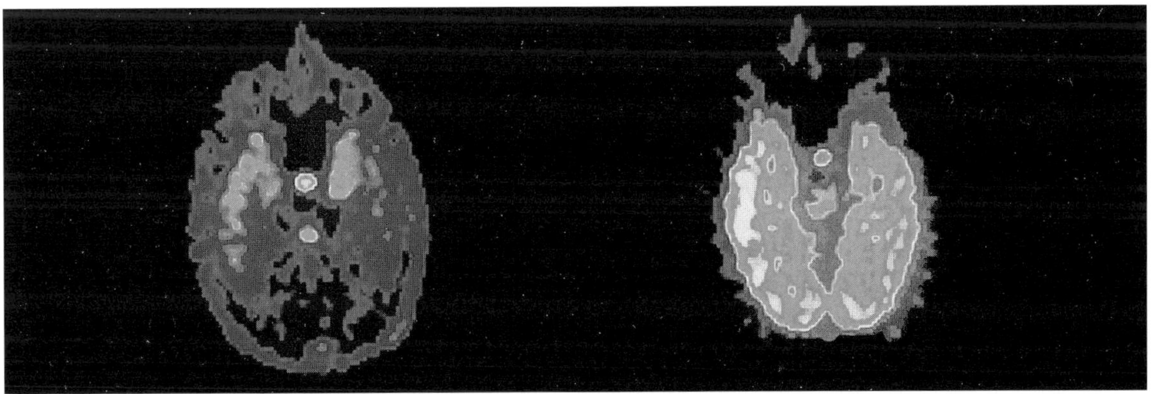

Fig. 2.6. Images of ^{11}C-carfentanil and ^{11}C-N-methyl naltrindole binding in a patient with right-sided temporal lobe seizure focus. Both ^{11}C-carfentanil and ^{11}C-N-methyl naltrindole binding are increased in the right temporal neocortex

sue are frequently altered markedly in neoplastic tissue. Alterations in the normal pattern of tracer accumulation can be due either to secondary events, commonly detectable by morphologic imaging, such as the disruption of the BBB, or perfusion modifications due to compression and dislocation of the cerebral structures. However, most interesting is the tracer accumulation due to biochemical modifications of the neoplastic tissue itself, as alterations of metabolic processes and their rates may be related to the rate of growth and cell type of the tumor, whereas the expression of specific antigens or receptors by the tumor may help in their histologic characterization and assist in treatment planning. Developments in morphologic imaging and concurrent advances in biochemical imaging have therefore completely modified the role of radiology and nuclear medicine in the assessment of patients with brain tumors.

The clinical use of radioactive tracers in neurooncology has followed their use for other purposes. This is the case of ^{18}F-fluorodeoxyglucose, developed for the assessment of neuronal functional activity, ^{11}C-methionine, developed for the assessment of amino acid transport and protein synthesis, followed by the development of ^{123}I-tyrosine. It also holds for ^{201}Tl and ^{99m}Tc-methoxy-isobutil-isonitrile (MIBI), both extensively used in nuclear cardiology. All of these tracers are relatively nonspecific, and some of them can also be used for the assessment of extracranial tumors. In other cases tracers have been developed for the assessment of tumors with very specific features, including the expression of antigens or receptors.

2.10.1 Imaging of Tumor Metabolic Processes

Tracers most commonly used for the assessment of cerebral tumors include ^{18}F-FDG, ^{11}C-methionine, ^{201}Tl, and ^{99m}Tc-MIBI. In various manners their uptake is dependent on basic processes, such as membrane permeability, to electrolytes by active and passive mechanisms, Na^+,K^+, ATP-ase activity, energy metabolism, and other metabolic variables such as protein synthesis, as well as on the presence of specific clearance mechanisms. The uptake and retention of tracer in tumor tissue depends also on cell type, extent of differentiation, immunogenicity, rate of growth, tissue mass perfusion pattern, BBB integrity, vascular neoformation, and maturation.

^{18}F-FDG is the most important tracer for PET oncologic studies (see Chap. 10). Relatively simple synthesis and long half-life along with extensive knowledge of the mechanisms determining its uptake and retention have made it very popular in neuro-oncology. Initial studies have related the grade of malignancy of gliomas to the rate of ^{18}F-FDG uptake, and have shown that while low-grade astrocytomas have low ^{18}F-FDG uptake, anaplastic astrocytomas and glioblastomas have markedly elevated tracer uptake (Di Chiro et al. 1982, 1988; Di Chiro and Brooks 1988). In tumor cells there is an overexpression of glucose transporters and enzymes related to glucose metabolism, and this causes an accumulation of tracer in tumor tissue that is generally higher than in normal tissue. As already stated, normal brain is avid of glucose, and therefore the accumulation of ^{18}F-FDG in tumor may in some cases be very close to that of normal tissue causing difficulties in the interpretation of the study. Based on these premises ^{18}F-FDG has been used for the assessment of tumor malignancy and prognosis, but the most important use is follow-up of patients with low-grade astrocytomas, possibly evolving into high-grade malignancy, and the differentiation between radiation necrosis and tumor recurrence in patients presenting with relapse of neurologic symptoms and nondiagnostic CT and/or MRI after radiation therapy. Problems related to the tumor/nontumor uptake ratio encountered with ^{18}F-FDG, and difficult differential diagnoses with other cerebral pathologies, i.e., infections, radiation necrosis, and edema, that may cause abnormal ^{18}F-FDG uptake, can be avoided by using ^{11}C-methionine, which uptake is related to amino acid transport and metabolic rate of the tumor (Bergstrom et al. 1987; Hatazawa et al. 1989).

An alternative to positron tracers neuro-oncology is ^{201}Tl (Elgazzar et al. 1993; Kim et al. 1990; Yoshi et al. 1993; Dierckx et al. 1994; Ricci et al. 1996). The discovery that ^{201}Tl accumulates in neoplastic tissue was serendipitous because it was observed in patients undergoing myocardial perfusion studies who also had tumors. The uptake of ^{201}Tl in brain tumors is related to blood flow, BBB integrity and malignant cell density, and is due to its similarities with potassium and thus on the Na^+,K^+, ATP-ase activity. ^{201}Tl uptake is also related to tumor type: as the rate of uptake differs, ^{201}Tl cannot be used as a partial substitute for histologic characterization and grading. It must be pointed out that, depending on the patient-selection process, ^{201}Tl sensitivity and specificity have been estimated to be approximately 70% and 80%, respectively, but sensitivity is lower in low-grade gliomas, whereas specificity is lower in cases with hemorrhagic infarction. The highest sensitivities have been observed in glioblastoma multiforme and metastatic lesions.

Another tracer that is amenable for imaging cerebral tumors with SPECT is ^{99m}Tc-MIBI (SOLER et al. 1998; MAFFIOLI et al. 1996), which was originally also developed for evaluating myocardial perfusion. This tracer is a cationic complex that is concentrated in cytoplasm and mitochondria as a result of passive diffusion across highly negative transmembrane potentials in relation to metabolic demand. Studies with this tracer have shown sensitivities similar to that of ^{201}Tl in malignant tumors and recurrence.

As for amino acid transport into tumor cells, the SPECT tracer ^{123}I-methyl-tyrosine has been evaluated in small patient series with promising results (BIERSACK et al. 1989; LANGEN et al. 1997).

2.10.2 Imaging of Cerebral Tumors by Antibodies and Receptor-Bound Tracers

Imaging modalities based on the use of SPECT and monoclonal antibodies is attracting increasing interest, in particular for those aimed at the signal amplification by tumor pretargeting techniques. This is best achieved by the administration of biotinylated monoclonal antibody, followed by administration of the radioactive tracer (two-step technique), or by the administration of avidin, after the monoclonal antibody, and then by the tracer administration (three-step technique). The additional steps are aimed at the enhancement of the signal-to-noise ratio, by allowing a longer time for the antibody localization on the tumor (two-step), and removal of free antibody by conjugation with avidin (three-step), prior to the administration of low doses of radioactive tracer.

The use of tracers, which specifically bind to receptors, has been applied mostly to pituitary adenomas, in particular in the assessment of nonsecreting tumors. Nonfunctioning pituitary adenomas, as well as meningiomas and craniopharyngiomas, do not cause any specific endocrine syndrome; thus, their presence is usually suggested by the evidence of compression of the parasellar nervous structures. Radiologic differential diagnosis may occasionally be difficult in primary parasellar lesions with presentation in the parasellar region. Diagnostic uncertainty after MRI investigation occurs in up to 10% of patients with hormonally inactive tumors of the sellar region. In these selected cases, the in vivo characterization of the biochemical and functional properties of the tissue may provide useful information about the nature of the pituitary mass.

The PET and SPECT techniques have been used for the assessment of adenomas and other parasellar tumors with ^{18}F-FDG, ^{11}C-methionine, ^{11}C-tyrosine, ^{11}C-deprenyl, ^{11}C, and ^{18}F labeled spiperone analogs, as well as ^{123}I-IBZM and ^{123}I-epidepride (MUHR et al. 1986; DAEMEN et al. 1991; BERGSTROM et al. 1992; PIRKER et al. 1996; LUCIGNANI et al. 1998; de HERDER et al. 1999). Some of the methods proposed for the assessment of sellar and parasellar tumors are based on measurements that are not specific to any particular type of neoplastic tissue, i.e., the rate of glucose metabolism or protein synthesis. These variables may indicate a neoplastic process when they are abnormally increased or decreased. Such methods have been shown to be useful for visualizing pituitary adenomas, for differentiating between viable neoplastic tissue and scar, and for assessing the response to pharmacologic treatment. Other methods are based on the use of radiopharmaceutical tracing processes in the normal and abnormal pituitary tissue, but neither in the other tumors of the sella nor in the nearest surrounding tissue.

Another approach to imaging pituitary adenomas is based on the presence of somatostatin receptors on pituitary tumors, which bind octreotide. For this purpose both ^{111}In-DTPA-pentetreotide and ^{123}I-Tyr3-octreotide have been used (KRENNING et al. 1993; see Chap. 9).

2.10.3 Differential Diagnosis of Lymphoma and Infectious Diseases in AIDS

Neurologic disorders occur in 40%–60% of patients with AIDS and approximately 10% develop focal lesions of the CNS. In these patients contrast-enhancing brain lesions are most frequently caused by infectious diseases (50–70% of patients), due to *Toxoplasma gondii, Candida albicans, Mycobacterium tuberculosis,* or by primary lymphomas (2%–10% of patients). Each type of lesion requires a timely, specific therapy, but it is a common practice to start antitoxoplasmosis therapy based on empirical evidence. In patients who do not respond to therapy a noninvasive diagnostic procedure, i.e., alternative to biopsy, is required for an appropriate therapeutic planning. In these patients ^{201}Tl, ^{18}F-FDG, or ^{99m}Tc-MIBI can be used to support the selection of a therapeutic approach, based on the evidence that in lymphomas the uptake of these tracers is generally higher than in focal infectious lesions (COSTA et al. 1995; D'AMICO et al. 1997).

2.11 Outlook for the Future

The state-of-the-art PET and SPECT techniques, which have been developed over the past 20 years, enable us to diagnose and evaluate CNS diseases, predominantly by measurement of cerebral blood flow and metabolism. Flow-metabolism methods permit identification of the areas of abnormal neuronal function and thus differentiation of distinct diseases due to cortical neuronal degeneration, such as the various forms of dementia that occur with cognitive impairment. However, as energy metabolism is a nonspecific process with respect to the activity of the neuronal subpopulations, radionuclide imaging of the brain is under continuous evolution as new methods are developed and applied also for the assessment of pre- and postsynaptic neurotransmitter function. These methods permit differentiation of syndromes occurring with motor impairment due to subcortical neuronal damage. Moreover, the use of neurochemical imaging, including the rate of synthesis and uptake of neurotransmitters, and their rate of binding to selective receptors, appears to be crucial for the assessment of neuronal viability and damage in cerebral vascular diseases and epilepsy. Finally, the assessment of neurochemical derangements is the only key to the understanding of psychiatric diseases.

The future of brain radionuclide imaging depends on the continuous development of devices to measure the radiotracer distribution, and on the search for new radiopharmaceuticals, along with improvements in the area of data processing. To this end, tomographic systems are being developed to improve the accuracy of measurements of radiotracer distribution with a concurrent reduction of the acquisition time, whereas radiopharmaceuticals that selectively tag the various receptor classes and subclasses are successfully manufactured. Last, but not least, analytical procedures are being implemented for faster and more accurate image and data processing.

The strategy for the assessment of neurologic patients will soon include the use of activation tasks with pharmacologic challenge, and the use of dedicated instruments that combine state-of-the-art X-ray CT and emission tomography imaging. This synergistic approach will overcome the spatial resolution limitations of emission tomography and add the power of biochemical imaging to morphologic imaging.

Part of this work was performed by Dr. Lucignani under Contract 14175-1998-07 F1PC ISP TI of the European Commission, Joint Research Center, Ispra, Institute for Health and Consumer Protection

References

Abou-Khalil BW, Siegel GJ, Sackellares JC, Gilman S, Hichwa R, Marshall R (1989) Positron emission tomography studies of cerebral glucose metabolism in chronic partial epilepsy. Ann Neurol 22:480–486

Albin RL, Minoshima S, D'Amato CJ, Frey KA, Kuhl DE, Sima AAF (1996) Fluoro-deoxyglucose positron emission tomography in diffuse Lewy body disease. Neurology 47:462–466

Alexandrov AV, Masdeu JC, Devous MD Sr, Black SE, Grotta JC (1997) Brain single-photon emission CT with HMPAO and safety of thrombolytic therapy in acute ischemic stroke. Proc Meeting of the SPECT Safe Thrombolysis Study Collaborators and the members of the Brain Imaging Council of the Society of Nuclear Medicine. Stroke28:1830–1834

Andersen AR, Gram L, Kjaer L, Fuglsang-Frederiksen A, Herning M, Lassen NA, Dam M (1988) SPECT in partial epilepsy: identifying side of the focus. Acta Neurol Scand (Suppl 117) 78:90–95

Antonini A, Schwarz J, Oertel WH, Pogarell O, Leenders KL (1997) Long-term changes of striatal dopamine D2 receptors in patients with Parkinson's disease: a study with positron emission tomography and [^{11}C]raclopride. Movement Disord 12:33–38

Arnett CD, Fowler JS, MacGregor RR (1987) Turnover of brain monoamine oxidase measured in vivo by positron emission tomography using L-^{11}C deprenyl. J Neurochem 49:522–527

Atlas SW (1991) Intraaxial brain tumours. In: Atlas SW (ed) Magnetic resonance imaging of the brain and spine. Raven Press, New York, pp 379–409

Baron JC, Bousser MG, Comar D, Soussaline F, Castaigne P (1981) Noninvasive tomographic study of cerebral blood flow and oxygen metabolism in vivo. Potentials, limitations, and clinical applications in cerebral ischemic disorders. Eur Neurol 20:273–284

Baronti F, Conant KE, Giuffra M, Davis TL, Brughitta G, Iadarola M, Berrettini WH, Chase TN, Mouradian MM (1991) Opioid peptides in Parkinson's disease: effects of dopamine repletion. Brain Res 560:92–96

Barrington SF, Koutroumanidis M, Agathonikou A, Marsden PK, Binnie CD, Polkey CE, Maisey MN, Panayiotopoulos CP (1998) Clinical value of "ictal" FDG-positron emission tomography and the routine use of simultaneous scalp EEG studies in patients with intractable partial epilepsies. Epilepsia 39:753–766

Bartenstein P, Ludolph A, Schober O, Lottes G, Scheidhauer K, Sciuk J, Beer H-F (1991) Benzodiazepine receptors and cerebral blood flow in partial epilepsy. Eur J Nucl Med 18:111–118

Baumgartner C, Serles W, Leutmezer F, Pataraia E, Aull S, Czech T, Pietrzyk U, Relic A, Podreka I (1998) Preictal SPECT in temporal lobe epilepsy: regional cerebral blood flow is increased prior to electroencephalography-seizure onset. J Nucl Med 39:978–982

Beer HF, Bläuenstein PA, Hasler PH, Delaloye B, Riccabona G, Bangerl I, Hunkeler W, Bonetti EP, Pieri L, Richards JG, Schubiger PA (1990) In vitro and in vivo evaluation of iodine-123-Ro16-0154: a new imaging agent for SPECT investigations of benzodiazepine receptors. J Nucl Med 31:1007–1014

Benson DF, Kuhl DE, Hawkins RA, Phelps ME, Cummings JL, Tsai SY (1983) The fluorodeoxyglucose-^{18}F scan in

Alzheimer's disease and multi-infarct dementia. Arch Neurol 40:711–714

Bergstrom M, Muhr C, Lundberg PO, Berstrom K, Lundqvist H, Antoni G, Fasth K-G, Langstrom B (1987) In vivo study of amino acid distribution and metabolism in pituitary adenomas using positron emission tomography with ^{11}C-D-methionine and ^{11}C-L-methionine. J Comput Assist Tomogr 11:384–389

Bergstrom M, Muhr C, Jossan S, Lilja A, Nyberg G, Langstrom B (1992) Differentiation of pituitary adenoma and meningioma: visualization with positron emission tomography and[^{11}C]-L-deprenyl. Neurosurgery 30:855–861

Berridge M, Comar D, Crouzel C, Baron JC (1983) ^{11}C-labelled ketanserin: a selective serotonin S2 antagonist. J Label Compounds Radiopharmacol 20:73

Biersack HJ, Coenen HH, Stocklin G, Reichmann K, Bockisch A, Oehr P, Kashab M, Rollmann O (1989) Imaging of brain tumors with L-3-[123I]iodo-alpha-methyl tyrosine and SPECT. J Nucl Med 30:110–112

Biousse V, Zilovicius M, De Recondo A, Woimant F, Amarenco P, Bousser MG et al. (1993) PET study of central benzodiazepine receptors (BZR) with [^{11}C]-flumazenil (Cflu) distinguishes "functional" from structural hypometabolism in stroke. Neurology 43:A381

Blum DE, Ehsan T, Dungan D, Karis JP, Fisher RS (1998) Bilateral temporal hypometabolism in epilepsy. Epilepsia 39:651–659

Bonte FJ, Stokely EM, Devous MD Jr, Homan RW (1983) Single-photon tomographic study of regional cerebral blood flow in epilepsy. A preliminary report. Arch Neurol 40:267–270

Brooks DJ, Salmon EP, Mathias CJ, Quinn N, Leenders KL, Bannister R, Marsden CD, Frackowiak RSJ (1990) The relationship between locomotor disability, autonomic dysfunction, and the integrity of the striatal dopaminergic system in patients with multiple system atrophy, pure autonomic failure, and Parkinson's disease, studied with PET. Brain 113:1539–1552

Brooks DJ, Ibanez V, Sawle GV, Quinn N, Lees AJ, Mathias CJ, Bannister R, Marsden CD, Frackowiak RSJ (1990) Differing patterns of striatal ^{18}F-dopa uptake in Parkinson's disease, multiple system atrophy, and progressive supranuclear palsy (see comments). Ann Neurol 28:547–555

Brooks DJ, Ilbanez V, Sawle GV, Plaayford ED, Quinn N, Mathias CJ, Lees AJ, Marsden CD, Bannister R, Frackowiak RSJ (1992a) Striatal D2 receptor status in patients with Parkinson's disease, striatonigral degeneration, and progressive supranuclear palsy, measured with 11C-raclopride and positron emission tomography. Ann Neurol 31:184–192

Brooks DJ, Playford ED, Ibanez V, Sawle GV, Thompson PD, Findley L, Masden CD (1992b) Isolated tremor and disruption of the nigrostriatal system: an 18F-dopa PET study (see comments). Neurology 42:1554–1560

Brucke T, Kornhuber J, Angelberger P, Asenbaum S, Frassine H, Podreka I (1993) SPECT imaging of dopamine and serotonin transporters with [^{123}I]beta-CIT. Binding kinetics in the human brain. J Neural Transm Gen Sect 94:137–146

Buck A, Westera G, Sutter M, Albani C, Kung HF, Schulthess GKJ von (1995) Iodine-123-IBF SPECT evaluation of extrapyramidal diseases. J Nucl Med 36:1196–1200

Chiro G di, Brooks RA (1988) PET-FDG of untreated and treated cerebral gliomas. J Nucl Med 29:421–422

Chiro G di, De LaPaz RL, Brooks RA, Sokoloff L, Kornblith PL, Smith BH, Patronas NJ, Kufta CV, Kessler RM, Johnson GS, Manning RG, Wolf AP (1982) Glucose utilization of cerebral gliomas measured by 18F-fluorodeoxyglucose and positron emission tomography. Neurology 32:1323–1329

Chiro G di, Oldfield E, Wright DC, Michele G de, Patronas N, Doppman JL, Larson SM, Masanori I, Kufta CV (1988) Cerebral necrosis after radiotherapy and/or intraarterial chemotherapy for brain tumours, PET and neuropathologic studies. Am J Roentgenol 150:189–197

Choksey MS, Costa DC, Iannotti F, Ell PJ, Chochard HA (1989) Tc-99m-HMPAO SPECT and cerebral blood flow: a study of CO2 reactivity. Nucl Med Commun 10:609–618

Coenen HH, Laufer P, Stocklin G, Wienhard K, Pawlik G, Bocker-Schwarz HG, Heiss WD (1987) 3-N-(2'[^{18}F]fluoroethyl)-spiperone: a new ligand for cerebral dopamine receptor studies with PET. Life Sci 40:81–88

Cordes M, Christe W, Henkes H, Delavier U, Eichstädt H, Schörner W, Langer R, Felix R (1990) Focal epilepsies: HM-PAO SPECT compared with CT, MR, and EEG. J Comput Assist Tomogr 14:402–409

Costa DC, Gacinovic S, Miller RF (1995) Radionuclide brain imaging in acquired immunodeficiency syndrome (AIDS). Q J Nucl Med 39:243–249

Crouzel C, Venet M, Irie T, Sanz G, Boullais C (1988) Labelling of a serotonergic ligand with ^{18}F: [^{18}F]setoperone. J Label Compounds Radiopharmacol 25:403

Cumming P, Gjedde A (1998) Compartmental analysis of dopa decarboxylation in living brain from dynamic positron emission tomograms. Synapse 29:37–61

Cutler NR, Haxby JV, Duara R, Grady CL, Kay AD, Kessler RM, Sundaram M, Rapoport SI (1985) Clinical history, brain metabolism, and neuropsychological function in Alzheimer's disease. Ann Neurol 18:298–309

Daemen BJ, Zwertbroek R, Elsinga PH, Paans AM, Doorenbos H, Vaalburg W (1991) PET studies with L-[^{11}C]tyrosine, L-[metyl-^{11}C]methionine and ^{18}F-fluorodeoxyglucose in prolactinomas in relation to bromocriptine treatment. Eur J Nucl Med 18:453–460

D'Amico A, Messa C, Castagna A, Zito F, Galli L, Pepe G, Lazzarin A, Lucignani G, Fazio F (1997) Diagnostic accuracy and predictive value of 201-Tl SPET for the differential diagnosis of cerebral lesions in AIDS patients. Nucl Med Commun 18:741–750

Dannals RF, Neumeyer JL, Milius RAJ, Ravert HT, Wilson AA, Wagner HN (1993) Synthesis of a radiotracer for studying dopamine uptake sites in vivo using PET: 2B-carbomethoxy-3B-(4-fluorophenyl)-[N-11C-methyl]-tropane (11 C)CFT or (11 C)-WIN 35,428. J Label Compounds Radiopharmacol 33:147–152

Davis S, Andrews J, Lichenstein M, Kaye A, Tress B, Rossiter S, Salehi N, Binns D (1990) A single-photon emission computed tomography study of hypoperfusion after subarachnoid hemorrhage. Stroke 21:252–259

Debets RM, Sadzot B, Brekelmans GJ, Meiners LC, Franck G (1997) Is 11C-flumazenil PET superior to 18FDG PET and 123I-iomazenil SPECT in presurgical evaluation of temporal lobe epilepsy. J Neurol Neurosurg Psychiatry 62:141–50

Herder WWA de, Reijs AEM, Swart J de, Kaandorp Y, Lamberts SWJ, Krenning EP, Kwekkeboom DJ (1999) Comparison of iodine-123 epidepride and iodine-123 IBZM for domapine D_2 receptor imaging in clinically non-functioning pituitary macroadenomas and macroprolactinomas. Eur J Nucl Med 26:46–50

Dey HM, Seibyl JP, Stubbs JB, Zoghbi SS, Baldwin RM, Smith EO, Zubal IG, Zea Ponce Y, Olson C, Charney DS (1994) Human biodistribution and dosimetry of the SPECT benzodiazepine receptor radioligand iodine-123 iomazenil. J Nucl Med 35:399–404

Devous MD Sr, Leroy RF (1989) Comparison of interictal and ictal regional cerebral blood flow findings with scalp and depth electrode seizure focus localization. J Cereb Blood Flow Metab 9:S91

Dierckx RA, Martin JJ, Dobbeleir A, Crols R, Neetens I, De Deyn PP (1994) Sensitivity and specificity of thallium-201 single-photon emission tomography in the functional detection and differential diagnosis of brain tumours. Eur J Nucl Med 21:621–633

Dubois B, Ruberg M, Javoy-Agid F, Ploska A, Agid Y (1983) A subcortico-cortical cholinergic system is affected in Parkinson's disease. Brain Res 288:213–218

Dubois B, Danze F, Pillon B, Cusimano G, Lhermitte F, Agid Y (1987) Cholinergic-dependent cognitive deficits in Parkinson's disease. Ann Neurol 22:26–30

Duncan JS (1997) Imaging and epilepsy. Brain 120:339–377

Duncan R, Patterson J, Roberts R, Hadley DM, Bone I (1993) Ictal/postictal SPECT in the pre-surgical localization of complex partial seizures. J Neurol Neurosurg Psychiatry 56:141–148

Eckelman WC, Reba RC, Rzeszotarski WJ, Gibson RE, Hill T, Holman BL, Budinger T, Conklin JJ, Eng R, Grissom MP (1984) Cerebral imaging of acetylcholine muscarinic receptors. Science 223:291–293

Elgazzar AH, Fernandez-Ulloa M, Silberstein EB (1993) 201-Tl as a tumour localizing agent: current status and future considerations. Nucl Med Commun 14:96–103

Engel J Jr (1988) Comparison of positron emission tomography and electroencephalography as measures of cerebral function in epilepsy. In: Pfurtscheller G, Lopes da Silva FH (eds) Functional brain imaging. Huber, Bern, pp 29–238

Engel J Jr, Brown WJ, Kuhl DE, Phelps ME, Mazziotta JC, Crandall PH (1982a) Pathological findings underlying focal temporal lobe hypometabolism in partial epilepsy. Ann Neurol 12:518–528

Engel J Jr, Kuhl DE, Phelps ME, Crandall PH (1982b) Comparative localization of epileptic foci in partial epilepsy by PCT and EEG. Ann Neurol 12:529–537

Engel J Jr, Kuhl DE, Phelps ME (1982c) Patterns of human local cerebral glucose metabolism during epileptic seizures. Science 218:64–66

Engel J Jr, Kuhl DE, Phelps ME, Rausch R, Nuwer M (1983) Local cerebral metabolism during partial seizures. Neurology 33:400–413

Engel J Jr, Henry TR, Risinger MW, Mazziotta JC, Sutherling WW, Levesque MF, Phelps ME (1990) Presurgical evaluation for partial epilepsy: relative contributions of chronic depth-electrode recordings versus FDG-PET and scalp-sphenoidal ictal EEG. Neurology 40:1670–1677

Feldman RS, Meyer JS, Quenzer LF (1997) Principles of neuropsychopharmacology. Sinauer Associates Inc., Sunderland, Maryland

Fieschi C, Argentino C, Lenzi GL, Sacchetti ML, Toni D, Bozzao L (1989) Clinical and instrumental evaluation of patients with ischemic stroke within the first six hours. J Neurol Sci 91:311–321

Fishbein DS (1988) Neuroradiologic work-up of brain tumours. In: Theodore WH (ed) Clinical neuroimaging. Alan R. Liss, New York, pp 111–137

Fowler JS, MacGregor RR, Wolf AP, Arnett CD, Dewey SL, Schlyer D, Christman D, Logan J, Smith M, Sachs H et al. (1987) Mapping human brain monoamine oxidase A and B with ^{11}C-labeled suicide inactivators and PET. Science 235:481–485

Fowler JS, Volkow ND, Logan J, Schlyer DJ, MacGregor RR, Wang GJ, Wolf AP, Pappas N, Alexoff D, Shea C (1993) Monoamine oxidase B (MAO B) inhibitor therapy in Parkinson's disease: the degree and reversibility of human brain MAO B inhibition by Ro 19 6327. Neurology 43:1984–1992

Frackowiak RSJ, Lenzi GL, Jones T, Heather JD (1980) Quantitative measurement of regional cerebral blood flow and oxygen metabolism in man using ^{15}O and positron emission tomography: Theory, procedure and normal values. J Comput Assist Tomogr 4:727–736

Franck G, Maquet P, Sadzot B, Salmon E, Debets R, Dive D, Grisar T, Guillaume D, Van Veelen C, Van Huffelen A, Van Emde Boas (1992) Contribution of positron emission tomography to the investigation of epilepsies of frontal lobe origin. In: Chauvel P, Delgado-Escueta AV et al. (eds) Advances in neurology, vol 57. Raven Press, New York, pp 471–485

Franck G, Sadzot B, Salmon E, Depresseux JC, Grisar T, Peters JM, Guillaume M, Quaglia L, Delfiore G, Delmotte D (1986) Regional blood flow and metabolic rates in human focal epilepsy and status epilepticus. In: Delgado-Escueta AV, Ward Jr AA, Woodbury DM, Porter RJ (eds) Advances in neurology, vol 44. Basic mechanisms of the epilepsies. Molecular and cellular approaches. Raven Press, New York, pp 935–948

Frey KA, Minoshima S, Kuhl DE (1998) Neurochemical imaging of Alzheimer's disease and other degenerative dementias. Q J Nucl Med 42:166–178

Friedland RP, Budinger TF, Ganz E, Yano Y, Mathis CA, Koss B, Ober BA, Muesman RH, Derenzo SE (1983) Regional cerebral metabolic alterations in dementia of the Alzheimer type: oositron emission tomography with [18F]fluorodeoxyglucose. J Comput Assist Tomogr 7:590–598

Friston KJ, Holmes AP, Worsley KJ, Poline JB, Frith CD, Frackowiak RS (1995) Statistical parametric maps in functional imaging: a general linear approach. Hum Brain Map 2:189–210

Frost JJ (1986) Measurement of neurotransmitter receptors by positron emission tomography: focus on the opiate receptor. NIDA Res Monogr 74:15–24

Frost JJ, Smith AC, Wagner HN Jr (1986) 3H-diprenorphine is selective for mu opiate receptors in vivo. Life Sci 38:1597–1606

Frost JJ, Mayberg HS, Fisher RS, Douglass KH, Dannals RF, Links JM, Wagner HN Jr (1988) Mu-opiate receptors measured by positron emission tomography are increased in temporal lobe epilepsy. Ann Neurol 23:231–237

Frost JJ, Mayberg HS, Sadzot B, Dannals RF, Lever JR, Ravert HT, Wilson AA, Wagner HN Jr, Links JM (1990) Comparison of [11 C]carfentanil binding to opiate receptors in humans by positron emission tomography. J Cereb Blood Flow Metab 10:484–492

Frost JJ, Rosier AJ, Reich SG, Smith JS, Ehlers MD, Snyder SH, Ravert HT, Dannals RF (1993) Positron emission tomographic imaging of the dopamine transporter with 11C-WIN 35,428 reveals marked declines in mild Parkinson's disease. Ann Neurol 34:423–431

Geraghty JJ, Jankovic J, Zetusky WJ (1985) Association between essential tremor and Parkinson's disease. Ann Neurol 17:329–333

Giobbe D, Castellano GC, Podio V (1993) Dopamine D2 receptor imaging with SPECT using IBZM in 16 patients with Parkinson's disease. Ital J Neurol Sci 14:165–169
Giubilei F, Lenzi GL, Piero V di, Pozzilli C, Pantano P, Bastianello S, Argentino C, Fieschi C (1990) Predictive value of brain perfusion single-photon emission computed tomography in acute ischemic stroke. Stroke 21:895–900
Gjedde A, Wong DF (1990) Modeling neuroreceptor binding of radioligands in vivo. In: Frost JJ, Wagner HN Jr (eds) Quantitative imaging: neuroreceptors, neurotransmitters, and enzymes. Raven Press, New York, pp 51–79
Goldberg HI (1991) Extraaxial brain tumours. In: Atlas SW (ed) Magnetic resonance imaging of the brain and spine. Raven Press, New York, pp 327–377
Grünwald F, Durwen HF, Bockisch A, Hotze A, Kersjes W, Elger CE, Biersack HJ (1991) Technetium-99m-HMPAO brain SPECT in medically intractable temporal lobe epilepsy: a postoperative evaluation. J Nucl Med 32:388–394
Hagglund J, Aquilonius SM, Eckernas SA, Hartvig P, Lundquist H, Gullberg P, Langstrom B (1987) Dopamine receptor properties in Parkinson's disease and Huntington's chorea evaluated by positron tomography using ^{11}C-N-methylspiperone. Acta Neurol Scand 75:87–94
Hajek M, Antonini A, Leonhard K, Wieser HG (1993) Mesiobasal versus lateral temporal lobe epilepsy: metabolic differences in the temporal lobe shown by interictal ^{18}F-FDG positron emission tomography. Neurology 43:79–86
Halldin C, Stone-Elander S, Farde L, Ehrin E, Fasth KJ, Langstrom B, Sedvall G (1986) Preparation of ^{11}C-labelled SCH 23390 for the in vivo study of dopamine D-1 receptors using positron emission tomography. Appl Radiat Isot 37:1039–1043
Halldin C, Farde L, Barnett A, Sedvall G (1990) Preparation of [^{11}C]SCH 39166, a new selective D_1 dopamine receptor ligand for PET. J Nucl Med 31:737
Hart J Jr, Lewis PJ, Lesser R, Fisher RS, Monsein LH, Schwerdt P, Bandeen-Roche K, Gordon B (1993) Anatomic correlates of memory from intracarotid amobarbital injections with technetium Tc-99m hexamethylpropyleneamine oxime SPECT. Arch Neurol 50:745–750
Hatazawa J, Shimosegawa J (1998) Imaging neurochemistry of cerebrovascular disease with PET and SPECT. Q J Nucl Med 42:196
Hatazawa J, Shimosegawa E, Okudera T, Inugami A, Ogawa T, Fujita H, Noguchi K, Kanno I, Miura S (1995) Evaluation of cerebral infarction with 123I-Iomazenil SPECT. J Nucl Med 36:2154–2161
Henry TR, Mazziotta JC, Engel J Jr, Christenson PD, Zhang JX, Phelps ME, Kuhl DE (1990) Quantifying interictal metabolic activity in human temporal lobe epilepsy. J Cereb Blood Flow Metab 10:748–757
Henry TR, Mazziotta JC, Engel J Jr (1992) The functional anatomy of frontal lobe epilepsy studied with PET. In: Chauvel P, Delgado-Escueta AV et al. (eds) Advances in neurology, vol 57. Raven Press, New York, pp 449–463
Herscovitch P, Markham J, Raichle ME (1983) Brain blood flow measured with intravenous $H_2{}^{15}0$. I. Theory and error analysis. J Nucl Med 24:782–789
Hicks BW, Rogers GA, Parsons SM (1991) Purification and characterization of a nonvesicular vesamicol-binding protein from electric organ and demonstration of a related protein in mammalian brain. J Neurochem 57:509–519
Hietala S-O, Silfvenius H, Aasly J, Olivecrona M, Johnson L (1990) Brain perfusion with intracarotid injection of ^{99m}Tc-HM-PAO in partial epilepsy during amobarbital testing. Eur J Nucl Med 16:683–687
Hoedt-Rasmussen L, Sveinsdottir E, Lassen NA (1966) Regional cerebral blood flow in man determined by intra-arterial injection of radioactive inert gas. Circ Res 18:237–247
Hornykiewicz O, Kish SJ (1984) Neurochemical basis of dementia in Parkinson's disease. Can J Neurol Sci 11:185–190
Hornykiewicz O, Kish SJ (1986) Biochemical pathophysiology of Parkinson's disease. Adv Neurol 45:19–34
Iinuma K, Yokoyama H, Otsuki T, Yanai K, Watanabe T, Ido T, Itoh M (1993) Histamine H_1 receptors in complex partial seizures. Lancet 341:238
Ilgin N, Zubieta JK, Reich SG, Ravert TH, Dannals RF, Frost JJ (1995) Differential diagnosis of Parkinson's disease and progressive supranuclear palsy with C11-WIN 35,248 PET imaging of the dopamine transporter. J Nucl Med 36:99
Ingvar DH, Lassen NA (1961) Quantitative determination of regional cerebral blood flow in man. Lancet 2:806–807
Innis RB, al-Tikriti MS, Zoghbi S, Baldwin RM, Sybirska EH, Laruelle MA, Malison RT, Seiby JP, Zimmermann RC, Johnson EW (1991) SPECT imaging of the benzodiazepine receptor: feasibility of in vivo potency measurements from stepwise displacement curves. J Nucl Med 32:1754–1761
Iyo M, Namba H, Fukushi K, Shinotoh H, Nagatsuka S, Suhara T, Nagatsuka S, Sumara T, Sudo Y, Suzuki K, Irie T (1997) Measurement of acetylcholinesterase by positron emission tomography in the brains of healthy controls and patients with Alzheimer's disease. Lancet 349:1805–1809
Jeffery PJ, Monsein LH, Szabo A, Hart JH, Fisher FS, Lesser RP, Debrun GM, Gordon B, Wagner HN Jr, Camargo EE (1991) Mapping the distribution of amobarbital sodium in the intracarotid Wada test by use of Tc-99m HMPAO with SPECT. Radiology 178:847–850
Jones AK, Luthra SK, Maziere B, Pike VW, Loc'h C, Crouzel C, Syrota A, Jones T (1988) Regional cerebral opioid receptor studies with [11 C]diprenorphine in normal volunteers. J Neurosci Methods 2:121–129
Jorgensen HS, Sperling B, Nakayama H, Raaschow HO, Olsen TS (1994) Spontaneous reperfusion of cerebral infarcts in acute stroke patients. Incidence, time course and clinical outcome: the Copenhagen Stroke study. Arch Neurol 57: 865–873
Kamo H, McGeer PL, Harrop R, McGeer EG, Calne DB, Martin WR, Pate BD (1987) Positron emission tomography and histopathology in Pick's disease. Neurology 37:439–445
Kanno I, Lassen NA (1979) Two methods for calculation of regional cerebral blood flow from emission computed tomography of emission tomography of inert gas concentration. J Comput Assist Tomogr 3:71–76
Kilbourn MR, Jung YW, Haka MS, Gildersleeve DL, Kuhl DE, Wieland DM (1990) Mouse brain distribution of a carbon-11 labeled vesamicol derivative: presynaptic marker of cholinergic neurons. Life Sci 47:1955–1963
Kilbourn MR, Snyder SE, Sherman PS, Kuhl DE (1996) In vivo studies of acetylcholinesterase activity using a labeled substrate, N-[11 C]methylpiperdin-4-yl propionate ([11 C]PMP). Synapse 22:123–131
Kim KT, Black KL, Marciano D, Mazziotta JC, Guze BH, Grafton S, Hawkins RA, Becker DP (1990) Thallium-201 SPECT imaging of brain tumors: methods and results. J Nucl Med 31:965–969
Koepp MJ, Labbe C, Richardson MP, Brooks DJ, Van PW, Cunningham VJ, Duncan JS (1997a) Regional hippocampal [11 C]flumazenil PET in temporal lobe epilepsy with uni-

lateral and bilateral hippocampal sclerosis. Brain 120:1865-1876

Koepp MJ, Richardson MP, Brooks DJ, Duncan JS (1998) Focal cortical release of endogenous opioids during reading-induced seizures. Lancet 352:952–955

Koepp MJ, Richardson MP, Brooks DJ, Cunningham VJ, Duncan JS (1997b) Central benzodiazepine/gamma-aminobutyric acid A receptors in idiopathic generalized epilepsy: an [11 C]flumazenil positron emission tomography study. Epilepsia 38:1089–1097

Koeppe RA, Frey KA, Mulholland GK, Kilbourn MR, Buck A, Lee KS, Kuhl DE (1994) [^{11}C]tropanyl benzilate-binding to muscarinic cholinergic receptors: methodology and kinetic modeling alternatives. J Cereb Blood Flow Metab 14:85–99

Krausz Y, Cohen D, Konstantini S, Meiner Z, Yaffe S, Atlan H (1991) Brain SPECT imaging in temporal lobe epilepsy. Neuroradiology 33:274–276

Krenning EP, Kwekkeboom DJ, Bakker WH, Breman WAP, Kooij PPM, Oei HJ, wan Haen M, Postema PTE, de Jong M, Reubi JC, Visser TJ, Reijs AEM, Hofland LJ, Koper JW, Lamberts SWJ (1993) Somatostatin receptor scintigraphy with ^{111}In-DTPA-D-Phe and ^{123}I-Tyr3-octeotride: the Rotterdam experience in more than 1000 patients. Eur J Nucl Med 20:716–731

Kuhl DE, Engel J Jr, Phelps ME, Selin C (1980) Epileptic patterns of local cerebral metabolism and perfusion in humans determined by emission computed tomography of ^{18}FDG and $^{13}NH_3$. Ann Neurol 8:348–360

Kuhl DE, Metter EJ, Riege WH (1984) Patterns of local cerebral glucose utilisation determined in Parkinson's disease by the 18F-fluorodeoxyglucose method. Ann Neurol 15:419–424

Kuhl DE, Koeppe RA, Fessler JA, Minoshima S, Ackermann RJ, Carey JE, Glidersleeve DL, Frey KA, Wieland DM (1994) In vivo mapping of cholinergic neurons in the human brain using SPECT and IBVM. J Nucl Med 35:405–410

Kuhl DE, Koeppe R, Snyder SE, Minoshima S, Frey KA, Kilbourn MR (1996a) Mapping acetylcholinesterase in human brain using PET an N-[C-^{11}]methylpiperidinyl propionate (PMP). J Nucl Med 37 (Suppl 5):21P

Kuhl DE, Minoshima S, Fessler JA, Frey KA, Foster NL, Ficaro EP, Wieland DM, Koeppe RA (1996b) In vivo mapping of cholinergic terminals in normal aging, Alzheimer's disease, and Parkinson's disease. Ann Neurol 40:339–410

Kung HF, Alavi A, Chang W, Kung MP, Keyes JW Jr, Velchik MG, Billings J, Pan S, Noto R, Rausch R et al. (1990) In vivo SPECT imaging of CNS D-2 dopamine receptors: initial studies with iodine-123-IBZM in humans. J Nucl Med 31:573–579

Kung MP, Stevenson DA, Plossl K, Meegalla SK, Beckwith A, Essman WD, Mu M, Lucki I, Kung HF (1997) [99mTc] TRODAT-1: a novel technetium-99m complex as a dopamine transporter imaging agent. Eur J Nucl Med 24:372–380

Lamusuo S, Ruottinen HM, Knuuti J, Harkonen R, Ruotsalainen U, Bergman J, Haaparanta M, Solin O, Mervaala E, Nousiainen U, Jaaskelainen S, Ylinen A, Kalviainen R, Rinne JK, Vapalahti M, Rinne JO (1997) Comparison of [18F]FDG-PET, [99mTc]-HMPAO-SPECT, and [123I]-iomazenil-SPECT in localising the epileptogenic cortex. J Neurol Neurosurg Psychiatry 63:743–748

Lang W, Podreka I, Suess E, Müller C, Zeitlhofer J, Deecke L (1988) Single photon emission computerized tomography during and between seizures. J Neurol 235:277–284

Langen K (1997) Evaluation of 123-I-a-L-methyltyrosine as a SPECT tracer of amino acid uptake in brain tumours. In: De Deyn PP, Dierckx RA, Alavi A, Pickut BA (eds) SPECT in neurology and psychiatry. Libbey, London, pp 387–405

Lassen NA (1966) The luxury-perfusion syndrome and its possible relation to acute metabolic acidosis localized within the brain. Lancet 2:1113–1115

Lee BI, Markand ON, Siddiqui AR, Park HM, Mock B, Wellman HH, Worth RM, Edwards MK (1986) Single photon emission computed tomography (SPECT) brain imaging using N,N,N'-trimethyl-N'-(2 hydroxy-3-methyl-5-^{123}I-iodobenzil)-1,3-propanediamine 2 HCl (HIPDM): intractable complex partial seizures. Neurology 36:1471–1477

Lee BI, Markand ON, Wellman HN, Siddiqui AR, Mock B, Krepshaw J, Kung H (1987) HIPDM single photon emission computed tomography brain imaging in partial onset secondarily generalized tonic-clonic seizures. Epilepsia 28:305–311

Lee BI, Markand ON, Wellman HN, Siddiqui AR, Park HM, Mock B, Worth RM, Edwards MK, Krepshaw J (1988) HIPDM-SPECT in patients with medically intractable complex partial seizures. Arch Neurol 45:397–402

Lee KS, Frey KA, Koeppe RA, Buck A, Mulholland GK, Kuhl DE (1996) In vivo quantification of cerebral muscarinic receptors in normal human aging using positron emission tomography and [^{11}C]tropanyl benzilate. J Cereb Blood Flow Metab 16:303–310

Leenders KL, Aquilonius SM, Bergstrom K, Bjurling P, Crossman AR, Eckernas SA, Gee AG, Hartuing P, Lundtquist H, Langstrom B (1988) Unilateral MPTP lesion in a rhesus monkey: effects on the striatal dopaminergic system measured in vivo with PET using various novel tracers. Brain Res 445:61–67

Lenzi GL, Frackowiak RSJ, Jones T (1982) Cerebral oxygen metabolism and blood flow in human cerebral ischemic infarction. J Cereb Blood Flow Metab 2:321–325

Leveille J, Demonceau G, Walovitch RC (1992) Intrasubject comparison between technetium-99m-ECD and technetium-99m-HMPAO in healthy human subjects. J Nucl Med 33:480–484

Lever JR, Scheffel U, Stathis M, Seltzman HH, Wyrick CD, Abraham P, Parkam K, Thomas BF, Boja JW, Fuhar MJ, Carroll FI (1996) Synthesis and in vivo studies of a selective ligand for the dopamine transporter: 3 beta-[4-(^{125}I)iodophenyl] tropan-2 beta-carboxylic acid isopropyl ester [(^{125}I)RTI-121]. J Nucl Med Biol 23:277–284

Limburg M, Royen EAV, Hijdra A, Verbeeten B Jr (1991) rCBF-SPECT in brain infarction: When does it predict outcome. J Nucl Med 3:382–387

Lucignani G, Losa M, Moresco RM, Del Sole A, Matarrese M, Bettinardi V, Mortini P, Giovanelli M, Fazio F (1998) Differentiation of clinically non-functioning pituitary adenomas from meningiomas and craniopharyngiomas by positron emission tomography with [18F]fluoro-ethyl-spiperone. Eur J Nucl Med 24:1149–1155

Madar I, Lever JR, Kinter CM, Scheffel U, Ravert HT, Musachio JL, Mathews WB, Dannals RF, Frost JJ (1996) Imaging of delta opioid receptors in human brain by N1'- ([^{11}C]-methyl)naltrindole and PET. Synapse 24:19–28

Madar I, Lesser RP, Krauss G, Zubieta JK, Lever JR, Kinter CM, Ravert HT, Musachio JL, Mathews WB, Dannals RF, Frost JJ (1997) Imaging of delta- and mu-opioid receptors in temporal lobe epilepsy by positron emission tomography. Ann Neurol 41:358–367

Maffioli L, Gasparini M, Chiti A, Gramaglia A, Mongoj V, Pozzi A, Bombardieri E (1996) Clinical role of thechnetium-99m sestamibi single-photon emission tomography in evaluating pretreated patients with brain tumours. Eur J Nucl Med 23:308–311

Magistretti PL, Uren RF (1983) Cerebral blood flow patterns in epilepsy. In: Nistico G, DiPerri R, Meinardi H (eds) Epilepsy: an update on research and therapy. Alan R. Liss, New York, pp 241–247

Marek KL, Seibyl JP, Zoghbi SS, Zea-Ponce Y, Baldwin RM, Fussell B, Charney DS, van Dyck C, Hoffer PB, Innis RP (1996) [1231] beta-CIT-SPECT imaging demonstrates bilateral loss of dopamine transporters in hemi-Parkinson's disease. Neurology 46:231–237

Markand ON, Salanova V, Worth R, Park HM, Wellman HN (1997) Comparative study of interictal PET and ictal SPECT in complex partial seizures. Acta Neurol Scand 95:129–136

Marks DA, Katz Am Hoffer P, Spencer SS (1992) Localization of extratemporal epileptic foci during ictal single photon emission computed tomography. Ann Neurol 31:250–255

Martin WRW, Stoessl AJ, Palmer M, Adam MJ, Ruth TJ, Grierson JR et al. (1988) Positron emission tomography in Parkinson's disease: glucose and dopa metabolism. Adv Neurol 50:223–229

Martin WR, Palmer MR, Patlak CS, Calne DB (1989) Nigrostriatal function in humans studied with positron emission tomography. Ann Neurol 26:535–542

Mayberg HS, Sadzot B, Meltzer CC, Fisher RS, Lesser RP, Dannals RF, Lever JR, Wilson AA, Ravert HT, Wagner HN Jr, Bryan RN, Cromwell CC, Frost JJ (1991) Quantification of mu and non-mu opiate receptors in temporal lobe epilepsy using positron emission tomography. Ann Neurol 30:3–11

Messa C, Perani D, Lucignani G, Zenorini A, Zito F, Rizzo G, Grassi F, Del Sole A, Franeschi M, Gilardi MC, Fazio F (1994) High resolution SPET/ [99mTc]HM-PAO in patients with probable Alzheimer's disease: comparison with PET/[18F]FDG. J Nucl Med 35:210–216

Messa C, Volonté MA, Fazio F, Zito F, Carpinelli A, D'Amico A, Rizzo G, Moresco RM, Paulesu E, Franceschi M, Lucignani G (1998) Differential distribution of striatal [^{123}I]bCIT in Parkinson's disease and progressive supranuclear palsy, evaluated with SPET. Eur J Nucl Med 25:1270–1276

Meyer M, Koeppe A, Frey KA, Foster NL, Kuhl DE (1995) Positron emission tomography measures of benzodiazepine binding in Alzheimer's disease. Arch Neurol 52:314–317

Miletich RS, Chan T, Gillespie M et al. (1988) Contralateral basal ganglia metabolism in abnormal in hemiparkinsonian patients. An FDG-PET study. Neurology 38:S260

Minoshima S, Frey KA, Koeppe RA, Chimowitz MI, McCune WJ, Kuhl DE (1993) Regional discordance between benzodiazepine receptor distribution and glucose metabolism in ischemic cerebral vascular disease. J Nucl Med 34:207

Minoshima S, Frey KA, Koeppe RA, Foster NL, Kuhl DE (1995) A diagnostic approach in Alzheimer's disease using three-dimensional stereotactic surface projections of fluorine-^{18}-FDG PET. J Nucl Med 36:1238–1248

Mueller-Gaertner HW, Mayberg HS, Fisher RS, Lesser RP, Wilson AA, Ravert HT, Dannals RF, Wagner HN, Uematsu S, Frost JJ (1993) Decreased hippocampal muscarinic cholinergic receptor binding measured by ^{123}I-iododexetimide and SPECT in epilepsy. Ann Neurol 34:235–238

Muhr C, Bergstrom M, Lundberg PO, Bergstrom K, Hartving P, Lundqvist H, Antoni G, Langstom B (1986) Dopamine receptors in pituitary adenomas: PET visualization with (^{11}C)-N-methyl-spiperone. J Comput Assist Tomogr 10:175–180

Mulholland GK, Otto CA, Jewett DM, Kilbourn MR, Koeppe RA, Sherman PS, Petry NA, Carey JE, Atkinson ER, Archer S, Frey KA, Kuhl DE (1992) Synthesis, rodent biodistribution, dosimetry, metabolism, and monkey images of carbon-11 labeled (+)-2a-tropanyl benzilate: a central muscarinic receptor imaging agent. J Nucl Med 33:423–430

Mulholland GK, Kilbourn MR, Sherman P, Carey JE, Frey KA, Koeppe RA, Kuhl DE (1995) Synthesis, in vivo biodistribution and dosimetry of [^{11}C]N-methylpiperidyl benzilate ([^{11}C]NMPB), a muscarinic acetylcholine receptor antagonist. Nucl Med Biol 22:13–17

Nadeau SE, Couch MW, Devane CL, Shukla SS (1995) Regional analysis of D2 dopamine receptors in Parkinson's disease using SPECT and iodine-123-iodobenzamide. J Nucl Med 36:384–393

Nahmias C, Garnett ES, Firnau G, Long A (1985) Striatal dopamine distribution in parkinsonian patients during life. J Neurol Sci 69:223–230

Neumeyer JL, Wang S, Milius RA, Baldwin RM, Zea Ponce Y, Hoffer PB, Sybirska E, al Tikriti M, Charney DS, Malison RT (1991) Iodine-123-2-b-carboxymethoxy -3-b-(4-iodophenyl)tropane (bCIT): high affinity SPECT radiotracer of monoamine reuptake sites in brain. J Med Chem 34:3144–3146.

Newton MR, Berkovic SF, Austin MC, Reutens DC, McKay WJ, Bladin PF (1992) Dystonia, clinical lateralization, and regional blood flow changes in temporal lobe seizures. Neurology 42:371–377

O'Brien TJ, Zupanc ML, Mullan BP, O'Connor MK, Brinkmann BH, Cicora KM, So EL (1998) The practical utility of performing peri-ictal SPECT in the evaluation of children with partial epilepsy. Pediatr Neurol 19:15–22

Obrist WD, Thompson HK Jr, Wang KS, Wilkinson WE (1975) Regional cerebral blood flow estimated by 133-Xenon inhalation. Stroke 6:245–256

Otsuka M, Ichiya Y, Hosokawa S (1991) Striatal blood flow, glucose metabolism, and ^{18}F-dopa uptake: difference in Parkinson's disease and atypical parkinsonism. J Neurol Neurosurg Psychiatry 54:898–904

Patlak C, Blasberg R, Fenstermacher J (1985) Graphical evaluation of blood-to-brain transfer constants from multiple-time uptake data. Generalizations. J Cereb Blood Flow Metab 5:584–590

Perlmutter JS, Raichle ME (1985) Regional blood flow in hemiparkinsonism. Neurology 35:1127–1134

Persson A, Ehrin E, Eriksson L, Farde L, Hedstrom CG, Litton JE, Mindus P, Sedvall G (1985). Imaging of [11 C]-labelled Ro 15-1788 binding to benzodiazepine receptors in the human brain by positron emission tomography. J Psychiatr Res 19:609–622

Phelps ME, Huang SC, Hoffman EJ, Selin C, Sokoloff L, Kuhl DE (1979) Tomographic measurement of local cerebral glucose metabolic rate in humans with (F-18)2-fluoro-2-deoxy-d-glucose: validation of method. Ann Neurol 6:371–388

Pirker W, Riedl M, Luger A, Czech T, Rossler K, Asenbaum S, Angelberger P, Kornhuber J, Deecke L, Podreka I, Brucke T (1996) Dopamine D_2 receptor imaging in pituitary adenomas using iodine-123-epidepride and SPECT. J Nucl Med 37:1931–1937

Ramsey SC, McLaughlin AF, Greenough R, Walsh J, Morris JG (1992) Comparison of independent aura, ictal and interictal cerebral perfusion. J Nucl Med 33:438–440

Reivich M, Kuhl D, Wolf A, Greenberg J, Phelps M, Ido T, Casella V, Fowler J, Hoffman E, Alavia A, Som P, Sokoloff L (1979). The ^{18}F-fluoro-deoxyglucose method for the measurement of local cerebral glucose utilization in man. Circ Res 44:127–137

Ricci M, Pantano P, Pieralini A, Stefano D di, Santoro A, Bozzao L, Lenzi GL (1996) Relationship between thallium-201 uptake by supratentorial glioblastomas and their morphological characteristics on magnetic resonance imaging. Eur J Nucl Med 23:524–529

Richardson MP, Friston KJ, Sisodiya SM, Koepp MJ, Ashburner J, Free SL, Brooks DJ, Duncan JS (1997) Cortical grey matter and benzodiazepine receptors in malformations of cortical development. A voxel-based comparison of structural and functional imaging data. Brain 120:1961-1973

Richardson MP, Koepp MJ, Brooks DJ, Duncan JS (1998) 11C-flumazenil PET in neocortical epilepsy. Neurology 51:485–492

Rinne JO, Laihinen A, Nagren K, Bergman J, Ruotsalainen U, Rinne UK (1990) PET demonstrates different behaviour of striatal dopamine D-1 and D-2 receptors in early Parkinson's disease. J Neurosci Res 27:494–499

Risinger MW, Engel J Jr, Van Ness PL, Henry TR (1989) Ictal localization of temporal lobe seizures with scalp/sphenoidal recordings. Neurology 39:1288–1293

Robitaille Y, Rasmussen T, Dubeau F, Tampieri D, Kemball K (1992) Histopathology of non-neoplastic lesions in frontal lobe epilepsy. Review of 180 cases with recent MRI and PET correlations. In: Chauvel P, Delgado-Escueta AV et al. (eds) Advances in neurology, vol 57. Raven Press, New York, pp 499–513

Rowe CC, Berkovic SF, Austin MC, McKay WJ, Bladin PF (1991a) Patterns of postictal cerebral blood flow in temporal lobe epilepsy: qualitative and quantitative analysis. Neurology 41:1096–1103

Rowe CC, Berkovic SF, Austin MC, Saling M, Kalnins RM, McKay WJ, Bladin PF (1991b) Visual and quantitative analysis of interictal SPECT with technetium-99m-HMPAO in temporal lobe epilepsy. J Nucl Med 32:1688–1694

Rowe CC, Berkovic SF, Sia STB, Austin M, McKay WJ, Kalnins RM, Bladin PF (1989) Localization of epileptic foci with postictal single photon emission computed tomography. Ann Neurol 26:660–668

Ryding E, Rosen I, Elmqvist B, Ingvar DH (1988) SPECT measurements with ^{99m}Tc-HMPAO in focal epilepsy. J Cereb Blood Flow Metab 8:S95–S100

Ryvlin P, Garcia-Larrea L, Philippon B, Froment JC, Fischer C, Revol M, Mauguière F (1992) High signal intensity on T2-weighted MRI correlates with hypoperfusion in temporal lobe epilepsy. Epilepsia 33:28–35

Sabatini U, Celsis P, Viallard G, Rascol A, Marc Vergnes JP (1991) Quantitative assessment of cerebral blood volume by single-photon emission computed tomography. Stroke 22:324–330

Sackellares JC, Siegel GJ, Abou-Khalil BW, Hood TW, Gilman S, McKeever PE, Hichwa RD, Hutchins GD (1990) Differences between lateral and mesial temporal metabolism interictally in epilepsy of mesial temporal origin. Neurology 40:1420–1426

Salanova V, Markand O, Worth R, Smith R, Wellman H, Hutchins G, Park H, Ghetti B, Azzarelli B (1998) FDG-PET and MRI in temporal lobe epilepsy: relationship to febrile seizures, hippocampal sclerosis and outcome. Acta Neurol Scand 97:146–153

Samson Y, Hantraye P, Baron JC, Soussaline F, Comar D, Maziere M (1985) Kinetics and displacement of 11C-Ro 15=1788, a benzodiazepine antagonist, studied in human brain in vivo by positron emission tomography. Eur J Pharmacol 110:247–251

Sanabria E, Chauvel P, Askienazy S, Vignal JP, Trottier S, Chodkiewicz JP, Bancaud J (1983) Single photon emission computed tomography (SPECT) using ^{123}I-isopropyl-iodo-amphetamine (IAMP) in partial epilepsy. In: Baldy-Moulinier M, Ingar D-H, Meldrum BS (eds) Current problems in epilepsy, vol 1. Cerebral blood flow, metabolism and epilepsy. Libbey, London, pp 82–87

Savic I, Persson A, Roland P, Pauli S, Sedvall G, Widen L (1988) In-vivo demonstration of reduced benzodiazepine receptor binding in human epileptic foci. Lancet 8616:863–866

Scheffel U, Dannals RF, Wong DF, Yokoi F, Carroll FI, Kuhar MJ (1992) Dopamine transporter imaging with novel, selective cocaine analogs. Neuroreport 3:969–972

Schwarz J, Antonini A, Tatsch K, Kirsch CM, Oertel WH, Leenders KL (1994) Comparison of ^{123}I-IBZM SPECT and ^{11}C-raclopride PET findings in patients with parkinsonism. Nucl Med Commun 15:806–813

Seibyl J, Wallace E, Smith E et al. (1994) Whole body biodistribution, radiation absorbed dose, and brain SPECT imaging with [^{123}I]b-CIT in healthy human subjects. J Nucl Med 35:764–770

Serrati C, Marchal G, Rioux P, Viader F, Petit Taboue MC, Lochon P, Luet D, Derlon JM, Baron JC (1994) Contralateral cerebellar hypometabolism: a predictor for stroke outcome? J Neurol Neurosurg Psychiatry 57:174–179

Shinotoh H, Yamasaki T, Inoue O, Itoh T, Suzuki K, Hashimoto K, Tateno Y, Ikehira H (1986) Visualization of specific binding sites of benzodiazepine in human brain. J Nucl Med 27:1593–1599

Shulkin BL (1997) PET applications in pediatrics. Q J Nucl Med 41:281–291

Siegel GJ, Agranoff BW, Wayne Albers R, Fisher SK, Uhler MD (1999) Basic Neurochemistry. Molecular, cellular and medical aspects, 6th edn. Lippincott-Raven, Philadelphia, New York

Sokoloff L (1960) The metabolism of the central nervous system in vivo. In: Field J, Magoun HW, Hall VE (eds) Handbook of physiology–neurophysiology, vol 3. American Physiological Society, Washington DC, pp 1843–1864

Soler C, Beauchesne P, Maatougui K, Schmitt T, Barral FG, Michel D, Dubois F, Brunon J (1998) Technetium-99m sestamibi brain single-photon emission tomography for detection of recurrent gliomas after radiation therapy. Eur J Nucl Med 25:1649–1657

Soucy JP, McNamara D, Mohr G, Lamoureux F, Lamoureux J, Danais S (1990) Evaluation of vasospasm secondary to subarachnoid hemorrhage with technetium-99m-hexamethylpropyleneamine oxime (HM-PAO) tomoscintigraphy. J Nucl Med 31:972–977

Stefan H, Kuhnen C, Biersack HJ, Reichmann K (1987a) Initial experience with ^{99m}Tc hexamethyl-propylene amine oxime (HM-PAO) single photon emission computed tomography (SPECT) in patients with focal epilepsy. Epilepsy Res1:134–138

Stefan H, Pawlik G, Böcher-Schwarz HG, Biersack HJ, Burr W, Penin H, Heiss W-D (1987b) Functional and morphological abnormalities in temporal lobe epilepsy: a comparison of interictal and ictal EEG, CT, MRI, SPECT and PET. J Neurol 234:377–384

Stocklin G (1992) Tracers for metabolic imaging of brain and heart. Eur J Nucl Med 19:527–551

Swartz BE, Halgren E, Delgado-Escueta AV, Mandelkern M, Gee M, Quinones N, Blahd WH, Repchan J (1989) Neuroimaging in patients with seizures of probable frontal lobe origin. Epilepsia 30:547–558

Swartz BE, Theodore WH, Sanabria E, Fisher RS (1992a) Positron emission and single photon emission computed tomographic studies in the frontal lobe with emphasis on the relationship to seizure foci. In: Chauvel P, Delgado-Escueta AV et al. (eds) Advances in neurology, vol 57. Raven Press, New York, pp 487–497

Swartz BE, Tomiyasu U, Delgado-Escueta AV, Mandelkern M, Khonsari A (1992b) Neuroimaging in temporal lobe epilepsy: test sensitivity and relationships to pathology and postoperative outcome. Epilepsia 33:624–634

Theodore WH, Fishbein D, Dubinsky R (1988) Patterns of cerebral glucose metabolism in patients with partial seizures. Neurology 38:1201–1206

Theodore WH, Newmark ME, Sato S, Paz R de la, Chiro G di, Brooks R, Patronas N, Kessler RM, Manning R, Margolin R, Channing M, Porter RJ (1984) ^{18}F-fluorodoxyglucose positron emission tomography in refractory complex partial seizures. Ann Neurol 14:429–437

Thomas P, Migneco O, Darcourt J, Chatel M (1992) Single photon emission computed tomography study of subclinical rhythmic electrographic discharge in adults. Electroencephalography and clinical neurophysiology 83:223–227

Tuomisto T, Tacke U (1986) Is histamine an anticonvulsive inhibitory transmitter? Neuropharmacology 25:955–958

Uhl GR, Hedreen JC, Price DL (1985) Parkinson's disease: loss of neurons from the ventral tegmental area contralateral to therapeutic surgical lesions. Neurology 35:1215–1218

Van Royen E, Verhoeff NF, Speelman JD, Wolters EC, Kuiper MA, Janssen AG (1993) Multiple system atrophy and progressive supranuclear palsy. Diminished striatal D2 dopamine receptor activity demonstrated by ^{123}I-IBZM single photon emission computed tomography. Arch Neurol 50:513–516

Vorstrup S, Brun B, Lassen NA (1986) Evaluation of the cerebral vasodilatory capacity by the acetazolamide test before EC-IC bypass surgery in patients with occlusions of the internal carotid artery. Stroke 17:1291–1298

Wagner HNJ, Burns HD, Dannals RF, Wong DF, Langstrom B, Duelfer T, Frost JJ, Ravert HT, Links JM, Rosenbloom SB, Lukas SE, Kramer AV, Kuhar MJ (1983) Imaging dopamine receptors in the human brain by positron emission tomography. Science 221:1264–1266

Wise RJS, Bernardi S, Frackowiak RSJ, Legg NJ, Jones T (1983) Serial observations on the pathophysiology of acute stroke: the transition from ischemia to infarction as reflected in regional oxygen extraction. Brain 106:197–222

Wolfson LI, Leenders KL, Brown LL, Jones T (1985) Alterations of regional cerebral blood flow and oxygen metabolism in Parkinson's disease. Neurology 35:1399–1405

Yamamoto YL, Ochs R, Gloor P, Ammann W, Meyer E, Evans AC, Cooke B, Sako K, Gotman J, Feindel WH, Diksic M, Thompson CJ, Robitaille Y (1983) Patterns of rCBF and focal energy metabolic changes in relation to electroencephalographic abnormality in the interictal phase of partial epilepsy. In: Baldy-Moulinier M, Ingar D-H, Meldrum BS (eds) Current problems in epilepsy, vol 1. Cerebral blood flow, metabolism and epilepsy. Libbey, London, pp 51–62

Yoshii Y, Satou M, Yamamoto T, Yamanda Y, Hyodo A, Nose T, Ishikawa H, Hatakeyama R (1993) The Role of thallium-201 single photon emission tomography in the investigation and characterisation of brain tumours in man and their response to treatment. Eur J Nucl Med 20:39–45

Zubieta JK, Frey KA, Koeppe RA, Kilbourn MR, Mulholland GK, Foster NL et al. (1994) Muscarinic receptor binding in aging and Alzheimer's disease determined with [^{11}C]n-methyl-4-piperidyl benzilate and PE. J Nucl Med 35:20P

3 Assessment of Myocardial Viability by Radionuclide Techniques

R. Campisi, F. Y. J. Keng, H. R. Schelbert

Contents

3.1 Introduction 37
3.2 Definition of Myocardial Viability 37
3.2.1 Myocardial Stunning 37
3.2.2 Myocardial Hibernation 38
3.3 Identification of Myocardial Viability 38
3.3.1 Thallium-201 Imaging of Blood Flow and Cell Membrane Integrity 38
3.3.1.1 Different Study Protocols 39
3.3.1.2 Clinical Implications 41
3.3.2 Technetium-99m Sestamibi and Relative Myocardial Blood Flow 42
3.3.3 Technetium-99m Tetrofosmin and Relative Myocardial Blood Flow 43
3.3.4 Myocardial Metabolism with Radio-Iodinated Fatty Acid Analogues 43
3.3.5 Myocardial Oxidative Metabolism with ^{11}C-Acetate 44
3.3.6 Perfusion and Metabolism by PET 45
3.3.6.1 Evaluation of Myocardial Blood Flow 45
3.3.6.2 Evaluation of Glucose Utilization 45
3.3.6.3 Myocardial FDG Imaging with SPECT-like Devices 47
3.3.6.4 Predicting Improvement in Regional and Global LV Function 47
3.3.6.5 Improvement in Congestive Heart Failure Symptoms and Exercise Capacity 48
3.3.6.6 Assessment of Cardiac Risk and Prediction of Cardiac Events 49
3.3.6.7 Myocardial Revascularization and Impact of PET, Timing of Surgery 50
3.4 Conclusion 51
References 51

3.1 Introduction

Ischemic cardiomyopathy associated with poor left ventricular (LV) function often presents a clinical management problem. There is overwhelming evidence that such patients have a poor prognosis when treated medically. Heart transplantation has now become a therapeutic alternative. However, the limited number of donor hearts makes this approach available to only the most qualified patients. On the other hand, it has been well documented that the long-term benefit of myocardial revascularization in this patient population is significantly better than medical treatment (Alderman et al. 1993). Because operative mortality remains high in these patients, the main concern is in the selection of those patients who will really benefit from revascularization.

Dysfunctional myocardium in patients with poor LV function can be due to one or a combination of the following: (a) necrosis followed by scar tissue formation (fibrosis); (b) chronic ischemia without necrosis; or (c) transient ischemia despite reperfusion. The last two mechanisms are usually referred to as "hibernation" and "stunning," respectively, which represent viable myocardium in these patients. Identifying "viable myocardium" from non-viable scar tissue is crucial because it is well known that revascularization in patients with substantial "viable myocardium" can improve LV function, symptoms, and survival.

3.2 Definition of Myocardial Viability

3.2.1 Myocardial Stunning

It has been documented in animal models as well as in humans that reversible abnormal wall motion in segments with normal or nearly normal resting blood flow represents myocardial stunning (Heyndrickx et al. 1975; Bolli 1992, 1998). Stunning has been demonstrated in patients with coronary artery disease in situations such as unstable angina, exercise-induced ischemia, acute myocardial infarction with early reperfusion, post-coronary artery bypass surgery, and heart transplantation (Kloner et al. 1998). Previously, myocardial stunning was considered as a regional contractile dysfunction that occurred after a brief episode of myocardial ischemia

R. Campisi, F. Y. J. Keng, H. R. Schelbert
Department of Molecular and Medical Pharmacology, UCLA School of Medicine, 10833 Le Conte Avenue, Los Angeles, CA 90095-1735, USA

(Braunwald and Cloner 1982). There is now evidence that recurrent episodes of ischemia in the same coronary territory may occur in patients with coronary artery disease (Kloner et al. 1998), resulting in chronic contractile dysfunction which is known as "repetitive stunning" (Bolli 1998). This mechanism is probably the most common form of myocardial stunning in patients with depressed ventricular function.

3.2.2 Myocardial Hibernation

Rahimtoola (1987) first described "hibernating" myocardium as a persistently impaired myocardial function in the setting of reduced coronary blood flow. This concept entails a perfusion-contraction match derived from clinical observations and, in contrast to stunned myocardium, still lacks definitive animal or human clinical models. Its original concept, however, has recently been questioned since measurements of blood flow with positron emission tomography (PET) have shown normal or near-normal flow at rest and a reduced coronary flow reserve in "hibernating segments" (Vanoverschelde et al. 1993; Marinho et al. 1996; Conversano et al. 1996). Vanoverschelde et al. (1993) reported that in patients with completely occluded left anterior descending coronary arteries but without prior myocardial infarction, collateral-dependent myocardium showed either severely reduced or normal wall motion. Both types of myocardium exhibited normal blood flow at rest. However, collateral-dependent myocardium with wall motion abnormalities showed an impaired coronary flow reserve, whereas collateral-dependent myocardium with normal wall motion exhibited normal flow reserve. Thus, recurrent episodes of transient ischemia (i.e., "repetitive stunning"), rather than a true existence of hibernating myocardium, might account for chronically impaired myocardial contractile function. It is important to note that PET only quantifies transmural myocardial blood flow, and that chronic subendocardial hypoperfusion might be enough to explain dysfunctional contraction. It would be seen as a mild transmural perfusion reduction and therefore might escape detection by PET imaging (Edwards et al. 1992). Another argument in favor of the existence of true hypoperfusion are studies in humans showing increased regional myocardial blood flow after coronary revascularization of reversibly dysfunctional myocardium (Maes et al. 1995; Wolpers et al. 1997).

Nevertheless, from a clinical standpoint, the "true mechanisms" of chronic poor LV dysfunction (i.e., hibernation or stunning) are not that relevant. Bolli (1992) described that a wide overlap of hibernation and stunning may occur. It is therefore very likely that in the majority of the clinical cases both mechanisms are present. Regardless of the mechanism(s) involved, the identification of dysfunctional myocardium in patients with chronic poor LV function that will improve after coronary revascularization is important.

3.3 Identification of Viable Myocardium

Different imaging modalities are available to assess myocardial viability such as SPECT, PET, MRI, and echocardiography. This chapter reviews the usefulness of radionuclide techniques in detecting viable myocardium, to select those patients with ischemic cardiomyopathy and poor LV function who will benefit most from revascularization. Critical for preserving viable myocardium is the amount of residual blood flow and preserved cell membrane function, which in turn is predicated upon some degree of sustained metabolic activity. Radionuclide techniques probe each of these critical components. Some approaches evaluate only a single aspect, whereas others explore several components of cell function in concert. Rather than reviewing how each of these components critical to cell survival can be assessed with radionuclide studies, for logistical reasons the various radionuclide approaches currently employed are discussed. For each radionuclide or imaging approach we describe the technical concepts and then implications for patient management. Throughout the chapter we refer at times to the metabolic evaluation of viability with ^{18}F-deoxyglucose (FDG), because this approach is often used for comparison by other techniques and is considered by many to be the gold standard of viability assessment.

3.3.1 Thallium-201 Imaging of Blood Flow and Cell Membrane Integrity

Thallium-201 (^{201}Tl) is the most widely used radionuclide for the assessment of myocardial viability by planar or SPECT imaging techniques. ^{201}Tl is a potassium analogue and its final distribution after intravenous administration is primarily intracellular.

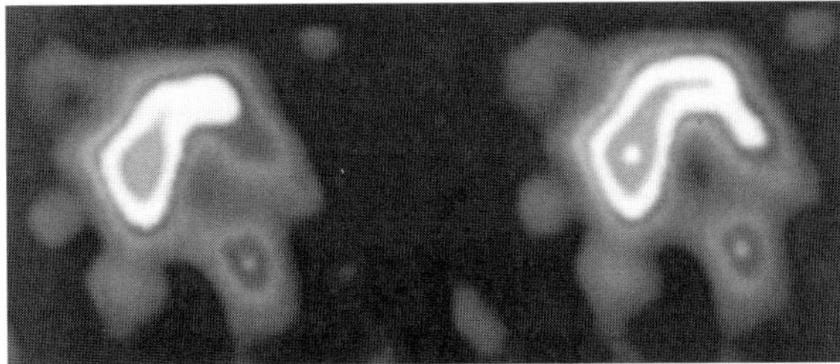

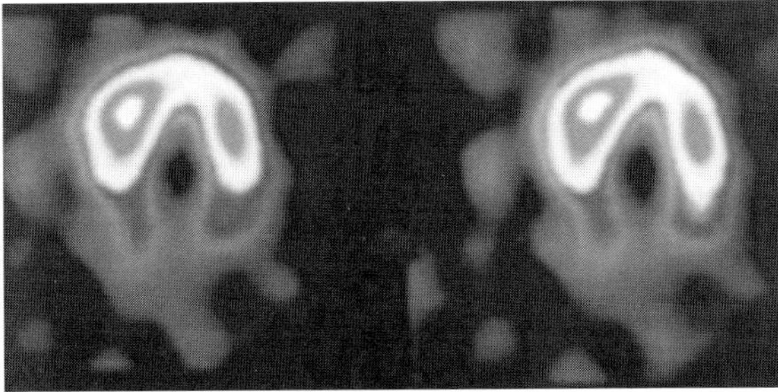

Fig. 3.1. Thallium-201 rest *(top)* and 4-h redistribution *(bottom)* images. Note the severe reduction in tracer uptake in the posterolateral wall on the initial images with almost complete defect resolution on the delayed images. (Courtesy of M. Hernandez Pampaloni)

Its early myocardial uptake is proportional to regional blood flow and the flow-dependent extraction fraction of ^{201}Tl as was confirmed by the microsphere technique (Weich et al. 1977). Following its initial distribution in the myocardium, ^{201}Tl concentration in the normal and ischemic regions changes as a function of time, known as the redistribution process (Pohost et al. 1977). Clinically, redistribution implies the partial or total resolution of initial perfusion defects at repeat imaging 2.5–4 h after ^{201}Tl administration (Fig. 3.1). The process of redistribution can be seen after transient underperfusion distal to a stenotic vessel with exercise, pharmacologic stress, or even in the resting state (Gimple et al. 1994). It is important to note that although the initial ^{201}Tl uptake represents myocardial blood flow, redistribution 3–4 h later reflects myocardial cellular membrane integrity and the intracellular potassium transport, which is indirect evidence of myocardial viability (Pohost et al. 1977).

Several imaging protocols have been employed for the evaluation of myocardial viability using ^{201}Tl: (a) stress/4-h redistribution; (b) stress/4-h redistribution/24-h redistribution; (c) stress/4-h redistribution/reinjection; and (d) rest/4-h redistribution. The most commonly employed are stress/4-h redistribution/reinjection, and rest/4-h redistribution.

3.3.1.1
Different Study Protocols

3.3.1.1.1
Stress 4-Hour Redistribution

Evaluation of stress-induced ischemia is usually a frequent and important question in patients with coronary artery disease. Inducible ischemia can be demonstrated when a perfusion defect improves from stress to rest images, whereas viability is determined by the change in tracer uptake between the resting and delayed images. When a perfusion defect demonstrates total resolution on the delayed images, it obviously implies stress induced ischemia and viability (Gibson et al. 1983). When ^{201}Tl is administered during exercise or pharmacologic stress, it is not possible to differentiate to what extent a reversible defect represents hibernating/stunned myocardium vs ischemia. Thus, reversible and irreversible stress/redistribution perfusion defects have a highly variable predictive value for recovery of regional LV dysfunction (Maddahi et al. 1994).

One technical aspect to enhance the detection of redistribution is the quantitative analysis of regional ^{201}Tl uptake (Beller 1996). Some perfusion defects that appear irreversible on visual analysis demonstrate redistribution when quantitative analysis is performed on initial and delayed images. The majority of studies have shown that a relative threshold of 50% of maximal count density can distinguish regions with ^{201}Tl perfusion defects that will have a high probability of improved function after revascularization (Gibson et al. 1983; Yamamoto et al. 1993). Persistent defects that are mild to moderate (25–50% relative reduction in ^{201}Tl activity) are also indicative of viability. In fact, these levels of activity have been shown to reflect a high prevalence of myocardial viability by FDG criteria (Bonow et al. 1991) and exhibit significant improvement in regional function following revascularization. In contrast, very few segments with persistent perfusion defects of more than 50% reduction in ^{201}Tl counts on post-stress and delayed images will improve function after revascularization (Gibson et al. 1983; Beller 1996). Recently, Kitsiou et al. (1998) using quantitative analysis, indicated that the identification of a reversible ^{201}Tl perfusion defects on stress images in an asynergic region more accurately predicted recovery of function after revascularization than mild to moderate irreversible thallium defects. The authors concluded that even at a similar mass of viable myocardium (as reflected by the final thallium content) the presence of inducible ischemia was associated with a significantly increased likelihood of functional recovery.

3.3.1.1.2 Stress, 4-Hour Redistribution, 24-Hour Redistribution

Redistribution imaging at 24 h after ^{201}Tl injection has been utilized to enhance detection of viability in persistent perfusion defects noted at 4 h (Gutman et al. 1983; Kiat et al. 1988). Kiat et al. (1988) reported that the presence of late redistribution at 18–24 h predicted enhanced regional perfusion after revascularization. They showed that 95% of myocardial segments with late redistribution showed such improvement as compared with only 37% of segments with persistent defects at 18–24 h.

This protocol, however, has limitations. A major problem is the suboptimal count statistics at 24 h following a standard 3-mCi dose, with poor target-to-background ratio making interpretation difficult. This could be overcome by a higher initial ^{201}Tl dose and longer acquisition times. Interestingly, Watson et al. (1990) have shown that by employing quantitative scintigraphy, most of the perfusion defects exhibiting late redistribution do already demonstrate some evidence of redistribution on the early images (2.5- to 4-h images). More recently, Perrone-Filardi et al. (1996) showed that 24-h ^{201}Tl redistribution images changed the interpretation of viable myocardium in only 2% of the 219 persistent perfusion defects analyzed by quantitative analysis. Also, Dilsizian et al. (1991) reported that late redistribution images after a resting injection of ^{201}Tl changed viability interpretation in only 4 of 127 segments that were interpreted as irreversible perfusion defects at 4 h. Thus, delayed 24-h redistribution imaging affects image interpretation and hence accuracy of detection of viability only minimally in a minimal amount of segments.

3.3.1.1.3 Stress 4-Hour Redistribution – Reinjection

Another approach to assess viable myocardium with ^{201}Tl is the injection of a second dose, 1–1.5 mCi of ^{201}Tl, which is administered following acquisition of the 2.5- to 4-h redistribution images. The purpose of the reinjection is to enhance the count statistics, and it provides better visual assessment of perfusion defect reversibility at rest.

Dilsizian et al. (1990) showed that, in 100 patients with coronary artery disease, 33% of abnormal segments demonstrated persistent defects on the 3- to 4-h images. Approximately half of these patients revealed improved or normal ^{201}Tl uptake after reinjection of a second dose of ^{201}Tl. Taking these observations together with other studies, ^{201}Tl reinjection immediately after 4-h SPECT imaging has been shown to improve the detection of viable myocardium in 30–50% of regions with fixed perfusion defects observed on 4-h redistribution images (Dilsizian et al. 1990; Tamaki et al. 1990; Ohtani et al. 1990).

Bonow et al. (1991) compared the reinjection protocol with myocardial uptake of FDG PET imaging in 16 patients with coronary artery disease and poor LV function and irreversible defects on the standard stress 4-h redistribution protocol. The FDG uptake was observed in 94% of perfusion defects on postexercise images that had partial or complete redistribution. Fifty-one percent of the persistent perfusion defects exhibited enhanced ^{201}Tl uptake after reinjection. The same percentage of such defects showed preserved FDG uptake. The investigators reported that detection of viability by enhanced ^{201}Tl uptake with the reinjection protocol and PET imaging of FDG uptake was concordant in 88% of defects. The authors concluded that the reinjection protocol was as sensitive as PET using FDG for detection of myocardial viability. However, post-revascularization results were not reported in this study.

The reinjection protocol was also compared with a reinjection-late 24-h redistribution approach (Dilsizian et al. 1990; Bobba et al. 1998). Dilsizian et al. (1990) showed that late 24-h imaging after reinjection did not seem to detect more viable segments compared with images acquired 10 min after reinjection. More recently, Bobba et al. (1998) reported the use of an imaging protocol without a delayed 4-h SPECT study prior to reinjection. Although the increased incidence of delayed 24-h reversibility compared with post-reinjection at 4 h was not frequent, it was most often seen in the absence of reversibility in the immediate post-reinjection images, and in the context of unstable angina or acute coronary syndromes, rather than in chronic ischemic heart disease.

3.3.1.1.4 Rest 4-Hour Redistribution

In the rest 4-h redistribution protocol, ^{201}Tl is injected with the patient at rest, the first set of images being obtained 10–20 min later and redistribution imaging 4 h later. This has been the preferred protocol for evaluation of myocardial viability in many centers. With this protocol, hibernating myocardium exhibits a reduced ^{201}Tl uptake on the initial images, but this initial perfusion defect is expected to improve on the redistribution images.

3.3.1.2
Clinical Implications

3.3.1.2.1
Predicting Improvement In Regional and Global LV Function

Various studies have shown that ^{201}Tl reversibility after reinjection predicts improvement in regional wall motion with an overall positive predictive accuracy of 69% and a negative predictive accuracy of 89% (Dilsizian et al. 1990; Tamaki et al. 1990; Ohtani et al. 1990; Haque et al. 1995; Vanoverschelde et al. 1996; Bax et al. 1996a,b). Dilsizian et al. (1990) reported that 87% of regions with enhanced ^{201}Tl uptake on reinjection images showed normal ^{201}Tl uptake and improved wall motion after angioplasty. In contrast, all regions without enhanced ^{201}Tl uptake after reinjection demonstrated abnormal ^{201}Tl uptake as well as abnormal wall motion both before and after PTCA. Similarly, Ohtani et al. (1990) reported that 47% of persistent perfusion defects observed at 3-h redistribution showed further increase in ^{201}Tl uptake after reinjection and the majority of these segments exhibited enhanced resting wall motion after coronary artery bypass surgery. Bax et al. (1996a) also assessed improvement of global LV function after revascularization in 17 patients with ^{201}Tl reinjection imaging. This protocol identified 5 of 6 patients who showed improvement in LVEF of at least 5% and identified non-viability in 6 of 11 patients without such improvement. It has also been reported that ^{201}Tl reinjection imaging has a sensitivity of 72% and specificity of 73% in predicting improvement in global LV function (Vanoverschelde et al. 1996).

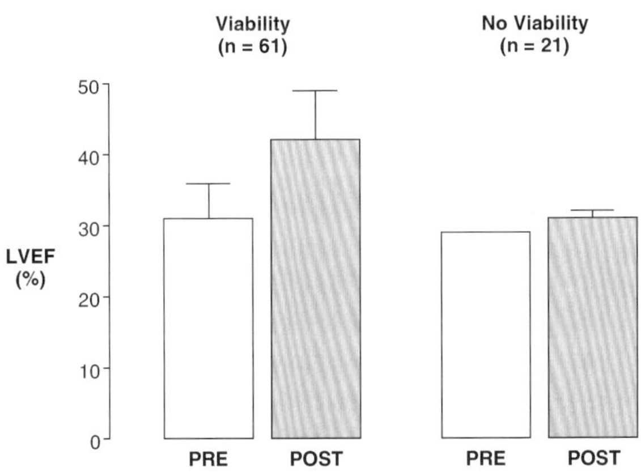

Fig. 3.2. Changes in left ventricular ejection fraction from baseline (*PRE*) to following interventional revascularization (*POST*). The data summarize the findings reported from three clinical investigations using ^{201}Tl redistribution imaging in a total of 82 patients: Ragosta et al. 1993, Iskandrian et al. 1983, and Gioia et al. 1995. The *left set of bars* indicate the patients with and the *right set of bars* the patients without evidence of viability

Several reports have shown that ^{201}Tl rest-redistribution imaging (planar and tomographic studies) predicts improvement in regional wall motion after revascularization with an overall sensitivity and specificity of 90 and 54%, respectively (Perrone-Filardi et al. 1996; Mori et al. 1991; Ragosta et al. 1993; Alfieri et al. 1993; Marzullo et al. 1993; Udelson et al. 1994; Charney et al. 1994; Qureshi et al. 1997). Sub-analysis of rest-redistribution SPECT studies (four reports with 83 patients) have shown cumulative positive and negative predictive values of 69 and 92%, respectively, for an improvement in regional function after revascularization (Perrone-Filardi et al. 1996; Bax et al. 1996a; Udelson et al. 1994; Charney et al. 1994). Three studies have reported on the prediction of functional recovery after revascularization with this protocol (Fig. 3.2; Mori et al. 1991; Ragosta et al. 1993; Iskandrian et al. 1983). The average positive and negative predictive accuracies of ^{201}Tl rest-redistribution scintigraphy for prediction improvement in global LVEF after revascularization (by at least 5%) was 70 and 77%, respectively.

It is of clinical relevance to consider how much viable myocardium is required to improve LV function after revascularization. Ragosta et al. (1993) using the rest-redistribution protocol have shown that in patients with depressed LV function the ejection fraction significantly increased (27±7 vs 41±11%; $p<0.01$) at 8 weeks after revascularization in patients with 7 of 14 myocardial segments being viable by ^{201}Tl (i.e., 50% of the left ventricle). In contrast, LVEF remained unchanged (27±5 vs 30±8%; not significant) in those with fewer than seven viable segments.

3.3.1.2.2
Assessment of Cardiac Risk and Prediction of Cardiac Events

The link between residual viability evaluated with ^{201}Tl imaging and improved clinical outcome after coronary bypass surgery in patients with ischemic cardiomyopathy remains largely unexplored. Gioia et al. (1995) assessed the prognostic value of ^{201}Tl rest-redistribution SPECT imaging in patients with coronary artery disease and depressed LV function. In that study, groups with viable and non-viable myocardium were comparable with respect to extent of coronary artery disease, LVEF, and extent of reversible and fixed perfusion defects. The authors reported a 13% annual mortality in those patients with myocardial viability treated medically vs 6% for those with comparable viability but undergoing revascularization. Pagley et al. (1997) reviewed the outcomes in 70 patients with multi-vessel coronary artery disease and an LVEF <40% who underwent planar quantitative rest ^{201}Tl imaging before coronary artery bypass surgery. Segmental viability scores were summed and divided by the number of segments visualized to determine a viability index. This viability index was significantly related to the 3-year survival free of cardiac events (cardiac death or heart transplantation) after bypass surgery (p=0.011) and was independent of age, ejection fraction, and number of diseased coronary vessels. There were six cardiac deaths and no transplants in patients with a higher viability index (>0.67) compared with 15 cardiac deaths and two transplants in patients with a lower viability index (0.67). Survival free of cardiac deaths or transplantation was significantly better in patients with greater viability by Kaplan-Meier analysis (Fig. 3.3). Thus, resting ^{201}Tl scintigraphy may be useful in the preoperative risk stratification for identification of patients most likely to benefit from revascularization.

3.3.2 Technetium-99m Sestamibi and Relative Myocardial Blood Flow

^{99m}Tc-sestamibi is a synthetic lipophilic cationic myocardial perfusion agent that is initially distributed in the myocardium according to blood flow. It actively and passively exchanges across sarcolemmal and mitochondrial membranes, and 90% of ^{99m}Tc-sestamibi activity is found in the mitochondria as the original free cationic complex, showing negligible redistribution over time (Carvalho et al. 1992). A negative mitochondrial charge gradient is essential for sestamibi accumulation and retention in the myocyte, which can only be maintained if the myocyte is viable (Beanlands et al. 1990). Therefore, delivery of ^{99m}Tc-sestamibi is dependent upon myocardial perfusion and its retention upon membrane integrity, and thus, upon myocardial viability (Rocco et al. 1989).

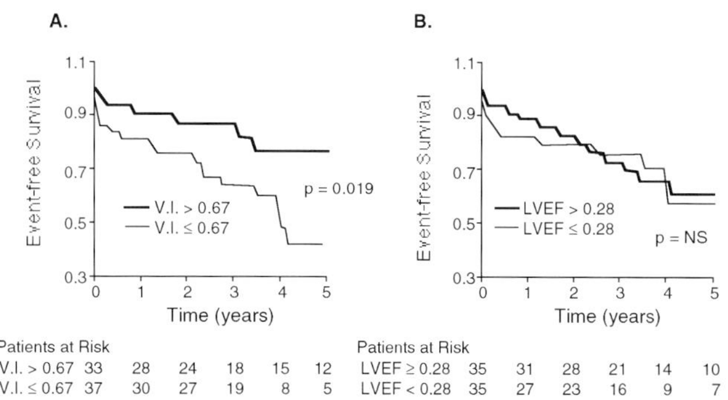

Fig. 3.3. Survival free from cardiac events such as, for example, cardiovascular death or cardiac transplantation by Kaplan-Meier Survival Analysis. **A** The event-free survival among patients with a viability index (*V.I.*) of greater than 0.67 and a survival index of less than 0.67. **B** In this group of patients with poor left ventricular ejection fraction, the event-free survival was largely independent of the ejection fraction (*LVEF*). (From Pagley et al. 1997)

The role of ^{99m}Tc-sestamibi as an agent to evaluate myocardial viability remains controversial. The major concern is that since distribution of ^{99m}Tc-sestamibi after resting injection is proportional to resting flow in low-flow regions, resting uptake of the tracer in these areas will be diminished and therefore will underestimate the extent of viability. In addition, its lack of significant redistribution could result in overestimation of non-reversibility (Caner et al. 1998).

Many studies have compared ^{99m}Tc-sestamibi imaging with other scintigraphic protocols, such as ^{201}Tl stress redistribution-reinjection (Cuocolo et al. 1992; Dilsizian et al. 1995), ^{201}Tl rest (Marzullo et al. 1993; Udelson et al. 1994; Dondi et al. 1993), ^{201}Tl rest redistribution (Dondi et al. 1993; Cuocolo et al. 1993; Kauffman et al. 1996), and FDG-PET imaging techniques (Altehoefer et al. 1992, 1994; Sawada et al. 1994; Soufer et al. 1995; Maes et al. 1997). These studies were consistent in showing that ^{99m}Tc-sestamibi was less accurate in detection of myocardial viability compared with the other modalities (Bax et al. 1997a).

In order to maximize the ability of ^{99m}Tc-sestamibi to detect viable myocardium, several approaches have been suggested. As with ^{201}Tl, quantitation of ^{99m}Tc-sestamibi imaging can be performed. It has been shown that relative ^{99m}Tc-sestamibi activity of more than 50–60% of maximal activity is usually indicative of myocardial viability (Fig. 3.4; Udelson et al. 1994; Kauffman et al. 1996; Maes et al. 1997). Due to the high count density of technetium, ^{99m}Tc-sestamibi imaging allows evaluation of regional and global LV function by first-pass radionuclide ventriculography or by gated acquisition of the SPECT perfusion images (Palmas et al. 1995; Chua et al. 1994). Wall motion data obtained from gated images can aid in the detection of viable myocardium because preserved function assessed by wall motion and thickening suggests preserved viability in the presence of diminished perfusion. Maunoury et al. (1997) have shown that indices of systolic LV function can also be derived also from gated ^{201}Tl perfusion images, which seems to offer similar

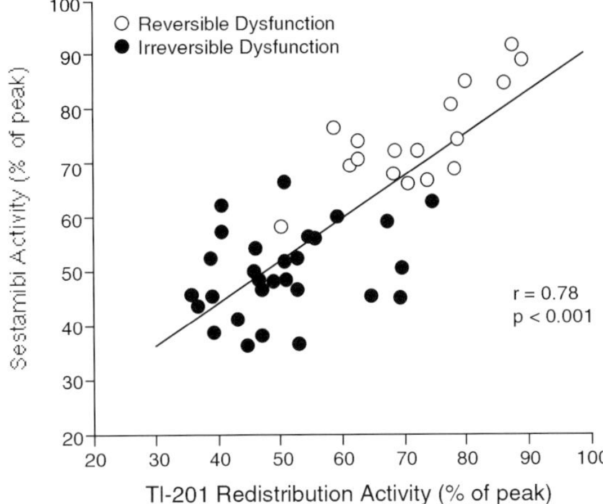

Fig. 3.4. Comparison between the relative ^{201}Tl redistribution and the ^{99m}Tc-sestamibi activity (both in percent of the peak myocardial activity) in segments with reversible and irreversible contractile dysfunction. (From UDELSON et al. 1994)

prognostic information as obtained with ^{99m}Tc-sestamibi-gated SPECT. Finally, investigations have described the use of nitrate infusion during ^{99m}Tc-sestamibi injection or acquisition of delayed redistribution ^{99m}Tc-sestamibi images in order to obtain information comparable to that of ^{201}Tl for evaluation of viable myocardium (DILSIZIAN et al. 1994; BISI et al. 1994; SCIAGRAA et al. 1996).

Most studies with ^{99m}Tc-sestamibi report a high sensitivity for predicting improvement in regional LV function (range 73–100%), whereas specificity was variable ranging from 35 to 86% (MARZULLO et al. 1993; UDELSON et al. 1994; MAES et al. 1997; MARZULLO et al. 1992; DAKIK et al. 1997). The accuracy of ^{99m}Tc-sestamibi can be enhanced by nitrate administration which improves mostly the specificity (BISI et al. 1994; SCIAGRAA et al. 1997). Recent data have also suggested that myocardial "counts" can predict improvement in LVEF. SCHNEIDER et al. (1998) used a rest ^{99m}Tc-sestamibi protocol with nitrate augmentation and showed that by using an infarct-location adjusted optimal threshold, the protocol had a positive predictive value of 90% and a negative predictive value of 91% for prediction of improvement of LVEF. FUJIWARA et al. (1998) showed that a reverse redistribution of ^{99m}Tc-sestamibi reflected recovery of LV function. Despite the promising results, further investigations are needed to validate the usefulness of ^{99m}Tc-sestamibi in evaluating myocardial viability as well as predicting outcome in patients with coronary artery disease and depressed ventricular function.

3.3.3 Technetium-99m Tetrofosmin and Relative Myocardial Blood Flow

Technetium-99m tetrofosmin is a cationic lipophilic myocardial perfusion agent with electrochemical properties similar to those of ^{99m}Tc-sestamibi. ^{99m}Tc-tetrofosmin has good diagnostic accuracy for detection of coronary artery disease when compared with ^{201}Tl (ZARET et al. 1995). Its uptake and retention depends on cellular metabolism, suggesting that cellular viability might be essential for the tracer uptake and its retention (PLATTS et al. 1995). Like ^{99m}Tc-sestamibi, it shows little redistribution over time and it has been suggested that this may have limitations for viability assessment. For example, in a low-flow ischemia animal model with profound systolic dysfunction, tetrofosmin uptake was quantitatively comparable to initial ^{201}Tl uptake. Delayed ^{201}Tl redistribution was slightly but significantly higher than ^{99m}Tc-tetrofosmin uptake (KOPLAN et al. 1996). In contrast, TAKAHASHI et al. (1996) reported that ^{99m}Tc-tetrofosmin uptake was a good indicator of myocardial viability.

Clinical studies that examined myocardial viability with this agent are lacking. It has been reported that ^{99m}Tc-tetrofosmin closely correlates with regional reinjection ^{201}Tl activity and that defect size on resting ^{99m}Tc-tetrofosmin images is similar to that obtained with reinjection ^{201}Tl images (MATSUNARI et al. 1995). GALASSI et al. (1998) reported a 90% concordance between ^{201}Tl redistribution and ^{99m}Tc-tetrofosmin uptake for the evaluation of myocardial viability by quantitative analysis of defect severity. The role of ^{99m}Tc-tetrofosmin in viability assessment, however, remains uncertain.

Prediction of regional and global wall motion improvement with ^{99m}Tc-tetrofosmin has been evaluated in only one study. MATSUNARI et al. (1997) showed that with a quantitative approach and SPECT imaging, rest ^{99m}Tc-tetrofosmin and rest redistribution of ^{201}Tl imaging were comparable in predicting functional recovery after revascularization.

3.3.4 Myocardial Metabolism with Radio-Iodinated Fatty Acid Analogs

Most of the clinical interest focused on two types of fatty acid tracers, 15-(*p*-[^{123}I]-iodophenyl)-pentadecanoic acid (IPPA), an aromatic fatty acid analog, and 15-(*p*-[^{123}I]-iodophenyl)-3-methylpentadecanoic acid

(BMIPP), a branched-chain fatty acid analog. These two agents can be employed in SPECT imaging for the assessment of myocardial viability (Machulla et al. 1978; Goodman et al. 1984). BMIPP has become more popular probably because of its longer retention in the myocardium leading to superior image quality (Knapp et al. 1986). Image acquisition protocols differ between the two agents. For IPPA, the protocol involves serial SPECT image acquisition at 4, 12, 20, 28, and 36 min after injection, whereas for BMIPP, a static image is usually acquired 20–30 min after injection (Hansen et al. 1988; Nishimura et al. 1998).

Studies with fatty acid imaging in patients with prior myocardial infarcts have reported discrepancies between relative myocardial blood flow and BMIPP uptake (Takahashi et al. 1996; Tamaki et al. 1996; Franken et al. 1994). This "mismatch" between regional myocardial blood flow and fatty acid uptake (i.e., fatty acid uptake reduced more severely than blood flow) has been taken to suggest the presence of myocardial viability (Fig. 3.5). Furthermore, it appears that the reduction in BMIPP uptake relative to perfusion correlates with the blood flow – FDG mismatch pattern by PET imaging (Kawamoto et al. 1994). These studies suggest an uncoupling of fatty acid uptake from blood flow in acutely injured but potentially viable myocardium. The significance of these findings needs to be explored further.

Some studies have examined the outcome of regional LV contractile function after revascularization. Most of these studies were performed in patients after acute myocardial infarction. They demonstrated that both IPPA (Iskandrian et al. 1995) and BMIPP (Nishimura et al. 1998; Franken et al. 1996) were of value in predicting recovery of ventricular function following revascularization. Furthermore, Tamaki et al. (1996) reported that the probability of cardiac events including cardiac death, non-fatal MI, unstable angina, and the need for revascularization was increased in patients with chronic coronary artery disease as a function of the extent of mismatches of BMIPP to ^{201}Tl. Finally, Nishimura et al. (1998) reported from a retrospective multicenter trial the potential usefulness of BMIPP and ^{201}Tl imaging in predicting recurrent ischemia in the chronic phase of myocardial infarction. The extent of BMIPP defect was correlated stronger with ejection fraction at the time of discharge and at 90 days after MI than the extent of ^{201}Tl defect, although this study did not report any significant prognostic value of fatty acid imaging.

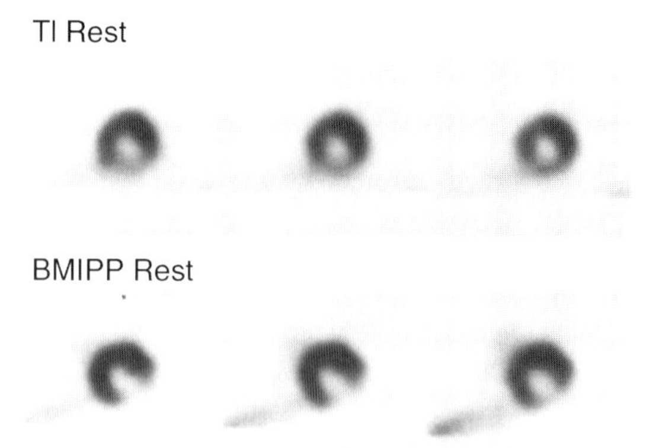

Fig. 3.5. Comparison of regional myocardial blood flow as assessed at rest with ^{201}Tl (TL REST) and fatty acid uptake (BMIPP REST). Note the more severely reduced BMIPP uptake in the inferolateral wall on the short-axis SPECT images in a patient with coronary artery disease. (From Tamaki et al. 1996)

3.3.5 Myocardial Oxidative Metabolism with ^{11}C Acetate

^{11}C-acetate allows the evaluation of flux through the tricarboxylic acid (TCA) cycle and because of its link to oxidative phosphorylation, it is an indicator of myocardial oxidative metabolism. After intravenous administration, the tracer becomes rapidly incorporated into the TCA cycle and is finally released from the cycle as $^{11}CO_2$. The rate of release from the myocardium parallels the rate of TCA cycle activity and by inference, estimates the rate of oxidative phosphorylation (for a detailed review of this tracer see Schelbert 1996). The net myocardial uptake, which reflects primarily delivery and extraction of tracer, also yields information on the distribution of regional myocardial blood flow. Both Gropler et al. (1993) and Rubin et al. (1996) have shown that the threshold criteria applied to ^{11}C-acetate images exhibited better predictive values for functional recovery than did the criteria with ^{18}F-deoxyglucose. These investigators therefore favor the use of ^{11}C-acetate for the identification of viable myocardium.

In reversibly dysfunctional myocardium, blood flow was initially thought to have a linear correlation with oxygen consumption. However, a non-linear biphasic correlation has been described between both variables (Wolpers et al. 1997; Feigl et al. 1990) which in fact might account for the above described observations with ^{11}C-acetate. Thus, measurements of oxygen consumption are more accurate than blood flow measurements alone in detecting viable tissue. However, the utility of ^{11}C-acetate for identifying viable tissue still remains uncertain. It has been reported that there is a considerable overlap in ^{11}C-acetate clearance rates between reversibly and irreversibly dysfunctional myocardium, whereas relative blood flow discriminated better between both types of myocardium in these studies (WOLPERS et al. 1997). Moreover, HATA et al. (1996) have shown that responses in ^{11}C-acetate clearance rates to low-dose dobutamine stimulation could differentiate both types of tissue. Further studies are needed to clarify the advantage of ^{11}C-acetate over estimates of blood flow for detecting viable myocardium.

3.3.6 Perfusion and Metabolism by PET

3.3.6.1 Evaluation of Myocardial Blood Flow

For the evaluation and quantitation of regional myocardial blood flow with PET, several tracers are available. Foremost are ^{13}N-ammonia, ^{82}Rb and ^{15}O-water (SCHELBERT 1996; SCHELBERT et al. 1996). The initial distribution of these flow tracers in myocardium parallels the distribution of myocardial blood flow. Quantitation of regional flows is possible with ^{13}N-ammonia employing dynamic image acquisition and two or three compartment tracer kinetic models, all validated in animal experiments. ^{15}O-water offers similarly accurate and extensively validated estimates of regional myocardial blood flow but requires subtraction of blood pool activity with ^{15}O-carbon-monoxide labeled red blood cells. Recent studies suggest that measurements can also be obtained by employing factor analysis of the serially acquired ^{15}O-water images, thus eliminating the need for additional blood pool imaging (HERMANSEN et al. 1998). Lastly, semiquantitative approaches have been used in the past with ^{82}Rb for obtaining estimates of regional flows, whereas more recent studies suggest the possibility of obtaining true estimates of blood flow with ^{82}Rb and an appropriate tracer kinetic model.

Assessment of regional blood flow in either relative or absolute terms may identify the presence of viable myocardium within dysfunctional regions. While normal blood flow in a dysfunctional region represents stunning, a severe blood flow deficit most likely represents non-viable tissue that is unlikely to improve function after revascularization (GEWIRTZ et al. 1994; BEANLANDS et al. 1997; KITSIOU et al. 1999). Absolute blood flow measurements have shown that viability will rarely be present in myocardium with flows below 0.25 ml/g/min (GEWIRTZ et al. 1994). Regional flow reductions of intermediate severity are more difficult to interpret. They may represent an admixture of subendocardial scar tissue with normal myocardial tissue, a condition unlikely to show improvement in function following revascularization. Conversely, such intermediate flow reduction could represent the coexistence of ischemic myocardium with either normal or scar tissue, which will likely improve function with revascularization. Some reports have shown that absolute measurements of blood flow alone are an unreliable measure of viability because of the considerable overlap in the values between reversibly and irreversibly damaged dysfunctional myocardium (WOLPERS et al. 1997; HATA et al. 1996; KITSIOU et al. 1999; VANOVERSCHELDE et al. 1992). Another study suggested that the late ^{13}N-ammonia retention, rather than estimates of regional flow, provided more useful information regarding functional recovery after revascularization (KITSIOU et al. 1999). However, it seems that this study pointed more to the limitation of absolute as compared with relative estimates of regional flows. In any event, evaluation of regional myocardial blood flow either in absolute or in relative terms appears to be of limited value for the accurate identification of viable myocardium especially when regional flow is only mildly to moderately reduced.

3.3.6.2 Evaluation of Glucose Utilization

Numerous studies have pointed out the incremental value of glucose metabolism assessments in addition to the evaluation of regional myocardial blood flow for identifying myocardial viability.

3.3.6.2.1 GENERAL CONSIDERATIONS

^{18}F-deoxyglucose (FDG) is an analog of glucose and is considered a marker of external glucose utilization. This tracer is transported into the myocyte by the same carrier as glucose and is phosphorylated to FDG-6-phosphate by the enzyme hexokinase (SCHELBERT 1996). This product is a poor substrate for glycogen synthesis, glycolysis and the fructose-pentose shunt. FDG-6-phosphate undergoes little dephosphorylation in the myocardium and therefore ^{18}F activity represents exogenous glucose uptake.

Rates of regional myocardial glucose utilization can be obtained from serially acquired FDG images using a two-compartment tracer kinetic model (Ratib et al. 1982; Krivokapich et al. 1982). This model assumes a mostly uni-directional tracer transport from blood into myocardium and, further, a fixed relationship between the transmembranous exchange and phosphorylation rate of glucose and of FDG as defined by the so-called lumped constant (Ratib et al. 1982; Krivokapich et al. 1982). However, studies in isolated heart preparations and in vivo experimental systems have suggested that this "lumped constant" may not be constant but varies depending on study conditions (Hariharan et al. 1995; Rhodes et al. 1999).

For the assessment of myocardial viability the finding of increased exogenous glucose utilization during mild acute myocardial ischemia served as the initial mechanistic underpinning. Yet, questions remain as to whether mechanisms accounting for the enhanced glucose utilization during acute ischemia can indeed be extrapolated to more chronic conditions such as hibernation and repetitive stunning. Translocation of glucose transporters GLUT 4 and GLUT 1 and increased expression of the mostly insulin-independent GLUT 1 as demonstrated in human dysfunctional myocardium may represent a flux generating step (Young et al. 1997; Brosius et al. 1997). As reviewed by Lopaschuk (1997), oxidation of glucose appears to be limited in "chronically" ischemic myocardium so that glycolysis and glucose oxidation are uncoupled. There is an excess in glycolysis with increased release of pyruvate in the form of lactate from the myocardium.

3.3.6.2.2 Flow-Metabolism Patterns in Dysfunctional Myocardium

For the detection of viable myocardium the most widespread approach is the evaluation of myocardial blood flow in conjunction with myocardial glucose uptake. With this protocol, three patterns are observed (Fig. 3.6): normal blood flow with normal FDG uptake, reduced blood flow with normal or increased FDG uptake (flow metabolism mismatch) and reduced blood flow with reduced FDG uptake (flow metabolism match). The pattern of *mismatch* between flow and metabolism detects reversibly dysfunctional myocardium (viable tissue), whereas the *match* pattern represents irreversibly dysfunctional myocardium (non-viable tissue).

It is important to consider some technical aspects of FDG studies. The plasma glucose level of the patient can influence myocardial glucose utilization. In the fasting state, normal myocardium preferentially consumes the fatty acid. In contrast, with increasing plasma glucose and insulin levels as, for example, after oral glucose loading, glucose becomes a major source of energy (Choi et al. 1993). Of note, ischemic myocardium preferentially utilizes glucose as energy substrate. Thus, FDG imaging can be performed either after glucose administration or in the fasting state. However, studies performed in the fasting state often result in inadequate tracer accumulation in the myocardium and poor target-to-background ratio (Choi et al. 1993; Berry et al. 1991). Therefore, the glucose loaded state is preferable for identifying viable myocardium. This can be achieved by oral glucose administration approximately 1 h prior to the tracer injection.

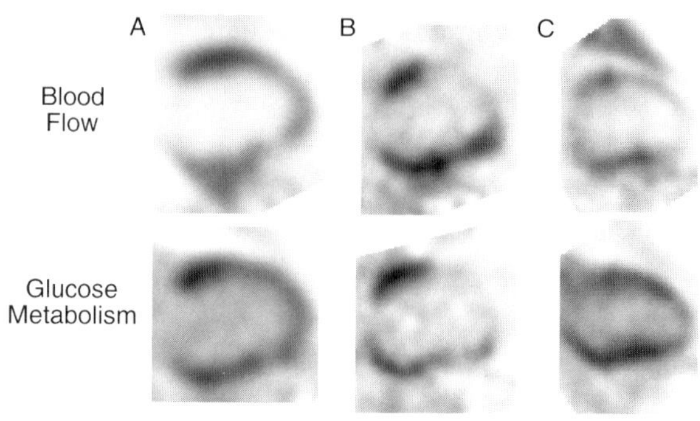

Fig. 3.6. Patterns of myocardial blood flow and glucose metabolism (as obtained with ^{13}N-ammonia and ^{18}F-deoxyglucose PET) in 3 patients with ischemic cardiomyopathy and poor left ventricular function. Only vertical long axis cuts through the mid-left ventricle are shown. Patient A demonstrates an enlarged left ventricular cavity with a mild decrease in perfusion in the anterior wall, apex, and the distal inferior wall. Glucose metabolism is homogeneous and exceeds perfusion in the anterior wall. In patient B there is a severe perfusion defect in the akinetic anterior wall that is matched to the glucose metabolic images by showing a decreased uptake of FDG referred to as "match" pattern. In contrast, in patient C, there is an extensive perfusion defect involving the anterior wall and the apex. However, the glucose metabolic images demonstrate preserved FDG uptake in the anterior and distal anterior wall. This pattern is referred to as a "blood flow / metabolism mismatch"

Patients with diabetes mellitus, many of whom have coronary artery disease, may also be challenging. Poorly controlled diabetics with high resting plasma glucose result in inadequate studies of limited diagnostic quality. The need for blood glucose standardization could thus be seen as a limitation for FDG imaging. Two alternatives can be considered in these patients to obtain high diagnostic quality images: the hyperinsulinemic-euglycemic glucose clamp technique (Hicks et al. 1991; Knuuti et al. 1992) or supplemental intravenous small doses of regular insulin (Schöder et al. 1999). Because the former is a very demanding procedure in the clinical setting, the latter is usually preferred. SCHÖDER et al. (1999) have reported that this protocol preserves the diagnostic accuracy of blood flow metabolism imaging in patients with type-II diabetes.

There has been concern that the quantitation of glucose uptake by FDG may underestimate regional glucose metabolism in vivo. HARIHARAN et al. (1995) showed in rat hearts that the uptake and retention of FDG in the myocardium was linearly related to glucose utilization only under steady-state conditions. The experimentally derived correction factor, the lumped constant that equates FDG uptake to glucose uptake was inaccurate when the physiological milieu of the heart was altered. These authors cautioned that estimates of regional rates of myocardial glucose utilization might be unreliable for the evaluation of myocardial viability. Whether these observations, to some extent obtained under extreme supra-physiologic conditions in isolated hearts, apply to human myocardium remains uncertain. If true, they may at least partially explain the limited value of absolute measurements of regional glucose metabolic rates for identifying dysfunctional myocardium. It is also possible that the variability of regional glucose metabolic rates as a function of variable circulating substrate in hormonal levels may similarly account for the limited value of absolute measurements. This variability further emphasizes the importance of relative regional FDG uptake values and the frequent need for simultaneous assessment of and comparison with regional myocardial blood flow.

3.3.6.3 Myocardial FDG Imaging with SPECT-like Devices

As an important technical aspect, FDG imaging was originally performed with dedicated PET only. However, recent studies have reported the feasibility of myocardial FDG imaging with modified or specifically designed SPECT systems (Fig. 3.7; BAX et al. 1996c; SANDLER et al. 1998). SPECT with high-energy collimator devices appears to yield diagnostic findings with an accuracy approaching that of PET (BAX et al. 1996c). Initial studies have demonstrated the feasibility of identifying blood flow-metabolism patterns with SPECT-like devices alone, with predictive accuracies approaching those previously reported by dedicated PET systems. BAX et al. (1996c) reported the agreement between ^{13}N-ammonia and FDG-PET and ^{201}Tl and FDG to detect viability in dyssynergic myocardium to be 76% with both techniques, yielding comparable results in 17 of 20 patients. CHEN et al. also reported an excellent statistical agreement (kappa=0.736) between the FDG-SPECT studies using a high-energy collimator and PET (BAX et al. 1996c; CHEN et al. 1997). One study in 17 patients with ^{201}Tl and FDG-SPECT imaging using high-energy photon collimators reported predictive accuracies similar to those for PET and exceeded those for low-dose dobutamine echocardiography (BAX et al. 1996a). The FDG-SPECT approach also appears to outperform the conventional ^{201}Tl-SPECT approach (BAX et al. 1997a). Image artifacts with apparent reductions in flow tracer uptake especially in the inferior wall of the left ventricle complicate the correlative interpretation of SPECT perfusion and FDG images (SAWADA et al. 1994). Correction for photon attenuation and scatter in SPECT imaging is now possible and is likely to overcome this limitation (MATSUNARI et al. 1998). With the anticipated widespread availability of FDG through regional distribution centers, flow-metabolism imaging for the identification of viable myocardium is likely to become clinically more widely accessible and at a lower cost.

3.3.6.4 Predicting Improvement in Regional and Global LV Function

The predictive accuracy of blood flow and glucose metabolism for detecting viable tissue has been evaluated in 13 studies totaling 422 patients using PET, the PET-SPECT hybrid technique (SPECT perfusion

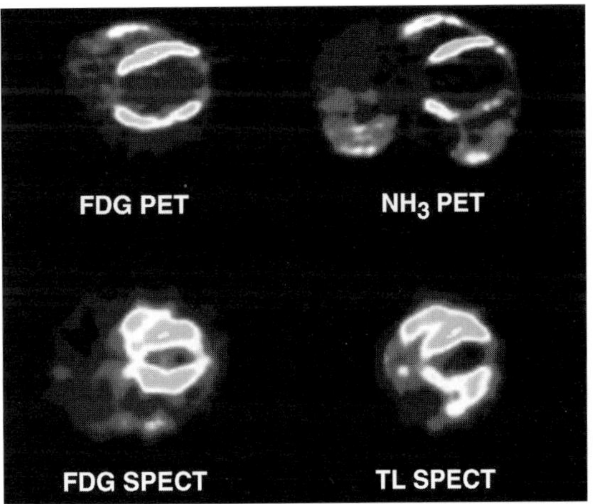

Fig. 3.7. Comparison of blood flow and metabolism imaging by PET and by SPECT. For the PET study, myocardial blood flow was evaluated with ^{13}N- ammonia (*NH_3*), whereas for the SPECT study myocardial perfusion was assessed with ^{201}Tl (TL). (From BAX et al. 1996c)

with PET-FDG imaging) or FDG-SPECT imaging (Gropler et al. 1993; Schöder et al. 1999; Tillisch et al. 1986; Tamaki et al. 1992; Lucignani et al. 1992; Carrel et al. 1992; Marwick et al. 1992; Knuuti et al. 1994; Paolini et al. 1994; vom Dahl et al. 1996a; Baer et al. 1996; Bax et al. 1997b). Wall motion abnormalities at rest were predicted to be reversible after revascularization in regions with normal flow and metabolism having a mismatched pattern, and irreversible in those having matched pattern. Based on these criteria, positive predictive accuracies ranged from 72 to 95% and negative predictive accuracies from 74 to 100%. The variability in predictive accuracies between studies might depend on patient selection, coronary anatomy, success of revascularization, criteria for image analysis and the time from revascularization to re-evaluation of regional myocardial wall motion.

Several investigators have reported the beneficial effect of revascularization of viable myocardium detected by blood flow-metabolism imaging on the global LV function. Average increases in ejection fraction ranged from 8% to 51% when PET had shown substantial amounts of viable dysfunctional myocardium (Maes et al. 1995; Schöder et al. 1999; Tillisch et al. 1986; Lucignani et al. 1992; Carrel et al. 1992; Marwick et al. 1992; Paolini et al. 1994; vom Dahl et al. 1996a; Depre et al. 1995; Schwarz et al. 1996; Haas et al. 1997; Flameng et al. 1997; Fath-Ordoubadi et al. 1998; Pagano et al. 1998; Beanlands et al. 1998) As shown in Fig. 3.8, when data were separately analyzed based on the LVEF prior to surgery, these studies showed a greater benefit in patients with ischemic cardiomyopathy and LVEF below 35% than those with EF greater than 35% (42% increase in EF vs 19%, respectively).

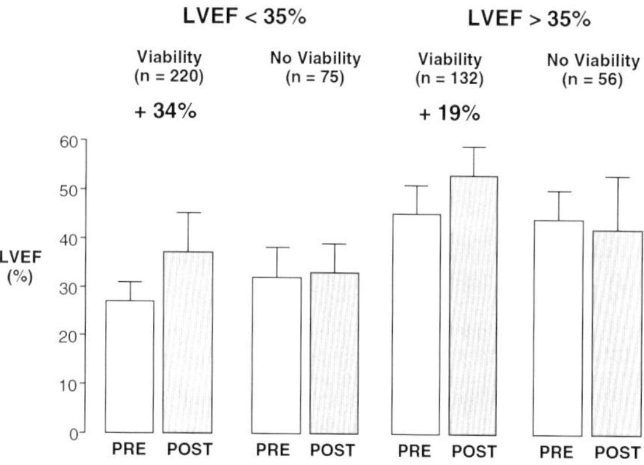

Fig. 3.8. Changes in left ventricular ejection fraction from baseline (*PRE*) to following revascularization (*POST*). The data represent the summary of 18 clinical studies in a total of 483 patients: Maes et al. 1995, Schöder et al. 1999, Tillisch et al. 1986, Lucignani et al. 1992, Carrel et al. 1992, Marwick et al. 1992, Paolini et al. 1994, Schwarz et al. 1996, Haas et al. 1997, Flameng et al. 1997, Fath-Ordoubadi et al. 1998, Pagano et al. 1998, Beanlands et al. 1998, vom Dahl et al. 1996b, Maes et al. 1994, vom Dahl et al. 1994, Depre et al. 1995, and Bax et al. 1997. Viability in these studies was determined with markers of metabolism using ^{11}C-acetate in two studies and ^{18}F-deoxyglucose in the remaining 16 studies

The magnitude of a post-revascularization improvement in global LV function depends on the relative amounts of normal and remodeled LV myocardium, scar tissue and fibrosis and, in particular, viable, i.e., reversibly dysfunctional, myocardium. Such dependence had already been demonstrated by previous studies on blood flow metabolism imaging where the LV ejection improved significantly only in patients with "mismatches" in at least two or more of a total of seven myocardial regions. More recent investigations provided additional support for such relationship and described a linear correlation between the extent of a mismatch (as the fraction of the LV myocardium) and the percent improvement in LVEF following revascularization (Fig. 3.9; Pagano et al. 1998).

3.3.6.5
Improvement in Congestive Heart Failure Symptoms and Exercise Capacity

With the exception of a few studies with single-photon-emitting tracers, mostly PET-based assessments of blood flow and metabolism have explored these important clinical endpoints. Several studies report significant post-revascularization changes in heart failure symptoms in patients with reversibly dysfunctional myocardium (Marwick et al. 1992; Haas et al. 1997; Eitzman et al. 1992; Di Carli et al. 1994). In one of these studies the percentage of patients with congestive heart failure classes III and IV declined significantly in only those patients with extensive blood flow metabolism mismatches who had been successfully revascularized (Di Carli et al. 1994). Revascularization of patients with mismatches were associated with substantial gains in LVEF during exercise (Carrel et al. 1992; Marwick et al. 1992, 1999). Peak rate-pressure product, maximal heart rate, and exercise capacity increased in those patients with multiple viable regions on preoperative PET imaging. There were no significant changes in exercise capacity and symptoms in patients with matched patterns only. The same investigators further showed that the improvement in exercise capacity correlated (r=0.63)

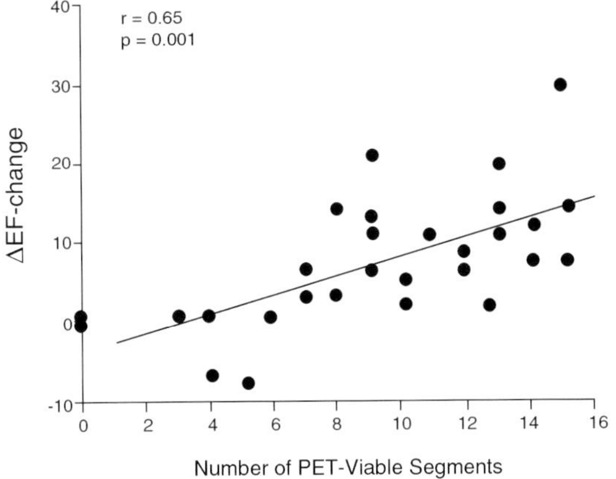

Fig. 3.9. Post-revascularization improvement in left ventricular ejection fraction (LVEF) as a function of the number of viable myocardial segments as determined by PET. (From PAGANO et al. 1998)

with the extent of viable myocardium (MARWICK et al. 1999). Other data have shown that by measuring physical activity with a specific activity scale, the post-revascularization gain in physical activity was found to correlate directly with the extent of the blood flow metabolism mismatch in 36 patients with ischemic cardiomyopathy (LVEF 28±6%; Fig. 3.10; DI CARLI et al. 1995). Large flow metabolism mismatches were associated with substantial gains in physical activity, whereas only small gains were achieved when no or only small amounts of flow metabolism mismatches were present. A flow metabolism mismatch involving 18% or more of the left ventricle was associated with a sensitivity and specificity of 76 and 78%, respectively, for predicting a significant improvement in heart failure class after bypass surgery.

Of interest is that one laboratory failed to observe significant differences in congestive heart failure symptoms following revascularization between patients with and without mismatches (MARWICK et al. 1992, 1999). Similarly, the LVEF at rest failed to increase significantly although there were significant gains in exercise performance and in LV function during exercise. As an important point, these investigations defined viability as disparities between regional myocardial uptake of FDG at rest and regional blood flow during pharmacologic stress. It is therefore likely that a substantial number of patients had only stress – rest mismatches. Revascularization in these patients would therefore not lead to an improvement in resting LV function, but rather during exercise, and augment the capacity for exercise.

3.3.6.6
Assessment of Cardiac Risk and Prediction of Cardiac Events

Lastly, evaluation of myocardial blood flow and glucose utilization in patients with coronary artery disease offers important clinical information about future cardiac events (EITZMAN et al. 1992; DI CARLI et al. 1994; 1998; TAMAKI et al. 1993; LEE et al. 1994; VOM DAHL et al. 1996b). Generally, follow-up after PET imaging indicates a higher incidence of cardiac events in patients with than in patients without blood flow metabolism mismatches. Three studies have examined the efficacy of revascularization over medical therapy in patients with moderate to severe LV dysfunction with and without evidence of viable myocardium (EITZMAN et al. 1992; DI CARLI et al. 1994; LEE et al. 1994). Despite not being randomized, these studies are the main source of understanding how to optimize treatment decisions in this patient population. The study population included patients with coronary artery disease and LVEF of less than 40%.

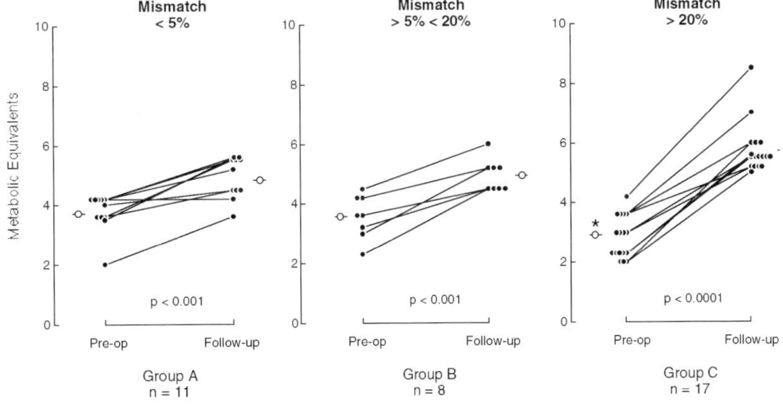

Fig. 3.10. Improvement in physical activity (measured in metabolic equivalents) as a function of the preoperative extent of a blood flow metabolism mismatch (in percent of the entire left ventricular myocardium). Note that the increase in physical activity was most striking in group-C patients with a blood flow metabolism mismatch occupying more than 20% of the left ventricular myocardium. (From DI CARLI et al. 1995)

Twenty to 68% of them had severe heart failure and approximately one third presented with angina. Survival and recurrent ischemic events (myocardial infarction, unstable angina and ventricular arrhythmia) were assessed for an average of 12–17 months. The patients were grouped based on the presence or absence of PET mismatch patterns. In patients with PET mismatch, 1-year event-free survival was poor with medical therapy. In contrast, 1-year event-free survival in these patients was significantly improved by revascularization. In patients without PET mismatch, 1-year event-free survival was similar with either medical therapy or revascularization. Thus, these studies show a clear benefit of revascularization over medical therapy for patients exhibiting a PET mismatch. Furthermore, the presence of blood flow metabolism mismatch and lack of revascularization were found to be the strongest predictors of cardiac death (Eitzman et al. 1992; Di Carli et al. 1994).

Di Carli et al. (1998) described the survival benefits of revascularization in patients with viable myocardium irrespective of symptoms (Fig. 3.11). In contrast, in patients without PET mismatch, coronary revascularization appeared to improve survival and symptoms only in patients with angina. Furthermore, long-term survival in patients with ischemic cardiomyopathy undergoing surgical revascularization appears to be similar to that achieved with cardiac transplantation. In 112 patients with ejection fractions below 35%, 5-year survival of patients with viable myocardium undergoing coronary artery bypass surgery was not different from that in patients who underwent transplantation (Duong et al. 1995).

3.3.6.7 Myocardial Revascularization and Impact of PET, Timing of Surgery

Recent observations have suggested that myocardial hibernation does not represent a steady state but rather an incomplete adaptation to ischemia (Elsässer et al. 1997). The precarious balance between perfusion and myocardial viability cannot be sustained indefinitely and necrosis, apoptosis, or both might occur if flow is not restored (Schwarz et al. 1996; Elsässer et al. 1997).

Dysfunctional myocardium characteristically exhibits "abnormal myocytes" (Flameng et al. 1981). Such myocytes reveal peri-nuclear loss of contractile protein and replacement by glycogen deposits. The structure of the cell nucleus is usually preserved; there are numerous small mitochondria of normal morphologic appearance (Borgers et al. 1995). Structural changes were correlated with the patterns of blood flow and metabolism which demonstrated a disproportionately greater fraction of abnormal myocytes in myocardium with flow metabolism mismatches (Vanoverschelde et al. 1993; Depre et al. 1995; Maes et al. 1994). In contrast, segments with normal flow and metabolism contained mostly normal myocytes with some abnormal cells and fibrosis, whereas myocardial segments with concordant reductions in flow and metabolism, considered as irreversibly dysfunctional, contained large amounts of fibrosis and scar tissue.

Some studies demonstrated a direct and statistically significant correlation between the fraction of abnormal myocytes and the relative FDG uptake (Depre et al. 1995), implicating such cells as the structural correlate of enhanced glucose uptake. However, the lack of such correlation between the severity of structural changes and FDG in another study (Schwarz et al. 1996) points to additional mechanisms of the enhanced glucose utilization.

The severity of morphological degeneration appears to correlate with the timing and the degree of functional recovery after revascularization (Schwarz et al. 1996; Elsässer et al. 1997). In fact, patients with mild morphological alterations showed faster and more complete recovery of LV function than those

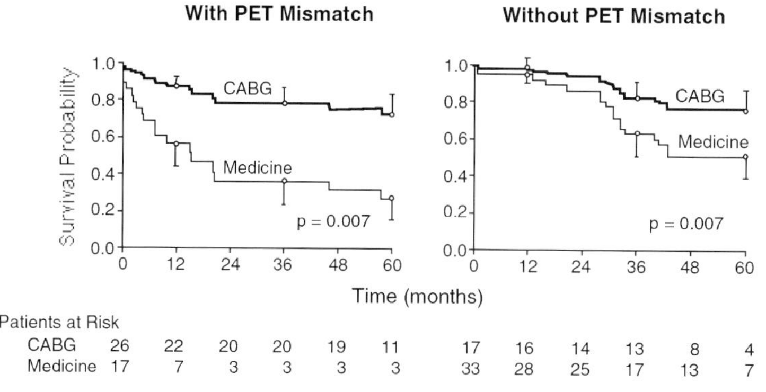

Fig. 3.11. Estimated survival probabilities by Kaplan-Meier analysis for patients with left ventricular function treated medically and with surgical revascularization based on the absence or presence of viability as determined by PET blood flow metabolism imaging. (From Di Carli et al. 1998)

with more severe changes (Elsässer et al. 1997). In support of this notion, the role of PET imaging for identification of high-risk patients with depressed ventricular function (ejection fraction less than 35%) was investigated (Beanlands et al. 1998). PET identified viable myocardium in 35 of 46 patients who were scheduled for revascularization. Preoperative mortality was significantly lower in patients undergoing early revascularization (<35 days) compared with those receiving late revascularization (>35 days; 0 vs 24%). Furthermore, LVEF improved significantly among patients in the early revascularization group (24±7 vs 31±11%) and not in those that underwent late revascularization (27±5 vs 28±6%).

3.4 Conclusion

This chapter emphasizes the considerable clinical evidence of the benefits of assessing myocardial viability prior to coronary revascularization. The various techniques highlighted and accompanying clinical data all point to the fact that viability assessment will lead to the correct use of resources for patients who would benefit the most from intervention, thus saving health care costs tremendously.

Each of the techniques mentioned has its strong points and its limitations. In selecting the type of test and tracer, one has to consider the temporal factors, availability of equipment, patient comfort and convenience, image quality, and costs involved. The authors consider perfusion-metabolic imaging with PET as the ideal choice. This is because assessment of myocardial viability is especially important in patients with ischemic cardiomyopathy when conventional SPECT-based imaging may be of limited diagnostic value because of the poor signal-to-noise ratios. Several studies have confirmed the higher diagnostic yield of FDG compared with conventional ^{201}Tl imaging in patients with markedly diminished LV function. However, if PET is unavailable, FDG-SPECT would come in a close second and we still consider ^{201}Tl imaging protocols an excellent choice for daily viability assessment. It is envisioned that with technological advancement, the costs for such tests and equipment will decrease and with widespread availability all modalities will approach each other in the degree of diagnostic accuracy.

Acknowledgements.
The authors thank D. Martin for assistance in preparing the figures and E. Rosenfeld for assistance in preparing the text. The Laboratory of Structural Biology and Molecular Medicine is operated for the U.S. Department of Energy by the University of California under contract no. DE-AC03-76-SF00012. This work was supported in part by the Director of the Office of Energy Research, Office of Health and Environmental Research, Washington D.C., by grant no. HL 33177, National Institutes of Health, Bethesda, Maryland, and by an Investigative Group Award by the Greater Los Angeles Affiliate of the American Heart Association, Los Angeles. R. Campisi is the recipient of the 1998 Society of Nuclear Medicine-DuPont Pharma Fellowship Grant.

References

Alderman EL, Corley SD, Fisher LD, Chaitman BR, Faxon DP, Foster ED, Killip T, Sosa JA, Bourassa MG. Five-year angiographic follow-up of factors associated with progression of coronary artery disease in the Coronary Artery Surgery Study (CASS). CASS Participating Investigators and Staff. J Am Coll Cardiol 1993;22:1141–1154

Alfieri O, La Canna G, Giubbini R, Pardini A, Zogno M, Fucci C. Recovery of myocardial function. The ultimate target of coronary revascularization. Eur J Cardiothorac Surg 1993;7:325–330

Altehoefer C, Kaiser HJ, Deorr R, Feinendegen C, Beilin I, Uebis R, Buell U. Fluorine-18 deoxyglucose PET for assessment of viable myocardium in perfusion defects in 99mTc-MIBI SPET: a comparative study in patients with coronary artery disease. Eur J Nucl Med 1992;19:334–342

Altehoefer C, Dahl J vom, Biedermann M, Uebis R, Beilin I, Sheehan F, Hanrath P, Buell U. Significance of defect severity in technetium-99m-MIBI SPECT at rest to assess myocardial viability: comparison with fluorine-18-FDG PET. J Nucl Med 1994;35:569–574

Baer FM, Voth E, Deutsch HJ, Schneider CA, Horst M, Vivie ER de, Schicha H, Erdmann E, Sechtem U. Predictive value of low dose dobutamine transesophageal echocardiography and fluorine-18 fluorodeoxyglucose positron emission tomography for recovery of regional left ventricular function after successful revascularization. J Am Coll Cardiol 1996;28:60–69

Bax JJ, Cornel JH, Visser FC, Fioretti PM, van Lingen A, Reijs AE, Boersma E, Teule GJ, Visser CA. Prediction of recovery of myocardial dysfunction after revascularization. Comparison of fluorine-18 fluorodeoxyglucose/thallium-201 SPECT, thallium-201 stress-reinjection SPECT and dobutamine echocardiography. J Am Coll Cardiol 1996a;28:558–564

Bax JJ, Cornel JH, Visser FC, Huybregts MA, Van Lingen A. Prediction of reversibility of wall motion abnormalities after revascularization using F18-fluorodeoxyglucose single photon emission computed tomography [letter]. Eur Heart J 1996b;17:480–481

Bax JJ, Visser FC, Blanksma PK, Veening MA, Tan ES, Willemsen TM, van Lingen A, Teule GJ, Vaalburg W, Lie KI, Visser CA. Comparison of myocardial uptake of fluorine-18-fluorodeoxyglucose imaged with PET and SPECT in dyssynergic myocardium. J Nucl Med 1996c;37:1631–1636

Bax JJ, Visser FC, Cornel JH, van Lingen A, Fioretti PM, Visser CA. Improved detection of viable myocardium with fluorodeoxyglucose-labeled single-photon emission computed tomography in a patient with hibernating myocardium: comparison with rest-redistribution thallium 201-labeled single-photon emission computed tomography. J Nucl Cardiol 1997a;4:178–179

Bax JJ, Cornel JH, Visser FC, Fioretti PM, van Lingen A, Huitink JM, Kamp O, Nijland F, Roelandt JR, Visser CA. Prediction of improvement of contractile function in patients with ischemic ventricular dysfunction after revascularization by fluorine-18 fluorodeoxyglucose single-photon emission computed tomography. J Am Coll Cardiol 1997b;30:377–383

Beanlands RS, Dawood F, Wen WH, McLaughlin PR, Butany J, D'Amati G, Liu PP. Are the kinetics of technetium-99 m methoxyisobutyl isonitrile affected by cell metabolism and viability? Circulation 1990;82:1802–1814

Beanlands RS, deKemp R, Scheffel A, Nahmias C, Garnett ES, Coates G, Johansen HL, Fallen E. Can nitrogen-13 ammonia kinetic modeling define myocardial viability independent of fluorine-18 fluorodeoxyglucose? J Am Coll Cardiol 1997;29:537–543

Beanlands RS, Hendry PJ, Masters RG, de Kemp RA, Woodend K, Ruddy TD. Delay in revascularization is associated with increased mortality rate in patients with severe left ventricular dysfunction and viable myocardium on fluorine 18-fluorodeoxyglucose positron emission tomography imaging. Circulation 1998;98:II51–II56

Beller GA. Comparison of 201Tl scintigraphy and low-dose dobutamine echocardiography for the noninvasive assessment of myocardial viability [editorial; comment]. Circulation 1996;94:2681–2684

Berry J, Baker J, Pieper K, Hanson M, Hoffman J, Coleman R. The effect of metabolic milieu on cardiac PET imaging using fluorine-18-deoxyglucose and nitrogen-13- ammonia in normal volunteers. J Nucl Med. 1991;32:1518–1525

Bisi G, Sciagraa R, Santoro GM, Fazzini PF. Rest technetium-99 m sestamibi tomography in combination with short-term administration of nitrates: feasibility and reliability for prediction of postrevascularization outcome of asynergic territories. J Am Coll Cardiol 1994;24:1282–1289

Bobba K, Botvinick EH, Sciammarella MG, Starsken NF, Zhu YY, Lapidus A, Dae MW. Is there any advantage to the acquisition of 24-hour thallium images, in the presence of persistent perfusion defects at 4 h after reinjection? Eur J Nucl Med 1998;25:509–514

Bolli R. Myocardial ‚stunning' in man. Circulation 1992; 86:1671–1691

Bolli R. Basic and clinical aspects of myocardial stunning. Prog Cardiovasc Dis 1998;40:477–516

Bonow RO, Dilsizian V, Cuocolo A, Bacharach SL. Identification of viable myocardium in patients with chronic coronary artery disease and left ventricular dysfunction. Comparison of thallium scintigraphy with reinjection and PET imaging with 18F-fluorodeoxyglucose [see comments]. Circulation 1991;83:26–37

Borgers M, Ausma J. Structural aspects of the chronic hibernating myocardium in man. Basic Res Cardiol 1995;90:44–46

Braunwald E, Kloner RA. The stunned myocardium: prolonged, postischemic ventricular dysfunction. Circulation 1982;66:1146–1149

Brosius FC, Nguyen N, Egert S, Lin Z, Deeb GM, Haas F, Schwaiger M, Sun D. Increased sarcolemmal glucose transporter abundance in myocardial ischemia. Am J Cardiol 1997;80:77A–84A

Caner B, Beller GA. Are technetium-99m-labeled myocardial perfusion agents adequate for detection of myocardial viability? Clin Cardiol 1998;21:235–242

Carli M di, Schelbert HR, Asgarzadie F, Rokshar S, Mody F, Czernin J, Brunken R, Laks H, Phelphs ME, Maddahi J. Is there a relationship between myocardial viability and change in heart failure post revascularization in patients with poor LV function? J Nucl Med 1994;35

Carli MF di, Asgarzadie F, Schelbert HR, Brunken RC, Laks H, Phelps ME, Maddahi J. Quantitative relation between myocardial viability and improvement in heart failure symptoms after revascularization in patients with ischemic cardiomyopathy. Circulation 1995;92:3436–3444

Carli MF di, Maddahi J, Rokhsar S, Schelbert HR, Bianco-Batlles D, Brunken RC, Fromm B. Long-term survival of patients with coronary artery disease and left ventricular dysfunction: implications for the role of myocardial viability assessment in management decisions. J Thorac Cardiovasc Surg 1998;116:997–1004

Carrel T, Jenni R, Haubold-Reuter S, Schulthess G von, Pasic M, Turina M. Improvement of severely reduced left ventricular function after surgical revascularization in patients with preoperative myocardial infarction. Eur J Cardiothorac Surg. 1992;6:479–484

Carvalho PA, Chiu ML, Kronauge JF, Kawamura M, Jones AG, Holman BL, Piwnica-Worms D. Subcellular distribution and analysis of technetium-99m-MIBI in isolated perfused rat hearts. J Nucl Med 1992;33:1516–1522

Charney R, Schwinger ME, Chun J, Cohen MV, Nanna M, Menegus MA, Wexler J, Franco HS, Greenberg MA. Dobutamine echocardiography and resting-redistribution thallium-201 scintigraphy predicts recovery of hibernating myocardium after coronary revascularization. Am Heart J 1994;128:864–869

Chen E, MacIntyre J, Go R, Brunken R, Saha G, Wong C, Neumann D, Cook S, Khandekar S. Myocardial viability studies using fluorine-18-FDG SPECT: a comparison with fluorine-18-FDG PET. J Nucl Med. 1997;38:582–586

Choi Y, Brunken RC, Hawkins RA, Huang S-C, Buxton DB, Hoh CK, Phelps ME, Schelbert HR. Factors affecting myocardial 2-[F-18]fluoro-2-deoxy-D-glucose uptake in positron emission tomography studies of normal humans. Eur J Nucl Med. 1993;20:308–318

Chua T, Kiat H, Germano G, Maurer G, van Train K, Friedman J, Berman D. Gated technetium-99 m sestamibi for simultaneous assessment of stress myocardial perfusion, postexercise regional ventricular function and myocardial viability. Correlation with echocardiography and rest thallium-201 scintigraphy. J Am Coll Cardiol 1994;23:1107–1114

Conversano A, Walsh JF, Geltman EM, Perez JE, Bergmann SR, Gropler RJ. Delineation of myocardial stunning and hibernation by positron emission tomography in advanced coronary artery disease. Am Heart J 1996;131:440–450

Cuocolo A, Maurea S, Pace L, Nicolai E, Nappi A, Imbriaco M, Trimarco B, Salvatore M. Resting technetium-99 m methoxyisobutylisonitrile cardiac imaging in chronic coronary artery disease: comparison with rest-redistribution thallium-201 scintigraphy. Eur J Nucl Med 1993;20:1186–1192

Cuocolo A, Pace L, Ricciardelli B, Chiariello M, Trimarco B, Salvatore M. Identification of viable myocardium in patients with chronic coronary artery disease: comparison of thallium-201 scintigraphy with reinjection and technetium-99m-methoxyisobutyl isonitrile [see comments]. J Nucl Med 1992;33:505–511

Dahl J vom, Eitzman D, Al-Aouar A, Kanter H, Hicks R, Deeb G, Kirsh M, Schwaiger M. Relation of regional function, perfusion, and metabolism in patients with advanced coronary artery disease undergoing surgical revascularization. Circulation 1994;90:2356–2366

Dahl J vom, Altehoefer C, Sheehan F, Buechin P, Uebis R, Messmer B, Buell U, Hanrath P. Recovery of regional left ventricular dysfunction after coronary revascularization: impact of myocardial viability assessed by nuclear imaging and vessel patency at follow-up angiography. J Am Coll Cardiol 1996a;28:948–958

Dahl J vom, Altehoefer C, Büchin P, Sheehan F, Schwarz E, Koch K, Schulz G, Uebis R, Schöndube F, Messmer B, Büll U, Hanrath P. Effect of myocardial viability and coronary revascularization on clinical outcome and prognosis: a follow-up study of 161 patients with coronary heart disease. Z Kardiol 1996b;85:868–881

Dakik HA, Howell JF, Lawrie GM, Espada R, Weilbaecher DG, He ZX, Mahmarian JJ, Verani MS. Assessment of myocardial viability with 99mTc-sestamibi tomography before coronary bypass graft surgery: correlation with histopathology and postoperative improvement in cardiac function. Circulation 1997;96:2892–2898

Depré C, Vanoverschelde J-LJ, Melin J, Borgers M, Bol A, Ausma J, Dion R, Wijns W. Structural and metabolic correlates of the reversibility of chronic left ventricular ischemic dysfunction in humans. Am J Physiol 1995;268:H1265–H1275

Dilsizian V, Rocco TP, Freedman NM, Leon MB, Bonow RO. Enhanced detection of ischemic but viable myocardium by the reinjection of thallium after stress-redistribution imaging [see comments]. N Engl J Med 1990;323:141–146

Dilsizian V, Smeltzer WR, Freedman NM, Dextras R, Bonow RO. Thallium reinjection after stress-redistribution imaging. Does 24-hour delayed imaging after reinjection enhance detection of viable myocardium? Circulation 1991;83:1247–1255

Dilsizian V, Arrighi JA, Diodati JG, Quyyumi AA, Alavi K, Bacharach SL, Marin-Neto JA, Katsiyiannis PT, Bonow RO. Myocardial viability in patients with chronic coronary artery disease. Comparison of 99mTc-sestamibi with thallium reinjection and [18F]fluorodeoxyglucose [published errata appears in Circulation 91:3026]. Circulation 1994;89:578–587

Dondi M, Tartagni F, Fallani F, Fanti S, Marengo M, DiTommaso I, Zheng QF, Monetti N. A comparison of rest sestamibi and rest-redistribution thallium single photon emission tomography: possible implications for myocardial viability detection in infarcted patients. Eur J Nucl Med 1993;20:26–31

Duong T, Hendi P, Fonarow G, Asgarzadie F, Stevenson L, Carli M di, Hage A, Moriguchi J, Kobashigawa J, Brunken R, Czernin J, Blitz A, Laks H, Phelps M, Schelbert H, Maddahi J. Role of positron emission tomographic assessment of myocardial viability in the management of patients who are referred for cardiac transplantation. Circulation 1995;92:1–123

Edwards NC, Sinusas AJ, Bergin JD, Watson DD, Ruiz M, Beller GA. Influence of subendocardial ischemia on transmural myocardial function. Am J Physiol 1992;262:H568–H576

Eitzman D, Al-Aouar Z, Dahl J vom, Kirsh M, Schwaiger M. Clinical outcome of patients with advanced coronary artery disease after viability studies with positron emission tomography. J Am Coll Cardiol 1992;20:559–565

Elsässer A, Schlepper M, Kleovekorn WP, Cai WJ, Zimmermann R, Meuller KD, Strasser R, Kostin S, Gagel C, Meunkel B, Schaper W, Schaper J. Hibernating myocardium: an incomplete adaptation to ischemia. Circulation 1997;96:2920–2931

Fath-Ordoubadi F, Pagano D, Marinho NV, Keogh BE, Bonser RS, Camici PG. Coronary revascularization in the treatment of moderate and severe postischemic left ventricular dysfunction. Am J Cardiol 1998;82:26–31

Feigl E, Neat G, Huang A. Interrelations between coronary artery pressure, myocardial metabolism and coronary blood flow. J Mol Cell Cardiol 1990;22:375–390

Flameng W, Suy R, Schwarz F, Borgers M, Piessens J, Thone F, Van Ermen H, De Geest H. Ultrastructural correlates of left ventricular contraction abnormalities in patients with chronic ischemic heart disease: determinants of reversible segmental asynergy post-revascularization surgery. Am Heart J 1981;102:846–857

Flameng WJ, Shivalkar B, Spiessens B, Maes A, Nuyts J, VanHaecke J, Mortelmans L. PET scan predicts recovery of left ventricular function after coronary artery bypass operation. Ann Thorac Surg 1997;64:1694–1701

Franken P, DeGeeter F, Dendale P, Demoor D, Block P, Bossuyt A. Abnormal free fatty acid uptake in subacute myocardial infarction after coronary thrombolysis: correlation with wall motion and inotropic reserve. J Nucl Med 1994;35:1758–1765

Franken P, Dendale P, DeGeeter F, Demoor D, Bossuyt A, Block P. Prediction of functional outcome after myocardial infarction using BMIPP and sestamibi scintigraphy. J Nucl Med 1996;37:718–722

Fujiwara S, Takeishi Y, Atsumi H, Chiba J, Takahashi K, Tomoike H. Quantitative assessment of myocardial 99mTc-sestamibi uptake during exercise: usefulness of response rate for assessing severity of coronary artery disease. Jpn Circ J 1998;62:592–598

Galassi AR, Tamburino C, Grassi R, Foti R, Mammana C, Virgilio A, Licciardello G, Musumeci S, Giuffrida G. Comparison of technetium 99m-tetrofosmin and thallium-201 single photon emission computed tomographic imaging for the assessment of viable myocardium in patients with left ventricular dysfunction. J Nucl Cardiol 1998;5:56–63

Gewirtz H, Fischman A, Abraham S, Gilson M, Strauss H, Alpert N. Positron emission tomographic measurements of absolute regional myocardial blood flow permits identification of nonviable myocardium in patients with chronic myocardial infarction. J Am Coll Cardiol 1994;23:851–859

Gibson RS, Watson DD, Taylor GJ, Crosby IK, Wellons HL, Holt ND, Beller GA. Prospective assessment of regional myocardial perfusion before and after coronary revascularization surgery by quantitative thallium-201 scintigraphy. J Am Coll Cardiol 1983;1:804–815

Gimple LW, Beller GA. Myocardial viability. Assessment by cardiac scintigraphy. Cardiol Clin 1994;12:317–332

Gioia G, Powers J, Heo J, Iskandrian AS. Prognostic value of rest-redistribution tomographic thallium-201 imaging in ischemic cardiomyopathy. Am J Cardiol 1995;75:759–762

Goodman M, Knapp F, Elmaleh D, Strauss H. Synthesis and evaluation of radioiodinated terminal p-iodophenyl-substituted alpha- and beta-methyl-branched fatty acids. J Med Chem 1984;25:390

Gropler RJ, Geltman EM, Sampathkumaran K, Perez JE, Schechtman KB, Conversano A, Sobel BE, Bergmann SR, Siegel BA. Comparison of carbon-11-acetate with fluorine-18-fluorodeoxyglucose for delineating viable myocardium by positron emission tomography. J Am Coll Cardiol 1993;22:1587–1597

Gutman J, Berman DS, Freeman M, Rozanski A, Maddahi J, Waxman A, Swan HJ. Time to completed redistribution of thallium-201 in exercise myocardial scintigraphy: relationship to the degree of coronary artery stenosis. Am H J 1983;106:989–995

Haas F, Haehnel CJ, Picker W, Nekolla S, Martinoff S, Meisner H, Schwaiger M. Preoperative positron emission tomographic viability assessment and perioperative and postoperative risk in patients with advanced ischemic heart disease [see comments]. J Am Coll Cardiol 1997;30:1693–1700

Hansen C, Corbett J, Pippin J. Iodine-123 phenylpentadecanoic acid and single photon emission computed tomography in identifying heart disease: comparison with thallium-201 myocardial tomography. J Am Coll Cardiol 1988;12:78

Haque T, Furukawa T, Takahashi M, Kinoshita M. Identification of hibernating myocardium by dobutamine stress echocardiography: comparison with thallium-201 reinjection imaging. Am Heart J 1995;130:553–563

Hariharan R, Bray M, Ganim R, Doenst T, Goodwin G, Taegtmeyer H. Fundamental limitations of [^{18}F]2-deoxy-2-fluoro-D-glucose for assessing myocardial glucose uptake. Circulation 1995;91:2435–2444

Hata T, Nohara R, Fujita M, Hosokawa R, Lee L, Kudo T, Tadamura E, Tamaki N, Konishi J, Sasayama S. Noninvasive assessment of myocardial viability by positron emission tomography with ^{11}C acetate in patients with old myocardial infarction: usefulness of low-dose dobutamine infusion. Circulation 1996;94:1834–1841

Hermansen F, Ashburner J, Spinks TJ, Kooner JS, Camici PG, Lammertsma AA. Generation of myocardial factor images directly from the dynamic oxygen-15-water scan without use of an oxygen-15-carbon monoxide blood-pool scan. J Nucl Med 1998;39:1696–1702

Heyndrickx G, Millard R, McRitchie R et al. Regional myocardial functional and electrophysiological alterations after brief coronary occlusion in conscious dogs. J Clin Invest 1975;56:978–985

Hicks R, Herman W, Kalff V, Molina E, Wolfe E, Hutchins G, Schwaiger M. Quantitative evaluation of regional substrate metabolism in the human heart by positron emission tomography. J Am Coll Cardiol 1991;18:101–111

Iskandrian A, Powers J, Cave V, Wasserleben V, Cassell D, Heo J. Assessment of myocardial viability by dynamic tomographic iodine 123 iodophenylpentadecanoic acid imaging: comparison with rest-redistribution thallium 201 imaging. J Nucl Cardiol. 1995;2:101–109

Iskandrian AS, Hakki AH, Kane SA, Goel IP, Mundth ED, Segal BL. Rest and redistribution thallium-201 myocardial scintigraphy to predict improvement in left ventricular function after coronary arterial bypass grafting. Am J Cardiol 1983;51:1312--1316

Kauffman GJ, Boyne TS, Watson DD, Smith WH, Beller GA. Comparison of rest thallium-201 imaging and rest technetium-99 m sestamibi imaging for assessment of myocardial viability in patients with coronary artery disease and severe left ventricular dysfunction [see comments]. J Am Coll Cardiol 1996;27:1592–1597

Kawamoto M, Tamaki N, Yonekura Y, Tadamura E, Fujibayashi Y, Magata Y, Nohara R, Sasayama s, Ikekubo K, Kato H et al. Combined study with I-123 fatty acid and thallium-201 to assess ischemic myocardium: comparison with thallium redistribution and glucose metabolism. Ann Nucl Med 1994;8:47–54

Kiat H, Berman DS, Maddahi J, De Yang L, Van Train K, Rozanski A, Friedman J. Late reversibility of tomographic myocardial thallium-201 defects: an accurate marker of myocardial viability. J Am Coll Cardiol 1988;12:1456–1463

Kitsiou AN, Srinivasan G, Quyyumi AA, Summers RM, Bacharach SL, Dilsizian V. Stress-induced reversible and mild-to-moderate irreversible thallium defects: are they equally accurate for predicting recovery of regional left ventricular function after revascularization? Circulation 1998;98:501–508

Kitsiou AN, Bacharach SL, Bartlett ML, Srinivasan G, Summers RM, Quyyumi AA, Dilsizian V. 13N-ammonia myocardial blood flow and uptake: relation to functional outcome of asynergic regions after revascularization. J Am Coll Cardiol 1999;33:678–686

Kloner RA, Bolli R, Marban E, Reinlib L, Braunwald E. Medical and cellular implications of stunning, hibernation, and preconditioning: an NHLBI workshop. Circulation 1998;97:1848–1867

Knapp F, Ambrose K, Goodman M. New radioiodinated methyl-branched fatty acids for cardiac studies. Eur J Nucl Med 1986;12:S39

Knuuti M, Nuutila P, Ruotsalainen U, Saraste M, Härkönen R, Ahonen A, Teräs M, Haaparanta M, Wegelius U, Haapanen A, Hartiala J, Voipio-Pulkki L-M. Euglycemic hyperinsulinemic clamp and oral glucose load in stimulating myocardial glucose utilization during positron emission tomography. J Nucl Med 1992;33:1255–1262

Knuuti M, Saraste M, Nuutila P, Härkönen R, Wegelius U, Haapanen A. Myocardial viability: fluorine-18-deoxyglucose positron emission tomography in prediction of wall motion recovery after revascularization. Am Heart J 1994;127:785–796

Koplan BA, Beller GA, Ruiz M, Yang JY, Watson DD, Glover DK. Comparison between thallium-201 and technetium-99m-tetrofosmin uptake with sustained low flow and profound systolic dysfunction. J Nucl Med 1996;37:1398–1402

Krivokapich J, Huang SC, Phelps ME, Barrio JR, Watanabe CR, Selin CE, Shine KI. Estimation of rabbit myocardial metabolic rate for glucose using fluorodeoxyglucose. Am J Physiol 1982;243:H884–H895

Lee K, Marwick T, Cook S, Go R, Fix J, James K, Sapp S, MacIntyre W, Thomas J. Prognosis of patients with left ventricular dysfunction, with and without viable myocardium after myocardial infarction. Circulation 1994;90:2687–2694

Lopaschuk G, Stanley W. Glucose metabolism in the ischemic heart. Circulation 1997;95:313–315

Lucignani G, Paolini G, Landoni C, Zuccari M, Paganelli G, Galli L, Credico G di, Vanoli G, Rossetti C, Mariani MA, Gilardi MC, Colombo F, Grossi A, Fazio F. Presurgical identification of hibernating myocardium by combined use of technetium-99 m hexakis 2-methoxyisobutylisonitrile single photon emission tomography and fluorine-18 fluoro-2-deoxy-D-glucose positron emission tomography in patients with coronary artery disease. Eur J Nucl Med 1992;19:874–881

Machulla HJ, Stocklin G, Kupfernagel CH, Freundlieb CH, Hock A, Vyska K, Feinendegen LE. Comparative evaluation of fatty acids with C-11, C1–34 m, Br-77, I-23, for metabolic studies of the myocardium: concise communication. J Nucl Med 1978;19:298–302

Maddahi J, Schelbert H, Brunken R, Di Carli M. Role of thallium-201 and PET imaging in evaluation of myocardial viability and management of patients with coronary artery disease and left ventricular dysfunction. J Nucl Med 1994;35:707–715

Maes A, Flameng W, Nuyts J, Borgers M, Shivalkar B, Ausma J, Bormans G, Schiepers C, De Roo M, Mortelmans L. Histological alterations in chronically hypoperfused myocardium. Correlation with PET findings. Circulation 1994;90:735–745

Maes A, Flameng W, Borgers M, Nuyts J, Ausma J, Bormans G, Van de Werf F, De Roo M, Mortelmans L. Regional myocardial blood flow, glucose utilization and contractile function before and after revascularization and ultrastructural findings in patients with chronic coronary artery disease. Eur J Nucl Med 1995;22:1299–1305

Maes AF, Borgers M, Flameng W, Nuyts JL, van de Werf F, Ausma JJ, Sergeant P, Mortelmans LA. Assessment of myocardial viability in chronic coronary artery disease using technetium-99 m sestamibi SPECT. Correlation with histologic and positron emission tomographic studies and functional follow-up. J Am Coll Cardiol 1997;29:62–68

Marinho NV, Keogh BE, Costa DC, Lammerstma AA, Ell PJ, Camici PG. Pathophysiology of chronic left ventricular dysfunction. New insights from the measurement of absolute myocardial blood flow and glucose utilization. Circulation 1996;93:737–744

Marwick T, Nemec J, Lafont A, Salcedo E, MacIntyre W. Prediction by postexercise fluoro-18 deoxyglucose positron emission tomography of improvement in exercise capacity after revascularization. Am J Cardiol 1992;69:854–859

Marwick T, Zuchowski C, Lauer M, Secknus M-A, Williams M, Lytle B. Functional status and quality of life in patients with heart failure undergoing coronary bypass surgery after assessment of myocardial viability. J Am Coll Cardiol 1999;33:750–758

Marzullo P, Sambuceti G, Parodi O. The role of sestamibi scintigraphy in the radioisotopic assessment of myocardial viability [see comments]. J Nucl Med 1992;33:1925–1930

Marzullo P, Parodi O, Reisenhofer B, Sambuceti G, Picano E, Distante A, Gimelli A, L'Abbate A. Value of rest thallium-201/technetium-99 m sestamibi scans and dobutamine echocardiography for detecting myocardial viability. Am J Cardiol 1993;71:166–172

Matsunari I, Fujino S, Taki J, Senma J, Aoyama T, Wakasugi T, Hirai J, Saga T, Ichiyanagi K, Hisada K. Myocardial viability assessment with technetium-99m-tetrofosmin and thallium-201 reinjection in coronary artery disease. J Nucl Med 1995;36:1961-1967

Matsunari I, Fujino S, Taki J, Senma J, Aoyama T, Wakasugi T, Hirai J, Saga T, Yamamoto S, Tonami N. Quantitative rest technetium-99 m tetrofosmin imaging in predicting functional recovery after revascularization: comparison with rest-redistribution thallium-201. J Am Coll Cardiol 1997;29:1226–1233

Matsunari I, Boening G, Ziegler S, Nekolla S, Stollfuss J, Kosa I, Ficaro E, Schwaiger M. Attenuation-corrected ^{99m}Tc-tetrofosmin single-photon emission computed tomography in the detection of viable myocardium: comparison with positron emission tomography using ^{18}F-fluorodeoxyglucose. J Am Coll Cardiol 1998;32:927–935

Maunoury C, Chen CC, Chua KB, Thompson CJ. Quantification of left ventricular function with thallium-201 and technetium-99m-sestamibi myocardial gated SPECT [published errata appears in J Nucl Med 38:1834]. J Nucl Med 1997;38:958–961

Mori T, Minamiji K, Kurogane H, Ogawa K, Yoshida Y. Rest-injected thallium-201 imaging for assessing viability of severe asynergic regions. J Nucl Med 1991;32:1718–1724

Nishimura T, Nishimura S, Kajiya T, Sugihara H, Kitahara K, Iamai K, Muramatsu T, Takahashi N, Yoshida H, Osada T, Terada K, Ito T, Narusa H, Iwabuchi M. Prediction of functional recovery and prognosis in patients with acute myocardial infarction by 123I-BMIPP and 201Tl myocardial single photon emission computed tomography: a multicenter trial. Ann Nucl Med 1998;12:237–248

Ohtani H, Tamaki N, Yonekura Y, Mohiuddin IH, Hirata K, Ban T, Konishi J. Value of thallium-201 reinjection after delayed SPECT imaging for predicting reversible ischemia after coronary artery bypass grafting. Am J Cardiol 1990;66:394–399

Pagano D, Townend JN, Littler WA, Horton R, Camici PG, Bonser RS. Coronary artery bypass surgery as treatment for ischemic heart failure: the predictive value of viability assessment with quantitative positron emission tomography for symptomatic and functional outcome. J Thorac Cardiovasc Surg 1998;115:791–799

Pagley PR, Beller GA, Watson DD, Gimple LW, Ragosta M. Improved outcome after coronary bypass surgery in patients with ischemic cardiomyopathy and residual myocardial viability. Circulation 1997;96:793–800

Palmas W, Friedman JD, Diamond GA, Silber H, Kiat H, Berman DS. Incremental value of simultaneous assessment of myocardial function and perfusion with technetium-99 m sestamibi for prediction of extent of coronary artery disease. J Am Coll Cardiol 1995;25:1024–1031

Paolini G, Lucignani G, Zuccari M, Landoni C, Vanoli G, Credico G di, Rossetti C, Mariani MA, Fazio F, Grossi A. Identification and revascularization of hibernating myocardium in angina-free patients with left ventricular dysfunction. Eur J Cardiothorac Surg 1994;8:139–144

Perrone-Filardi P, Pace L, Prastaro M, Squame F, Betocchi S, Soricelli A, Piscione F, Indolfi C, Crisci T, Salvatore M, Chiariello M. Assessment of myocardial viability in patients with chronic coronary artery disease. Rest-4-hour-24-hour 201Tl tomography versus dobutamine echocardiography [see comments]. Circulation 1996;94:2712–2719

Platts EA, North TL, Pickett RD, Kelly JD. Mechanism of uptake of technetium-tetrofosmin. I. Uptake into isolated adult rat ventricular myocytes and subcellular localization [published errata appears in J Nucl Cardiol 2:560]. J Nucl Cardiol 1995;2:317–326

Pohost G, Zir L, Moor R. Differentiation of transiently ischemic from infarcted myocardium by serial imaging after single dose of Tl-201. Circulation 1977;55:294

Qureshi U, Nagueh SF, Afridi I, Vaduganathan P, Blaustein A, Verani MS, Winters WL Jr, Zoghbi WA. Dobutamine echocardiography and quantitative rest-redistribution 201Tl tomography in myocardial hibernation. Relation of contractile reserve to 201Tl uptake and comparative prediction of recovery of function. Circulation 1997;95:626–635

Ragosta M, Beller GA, Watson DD, Kaul S, Gimple LW. Quantitative planar rest-redistribution ^{201}Tl imaging in detection of myocardial viability and prediction of improvement in left ventricular function after coronary bypass surgery in patients with severely depressed left ventricular function. Circulation 1993;87:1630–1641

Rahimtoola SH. A perspective on the three large multicenter randomized clinical trials of coronary bypass surgery for chronic stable angina. Circulation 1987;72:V123–V135

Ratib O, Phelps ME, Huang SC, Henze E, Selin CE, Schelbert HR. Positron tomography with deoxyglucose for estimating local myocardial glucose metabolism. J Nucl Med 1982;23:577–586

Rhodes CG, Camici PG, Taegtmeyer H, Doenst T. Variability of the lumped constant for [18F]2-deoxy-2-fluoroglucose and the experimental isolated rat heart model: clinical perspectives for the measurement of myocardial tissue viability in humans [letter]. Circulation 1999;99:1275–1276

Rocco TP, Dilsizian V, Strauss HW, Boucher CA. Technetium-99 m isonitrile myocardial uptake at rest. II. Relation to clinical markers of potential viability [see comments]. J Am Coll Cardiol 1989;14:1678–1684

Rubin P, Lee D, Davila-Roman V, Geltman E, Schechtman K, Bergmann S, Gropler R. Superiority of C-11 acetate compared with F-18 fluorodeoxyglucose in predicting myocardial functional recovery by positron emission tomography in patients with acute myocardial infarction. Am J Cardiol 1996;78:1230–1236

Sandler MP, Bax JJ, Patton JA, Visser FC, Martin WH, Wijns W. Fluorine-18-fluorodeoxyglucose cardiac imaging using a modified scintillation camera. J Nucl Med 1998;39:2035–2043

Sawada SG, Allman KC, Muzik O, Beanlands RS, Wolfe ER Jr, Gross M, Fig L, Schwaiger M. Positron emission tomography detects evidence of viability in rest technetium-99 m sestamibi defects. J Am Coll Cardiol 1994;23:92–98

Schelbert H. Principles of positron emission tomography. In: Skorton D, Schelbert H, Wolf G, Brundage B (eds) Marcus' cardiac imaging, 2nd edn. Saunders, Philadelphia, 1996, pp 1063–1092

Schelbert H, Demer L. Evaluation of myocardial blood flow in cardiac disease. In: Skorton D, Schelbert H, Wolf G, Brundage B (eds) Marcus' cardiac imaging, 2nd edn. Saunders, Philadelphia, 1996, pp 1093–1112

Schneider CA, Voth E, Gawlich S, Baer FM, Horst M, Schicha H, Erdmann E, Sechtem U. Significance of rest technetium-99 m sestamibi imaging for the prediction of improvement of left ventricular dysfunction after Q wave myocardial infarction: importance of infarct location adjusted thresholds. J Am Coll Cardiol 1998;32:648–654

Schöder H, Campisi R, Ohtake T, Hoh CK, Moon DH, Czernin J, Schelbert HR. Blood flow-metabolism imaging with positron emission tomography in patients with diabetes mellitus for the assessment of reversible left ventricular contractile dysfunction. J Am Coll Cardiol 1999;33:1328–1337

Schwarz ER, Schaper J, Dahl J vom, Altehoefer C, Grohmann B, Schoendube F, Sheehan FH, Uebis R, Buell U, Messmer BJ, Schaper W, Hanrath P. Myocyte degeneration and cell death in hibernating human myocardium. J Am Coll Cardiol 1996;27:1577–1585

Sciagraa R, Bisi G, Santoro GM, Agnolucci M, Zoccarato O, Fazzini PF. Influence of the assessment of defect severity and intravenous nitrate administration during tracer injection on the detection of viable hibernating myocardium with data-based quantitative technetium 99m-labeled sestamibi single-photon emission computed tomography. J Nucl Cardiol 1996;3:221–230

Sciagraa R, Bisi G, Santoro GM, Zerauschek F, Sestini S, Pedenovi P, Pappagallo R, Fazzini PF. Comparison of baseline-nitrate technetium-99 m sestamibi with rest-redistribution thallium-201 tomography in detecting viable hibernating myocardium and predicting postrevascularization recovery. J Am Coll Cardiol 1997;30:384–391

Soufer R, Dey HM, Ng CK, Zaret BL. Comparison of sestamibi single-photon emission computed tomography with positron emission tomography for estimating left ventricular myocardial viability. Am J Cardiol 1995;75:1214–1219

Takahashi N, Reinhardt CP, Marcel R, Leppo JA. Myocardial uptake of 99mTc-tetrofosmin, sestamibi, and 201Tl in a model of acute coronary reperfusion. Circulation 1996;94:2605–2613

Tamaki N, Ohtani H, Yonekura Y, Nohara R, Kambara H, Kawai C, Hirata K, Ban T, Konishi J. Significance of fill-in after thallium-201 reinjection following delayed imaging: comparison with regional wall motion and angiographic findings [see comments]. J Nucl Med 1990;31:1617–1623

Tamaki N, Ohtani H, Yonekura Y, Shindo M, Nohara R, Kambara H, Kawai C, Hirata K, Ban T, Konishi J. Viable myocardium identified by reinjection thallium-201 imaging: comparison with regional wall motion and metabolic activity on FDG-PET. J Cardiol 1992;22:283–293

Tamaki N, Kawamoto M, Takahashi N, Yonekura Y, Magata Y, Nohara R, Kambara H, Sasayama S, Hirata K, Ban T, Konishi J. Prognostic value of an increase in fluorine-18 deoxyglucose uptake in patients with myocardial infarction: comparison with stress thallium imaging. J Am Coll Cardiol 1993;22:1621–1627

Tamaki N, Tadamura E, Kudoh T, Hattori N, Yonekura Y, Nohara R, Sasayama S, Ikekubo K, Kato H, Konishi J. Prognostic value of iodine-123 labelled BMIPP fatty acid analogue imaging in patients with myocardial infarction. Eur J Nucl Med 1996;23:272–279

Tillisch J, Brunken R, Marshall R, Schwaiger M, Mandelkern M, Phelps M, Schelbert HR. Reversibility of cardiac wall motion abnormalities predicted by positron tomography. N Engl J Med 1986;314:884–888

Udelson JE, Coleman PS, Metherall J, Pandian NG, Gomez AR, Griffith JL, Shea NL, Oates E, Konstam MA. Predicting recovery of severe regional ventricular dysfunction. Comparison of resting scintigraphy with 201Tl and 99mTc-sestamibi. Circulation 1994;89:2552–2561

Vanoverschelde JL, Melin JA, Bol A, Vanbutsele R, Cogneau M, Labar D, Robert A, Michel C, Wijns W. Regional oxidative metabolism in patients after recovery from reperfused anterior myocardial infarction. Relation to regional blood flow and glucose uptake. Circulation 1992;85:9–21

Vanoverschelde JL, Wijns W, Deprae C, Essamri B, Heyndrickx GR, Borgers M, Bol A, Melin JA. Mechanisms of chronic regional postischemic dysfunction in humans. New insights from the study of noninfarcted collateral-dependent myocardium [see comments]. Circulation 1993;87:1513–1523

Vanoverschelde JL, D'Hondt AM, Marwick T, Gerber BL, De Kock M, Dion R, Wijns W, Melin JA. Head-to-head comparison of exercise-redistribution-reinjection thallium single-photon emission computed tomography and low dose dobutamine echocardiography for prediction of reversibility of chronic left ventricular ischemic dysfunction [see comments]. J Am Coll Cardiol 1996;28:432–442

Watson D. Quantitative analysis of Tl-201 redistribution at 24 hours compared to 2 and 4 hours post-injection (Abstract). J Nucl Med 1990;31:763

Weich HF, Strauss HW, Pitt B. The extraction of thallium-201 by the myocardium. Circulation 1977;56:188–191

Wolpers H, Burchert W, van den Hoff J, Weinhardt R, Meyer G, Lichtlen P. Assessment of myocardial viability by use of ^{11}C-acetate and positron emission tomography. Circulation 1997;95:1417–1424

Yamamoto K, Asada S, Masuyama T, Nanto S, Matsumura Y, Naito J, Hirayama A, Mishima M, Naka M, Sasaki J et al. Myocardial hibernation in the infarcted region cannot be assessed from the presence of stress-induced ischemia: usefulness of delayed image of exercise thallium-201 scintigraphy. Am Heart J 1993;125:33–40

Young L, Renfu Y, Russell R, Hu X, Caplan M, Ren J, Shulman G, Sinusas A. Low-flow ischemia leads to translocation of canine heart GLUT-4 and GLUT-1 glucose transporters to the sarcolemma in vivo. Circulation 1997;95:415--422

Zaret BL, Rigo P, Wackers FJ, Hendel RC, Braat SH, Iskandrian AS, Sridhara BS, Jain D, Itti R, Serafini AN et al. Myocardial perfusion imaging with 99mTc tetrofosmin. Comparison to 201Tl imaging and coronary angiography in a phase III multicenter trial. Tetrofosmin International Trial Study Group [see comments]. Circulation 1995;91:313–319

4 Thromboembolism Imaging

H. D. Royal, D. A. Hillier

Contents

4.1 Introduction 57
4.2 Clinical Issues 58
4.2.1 Importance of Risk Stratification 58
4.2.2 Medical Decision Making 59
4.2.3 Pre-Test Probability 59
4.2.4 Utility Analysis 60
4.2.5 Patient Outcome 63
4.3 Ventilation-Perfusion Imaging 63
4.3.1 Technical Issues 63
4.3.2 Interpretation Criteria 64
4.3.2.1 PIOPED 64
4.4. Other Diagnostic Tests 68
4.4.1 Chest Radiograph 68
4.4.2 D-dimer 69
4.4.3 Detection of Deep Venous Thrombosis 69
4.4.4 Pulmonary Arteriogram 70
4.4.5 Spiral-CT Angiography 70
4.5 Conclusion 71
4.6 Appendix: Medical Decision Making 72

4.1 Introduction

Dramatic developments regarding the diagnosis and treatment of pulmonary embolism occurred in the 1960s. Anticoagulants were introduced into clinical practice (Barritt and Jordan 1960) and techniques for pulmonary arteriography were refined (Wiener et al. 1966; Dalen et al. 1971; Stein 1971). With the advent of Anger cameras and the availability of appropriate radiopharmaceuticals, ventilation-perfusion imaging for the diagnosis of pulmonary embolism became widely available in the 1970s. Shortly thereafter, the foundations of the current criteria used to interpret ventilation-perfusion studies were laid (McNeil 1976; Biello et al. 1979). From the very beginning, the diagnosis and treatment of pulmonary embolism was surrounded by controversy. One of the more controversial papers from these early days claimed that pulmonary embolism was overdiagnosed and overtreated, particularly in young otherwise healthy adults. The unreliability of ventilation-perfusion imaging was partly to blame for this problem (Robin 1977).

Twenty-five years after the widespread introduction of ventilation-perfusion imaging, little seems to have changed. A few technical advances have occurred and minor refinements in the criteria used to interpret ventilation-perfusion studies have been made. Conventional dogma continues to be that pulmonary embolism kills and these fatalities can be readily prevented if the diagnosis of pulmonary embolism is made and the patient is treated (Dalen and Alpert 1975). Given the apparent stagnant state of affairs, why read yet another chapter on the diagnosis and treatment of this common, familiar disease?

With current emphasis on evidence-based medicine (Anonymous 1992; Oxman et al. 1993) and patient outcomes (Eddy 1990), pressure is building for significant changes in how we think about the diagnosis and treatment of pulmonary embolism. Heretical questions such as "Does all pulmonary embolism need to be treated?" are being asked (Kelley et al. 1991; Stein et al. 1995). As more and more diagnostic tests are developed to detect pulmonary embolism, the concept of diagnostic "truth" becomes more complicated. Emphasis on patient outcomes have transformed diagnostic truth from the simple "If the pulmonary arteriogram was positive, the patient had pulmonary embolism" to the more complicated "How do we identify patient's in whom the risk of treatment is less than the risk of no treatment?"

In this chapter the conventional, comfortable, and sometimes mythological views of pulmonary embolism are, whenever possible, contrasted with alternative views. Only new thinking will allow us to finally make needed progress in how we diagnose and manage patients suspected of pulmonary embolism.

H. D. Royal, D. A. Hillier
Division of Nuclear Medicine, Mallinckrodt Institute of Radiology, 510 S. Kingshighway Blvd., Saint Louis, MO 63110, USA

This chapter consists of four sections. The first section, on clinical issues, reviews basic medical decision-making principles that are used in order to understand the complicated problems involved with the diagnosis and management of patients suspected of having pulmonary embolism. The importance of estimating the pre-test probability of pulmonary embolism and of risk stratification is emphasized. The next section discusses ventilation-perfusion imaging, the strengths and weaknesses of the PIOPED study, and the current state of the criteria used to interpret ventilation-perfusion studies. The third section delineates the role of other diagnostic tests in the diagnosis of pulmonary embolism with particular emphasis on the role of spiral CT and pulmonary arteriography. The final section summarizes the current state of affairs and proposes future advances.

4.2 Clinical Issues

In the 1960s and 1970s, when tools became available for the diagnosis (ventilation-perfusion imaging and pulmonary arteriography) and treatment (heparin and warfarin) of pulmonary embolism, efforts were made to make clinicians aware of this potentially lethal disease that now could be identified and treated. One of the most often quoted articles estimated that 200,000 deaths were caused in the United States every year from pulmonary embolism and implied that 88,000 of these deaths could be prevented if pulmonary embolism were diagnosed and treated (Dalen and Alpert 1975). In addition, autopsy studies then and since have demonstrated that the prevalence of undiagnosed pulmonary embolism is high in this very select population (Morpurgo and Schmid 1995; Cohen et al. 1996; Goldhaber et al. 1982). These factors have led to the conventional view that pulmonary embolism is a relatively common cause of preventable death. Even today, an often quoted statistic is that untreated pulmonary embolism has a mortality rate of 30% that could be reduced to 8% if the patient were treated.

What is the scientific basis for these seminal ideas, i.e., pulmonary embolism is a relatively common, treatable, often undiagnosed cause of death, which have so greatly influenced our thinking about pulmonary embolism over the past 30 years? As with many other diseases, early reports on the importance and effectiveness of treatment of pulmonary embolism are probably inflated. The 88,000 preventable deaths cited above are based on several very speculative estimates. Firstly, accurately determining the prevalence of pulmonary embolism is a very difficult task. Factors that will have major effects on the measured prevalence include the intensity of the diagnostic work-up, the diagnostic criteria used, and the population studied. Secondly, the natural history of treated and untreated pulmonary embolism has been poorly studied. There is reasonably good scientific evidence that the prognosis of untreated (Stein et al. 1995) and treated pulmonary embolism (Carson et al. 1992; Douketis et al. 1998) is better than the 30 and 8% mortality figures given by Dalen and Alpert (1975).

The results of autopsy studies are often cited as evidence that clinically important pulmonary embolism is frequently undiagnosed (Morpurgo and Schmid 1995; Rubinstein et al. 1988). Unfortunately, extrapolating the results of autopsy studies to living patients is fraught with errors. Not only are the deceased subjects a very select group of patients, it is also difficult to reliably determine if the emboli were simply agonal events or whether they significantly shortened patient life expectancy. It is likely that the incidence of undiagnosed pulmonary embolism is decreasing (Cohen et al. 1996; Dismuke and Wagner 1986).

Even the effectiveness of anticoagulation has only been studied in one small, quite old, randomized controlled study (Barritt and Jordan 1960). In this study, the diagnosis of pulmonary embolism was made based solely on clinical grounds. No pulmonary arteriography or ventilation-perfusion imaging was available at the time of this study. Presumably, these patients had massive pulmonary embolism, and in patients with massive pulmonary embolism mortality rates of 30% untreated and 8% treated may be reasonable. Dalen and Alpert (1975) used these mortality rates derived from patients with presumed massive pulmonary embolism to estimate the annual mortality due to pulmonary embolism in the United States.

4.2.1 Importance of Risk Stratification

Fortunately, the simple monolithic view of pulmonary embolism is crumbling. Increasingly it is being recognized as a complex, multifaceted disease, often the complication of other diseases, which ultimately are major determinants in the patient's survival. The patients at greatest risk for sudden preventable death due to pulmonary embolism are postoperative patients. Given the current emphasis on prophylaxis, it is not surprising that decreases in deaths due to post-operative pulmonary embolism have been well documented. Pulmonary embolism in healthy ambulatory patients rarely occurs.

The next quantum advance that we must make in our thinking about pulmonary embolism is that the diagnosis is not simply a binary (present or not present) task. Our level of sophistication when making the diagnosis of coronary artery disease is much greater than our level of sophistication when making the diagnosis of pulmonary embolism. The importance of risk stratification with coronary artery disease is universally recognized. Risk stratification for pulmonary embolism will have to account for (a) the physiological impact of pulmonary emboli that have already occurred, (b) the potential for future emboli, and (c) the overall medical condition of the patient. Ventilation-perfusion imaging cannot be used to assess the last two factors. Patients who have extensive, documented deep venous thrombosis are at higher risk than patients who have limited or no documented deep venous thrombosis. Patients with underlying cardiopulmonary disease are likely not to be able to tolerate pulmonary embolism as well as otherwise healthy patients.

4.2.2 Medical Decision Making

At a time when interest in the diagnosis and treatment of pulmonary embolism was growing, interest in medical decision making was also growing. In 1975 the *New England Journal of Medicine* devoted an entire issue to the topic of medical decision making (McNeil and Adelstein 1975; McNeil et al. 1975). The editors for this unique issue were two nuclear medicine physicians from the Brigham and Women's Hospital in Boston. Not surprisingly, medical decision making was quickly applied to the use of diagnostic tests in diseases such as pulmonary embolism.

Few disciplines in medicine have provoked as strong a reaction from the medical community as medical decision making. Individuals in the medical community appear to either love or hate the concepts, which provide the foundation for medical decision making. Some individuals shun medical decision making as an oversimplified impractical construct that has no clinical relevance; others believe that medical decision making provides some basic tools that can help further our understanding of the complexities of making decisions in medicine (Jaeschke et al. 1994a,b). For a summary of concepts, definitions, and applications, see the Appendix 4.6.

4.2.3 Pre-Test Probability

It should be clear that it is not possible to determine the post-test probability of disease solely based on the test result (see Appendix). The pre-test probability plays an equally important role in this assessment. For pulmonary embolism some experts argue that it is not possible to determine the pre-test probability for particular patients. This pessimism is not supported by the literature. In the PIOPED study, patients were stratified not only by the result of ventilation-perfusion imaging, but also by the clinician's pre-test assessment of the probability for pulmonary embolism (PIOPED Investigators 1990). Pre-test probability was broadly categorized as low (0–19%), intermediate (20–79%), or high (80–100%). Examination of the results of the PIOPED study clearly show that for the same test results the post-test probability of disease varied depending on the clinician's assessment of the pre-test probability (Fig. 4.1).

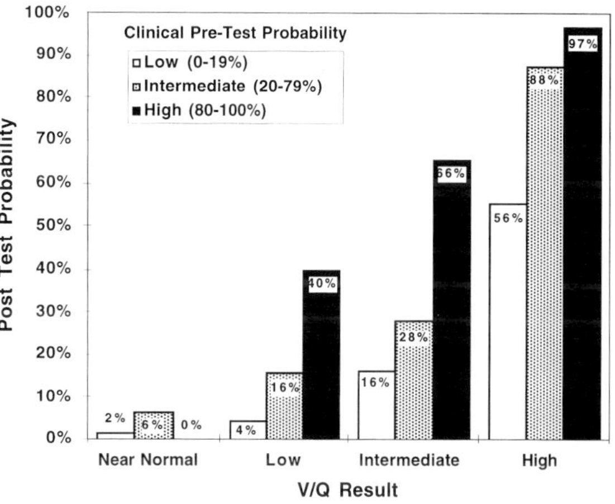

Fig. 4.1. The effect of the clinicians' estimate of pre-test probability on the post-test probability for each category of test results in the PIOPED study. The pre-test probability clearly had an effect on the post-test probability of disease (PIOPED Investigators 1990)

The difficulty with assessing the pre-test probability of pulmonary embolism is that there is no simple clinical rule that has been widely accepted to produce a valid result. Most recently, Wells et al. (1998)

demonstrated that the risk for thromboembolic disease could be accurately assessed by using the clinical history, the results of ventilation-perfusion imaging, and the results of serial compression ultrasound of the lower extremities. Using a simple scheme, these authors proposed a method for accurately assessing pre-test probability (Fig. 4.2).

4.2.4 Utility Analysis

Once the post-test probability of disease is known, the clinician must decide what to do next. Management of patients with pulmonary embolism can be simply modeled using utility analysis, which provides some useful insight into why we do the things that we do.

Utility analysis considers the expected outcome for patients based on different patient management decisions. There are six major outcomes in patients suspected of pulmonary embolism. These outcomes and their utility are listed in Table 4.1. These six outcomes can be divided into two groups of three. The first group is the outcome from patients who do not have pulmonary embolism, and the second group is the outcome from patients who do have pulmonary embolism. For patients without pulmonary embolism, the best outcome is that they are not treated with anticoagulation; therefore, they are not unnec-

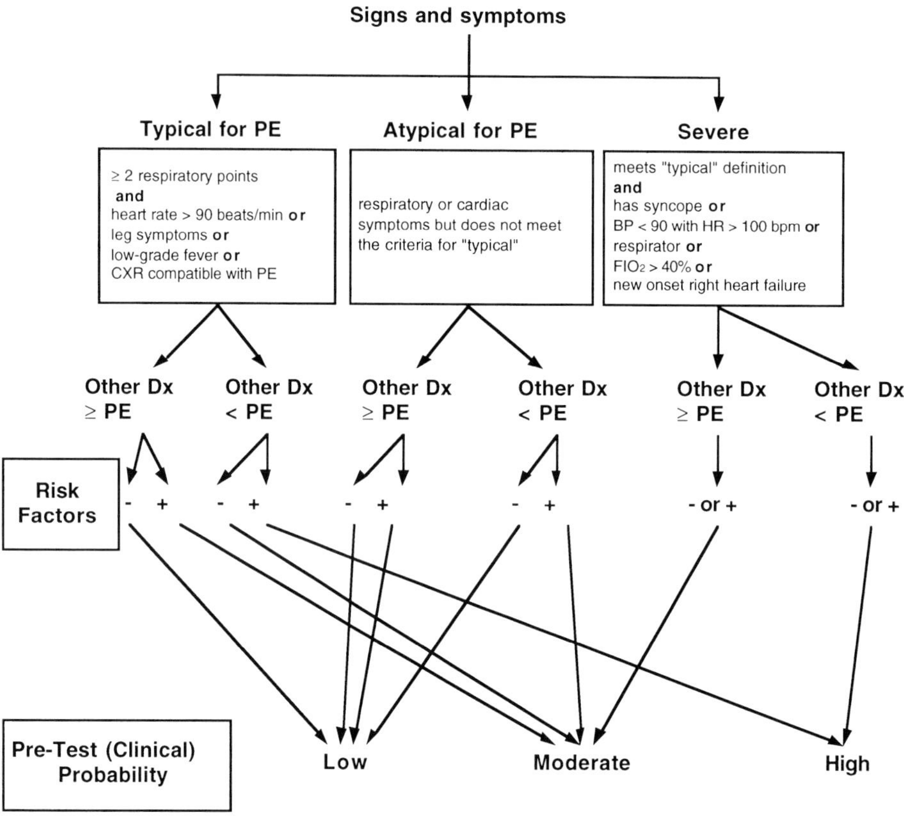

Fig. 4.2. An algorithm for the assessment of the pre-test probability of disease. Respiratory points consist of dyspnea or worsening of chronic dyspnea, pleuritic chest pain, chest pain that is non-retrosternal and non-pleuritic, and arterial oxygen saturation less than 92% while breathing room air that corrects with oxygen supplementation less than 40%, hemoptysis, and pleural rub. Risk factors are surgery within 12 weeks, immobilization (complete bedrest) for 3 or more days in the 4 weeks before presentation, previous deep venous thrombosis or objectively diagnosed pulmonary embolism, fracture of a lower extremity and immobilization of the fracture within 12 weeks, strong family history of deep venous thrombosis or pulmonary embolism (two or more family members with objectively proven events or a first-degree relative with hereditary thrombophilia), cancer (treatment ongoing, within the past 6 months, or in the palliative stages), the postpartum period, and lower-extremity paralysis. (Modified from Wells 1998)

Table 4.1. Expected utilities (outcomes)

Patients without pulmonary embolism		Patients with pulmonary embolism	
Management strategy	Expected utility	Management strategy	Expected utility
No therapy; no pulmonary angiogram	1.00	Therapy	0.84
Pulmonary angiogram; no therapy	0.98	Pulmonary angiogram, therapy	0.82
Therapy	0.92	No therapy	0.70

essarily exposed to the risk of anticoagulation. The next best outcome is that they are exposed to the morbidity of having a pulmonary arteriogram to prove that they do not have pulmonary embolism and they thus avoid the risk of anticoagulation. The worst outcome for patients without pulmonary embolism is that they are needlessly anticoagulated. Typically, the best outcome is given a value of 1. Less good outcomes are given values less than 1, and these values should be directly related to the loss of health. Although exact quantification is difficult, it is easy to agree about the hierarchy of outcomes. Clearly, not receiving anticoagulation if it is unnecessary is the best outcome. Traditionally, the risk of pulmonary arteriography is viewed as being less than the risk of anticoagulation; therefore, pulmonary arteriography is often done in order to prove that the patient does not have pulmonary embolism.

For patients who have pulmonary embolism, there are also three major outcomes. The outcome with the highest utility would be patients who are treated with anticoagulants but who do not get subjected to the morbidity of pulmonary arteriography. The second best outcome is to require a pulmonary arteriography in order to accurately make the diagnosis of pulmonary embolism, and thus, be anticoagulated. The worst outcome is to have untreated pulmonary embolism. Again, these three outcomes have a natural hierarchy even though their exact values may be questioned. Another important thing to note is that the best outcome for patients with pulmonary embolism has to be worse than the worst outcome for patients without pulmonary embolism, because patients with pulmonary embolism are not only subjected to the risk of anticoagulation, but they have the additional risk of treated thromboembolic disease.

If these six outcomes in patients with pulmonary embolism are plotted on a graph of utilities and prevalence of pulmonary embolism (Fig. 4.3), the three utilities in patients without the pulmonary embolism are plotted on the y-axis where the prevalence is 0% and the three utilities for patients with pulmonary embolism can be plotted on the y-axis where the prevalence of pulmonary embolism equals 100%. Mathematically, it can be shown that the expected utility for the three major patient management options (treatment, no treatment, and pulmonary arteriography) fall on a line connecting the points that represent each of these management strategies.

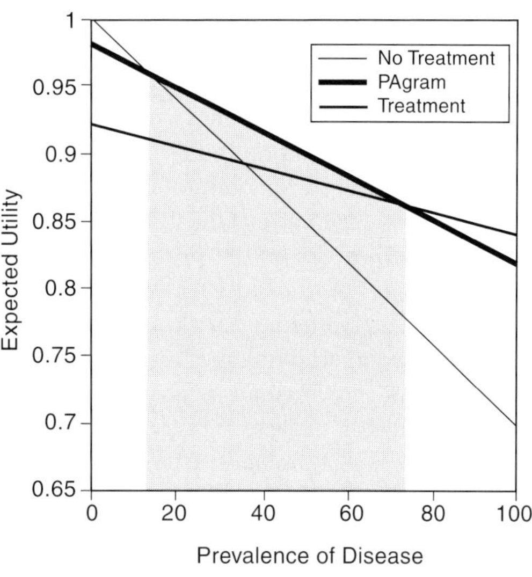

Fig. 4.3. The traditional expected utilities of three different management strategies for patients suspected of pulmonary embolism are plotted as a function of the prevalence of disease. The *shaded area* shows that the greatest expected utility can be obtained by performing a pulmonary arteriogram in patients who have a prevalence of disease ranging between 15 and 75%. Note that at the extremes of this range, there is very little difference in the expected utility of the alternative management strategy

When the traditional values for the six outcomes discussed previously are used, it is apparent that the expected utility from performing a pulmonary arteriogram is higher than the expected utility for the other two management strategies when the prevalence of pulmonary embolism in the population ranges from approximately 15–75% (shaded area under the curve in Fig. 4.3). Hence, the often quoted statement that if the result of a pulmonary ventilation-perfusion study is intermediate, the patient management option with the greatest utility is to perform pulmonary arteriography; if the prevalence of pulmonary embolism is greater than approximately 75%, the best strategy is to treat the patient, and if the prevalence is less than approximately 15%, the best strategy is to not treat the patient.

In clinical practice there is an apparent discordance between what the foregoing utility analysis would indicate (obtain a pulmonary arteriogram when the prevalence of disease is between 15 and 75%) and what actually happens. In our institution, only approximately 14% of patients with an intermediate likelihood ratio result on their ventilation-perfusion study are referred for pulmonary arteriography. There are two explanations for this discordance. The first explanation is that the prevalence of pulmonary embolism (or the post-test probability of disease) is not determined from the results of the ventilation-perfusion study alone. In fact, the likelihood ratio for an intermediate probability ventilation-perfusion study is close to 1; therefore, as shown in Fig. 4.3, the post-test probability will be very similar to the pre-test probability. The average prevalence of pulmonary embolism in patients referred for pulmonary embolism in our hospital is approximately 15%, so not treating the patient and not obtaining a pulmonary arteriogram in patients with an intermediate likelihood ratio result is not inconsistent with optimizing the expected utility as shown in Fig. 4.3. With a prevalence of 15%, the expected utility of not treating the patient and of obtaining a pulmonary arteriogram is similar. Maybe this helps explain why it often seems that the decision to obtain a pulmonary arteriogram in patients with intermediate likelihood ratio results on their ventilation-perfusion study is based on the flip of a coin.

Unfortunately, current interpretation criteria for ventilation-perfusion imaging blur the distinction between the test result and post-test probability of disease (which necessarily includes an assessment of the pre-test probability). To make a management recommendation based solely on the test results without accounting for pre-test probability is wrong. At our institution, we have tried to emphasize the importance of incorporating the pre-test probability with the test results in order to calculate the post-test probability by reporting the ventilation-perfusion imaging results as likelihood ratios rather than probabilities which are easily confused with post-test probabilities.

A second, and equally important, reason why only a few patients with an intermediate probability for pulmonary embolism are referred to pulmonary arteriography is that the expected utilities for different management strategies may vary greatly with individual patients. For example, it is likely that an otherwise healthy patient who has a removable risk factor for thromboembolic disease (surgery) who is now ambulating and has a negative lower-extremity compression ultrasound is at low risk for recurrent thromboembolic disease, even if they are untreated. The expected utilities for such a patient are shown in Fig. 4.4. Note that no treatment and no pulmonary arteriogram would be indicated for any prevalence of pulmonary embolism. The only assumption that has changed is that the expected utility for treated and untreated pulmonary embolism is now 0.98 and 0.9, respectively. Expected utilities of 0.92 and 0.7 were used in Fig. 4.3. When the morbidity from recurrent thromboembolic disease is lower than the risk from anticoagulation, the preferred option is no treatment.

The most important point in the preceding decision is that the management of patients suspected of pulmonary embolism cannot be rationally determined based on the results of the ventilation-perfusion study alone. The risks of pulmonary arteriography, anticoagulation, and untreated pulmonary embolism for each patient must be considered, as well.

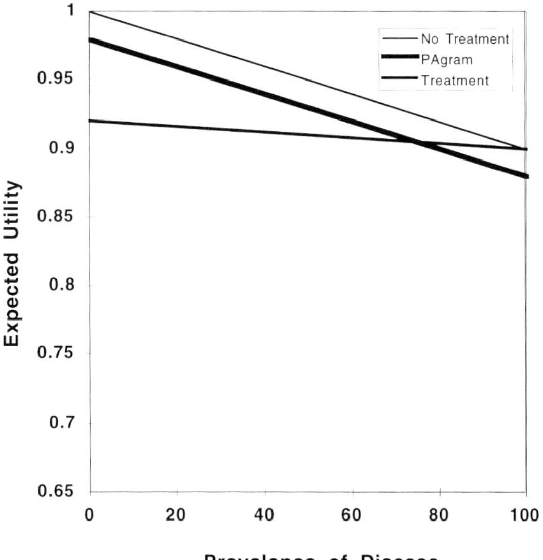

Fig. 4.4. Expected utilities of three different management strategies in patients suspected of pulmonary embolism who are at low risk for recurrent disease if untreated. If the risk of recurrent thromboembolic disease is less than the risk from treatment, the expected utility of no treatment is always greater than the expected utility of treatment

4.2.5
Patient Outcome

Patient outcome has become increasingly recognized as the most important factor in determining the best diagnostic and management strategy (EDDY 1990a,b). Utility analysis, as described previously, provides a mathematical model that can be used to predict patient outcome. An alternative approach is to directly measure patient outcome. One possible design for a patient outcome study for a diagnostic test is shown in Fig. 4.5. This study design is similar to the study design typically used to measure the effects of a therapeutic intervention. Key elements are that patients are randomized to have or not have the diagnostic test that is being evaluated and the study endpoints are outcomes that are important to patients and society rather than diagnostic accuracy (e.g., sensitivity, specificity). Outcomes of interest would include mortality, morbidity, and costs. Using this paradigm, diagnostic tests would only be recommended if they have some measurable effect on patient or societal outcomes. Patient outcome studies are more difficult to perform than simple diagnostic accuracy studies, but they provide far more valuable information.

Diagnostic strategies that do not include pulmonary arteriography have been shown to accurately identify patients who are at low risk for recurrent thromboembolic disease when they are not treated (WELLS et al. 1998; PERRIER et al. 1999). In a well-designed study, WELLS et al. (1998) showed that the occurrence of recurrent thromboembolic disease in a large portion of patients who were evaluated using only clinical history and non-invasive studies was as low as the recurrent thromboembolic rate in populations who had negative pulmonary arteriograms. Several older studies have also shown that ventilation-perfusion studies can be used to identify groups of patients with low incidence of recurrent thromboembolic disease, even when anticoagulation is not given (LEE et al. 1985; SMITH et al. 1987; KAHN et al. 1989; HULL et al. 1990; JACOBSON et al. 1997). In the future, it will be difficult to justify recommendations for more invasive, more costly diagnostic and managing strategies if a change in patient outcomes cannot be documented.

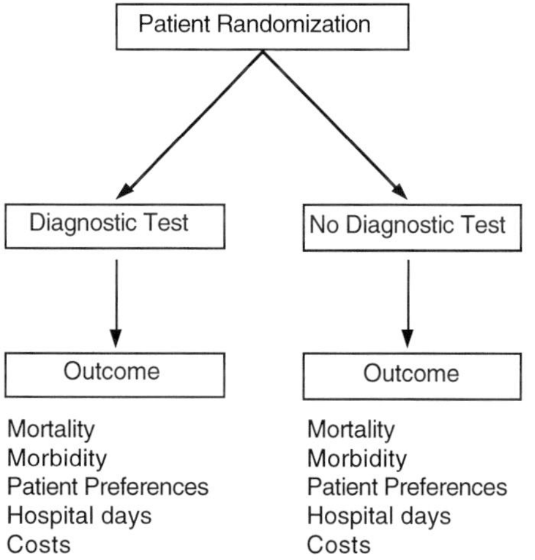

Fig. 4.5. Study design to determine the impact of a diagnostic test on patient outcome. The most reliable way to determine if a diagnostic test uniquely contributes to improved patient outcome is to randomize eligible patients to have or not have the diagnostic test. Justifying the use of diagnostic tests that have no measurable effects on patient outcomes will become increasing difficult as health care resources become more limited

4.3
Ventilation-Perfusion Imaging

4.3.1
Technical Issues

Several radiopharmaceuticals are available to study regional ventilation. In the United States, ^{99m}Tc-aerosols and ^{133}Xe-xenon ventilation studies are most common because of the unavailability of pertechnegas and the cost of ^{81m}Kr-krypton. Despite their differences, all of these agents are suitable for studying regional ventilation.

Currently, it is common practice to perform both a ventilation and perfusion study on patients suspected of pulmonary embolism. The motivation for performing a dual study is partly due to the fact that the technical quality of a ventilation study performed with the xenon or a technetium-labeled agent ventilation study is better when performed prior to the injection of ^{99m}Tc-macro-aggregated-albumen (MAA).

When the ventilation study is performed first, it has to be performed in all patients since patients cannot be selected based on the results of their perfusion study. If the ventilation study were performed after the perfusion study, the ventilation study could probably be avoided in one half to two thirds of patients who do not have any significant discrete perfusion abnormalities. Avoiding unnecessary ventilation studies may have a higher priority in managed care system than in a fee-for-service system. Performing the ventilation study after the perfusion study in selected patients has several advantages including: (a) avoiding unnecessary ventilation studies; and (b) being able to perform the ventilation study in the view in which the perfusion abnormality is best seen. The disadvantages of performing the ventilation study after the perfusion study include: (a) a technically less satisfactory study due to downscatter (or crosstalk) from ^{99m}Tc; and (b) each perfusion study takes longer because a smaller dose of ^{99m}Tc-MAA should be used. Whatever technique is used, our technical ability to detect perfusion abnormalities is better than our ability to detect ventilatory abnormalities; therefore, technical mismatches (positive perfusion with apparently negative ventilation defects) can occur.

Imaging technology has improved significantly since the mid-1970s. SPECT imaging of perfusion and ventilation is now possible. These technical advances, however, do not solve inherent problems of ventilation-perfusion imaging. Firstly, diseases other than pulmonary embolism sometimes present with ventilation-perfusion mismatches and pulmonary embolism can sometimes cause ventilation-perfusion matches. Secondly, ventilation-perfusion imaging can only reliably detect acute pulmonary embolism. Emboli may resolve quickly, especially in younger patients without pre-existing cardiopulmonary disease. Older, partially lysed emboli that are adherent to the vessel wall may not decrease regional pulmonary perfusion and therefore may not be detectable with perfusion imaging. In contrast, these older, partially lysed emboli may still cause intraluminal filling defects demonstrable with pulmonary arteriography or spiral CT. Given the apparently good outcome in a patient with a low likelihood ratio result on a ventilation-perfusion study, the clinical significance of partially lysed emboli that do not cause a perfusion abnormality can be questioned. Thirdly, ventilation perfusion imaging can only provide information about what has already happened in the lungs. The patient's ultimate prognosis will depend on the occurrence of future emboli. Evaluating venous structures that are likely sources of emboli can only accurately assess the risk for future emboli.

4.3.2 Interpretation Criteria

The interpretation criteria for ventilation-perfusion scintigraphy have been codified by numerous groups (Table 4.2; Kwok et al. 1996). These interpretation criteria provide a useful framework for inexperienced physicians to use and to learn how to interpret ventilation-perfusion studies. By necessity, the interpretation criteria are overly simplistic and cannot replace the judgment of an experienced physician. Experience is important because of the ambiguity and simplicity of the interpretation criteria. For example, the interpretation criteria only allow for a binary (matched or mismatched) classification of ventilation and perfusion defects. In practice, degree to which a perfusion defect has an associated ventilatory abnormality varies on a continuum. Deciding when to consider a perfusion defect as matched or mismatched requires some judgment. The significance of a perfusion abnormality is also affected by additional characteristics such as how well the abnormality conforms to the segmental anatomy of the lung, how distinct the borders of the abnormality are, and the severity of the perfusion abnormality. The patient's presentation and the time that has elapsed since the event that raised the suspicion of pulmonary embolism need to be considered. If a ventilation-perfusion study is obtained within hours of a patient having syncope, it is unlikely that one or two moderate-size perfusion defects could account for the patient's presentation. On the other hand, if the syncopal episode was days ago, these same findings would need to be interpreted more cautiously since considerable lysis of the patient's emboli may have occurred. None of these nuances are incorporated into the simple interpretation criteria as shown in Table 4.2.

4.3.2.1 PIOPED

Ventilation-perfusion imaging was the subject of a rigorous prospective multicenter study known as the PIOPED (Prospective Investigation of Pulmonary Embolic Disease) study (PIOPED Investigators 1990). The motivation for this study came from concerns that prior retrospective single institution studies comparing the results of ventilation-perfusion imaging with pulmonary arteriography were biased because only a small subset of patients who had ventilation-perfusion imaging were referred for pulmonary arteriography. In the major arm of the PIOPED study, all patients with any perfusion abnormality on ventilation-perfusion imaging were required to have a pulmonary arteriogram. This requirement for pulmonary arteriography undoubtedly resulted in some selection bias since clinicians presumably would only allow their patients to enroll in a study in which a high percentage would have a mandatory pulmonary arteriogram if they had a relatively high suspicion for pulmonary embolism. This supposition is supported by the fact that the preva-

Table 4.2. V/Q criteria for categorizing probability of pulmonary embolism. (From Kwok 1996). *V*, ventilation; *Q*, perfusion; *CXR*, chest radiograph; *OPD*, obstructive pulmonary disease; <<, substantially smaller than; >>, substantially larger than; *non-segmental Q defect* means very small effusion, cardiomegaly, enlarged aorta, hila, or mediastinum, elevated diaphragm

Probability	Sullivan (based on McNeil 1976)	Biello et al. (1979)	PIOPED (1990)	Revised PIOPED
Normal	No Q defects	No Q defects	No Q defects Q outlines exactly the shape of the lungs on CXR	Same as PIOPED
Very low			≤3 small Q defects with normal CXR	
Low	Multiple V/Q matches Single subsegmental V/Q mismatch	Small V/Q mismatches V/Q matches without corresponding CXR changes Q defect<<CXR density	Nonsegmental Q defect 1 moderate V/Q mismatch, with normal CXR Q defect<<CXR density Large or moderate V/Q matches, involving ≤4 segments in 1 lung and ≤3 segments in 1 lung region with normal CXR or CXR findings<<Q defects >3 small Q defects with normal CXR	Non-segmental Q defect Any Q defect<<CXR abnormality V/Q matches provided that the CXR is normal and perfusion in some areas of the lungs is normal[a] Any number of small Q defects with a normal CXR
Intermediate	Q defect with matched density on CXR Mixed V/Q mismatches and matches Single segment, lobe or lung V/Q mismatch Multiple subsegmental V/Q mismatches	Severe diffuse OPD with Q defects Single medium or large V/Q mismatch Q defect same size as CXR change	Anything not falling into normal, very low, low, or high-probability categories Borderline high or borderline low Difficult to categorize as low or high	1 moderate to 2 large V/Q mismatches or the arithmetic equivalent in moderate or large and moderate defects[b] Single V/Q match and normal CXR Difficult to categorize as low or high, or not described as low or high
High	Multiple segmental or larger V/Q mismatches	≥2 medium or large V/Q mismatches Q defect>>CXR density	≥2 large V/Q mismatches, with normal CXR or findings<<Q defects ≥2 moderate V/Q mismatches and 1 large V/Q mismatch without CXR findings ≥4 moderate V/Q mismatches without CXR findings	≥2 large V/Q mismatches or the arithmetic equivalent in moderate or large and moderate defects[b]

Biello criteria: *small*, <25% of a segment; *medium*, 25–90% of a segment; *large*, >90% of a segment
PIOPED criteria: *small*, <25% of a segment; *moderate*, 25–75% of a segment; *large*, >75% of a segment

[a] Very extensive defects can be categorized as low probability. Single V/Q matches are borderline for low probability and thus should be categorized as intermediate in most circumstances by most readers, although individual readers may correctly interpret individual scans with this pattern as showing low probability

[b] Two large V/Q mismatches are borderline for high probability. Individual readers may correctly interpret individual scans with this pattern as showing high probability for pulmonary embolism. In general, it is recommended that more than this degree of mismatch be present for inclusion in the high-probability category

lence of pulmonary embolism in the PIOPED study is high (33%).

This study had a few strengths and several major weaknesses. One of its greatest strengths was that it clearly showed that clinicians can assess pre-test probability. For the same ventilation perfusion imaging result, the post-test probability of pulmonary embolism changed as expected when the clinician's assessment of pre-test probability was considered (Fig. 4.1). Another strength of the PIOPED study is that information about observer variability for both ventilation-perfusion imaging and pulmonary arteriography was obtained (Table 4.3). Ordinarily, we think of the results of pulmonary arteriography as being positive or negative. In the PIOPED study, the interpretation of the pulmonary arteriogram was read as positive, negative, or uncertain in 33, 64, and 3% of patients, respectively. Technically unsatisfactory pulmonary arteriograms that were uninterpretable occurred in 5% of patients. Blinded independent observers agreed that the pulmonary arteriogram was positive, negative, or uncertain 92, 83, and 89% of the time, respectively. The fact that there is considerable observer variability in the reading of pulmonary arteriograms is often overlooked. It is unrealistic to expect that a completely independent test for pulmonary embolism (ventilation-perfusion imaging) would agree with the reading of the pulmonary arteriogram better than two blinded readings of the same pulmonary arteriogram would agree. Given that 17% of negative pulmonary arteriograms will be read as positive by one of two blinded readers, it is remarkable that low likelihood ratio results on ventilation-perfusion imaging agree with negative pulmonary arteriography 85–90% of the time.

Table 4.3. Observer agreement: PIOPED Investigators (1990)

Ventilation-perfusion study		Pulmonary arteriogram	
High	95%	Present	92%
Intermediate	75%	Absent	83%
Low	70%	Uncertain	89%
Very low	92%		
Normal	94%		

There are several major flaws with PIOPED. Firstly, the endpoint was diagnostic accuracy (How often does ventilation-perfusion imaging agree with the pulmonary arteriogram?) rather than patient outcome. A much more valuable study would have been to randomize patients with low and/or intermediate likelihood ratio results on their ventilation-perfusion study to have or not have a pulmonary arteriogram. Would there have been any measurable difference in outcome between the patients with and without a pulmonary arteriogram? The costs and patient discomfort would be more in the pulmonary arteriogram group. What would have been the offsetting benefits? Would fewer or more patients be anticoagulated? Would there be a change in mortality or morbidity?

Secondly, PIOPED perpetuated the use of discrete categories for the interpretation of ventilation-perfusion studies, when in fact the results of any complex imaging test are better represented as a continuum and should be reported as likelihood ratios (Jaeschke et al. 1994a,b). Use of discrete categorizations also distorts any analysis of observer variability. For example, as shown in Fig. 4.6, the results of any complex imaging test naturally falls on a continuum from definitely normal to definitely abnormal. When this continuum is broken up into discrete segments such as normal, low, intermediate, and high likelihood ratio results, this artificially creates some apparent observer disagreement. As shown in Fig. 4.6, using a continuous scale, readers A and B disagree more on

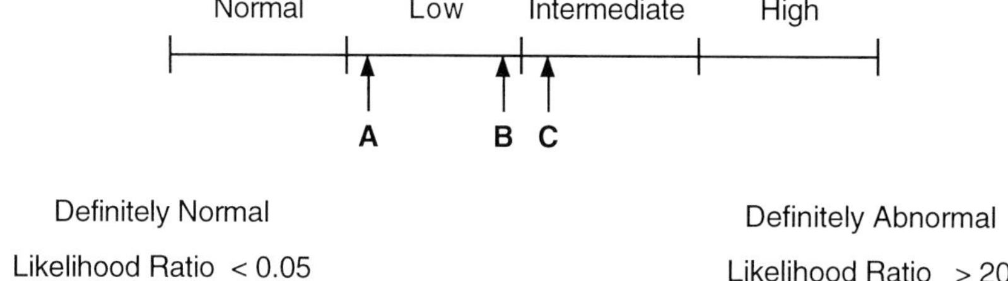

Fig. 4.6. Continuous vs discrete results. Forcing readers to use a discrete scale, rather than a continuous scale, often distorts studies of observer agreement. The results of observers B and C would be classified as disagreements when a discrete scale is used, even though they are more in agreement than are observers A and B

the interpretation of the study, but since both readers A and B's interpretations fall within the category of low they are said to agree. In contrast, readers B and C are closer together on the continuous scale, yet when forced to put their results into these discrete categories, they appear to disagree. The creation of discrete category introduces the problem of exactly how to identify the line dividing each of the categories on the continuous scale. For example, the dividing line between normal and low is difficult to define unambiguously. Discrete categories can also frustrate readers since they may have to agonize about which side of the artificial line they must choose to categorize the result. Allowing readers to give an approximate likelihood ratio for the results of ventilation imaging studies would (a) help identify true observer variability, (b) decrease the artificial mental anguish induced by an arbitrary discrete scale, and (c) more clearly convey the results of the test.

A third major problem with PIOPED is that it has continued to confuse the test result with the post-test probability of disease. As previously shown in Fig. 4.1, the clinical history and other information must be combined with the test result in order to come up with a true post-test probability. Failure to distinguish the test result from post-test probability has resulted in enormous confusion in the literature where management recommendations are based on test results that are mistakenly interpreted as post-test probabilities. For example, in Fig. 4.1, note that the post-test probability for pulmonary embolism was less for a patient with a high result and a low pre-test probability (56%) than it was for a patient with an intermediate result and a high pre-test probability (66%). Likewise, the post-test probability for a patient with an intermediate result and a low pre-test probability (16%) was the same as for a patient with a low result and an intermediate pre-test probability (16%).

Another major shortcoming of the current interpretation criteria is that no distinction is made between intermediate likelihood ratio results for mild, moderate, or massive pulmonary embolism. More risk stratification information is available from ventilation-perfusion imaging than is conveyed by the simple categories of normal, low, intermediate, and high.

Finally, the PIOPED INVESTIGATORS (1990) reported the results of their study using sensitivity and specificity (Table 4.4). These measures are only appropriate if the simple binary test results are obtained. It is virtually impossible to interpret the results of complex imaging results that have multiple outcomes when they are presented in this way. A much better way to present the results is as likelihood ratios (Table 4.5). As explained in the Appendix, the likelihood ratio is calculated by dividing the P(T-|D+) by P(T-|D-). The likelihood ratios listed in Table 4.5 provide much more useful information (JAESCHKE et al. 1994a,b) than the sensitivities and specificities that were provided by the PIOPED INVESTIGATORS and that are listed in Table 4.4. A high likelihood ratio result increases the pre-test odds of disease by a factor of almost 14. An intermediate likelihood ratio result does not change the pre-test odds of disease; therefore, if the pre-test odds were low before performing ventilation-perfusion imaging, they remain low after imaging. Low likelihood ratio results and near-normal/normal results decrease the pre-test odds by a factor of 0.37 and 0.19, respectively. These last two likelihood ratios are not as low as desirable, but it must be remembered that the observer agreement for a negative pulmonary arteriogram was only 83% (Table 4.3). That means that 17% of the time, the sec-

Table 4.4. PIOPED results

Scan category	Sensitivity (%)	Specificity (%)
High	41	97
High or intermediate	82	52
High, intermediate, or low	98	10

Table 4.5. PIOPED results. *PE* pulmonary embolism; $P(T_n|D+)$ probability of the nth test result with presence of disease; LR_n likelihood ratio of the nth test result

Scan category	PE+	PE–	$P(T_n\|D+)$	$P(T_n\|D-)$	LR_n
High	102	14	0.4064	0.0292	13.93
Intermediate	105	217	0.4183	0.4521	0.93
Low	39	199	0.1554	0.4146	0.37
Near normal/normal	5	50	0.0199	0.1042	0.19
Total	251	480			

ond observer reads the pulmonary arteriogram as (falsely) positive. This observer variability with negative pulmonary arteriograms partly explains the less than desirable likelihood ratios for low and near-normal/normal results. When clinical follow-up is used to classify the disease status of patients, the values for the likelihood ratios for low and near-normal/normal results are much lower.

4.4 Other Diagnostic Tests

The diagnosis and management of patients suspected of pulmonary embolism requires information from several sources. The clinical evaluation of the patient and the role of ventilation-perfusion imaging have already been discussed. This section describes the other diagnostic tests. The chest radiograph has long been used in conjunction with ventilation-perfusion imaging. Likewise, pulmonary arteriography has long been regarded as the reference standard for diagnosis of pulmonary embolism. Three newer diagnostic tests that are available to evaluate patients include serum D-dimer levels, compression ultrasound of the lower extremities, and spiral CT of the pulmonary arteries.

4.4.1 Chest Radiograph

The chest radiograph is routinely obtained in all patients suspected of pulmonary embolism. Because the findings on the chest radiograph are non-specific for pulmonary embolism (Worsley et al. 1993; Stein et al. 1991), the chest radiograph is useful mainly for discovering other causes for the patient's signs and symptoms such as pneumonia, pneumothorax, congestive heart failure, and pleural effusions.

The non-specificity of radiographic abnormalities is illustrated in Table 4.6 (Elgazzar 1997). The likelihood ratio for most findings is close to 1; therefore, the chest radiograph findings do not increase or decrease the pre-test odds for pulmonary embolism, except for the presence of Westermark's sign (likelihood ratio: 4) and pulmonary edema (likelihood ratio: 0.3).

There is almost universal agreement that a chest radiograph is needed to interpret ventilation-perfusion studies, although one group of investigators recently reported that the availability of the chest radiograph did not affect their interpretations of ventilation-perfusion studies (Denton et al. 1998). These investigators acknowledged that their inability to demonstrate the need for a chest radiograph was likely due to the fact that few of their patients had abnormalities on their chest radiograph. Occasionally, with a low or near-normal ventilation-perfusion study, one is tempted not to obtain a chest radiograph since the chest radiograph is very unlikely to change the interpretation of the ventilation-perfusion study. Not obtaining a chest radiograph under these circumstances is a mistake, because alternative explanations for the patient's symptoms may be apparent on the chest radiograph.

Another issue that always arises is how close in time the chest radiograph needs to be to the ventilation-perfusion studies. There is a common, simple, less accurate answer and an uncommon, complicated, longer, more accurate answer. The simple answer is the chest radiograph should be obtained within 24 h of the ventilation-perfusion study. The complicated answer is that it depends on the clinical circumstances. If a patient has acute onset of shortness of breath 1 h prior and the most recent chest radiograph was 2 h prior, a repeat chest radiograph should be obtained. The rationale for this recommendation is that there are acute processes such as small pneumothoraces that can be seen on a chest radiograph that may not be detected by ventilation-perfusion imaging. On the other hand, if a patient with no intervening pulmonary symptoms has a near-normal chest radiograph that is 48–72 h old, and if the results of the ventilation-perfusion imaging are normal or low likelihood ratio, no repeat chest radiograph is needed. If there are unexpected findings on the ventilation-perfusion study, the chest radiograph should be repeated.

Table 4.6. Chest radiograph findings in suspected pulmonary embolism

Finding	$P(T_n\|D+)$	$P(T_n\|D-)$	LR_n
Atelectasis	0.71	0.46	1.54
Pleural effusion	0.54	0.37	1.46
Pleural-based opacity	0.35	0.21	1.67
Elevated hemidiaphragm	0.30	0.23	1.30
Oligemia	0.21	0.12	1.75
Prominent pulmonary artery	0.26	0.23	1.13
Cardiomegaly	0.14	0.13	1.08
Pulmonary edema	0.04	0.13	0.31
Westermark's sign[a]	0.13	0.03	4.33

[a] Prominent pulmonary artery and decreased pulmonary vascularity

Our current interpretation criteria are vague about how to use the results of chest radiographs. All chest radiograph abnormalities are lumped together in the generic term "chest radiograph abnormality." There are conflicting reports about how to interpret ventilation-perfusion studies in patients with pleural effusions (Bedont and Datz 1985; Goldberg et al. 1996). In truth, different radiographic abnormalities should likely affect our interpretation of ventilation-perfusion imaging differently. Chronic radiographic abnormalities must have a different meaning than acute abnormalities since chronic abnormalities cannot explain a patients acute symptoms. Finally, should chest radiographic abnormalities that are clearly caused by a disease process other than pulmonary embolism (e.g., pneumonia, cancer) be interpreted as an intermediate likelihood ratio for pulmonary embolism simply because they cause a triple match?

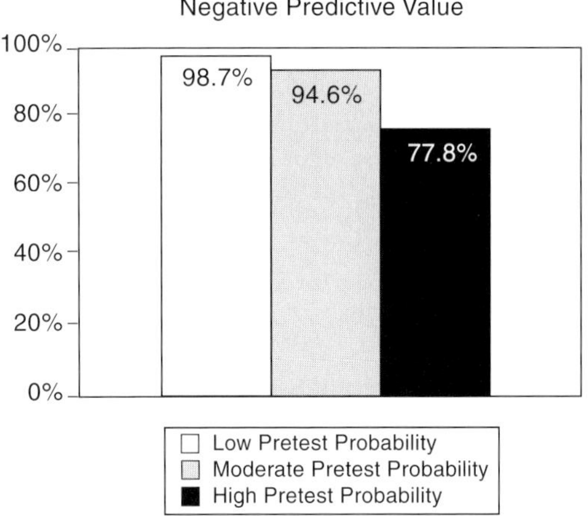

Fig. 4.7. Negative predictive value for patients with a low or intermediate result on the ventilation-perfusion study and a negative serum D-dimer test. The negative predictive value is acceptably low with a low or intermediate probability for recurrent thromboembolic disease, a negative serum D-dimer, and a low or moderate pre-test probability (Ginsberg 1998)

4.4.2 D-dimer

A rapid assay for testing of whole-blood D-dimer is now available. D-dimer is a fibrin degradation product that is highly sensitive for the detection of thromboembolic disease; however, it is non-specific since it also can be elevated in patients with a variety of other diseases including myocardial infarction, pneumonia, heart failure, cancer, and recent surgery (Goldhaber 1998). An elevated D-dimer level is not helpful in making the diagnosis of pulmonary embolism; however, a normal D-dimer level is helpful in excluding the diagnosis.

In one large study (Ginsberg et al. 1998), the combination of a non-diagnostic lung scan (low or intermediate likelihood ratio) and a normal D-dimer test result had a negative predictive value of 97.2%. Sixty-two percent of all patients with non-diagnostic lung scan results (i.e., intermediate probability for pulmonary embolism) had normal D-dimer test results; therefore, pulmonary embolism could be excluded in a large percentage of patients with the addition of this simple test. When the authors also included the pre-test probability of the disease, the negative predictive value of a non-diagnostic lung scan and a normal D-dimer test were 98.7, 94.6, and 77.8% in patients with low, moderate, and high pre-test probabilities, respectively (Fig. 4.7). The authors concluded that in low and intermediate pre-test probability patients a non-diagnostic lung scan and normal D-dimer test results had a high enough negative predictive value to exclude clinically significant pulmonary embolism.

4.4.3 Detection of Deep Venous Thrombosis

Several non-invasive tests have been recommended for detecting deep venous thrombosis. Impedance plethysmography, a test that measures reserve venous capacity in the rapidity of outflow from the deep venous system of the lower extremities, has largely been replaced by the use of compression ultrasound. Compression ultrasound involves a meticulous examination of the major deep venous structures of the lower extremities. Thrombosis is identified by the inability to compress the vein. Compression ultrasound has numerous limitations including the fact that it is very operator dependent, it can only reliably detect thrombosis in the thigh and knee, and there is considerable difficulty in differentiating new from old thrombi. Because of the difficulty in assessing thrombosis below the knee, serial compression ultrasound has been recommended in order to improve the sensitivity of this technique in detecting clinically significant disease (Kearon et al. 1998a,b). When serial ultrasound is negative the risk for recurrent thromboembolic disease in patients with a low or intermediate result on the ventilation-perfusion study was <2% during a 6-month follow-up period. Doppler ultrasound that looks at venous flow patterns in the vein is less reliable in detecting deep venous thrombosis.

4.4.4 Pulmonary Arteriogram

Pulmonary arteriography is regarded as the reference standard for the diagnosis of pulmonary embolism. Its limitations are rarely emphasized. In the PIOPED study (STEIN et al. 1992), there were 5 deaths among the 1111 patients who had had a pulmonary arteriogram. In addition, there were 9 major non-fatal complications that included respiratory distress, renal failure, and bleeding requiring transfusions. There were minor complications in an additional 60 patients.

As discussed previously, observer agreement for a complex imaging test, such as pulmonary arteriography, is less than perfect. Observer agreement depends on the quality of the pulmonary arteriogram. In the PIOPED study, 691 of the 1099 pulmonary arteriograms were rated as good quality, 355 were rated as fair quality, and 46 were rated as poor quality. Observer agreements on positivity were 93, 90, and 98% for good-, fair-, and poor-quality arteriograms, respectively. Agreement on negativity was less good. There was 88% agreement for good-quality arteriograms, 77% agreement for fair quality, and 54% for poor-quality arteriograms.

It is important to recognize that the phenomenon demonstrated by pulmonary arteriography is very different from the pathology that is detected by regional perfusion studies. The detection task for pulmonary arteriography is to identify an intraluminal filling defect. The detection task becomes more and more difficult as the vessel size gets smaller and there are more and more vessels. Observer agreement clearly decreases as vessel size gets smaller.

The ability of pulmonary arteriography to distinguish acute from chronic emboli is not well documented since there is no independent reference standard. It is likely that acute emboli cause complete occlusion of a vessel since a soft, freely mobile embolus is likely to completely obstruct the vessel. Once the embolus becomes adherent to the vessel wall and once some thrombolysis has occurred, tracking of contrast can be seen around the embolus. This finding is regarded as being the most reliable finding for acute pulmonary embolism. It remains to be seen whether or not the presence of intraluminal filling defects on pulmonary arteriography or the presence of regional perfusion abnormalities on a perfusion study have greater prognostic significance. Interestingly, the best validation for pulmonary arteriography has been follow-up of patients who have had negative pulmonary arteriograms and who have not been anticoagulated (NOVELLINE et al. 1978). In this retrospective analysis, 180 patients with suspected pulmonary embolus and negative arteriograms were followed for a minimum of 6 months. Of the 167 patients who did not undergo therapy, none died as a result of thromboembolic disease. Twenty patients died of other causes. None of the 147 remaining patients suffered a recurrent embolus. This suggests that, indeed, the pulmonary emboli that are missed with pulmonary angiography are not of great health risk, and that a negative pulmonary arteriogram can be regarded as adequate information to not introduce therapy. It is somewhat surprising that such good prognostic information can be obtained solely from examining the pulmonary arteries.

4.4.5 Spiral-CT Angiography

Early anecdotal reports revealed that pulmonary emboli may be seen with contrast-enhanced computed tomography (BREATNACH and STANLEY 1984; CHINTAPALLI et al. 1988; GOODMAN et al. 1997). However, motion artifacts due to respiratory motion and sampling error prevented the use of CT as a primary diagnostic tool for pulmonary embolus. Technological advances manifested by spiral CT and electron-beam CT now enable the acquisition of a study in a single breath-hold. Subsegmental pulmonary emboli may be detected with this technology (GERAGHTY et al. 1992). Magnetic resonance angiography protocols utilizing gadolinium enhancement also have been developed to acquire images of the pulmonary vasculature in a single breath-hold, which can detect subsegmental pulmonary emboli (MEANEY et al. 1997).

Computed tomography is minimally invasive, an advantage over pulmonary angiography. Spiral CT provides a significant additional benefit of imaging the thorax, potentially facilitating a diagnosis to explain the patient's symptoms other than pulmonary embolus. Numerous early studies have suggested that spiral CT is more "accurate" than ventilation-perfusion scintigraphy in diagnosing pulmonary embolism. These early studies should be interpreted with caution since they involve a small number of selected patients. Technically inadequate studies and patients in whom the exam could not be performed are commonly excluded from the result tabulations.

One prospective study (MAYO et al. 1997) evaluated spiral-CT angiography and ventilation-perfusion scintigraphy in 139 patients. Final diagnosis was established by concordant interpretation of the spiral CT and ventilation-perfusion studies. If the ventilation-perfusion scintigraphy was interpreted as low or very-low probability for pulmonary embolism and the CT was negative and the clinical suspicion was high, a pulmonary arteriogram was performed. If the ventilation-perfusion scintigraphy or spiral-CT results were intermediate, or if they were discordant, a pulmonary arteriogram was performed. In negative cases a 3-month follow-up was undertaken via a phone call to the patient's physician. The results showed that spiral CT yielded a true-positive reading in 40 cases, false positive in 2 cases, true negative in 88 cases, false negative in 5 cases, and was indeterminate in 4 cases. Positive predictive value was therefore 95% and negative predictive value also 95%. By comparison, pulmonary embolus was present in 30 of 36 high-probability results on their ventilation-perfusion studies, 6 of 20 intermediate probability exams, 8 of 58 low probability exams, and 2 of 25 very low probability or normal exams. The positive predictive value of a high probability exam was therefore 83% and the negative predictive value of a normal, low- or very low-probability exam was 88%.

There are several limitations to the use of spiral-CT angiography. Relative contraindications to spiral CT include marginal renal function, history of contrast reaction, hemodynamic instability and severe dyspnea. In one study (GARG et al. 1998), 4.9% of patients were excluded from spiral CT for such reasons. An additional 13% had suboptimal studies and were excluded from calculations of sensitivity, specificity, and predictive values. It is estimated that approximately 5–10% of spiral-CT studies are technically inadequate (KUZO and GOODMAN 1997; GOODMAN et al. 1997).

Some vessels are not well seen or could not be visualized at all on spiral CT (REMY-JARDIN et al. 1992). These were predominantly vessels oriented obliquely in the right middle lobe and lingula. However, given the nature of pulmonary emboli (which tend to be multiple), this was not thought to be a major limitation. Current interpretation criteria for pulmonary embolus and potential pitfalls in the evaluation of spiral-CT exams have been described (BEIGELMAN et al. 1998). A good understanding of the vascular anatomy of the lung (e.g., arteries run with bronchi, whereas veins run independently) is necessary. Pitfalls include the external compression of arteries by lymph nodes, which may mimic a mural thrombus. Volume averaging may be confusing when vessels run obliquely. Perivascular edema may produce a collar of low attenuation simulating an embolus. Motion artifact is frequently a problem. Streak artifacts originating from the superior vena cava (SVC) due to high rate of injection into the SVC can mimic pulmonary embolism. Insufficient enhancement can occur due to delayed injection, SVC obstruction, shunts, increased pulmonary vascular resistance from consolidation, or large pleural effusion. The display-window setting can adversely affect interpretation.

4.5 Conclusion

The prevailing view is that pulmonary embolism is a monolithic disease. Diagnostic strategies are based on studies that have imperfect binary diagnostic endpoints. Since the dogma has been that all patients with pulmonary embolism need to be treated, there have been few attempts to overtly risk-stratify patients.

A great deal of the shortcomings of how we currently diagnose and manage patients with suspected pulmonary embolism are due to how we have evaluated diagnostic tests in the past. Diagnostic accuracy tests which compare the results of one imperfect diagnostic test (e.g., ventilation-perfusion imaging) to another imperfect test (e.g., pulmonary arteriography) are inevitably misleading. What is needed is patient outcome studies that determine which diagnostic strategies result in the best patient outcomes. One reason for accepting a negative pulmonary arteriogram as a strong indicator of a good prognosis is that there are a few patient outcome studies that show that the risk of recurrent thromboembolism is low in these patients, even when they are not anticoagulated. Similarly, other diagnostic strategies that use readily available non-invasive diagnostic tests have been shown to identify low-risk patients.

In order to be optimized, diagnostic and management strategies must account for information from a variety of sources. Management strategies that are based on the results of a single test (e.g., all patients with an intermediate likelihood ratio result on their ventilation should have a pulmonary arteriogram) are naive and doomed to failure. Rational decisions can only be made on the basis of the patient's post-test probability of disease (which means the test result must be combined with an estimate of the pre-test probability of disease), the risk of invasive diagnostic tests, and the risk of treatment and no treatment. The risk of no treatment likely depends on the clot burden in the lung, the potential for future emboli, and the overall medical condition of the patient. It is unclear whether the clot burden in the lung is best assessed by regional perfusion abnormalities detected by ventilation-perfusion imaging or by the presence of intraluminal filling defects detected by pulmonary arteriography or spiral-CT angiography. One could argue that the presence of regional perfusion abnormalities has more prognostic significance than the presence of intraluminal filling defects that have no effect on regional perfusion. In the former instance, the lung is overwhelmed by the embolic burden, whereas in the latter case, the lungs' own potent thrombolytic mechanisms are able to keep up with the embolic burden. The risk of future emboli cannot be assessed by any test that looks solely at the lungs.

4.6 Appendix: Medical Decision Making

A very basic need in medical decision making is a way to quantify the accuracy of diagnostic tests. The most common and simplest approach assumes that test outcomes and disease states are binary (positive or negative). A 2+2 table, in which the columns usually represent the disease states and the rows represent the test results (Table A4.1), is usually used to calculate several ratios (accuracy, sensitivity, specificity, predictive value of a positive test, predictive value of a negative test, likelihood of a positive test, and the likelihood ratio of a negative test) related to the accuracy of diagnostic tests (Table A4.1). These ratios can also be written more concisely in probability notation. When using probability notation, the vertical bar "|" is read as "given the condition that" so the notation P(T+|D+) is read as "the probability of having a positive test result given the condition that the patient has the disease."

In this simplified binary world, sensitivity and specificity are regarded as the best measures of test performance since, unlike accuracy and the predictive value of the test, these values are not effected by the prevalence of disease. Unfortunately, sensitivity and specificity have many other shortcomings including the fact that disease states and test outcomes are not binary and sensitivity or specificity can be artificially inflated or deflated depending on the threshold which is used to divide positive and negative disease states (Royal 1994).

Table A4.1. 2+2 Decision matrix

Test Results	Disease State D+	Disease State D−
T+	TP	FP
T−	FN	TN

T+ = Test Positive
T− = Test Negative
D+ = Diagnosis Positive
D− = Diagnosis Negative

TP = True Positive
FP = False Positive
TP = False Negative
TP = True Negative

Derived Ratios

$$\text{Accuracy} = \frac{TP + TN}{TP + TN + FP + FN}$$

$$\text{Sensitivity} = \frac{TP}{TP + FN}$$

$$\text{Specificity} = \frac{TN}{TN + FP}$$

$$\text{Predictive Value of a Positive Test} = \frac{TP}{TP + FP}$$

$$\text{Predictive Value of a Negative Test} = \frac{TN}{TN + FN}$$

$$\text{Likelihood Ratio of a Positive Test} = \frac{\text{Sensitivity}}{\text{1-Specificity}}$$

$$\text{Likelihood Ratio of a Negative Test} = \frac{\text{1-Sensitivity}}{\text{Specificity}}$$

Probability Notation

Sensitivity = $P(T+|D+)$
Specificity = $P(T-|D-)$
Predictive Value of a Positive Test = $P(D+|T+)$
Predictive Value of a Negative Test = $P(D-|T-)$
Likelihood Ratio for the nth Test Result = $\frac{P(T_n|D+)}{P(T_n|D-)}$

The effects of the choice of the threshold on sensitivity and specificity is illustrated in Fig. A4.1. The results of complex imaging tests do not naturally fit into the binary world of sensitivity and specificity. These results are more realistically viewed as a continuum that ranges from very normal results to very abnormal results. In order to capture the range of possible test results, they are typically categorized as definitely normal, probably normal, possibly abnormal, probably abnormal, and definitely abnormal, rather than simply as positive or negative. When test results are tabulated in this way, a family of sensitivi-

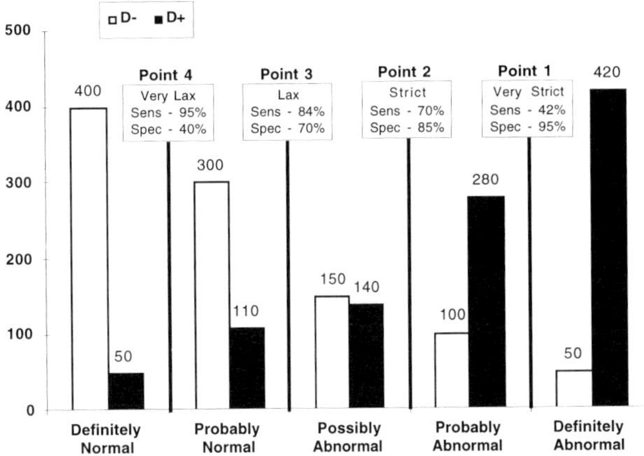

Fig. A4.1. A frequency histogram showing the distribution of test results that might be obtained in a diseased (*filled bar*) and a non-diseased (*open bar*) population. The number of subjects having each of the test results is shown *above the bars*. As would be expected, test results from the diseased population are more likely to be abnormal. In order to construct an ROC curve (see Fig. A4.2), a family of sensitivity and specificity pairs is generated by calculating the sensitivity and specificity for four possible thresholds (Points 1–4). For each threshold, all results to the left of the threshold are considered normal and all of the results to the right are considered abnormal

ty and specificity pairs can be generated depending on the threshold that is used to distinguish "positive" from "negative" test results. If a very strict threshold is used (Point 1 in Figs. 4.1 and 4.2), the test will have

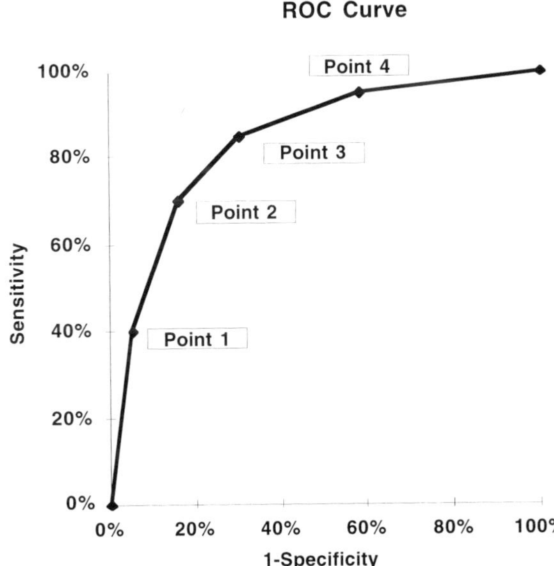

Fig. A4.2. The sensitivity/specificity pairs generated from Fig. A4.1 are plotted. Note that any sensitivity or specificity can be achieved by varying the threshold (Points 1–4); however, there is a trade-off between sensitivity and specificity

a low sensitivity (because the test result needs to be "definitely abnormal" in order to consider it a positive result) but a high specificity (since few non-diseased patients will have that test result). The family of sensitivity and specificity pairs can be plotted on a graph where the y-axis is sensitivity and the x-axis is 1-specificity (Fig. A4.2). This graph is called a receiver-operating-characteristics (ROC) curve.

More recently, likelihood ratios have gained in popularity. Likelihood ratios have several major advantages over sensitivity and specificity. Once their meaning is understood, this one value provides more meaningful information about the meaning of a particular test result than does sensitivity or specificity. In addition, their use is more appropriate with complex non-binary test outcomes such as the results of imaging tests. The general formula for the likelihood ratio is:

$$LR_n = \frac{P(T_n|D+)}{P(T_n|D+)}$$

where LR_n is the likelihood ratio of the nth test result, $P(T_n|D+)$ is the probability of getting the nth test result in patients with the disease, and $P(T_n|D-)$ is the probability of getting the nth test result in patients without the disease.

If the nth test result is more common in patients with the disease, the likelihood ratio will be greater than 1; if the nth test result is more common in patients without the disease, the likelihood ratio will be less than 1; if the nth test result occurs with the same frequency in patients with and without the disease, the likelihood ratio will be close to 1. Test results that are useful for ruling in a disease typically have likelihood ratios greater than 10; test results that are useful for ruling out the disease typically have likelihood ratios of less than 0.1. The likelihood ratio for the test results shown in Fig. A4.1 are listed in Table A4.2. Note how likelihood ratios better capture the mean-

Table A4.2. Likelihood ratios

Test result	D+	D−	$P(T_n\|D+)$	$P(T_n\|D-)$	LR_n
Definitely normal	50	400	0.05	0.40	0.125
Probably normal	110	300	0.11	0.30	0.367
Possibly abnormal	140	150	0.14	0.15	0.933
Probably abnormal	280	100	0.28	0.10	2.80
Definitely abnormal	420	50	0.42	0.05	8.40

ing of each individual test result. When a family of sensitivity and specificity pairs is generated as was done to construct the ROC curve, the test results in different categories are summed, so important information about the meaning of each test result is lost. As is shown below, another important advantage of likelihood ratios is that they simplify the calculation of the post-test probability of disease.

Measures of test performance, such as sensitivity and specificity, tell us how often a patient with the disease (or without the disease) will have positive (or negative) test results (P(T+|D+), P(T-|D-), respectively). This is not the clinically relevant question. The clinician wants to know how often a patient with a positive test result will have the disease, P(D+|T+), and how often the patient with a negative test result will not have the disease, P(D-|T-). In order to determine the predictive value of a positive or negative test, information about the prevalence of disease or pre-test probability, P(D+), in the population studied is needed. If the test result, the performance characteristics of the test, and the pre-test probability are known, the post-test probability can be calculated. There are three ways in which to make this calculation. These three ways are illustrated in the following example: the effects of pre-test probability on post-test probability for a range of likelihood ratios is shown in Table A4.3. Assume that the prevalence of disease is 10% and that the sensitivity of the test is 87% and the specificity 75%. The first way to calculate the post-test probability is to use an intuitive method (Table A4.3). Based on the prevalence of disease, the sums of the columns in a 2+2 matrix can be calculated (Table A4.3, Step 1). An arbitrary but large number is used to minimize round-off error. If the prevalence of disease is 10%, and if the arbitrary large number of studied patients is 1000, the sum of the disease-positive results would be 100 and the sum of the disease-negative results would be 900. Once the sums of the disease-positive and disease-negative columns are known, the values of the 2+2 matrix can be calculated. If the sensitivity of the test is 87%, 87 of the 100 patients with the disease will have a positive test result and 13 will have a negative test result (Table A4.3, Step 2). If the specificity is 75%, 730 of the 900 patients without disease will have a negative test result and 170 will have a positive test result (Step 3). Once the squares of the 2+2 matrix have been filled in, then the predictive value of a positive and negative test result can be calculated. If the test results are positive, 87 of the 210 patients who had positive test results will actually have the disease (Step 4). Likewise, 730 of the 750 patients with negative test results will not have the disease (Step 5).

A second method (Table A4.4) used to calculate the predictive value of a positive test and the predictive value of a negative test is to use Bayes' theorem. Bayes' theorem uses the same simple formula (true positives divided by true positives plus false positives) as the intuitive method described previously but the formula is rewritten using probability notation. The formula for Bayes' theorem appears to be more complicated than it really is. The advantage of Bayes' theorem is that the post-test probability of disease can be determined in one step.

Finally, the simplest way to calculate post-test probability is to use odds rather than probabilities

Table A4.3. Post-test probability: intuitive method

Assumptions
P(D+) = 0.1
P(T+|D+) = 0.87
P(T−|D−) = 0.75

Test Results	Disease State D+	Disease State D−	
	Step 2	Step 3	Step 4
T+	**87** (0.87×100)	**225** (900−675)	$P(D+\|T+) = \frac{87}{87+225} = 27.9\%$
			Step 5
T−	**13** (100−87)	**675** (0.75×900)	$P(D-\|T-) = \frac{675}{13+675} = 98.1\%$
Step 5 **Column Totals**	**100**	**900**	

Table A4.4. Post-test probability: Bayes theorem

Assumptions
P(D+) = 0.1
P(T+|D+) = 0.87
P(T−|D−) = 0.75

Predictive value of a positive test:

$$P(D+|T+) = \frac{TP}{TP + FP} = \frac{P(T+|D+) \times P(D+)}{P(T+|D+) \times P(D+) + P(T+|D- \times (1\text{-}P(D+))}$$

$$P(D+|T+) = \frac{87}{87 + 225} = \frac{0.87 \times 0.1}{0.87 \times 0.1 + 0.25 \times 0.9} = 27.9\%$$

Predictive value of a negative test:

$$P(D-|T-) = \frac{TN}{TN + FN} = \frac{P(T-|D-) \times P(D-)}{P(T-|D-) \times P(D-) + P(T-|D- \times (1\text{-}P(D-))}$$

$$P(D-|T-) = \frac{675}{675 + 13} = \frac{0.75 \times 0.9}{0.75 \times 0.9 + 0.13 \times 0.1} = 98.1\%$$

and to use the likelihood ratios (Table A4.5). The mathematical manipulations, which are necessary, are considerably simpler than those required for Bayes' theorem. Once familiar with likelihood ratios and odds, post-test probabilities can easily be calculated in one's head. The first step in this method is to convert the pre-test probability to pre-test odds. A 10% chance of having the disease is the same as one chance of having the disease and nine chances of not having the disease. Using odds notation this is written as 1:9. Using the likelihood ratio, the post-test odds of disease can be calculated simply by multiplying the chances of having disease by the likelihood ratio (Table A4.5, Step 3). If desired, odds can then be converted back to probabilities (Table A4.5, Step 4). The effect of pre-test probability on post-test probability for a range of likelihood ratios is shown in Fig. A4.3.

Table A4.5. Post-test probability: likelihood ratio

Assumptions

$P(D+) = 0.1$
$P(T+|D+) = 0.87$
$P(T-|D-) = 0.75$

Step 1: Convert probabilities to odds
If $P(D+) = 0.1$ then Odds $= 1:9$

Step 2: Calculate the likelihood ratios
For a test with binary outcomes:
Likelihood Ratio of a Positive Test =

$$\frac{\text{Sensitivity}}{\text{1-Specificity}} = \frac{0.87}{1-0.75} = 3.48$$

Step 3: Calculate the post-test odds
Post-test odds = pre-test odds × likelihood ratio

For a positive test:
Post-test odds $= 1:9 \times 3.48 = 3.48:9$

For a negative test:
Post-test odds $= 1:9 \times 0.17333 = 0.17333:9$

Step 4: Convert post-test odds to post-test probability
For a positive test

$$P(D+|T+) = \frac{\text{Odds}(D+)}{\text{Odds}(D+) + \text{Odds}(D-)} = \frac{3.48}{3.48+9} = 27.9\%$$

For a negative test

$$P(D-|T-) = \frac{\text{Odds}(D-)}{\text{Odds}(D-) + \text{Odds}(D+)} = \frac{9}{0.17333+9} = 98.1\%$$

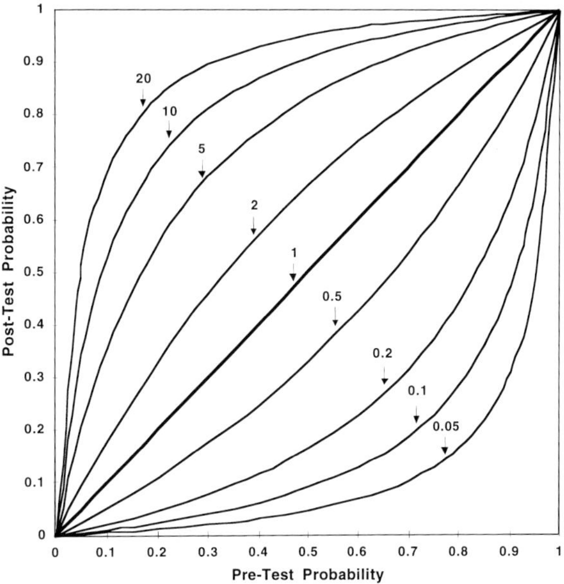

Fig. A4.3. Effects of likelihood ratios and pre-test probability on the post-test probability of disease. Each line on this graph shows the effects of a test result with a particular likelihood ratio on post-test probability for a given pre-test probability

References

Anonymous (1992) Evidence-based medicine. A new approach to teaching the practice of medicine. Evidence-Based Medicine Working Group [see comments]. J Am Med Assoc 268: 2420–2425

Barritt DW, Jordan SC (1960) Anticoagulant drugs in the treatment of pulmonary embolism: a controlled trial. Lancet 1: 1309–1312

Bedont RA, Datz FL (1985) Lung scan perfusion defects limited to matching pleural effusions: low probability of pulmonary embolism. Am J Roentgenol 145: 1155–1157

Beigelman C, Chartrand-Lefebvre C, Howarth N, Grenier P (1998) Pitfalls in diagnosis of pulmonary embolism with helical CT angiography. Am J Roentgenol 171: 579–585

Biello DR, Mattar AG, McKnight RC, Siegel BA (1979) Ventilation-perfusion studies in suspected pulmonary embolism. Am J Roentgenol 133: 1033–1037

Breatnach E, Stanley RJ (1984) CT diagnosis of segmental pulmonary artery embolus. J Comput Assist Tomogr 8: 762–764

Carson JL, Kelley MA, Duff A, Weg JG, Fulkerson WJ, Palevsky HI, Schwartz JS, Thompson BT, Popovich J Jr, Hobbins TE et al. (1992) The clinical course of pulmonary embolism [see comments]. N Engl J Med 326: 1240–1245

Chintapalli K, Thorsen MK, Olson DL, Goodman LR, Gurney J (1988) Computed tomography of pulmonary thromboembolism and infarction. J Comput Assist Tomogr 12: 553–559

Cohen AT, Edmondson RA, Phillips MJ, Ward VP, Kakkar VV (1996) The changing pattern of venous thromboembolic disease. Haemostasis 26: 65–71

Dalen JE, Alpert JS (1975) Natural history of pulmonary embolism. Prog Cardiovasc Dis 17: 257–270

Dalen JE, Brooks HL, Johnson LW, Meister SG, Szucs MM Jr, Dexter L (1971) Pulmonary angiography in acute pul-

monary embolism: indications, techniques, and results in 367 patients. Am Heart J 81: 175–185
Denton ER, Barrington SF, Kettle AG, Morrison ID, O'Doherty MJ (1998) The value of the chest radiograph in reporting aerosol ventilation-perfusion scans. Nucl Med Commun 19: 71–76
Dismuke SE, Wagner EH (1986) Pulmonary embolism as a cause of death. The changing mortality in hospitalized patients. J Am Med Assoc 255: 2039–2042
Douketis JD, Kearon CK, Bates S, Duku EK, Ginsberg JS (1998) Risk of fatal embolism in patients with treated venous thromboembolism. J Am Med Assoc 279: 458–462
Eddy DM (1990a) Clinical decision making: from theory to practice. Anatomy of a decision. J Am Med Assoc 263: 441–443
Eddy DM (1990b) Clinical decision making: from theory to practice. Practice policies –What are they? [see comments]. J Am Med Assoc 263: 877–878, 880
Elgazzar AH (1997) Scintigraphic diagnosis of pulmonary embolism: unraveling the confusion seven years after PIOPED. Nucl Med Annu 1997: 69–101
Garg K, Welsh CH, Feyerabend AJ, Subber SW, Russ PD, Johnston RJ, Durham JD, Lynch DA (1998) Pulmonary embolism: diagnosis with spiral CT and ventilation-perfusion scanning: correlation with pulmonary angiographic results or clinical outcome. Radiology 208: 201–208
Geraghty JJ, Stanford W, Landas SK, Galvin JR (1992) Ultrafast computed tomography in experimental pulmonary embolism. Invest Radiol 27: 60–63
Ginsberg JS, Wells PS, Kearon C, Anderson D, Crowther M, Weitz JI, Bormanis J, Brill-Edwards P, Turpie AG, MacKinnon B, Gent M, Hirsh J (1998) Sensitivity and specificity of a rapid whole-blood assay for D-dimer in the diagnosis of pulmonary embolism. Ann Intern Med 129: 1006–1011
Goldberg SN, Richardson DD, Palmer EL, Scott JA (1996) Pleural effusion and ventilation/perfusion scan interpretation for acute pulmonary embolus. J Nucl Med 37: 1310–1313
Goldhaber SZ (1998) Pulmonary embolism. N Engl J Med 339: 93–104
Goldhaber SZ, Hennekens CH, Evans DA, Newton EC, Godleski JJ (1982) Factors associated with correct antemortem diagnosis of major pulmonary embolism. Am J Med 73: 822–826
Goodman LR, Lipchik RJ, Kuzo RS (1997) Acute pulmonary embolism: the role of computed tomographic imaging. J Thorac Imaging 12: 83–102
Hull RD, Raskob GE, Coates G, Panju AA (1990) Clinical validity of a normal perfusion lung scan in patients with suspected pulmonary embolism. Chest 97: 23–26
Jacobson AF, Patel N, Lewis DH (1997) Clinical outcome of patients with intermediate probability lung scans during six-month follow-up. J Nucl Med 38: 1593–1596
Jaeschke R, Guyatt G, Sackett DL (1994a) Users' guides to the medical literature. III. How to use an article about a diagnostic test. A. Are the results of the study valid? Evidence-Based Medicine Working Group. J Am Med Assoc 271: 389–391
Jaeschke R, Guyatt GH, Sackett DL (1994b) Users' guides to the medical literature. III. How to use an article about a diagnostic test. B. What are the results and will they help me in caring for my patients? The Evidence-Based Medicine Working Group. J Am Med Assoc 271: 703–707
Kahn D, Bushnell DL, Dean R, Perlman SB (1989) Clinical outcome of patients with a "low probability" of pulmonary embolism on ventilation-perfusion lung scan. Arch Intern Med 149: 377–379
Kearon C, Ginsberg JS, Hirsh J (1998) The role of venous ultrasonography in the diagnosis of suspected deep venous thrombosis and pulmonary embolism. Ann Intern Med 129: 1044–1049
Kearon C, Julian JA, Newman TE, Ginsberg JS (1998) Noninvasive diagnosis of deep venous thrombosis. Ann Intern Med 129: 425
Kelley MA, Carson JL, Palevsky HI, Schwartz JS (1991) Diagnosing pulmonary embolism: new facts and strategies [see comments]. Ann Intern Med 114: 300–306
Kuzo RS, Goodman LR (1997) CT evaluation of pulmonary embolism: technique and interpretation. Am J Roentgenol 169: 959–965
Kwok CG, Skibo LK, Segall GM (1996) Low probability lung scan in a patient at high risk for pulmonary embolism [clinical conference]. J Nucl Med 37: 165–170
Lee ME, Biello DR, Kumar B, Siegel BA (1985) "Low-probability" ventilation-perfusion scintigrams: clinical outcomes in 99 patients. Radiology 156: 497–500
Mayo JR, Remy-Jardin M, Muller NL, Remy J, Worsley DF, Hossein-Foucher C, Kwong JS, Brown MJ (1997) Pulmonary embolism: prospective comparison of spiral CT with ventilation-perfusion scintigraphy. Radiology 205: 447–452
McNeil BJ (1976) A diagnostic strategy using ventilation-perfusion studies in patients suspect for pulmonary embolism. J Nucl Med 17: 613–619
McNeil BJ, Adelstein SJ (1975) Measures of clinical efficacy. The value of case finding in hypertensive renovascular disease. N Engl J Med 293: 221–226
McNeil BJ, Keller E, Adelstein SJ (1975) Primer on certain elements of medical decision making. N Engl J Med 293: 211–215
Meaney JF, Weg JG, Chenevert TL, Stafford-Johnson D, Hamilton BH, Prince MR (1997) Diagnosis of pulmonary embolism with magnetic resonance angiography [see comments]. N Engl J Med 336: 1422–1427
Morpurgo M, Schmid C (1995) The spectrum of pulmonary embolism. Clinicopathologic correlations. Chest 107: 18S–20S
Novelline RA, Baltarowich OH, Athanasoulis CA, Waltman AC, Greenfield AJ, McKusick KA (1978) The clinical course of patients with suspected pulmonary embolism and a negative pulmonary arteriogram. Radiology 126: 561–567
Oxman AD, Sackett DL, Guyatt GH (1993) Users' guides to the medical literature. I. How to get started. The Evidence-Based Medicine Working Group. J Am Med Assoc 270: 2093–2095
Perrier A, Desmarais S, Miron MJ, Moerloose P de, Lepage R, Slosman D, Didier D, Unger PF, Patenaude JV, Bounameaux H (1999) Non-invasive diagnosis of venous thromboembolism in outpatients. Lancet 353: 190–195
PIOPED Investigators (1990) Value of the ventilation/perfusion scan in acute pulmonary embolism. Results of the prospective investigation of pulmonary embolism diagnosis (PIOPED). (see comments) J Am Med Assoc 263: 2753–2759
Remy-Jardin M, Remy J, Wattinne L, Giraud F (1992) Central pulmonary thromboembolism: diagnosis with spiral volumetric CT with the single-breath-hold technique: comparison with pulmonary angiography. Radiology 185: 381–387
Robin ED (1977) Overdiagnosis and overtreatment of pulmonary embolism: the emperor may have no clothes. Ann Intern Med 87: 775–781

Royal HD (1994) Technology assessment: scientific challenges. Am J Roentgenol 163: 503–507

Rubinstein I, Murray D, Hoffstein V (1988) Fatal pulmonary emboli in hospitalized patients. An autopsy study. Arch Intern Med 148: 1425–1426

Smith R, Maher JM, Miller RI, Alderson PO (1987) Clinical outcomes of patients with suspected pulmonary embolism and low-probability aerosol-perfusion scintigrams. Radiology 164: 731–733

Stein PD (1971) Wedge arteriography for the identification of pulmonary emboli in small vessels. Am Heart J 82: 618–623

Stein PD, Athanasoulis C, Alavi A, Greenspan RH, Hales CA, Saltzman HA, Vreim CE, Terrin ML, Weg JG (1992) Complications and validity of pulmonary angiography in acute pulmonary embolism. Circulation 85: 462–468

Stein PD, Henry JW, Relyea B (1995) Untreated patients with pulmonary embolism. Outcome, clinical, and laboratory assessment [see comments]. Chest 107: 931–935

Stein PD, Terrin ML, Hales CA, Palevsky HI, Saltzman HA, Thompson BT, Weg JG (1991) Clinical, laboratory, roentgenographic, and electrocardiographic findings in patients with acute pulmonary embolism and no pre-existing cardiac or pulmonary disease [see comments]. Chest 100: 598–603

Wells PS, Ginsberg JS, Anderson DR, Kearon C, Gent M, Turpie AG, Bormanis J, Weitz J, Chamberlain M, Bowie D, Barnes D, Hirsh J (1998) Use of a clinical model for safe management of patients with suspected pulmonary embolism. Ann Intern Med 129: 997–1005

Wiener SN, Edelstein J, Charms BL (1966) Observations on pulmonary embolism and the pulmonary angiogram. Am J Roentgenol Radium Ther Nucl Med 98: 859–873

Worsley DF, Alavi A, Aronchick JM, Chen JT, Greenspan RH, Ravin CE (1993) Chest radiographic findings in patients with acute pulmonary embolism: observations from the PIOPED Study. Radiology 189: 133–136

5 Renal Imaging

F. JAMAR

CONTENTS

5.1 Introduction 79
5.2 Renal Tracers 79
5.3 Measurement of Absolute Renal Function 81
5.4 Renography and Pharmacological Intervention 82
5.4.1 Standard Renography 82
5.4.2 ACE Inhibition and Renovascular Hypertension 84
5.4.3 Diuretic Renography and Obstructive Uropathy 87
5.5 Renal Cortical Imaging 89

5.1 Introduction

The use of radiopharmaceuticals in studies of the urinary system is dedicated to three major goals: quantification of renal function, dynamic imaging (i.e., renography) and parenchymal scintigraphy. This chapter deals with the current status and recent achievements in these fields with particular emphasis on pharmacological interventions.

5.2 Renal Tracers

Two types of radioactive tracer are in use for renal studies: tracers cleared from plasma by glomerular filtration and those cleared by tubular secretion. The first class comprises ^{99m}Tc-labeled diethylenetriamine pentaacetic acid (^{99m}Tc-DTPA), ^{125}I-iothalamate and ^{51}Cr-labeled ethylenediamine tetraacetic acid (^{51}Cr-EDTA). Several other agents, such as ^{169}Yb-DTPA, were tested in the past without reaching the clinical arena. Glomerular filtration is a passive mechanism through which plasma is cleared from water and solutes. Glomerular filtration rate (GFR) amounts to 20% of renal plasma flow and is ideally reflected by the clearance of (non-radioactive) inulin. Renal clearance of the listed radioactive tracers approaches the clearance of inulin, indicating almost complete glomerular filtration without significant tubular reabsorption and extrarenal clearance. ^{99m}Tc-DTPA is commonly used for both imaging studies and clearance measurements while ^{125}I-iothalamate and ^{51}Cr-EDTA do not produce adequate photons for imaging and are therefore less widely used. Furthermore, although being recognized as the tracer of choice for GFR measurements because its clearance is virtually identical with that of inulin, ^{51}Cr-EDTA is not available in the USA (BLAUFOX 1991). ^{99m}Tc-DTPA is minimally bound to plasma proteins, resulting in a small error (<5%) in the measurement of the glomerular filtration rate (RUSSELL et al. 1986). ^{99m}Tc-DTPA is widely used because it not only allows the measurement of absolute renal function but also imaging in a variety of renal disorders. Furthermore, it is inexpensive, fairly stable and has a low radiation dose.

Tubular tracers include those cleared in urine after tubular uptake and ^{99m}Tc-dimercaptosuccinic acid (DMSA), which is retained in the renal cortex and minimally excreted in urine, hence providing an ideal way to perform parenchymal scanning (Fig. 5.1). Up to 40% of the injected dose is retained in tubular cells (proximal tubule and loop of Henle), which enables imaging of the cortex with fine resolution (MORETTI et al. 1984). DMSA uptake also reflects effective renal plasma flow (ERPF) and can be used as a marker of tubular dysfunction in rare disorders such as congenital tubular acidosis and in more common applications such as chemotherapy-induced renal toxicity (ANNINGA et al. 1994).

The other tubular agents are excreted in urine. Their prototype is radioiodinated orthoiodohippurate (^{123}I- or ^{131}I-hippuran, OIH), which is cleared from plasma by tubular secretion (NORDYKE et al. 1960). Its clearance is 81–96% of the clearance of the reference agent *para*-aminohippuric acid (PAH), which makes it suitable for the estimation of ERPF.

F. JAMAR
Center of Nuclear Medicine, University of Louvain Medical School, UCL 54.30, Avenue Hippocrate 54, B-1200 Brussels, Belgium

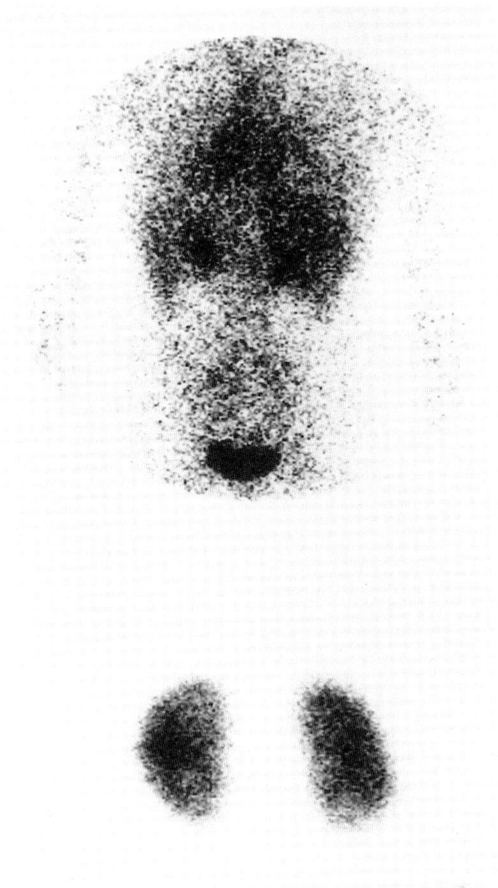

Fig. 5.1. ^{99m}Tc-DMSA scans, posterior view. *Top* patient with congenital tubular acidosis and almost no cortical retention of the tracer. *Bottom* patient with acute pyelonephritis showing globally homogeneous cortical uptake with little background activity and a small defect in the lower pole of the right kidney

Labeled with either ^{123}I or ^{131}I, OIH can be used for renographic studies. However, ^{131}I is far from optimal with regard to physical properties and hence to image quality and radiation burden. ^{123}I has therefore been introduced as label. It provides high quality renograms but is more expensive and not readily available. Due to these limitations, since the early eighties, efforts were directed to design a ^{99m}Tc-labeled tracer which would have a higher extraction fraction than ^{99m}Tc-DTPA and would overcome the practical drawbacks of OIH as listed above. This search has mainly focused on two families of donor ligand systems: the diamine dithiolate (N_2S_2) and triamide mercaptide (N_3S) (Eshima et al. 1990). The availability of one of the latter, ^{99m}Tc-mercaptoacetyltriglycine (MAG_3), in a kit formulation, is one of the major achievements of the last decade in renal nuclear medicine. It provides high quality imaging with an extraction efficiency two- to threefold that of ^{99m}Tc-DTPA and has become the most widely used agent for renography. The dosimetry is more favorable than with hippuran and the tracer is readily available (Taylor et al. 1987). Its extraction by the tubular cells is only 50–60% of that of PAH because of a high protein binding (Müller-Suur et al. 1990; Jafri et al. 1988). Therefore, it is an almost perfect tubular agent since there is hardly any glomerular filtration (Müller-Suur and Müller-Suur 1989). Some limitations include the boiling step in the labeling process, the presence of several potential species depending on the kit formulation and some liver activity and hepatobiliary clearance, especially with decreased renal function (Shattuck et al. 1994).

Further developments were made by Verbruggen et al. (1992), who synthesized L,L-ethylenedicysteine and labeled it with ^{99m}Tc. This compound is the more polar metabolite of the brain agent ^{99m}Tc-L,L-ethylenedicysteine diethylester (^{99m}Tc-ECD). In alkaline conditions, its advantage over MAG_3 is the labeling efficiency and high stability at room temperature. Several validation studies were undertaken in animals and humans and the physiological properties of ^{99m}Tc-L,L-ethylene dicysteine (^{99m}Tc-EC) are now well characterized (Table 5.1) (Van Nerom et al. 1993; Stoffel et al. 1994). Major differences with MAG_3 are the higher extraction fraction, lower protein binding and lack of hepatobiliary

Table 5.1. Pharmacokinetic properties of OIH, ^{99m}Tc-MAG_3 and ^{99m}Tc-EC

Property	^{123}I- or ^{131}I-OIH	^{99m}Tc-MAG_3	^{99m}Tc-EC
Molecular weight (Da)	303	374	379
Extraction efficiency (%)	66–87	50	53
Glomerular filtered fraction (%)	<20	<5	17
Protein binding (%)	53–70	79–90	24
RBC binding (%)	15–29	5	<5
Distribution volume (ml/kg)	190	125	192
Clearance (% of OIH)	100	49–67	70

RBC, red blood cells.

clearance. Clearance of EC amounts to 70% of the clearance of OIH as compared to 51% for MAG_3 (STOFFEL et al. 1994). Initial clinical studies indicated that ^{99m}Tc-EC is a valid alternative to MAG_3 for the coming years (KABASAKAL et al. 1995; GUPTA et al. 1995; PRVULOVICH et al. 1997). Recently, TAYLOR et al. (1997) showed that the clearance of the stereoisomer ^{99m}Tc-D,D-EC might be even closer to that of OIH.

5.3 Measurement of Absolute Renal Function

Two major parameters of renal function are currently used as indicators of clinical function: renal blood flow (RBF) and glomerular filtration rate (GFR). Glomerular filtration is related to RBF, and the integrity of the glomeruli (expressed as the filtration fraction) and, in routine applications, the GFR is reflected by serum creatinine. However, the relationship between endogenous creatinine clearance and GFR is affected by several factors, including poor renal function. With decreasing renal function, there is a compensatory increase in tubular reabsorption of creatinine. Thus, creatinine clearance is inaccurate and relatively insensitive to detect subtle to moderate changes of renal function (WALSER et al. 1988; LEVEY et al. 1988). The reference method for measuring GFR is the clearance of continuously infused – steady state – inulin, which is exclusively excreted by glomerular filtration without reabsorption at the tubular level. However, the technique is time-consuming, cumbersome and expensive and, therefore, no longer in use. Many methods using radioactive tracers such as ^{99m}Tc-DTPA or ^{51}Cr-EDTA have been proposed. The continuous infusion method is probably the most accurate but again is time-consuming and only used for research purposes (DONKER et al. 1977). For all agents the most often used way to measure GFR is the single-injection method and withdrawal of typically two to four blood samples, between 2 and 4 h (CHANTLER et al. 1969; BRÖCHNER-MORTENSEN and RÖDBRO 1976). The plasma clearance is assumed to be mono-exponential from 90 to 120 min following injection, although compartmental analysis describes plasma clearance as bi-exponential (SAPIRSTEIN et al. 1955) (Fig. 5.2). Sapirstein's equation, however, necessitates multiple blood samples. Assuming a mono-exponential clearance simplifies the equation, and two samples suffice, resulting in a systematic overestimation by neglecting the first exponential, which is corrected for

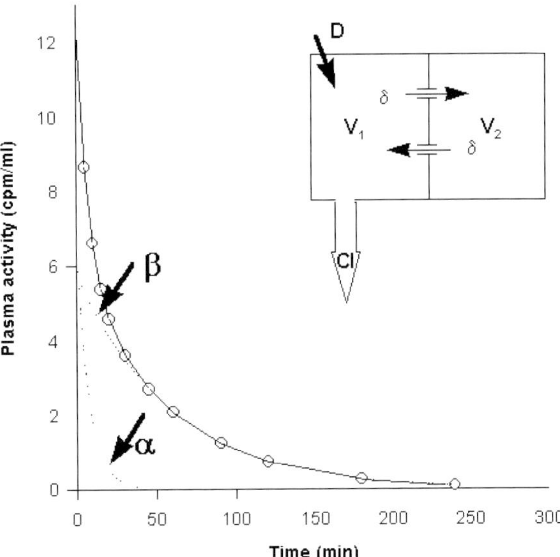

Fig. 5.2. Schematic representation of the open bi-compartmental model of Sapirstein. V_1 and V_2 represent the plasma and interstitial fluid volumes respectively; *D* and *Cl* indicate dose and renal clearance. *The continuous line* shows the bi-exponential curve fitted to the original data (*open circles*). *The dotted lines* represent the two components of this bi-exponential curve. In the simplified mono-exponential model, only curve β is considered with samples between 2 and 4 h

empirically. GFR can be estimated according to the general formula:

$$GFR = k \times \hat{Vd} \times a \quad (5.1)$$

In Eq. (5.1) $\hat{Vd}$ is the volume of distribution, calculated from the injected dose and intercept of plasma activity at t_0, *a* is the slope of the exponential function and *k* is a correction factor which varies according to the method used.

More simplified methods using only one sample have been proposed especially for pediatric purposes. Some even use capillary blood (FJELDBORG and BRÖCHNER-MORTENSEN 1986). HAM and PIEPSZ (1991) use a single sample at 120 min, and apply a method based on the distribution volume. They were able to derive a formula for calculating ^{51}Cr-EDTA clearance in children regardless of age and for determining reference values (PIEPSZ et al. 1994). A multitude of other methods for calculating the ^{99m}Tc-DTPA clearance were introduced over the last two decades. Following the approach by GATES (1982), some of these techniques are based on gamma camera imaging and may necessitate the calibration of the camera response to external standards, heart activity or one blood sample. Critical analysis of these methods is beyond the scope of this chapter. As an example, Fawdry et al. (1985) compared five simplified methods, including three with camera uptake measurements, and found that a patient with a GFR of 80 ml/min, measured by the single-injection multiple-sample technique, would have a predicted GFR in the range of 30–136 ml/min (95% confidence interval). In this study, the most accurate method gave a predicted GFR of 67–81 ml/min. In general, the simplified methods have proven not to be accurate, especially for a GFR below 30 ml/min (Li et al. 1997). Gamma camera based methods, however, offer the advantage of being a complement to renographic studies and of allowing the determination of relative, i.e., split, renal function. In view of the difficulty of analyzing the relative merits and drawbacks of the multiple methods available, a consensus report was published by the Radionuclides in Nephrourology Committee on Renal Clearance (Blaufox et al. 1996a). They recommend the Groth 4-h methodology (single-sample) for patients with GFR >30 ml/min and urinary clearances for GFR <30 ml/min; two-sample methods should be used for investigational purposes. Finally, an elegant technique was devised by Rabito et al. (1993) for continuous monitoring of renal function. Using a Cd-Te detector they made up a battery-operated arm probe (Ambulatory Renal Monitor, "ARM") that could be used to identify real-time changes in renal function. The use of this relatively simple equipment may lead to an improved management of patients in whom critical changes of renal function require rapid measurement, such as patients in the intensive care unit or following major surgery.

Although indirect measurements have been performed (Peters et al. 1990), direct measurement of RBF requires complicated methods such as the indicator-dilution or inert gas washout techniques (Schillig 1964; Ladegofed 1966). Smith et al. (1938) introduced the concept of Effective Renal Plasma Flow (ERPF), which describes the fraction of the plasma flow that goes to the nephrons (i.e., for urine formation) since about 10% of the RBF is used for the renal capsule, perirenal fat and interstitial tissue. ERPF can be measured with the clearance method. The reference method uses PAH with an extraction coefficient which is close to 100% (Smith et al. 1945). As for GFR, many scintigraphic methods have been devised to substitute for PAH clearance. Most used radioiodinated OIH and again two-sample or single-sample simplified techniques were proposed. One of the most popular was devised by Tauxe et al. (1982) and is based on a single sample obtained at 44 min: this method was recommended in the consensus report of the Radionuclides in Nephrourology Committee on Renal Clearance (Blaufox et al. 1996a). Methods based on fractional uptake can also be used to estimate the relative renal function (Chachati et al. 1987). Since the early nineties, substitution of ^{99m}Tc-MAG_3 for OIH has called for methods and algorithms for estimating ERPF using MAG_3 clearance (Russell et al. 1988, 1996; Müller-Suur et al. 1991). Simplified methods, based on plasma samples or on gamma camera images, did not appear entirely satisfactory due to the variable extraction fraction of the tracer. Nonetheless, some were implemented in clinical settings, especially in pediatrics, using the gamma camera (Gordon et al. 1991) or single-sample approach (Piepsz et al. 1993). The latter method, applied in a multicenter study, allowed the determination of reference values in *children with minimal renal disease* (Meyer et al. 1998).

A completely different concept was applied by Bubeck (1993). This principle is based on the theoretical volume of distribution determined by normalizing the plasma concentration in one sample to the individual body dimensions. More importantly, the principle can be applied to both adults and children and does not require imaging. This methodology measures a "tubular extraction rate" (TER), instead of ERPF, and does not take into account the variability between OIH and MAG_3 clearances. A significant concern that has been raised for MAG_3 clearance is the relatively high day-to-day variation in the measurements (Piepsz et al. 1996). Finally, simplified methods were proposed to derive ERPF from plasma clearance of ^{99m}Tc-EC (Stoffel et al. 1996).

5.4 Renography and Pharmacological Intervention

5.4.1 Standard Renography

A dynamic study of renal function, using the gamma camera, allows the evaluation of three distinct phases: perfusion, concentration and excretion. This can be achieved with GFR (DTPA) or tubular (OIH and MAG_3) tracers. There are relatively few indications in nephrology, and baseline scans have been progressively replaced by renographic studies augmented by pharmacological interventions, especially furosemide-induced diuresis in the study of dilated excretion systems, angiotensin-converting enzyme inhibitors (ACEI) for the diagnosis of renovascular hypertension and stress renography in assessing essential hypertension (CLORIUS and SCHMIDLIN 1983).

There are two exceptions to performing augmentations. First, standard renography remains very useful in acute renal failure (BLAUFOX 1991). Ultrasonography remains the method of choice, but other radiological studies with contrast media are not advisable since they can precipitate azotemia in these patients, particularly in diabetic patients. It was shown years ago that non-visualization of one or both kidneys had a negative prognostic value, provided acute obstruction could be ruled out (SHERMAN and BLAUFOX 1980). Other indications in acute renal diseases include acute tubular necrosis, renal emboli or renal vein thrombosis.

The second widely accepted exception is the evaluation of renal transplants. Renal transplantation has been successfully performed for over 30 years and has become the treatment of choice for end-stage renal failure (EGGERS 1988). The high success rate of the technique is not only due to improvements in the surgical management but also to a better selection of donors (including HLA-matched living-related donors and living-non-related donors). Immunosuppressive therapy is the major contributor to the long-term success of transplantation (CARPENTER 1990). Nevertheless, acute and chronic complications of renal grafts frequently occur and nuclear medicine procedures are routinely performed because they are non-invasive and do not have the risk of jeopardizing renal function as do contrast media. The most common indications are acute tubular necrosis (ATN), acute rejection, arterial thrombosis and chronic rejection. Differential diagnosis of transplant dysfunction now also includes cyclosporin-induced nephrotoxicity (MYERS et al. 1984). Transplant infarcts can be studied with ^{99m}Tc-DMSA. For renographic studies, ^{99m}Tc-MAG$_3$ is the agent of choice, although the typical back-diffusion pattern observed in ATN with ^{99m}Tc-DTPA is a major advantage for this tracer. Interpretation of the renograms is usually by visual criteria and renographic curve analysis, following the three classical phases described by TAPLIN (1971) (Fig. 5.3). Semiquantitative indices have been derived such as the perfusion index proposed by HILSON et al. (1978). Interested readers are referred to the literature (DUBOVSKY et al. 1995). In summary, MAG$_3$ (or OIH) renograms are particularly useful in kidney transplants to identify: (1) absence of perfusion in acute rejection and arterial thrombosis (Fig. 5.4), (2) maintained perfusion and parenchymal retention in ATN (Fig. 5.5), and (3) progressive degradation of uptake parameters in chronic rejection (Fig. 5.6). Finally, it must be stressed that there is no absolute criteri-

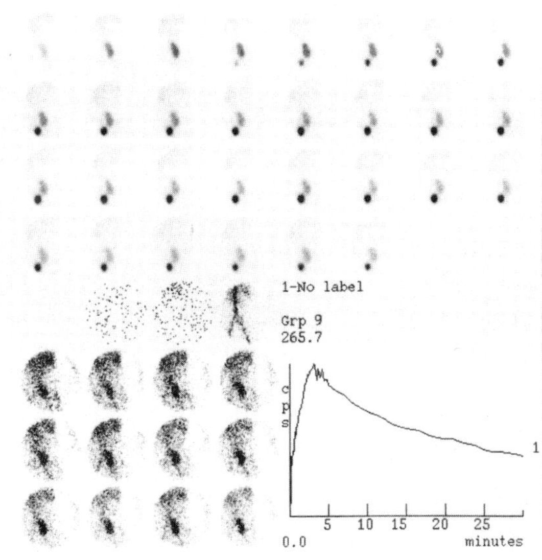

Fig. 5.3. Normal transplant study with ^{99m}Tc-MAG$_3$. The first-pass study (*left lower panel*) shows excellent perfusion and the renographic study (*upper panel*) good tracer uptake with a short parenchymal transit time (3–4 min). The transplant curve is normal (*right lower panel*)

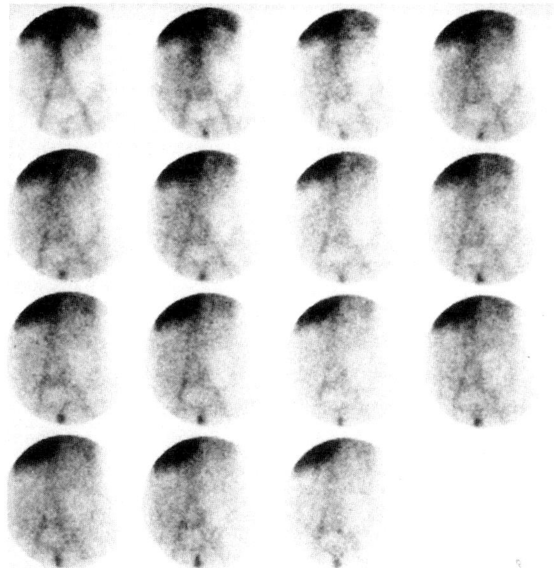

Fig. 5.4. Vascular phase study with ^{99m}Tc-MAG$_3$ showing no perfusion at all in the left-sided transplant, indicating acute arterial thrombosis. The transplant appears as a "background defect"

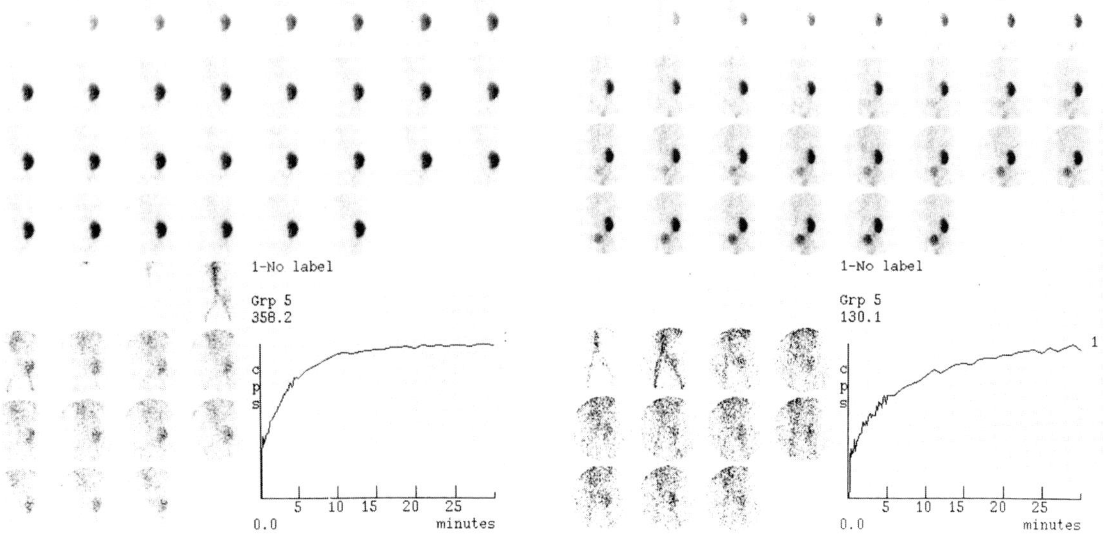

Fig. 5.5. Typical study with ^{99m}Tc-MAG$_3$ in acute tubular necrosis showing good perfusion (*left lower panel*), good tubular uptake and parenchymal retention (*upper panel*). The renographic curve shows good uptake which plateaus 10 min postinjection

Fig. 5.6. ^{99m}Tc-MAG$_3$ study in chronic rejection showing impaired flow phase (*left lower panel*), delayed uptake and altered washout of the tracer (*upper panel*). The curve shows delayed concentration and impaired excretion

on of the normal renal transplant's function. In evaluating chronic rejection, the patient is his/her own control and changes over time are more important than any parameter taken individually (Hilson 1991).

5.4.2 ACE Inhibition and Renovascular Hypertension

Renovascular hypertension (RVH) caused by renal artery stenosis (RAS) accounts for approximately 1% of all cases of hypertension. Since angioplasty is often curative, it must be recognized early, as part of primary management of hypertensive disease. Thus, there is a need for a screening method that is highly sensitive, but also has enough specificity in view of the low prevalence of the disease. Hypertension is common in the general population; therefore screening must be non-invasive and inexpensive. First of all, clinical clues suggesting RVH must be considered, including abrupt onset of hypertension at any age, severe or malignant hypertension, difficult to control hypertension with medical treatment (three-drug regimen), unexplained impairment of renal function and physical signs such as an abdominal bruit, evidence of vascular occlusive disease and retinopathy (Vidt 1991); a small unilateral kidney is also suggestive. Beyond these suggestive features, most tests developed for diagnosing RVH are rather invasive (e.g., arteriography or renal vein renin sampling) or insufficiently sensitive and/or specific (e.g., peripheral renin assay and "captopril test"). RAS is demonstrated by direct arteriography or less invasively by intravenous digital subtraction angiography; these tests, however, do not provide functional information and do not establish whether hypertension in a particular individual is related to RAS: only successful revascularization followed by disappearance of hypertension is final proof.

Another clinical feature of RVH, which was deliberately omitted in the above list of clues, is impairment of renal function as a consequence of angiotensin-converting enzyme inhibitors and, to a lesser extent, poor antihypertensive effect. This clinical fact, along with the serendipitous finding by Majd et al. (1983), led several groups to develop protocols to study the effect of ACEI (essentially captopril) on nephroscintigraphy in RVH. The effects and mechanisms involved can be summarized as follows: RAS leads to a decrease in the periglomerular arterial gradient: transglomerular filtration pressure, hence GFR, is maintained by vasoconstriction of the efferent arteriole, secondary to increased intrarenal angiotensin II. When angiotensin II production is blocked in the presence of captopril, this compensa-

Table 5.2. Recommended protocol for ACEI renography (adapted from TAYLOR et al. 1996)

Discontinue ACEI (24 h) and diuretics (48 h), when possible
Four hours fasting before captopril; no fasting if enalaprilat i.v.
Good oral hydration (500 ml 30–60 min before test)
Place i.v. line if hypotension anticipated (high-risk patients, enalaprilat)
DTPA, MAG_3, or OIH are all adequate
Captopril (25 mg or 50 mg) p.o. 60 min before tracer injection
Or enalaprilat 40 μg/kg slow i.v., 15 min before tracer injection
Thirty-minute renogram study usually sufficient (1- to 3-s images for flow study optional)

tory mechanism is extinguished: glomerular pressure falls, leading to decreased GFR and urine formation. These pathophysiological phenomena explain the findings on renography. With a filtered agent such as DTPA, the drop in GFR results in moderate to severe reduction of tracer uptake by the affected kidney which in extreme cases can be complete, i.e., only background activity and no appearance of tracer in the collecting system. The tubular tracers, MAG_3 and OIH, typically reveal progressive accumulation of the tracer in tubular cells with modest or no decrease in uptake in time, i.e., retention of the tracer in the renal parenchyma and prolonged renal transit time can be explained by decreased urine formation following GFR reduction.

Since the introduction of captopril renography, a number of different protocols were proposed. Standardization was achieved by the Consensus Report on ACE Inhibitor Renography, published after the Ninth Symposium on Radionuclides in Nephrourology held in Santa Fe in 1995 (TAYLOR et al. 1996). The recommendations are summarized in Table 5.2.

MAG_3 is preferred in case of reduced renal function (PRIGENT 1993). ACEI and diuretic treatment should ideally be stopped before scanning. However, in some cases this must be discussed with the referring physician. Both concurrent therapies are known to slightly alter the diagnostic value of the test (VISSCHER et al. 1995; SETARO et al. 1991; KOPECKY et al. 1987). In addition, ACEI renography with chronic diuretic treatment may result in hypotension, especially in dehydrated patients (SVETKEY et al. 1989; DONDI et al. 1989; ELLIOT et al. 1993). Conversely, some authors have proposed enhancing parenchymal (i.e., tubular) retention of MAG_3 or OIH by furosemide administration, which results in washout of the pelvicaliceal activity (BOURGOIGNIE et al. 1994; ERBSLOH-MÖLLER et al. 1991). It is, however, not considered "an essential component of ACEI renography" (TAYLOR et al. 1996) and may be proposed if stasis is observed in the collecting system (FINE 1994). A last practical issue is whether scanning with and without ACEI should or could be performed on the same day. Both the 1-day, i.e., baseline study followed by ACEI study, and 2-day protocols are acceptable. If the 1-day protocol is chosen, care must be taken to increase the tracer dose for the second study, i.e., 40–80 MBq (1–2 mCi) followed by 185–375 MBq (5–10 mCi). Such a protocol is appropriate for patients with a relatively high likelihood of RVH, whereas, in my opinion, in patients with a relatively low likelihood of having the disease, renography can be started with ACEI since a normal study will avoid the need for a baseline study.

A more important issue is to determine which patients do need a ACEI renogram. To be cost-effective, the test should not be used as a general screening test in a hypertensive population but rather focus on moderate- to high-risk patients (BLAUFOX et al. 1996b). These groups are defined by clinical features as listed previously and include patients with "typical presentation" of RVH (abrupt onset, abdominal bruits, small kidney, malignant course and unexplained azotemia) or patients with a milder course who are unresponsive to closely monitored antihypertensive treatment or who display worsening of renal function when started on ACEI therapy. Diabetic patients, in whom contrast media injection should be avoided, are also candidates for ACEI renography.

Interpretation of the test not only relies on the comparison of renographic images, but also on the comparison of curves, and looking for worsening of the pattern (flattening, delayed peak, reduced uptake) under ACEI as compared with the baseline study (Fig. 5.7a,b). Changes in relative renal function are also important to consider. Evaluation of the flow phase (first-pass angiography) is not reliable (SCHREIJ et al. 1996). Diagnostic criteria have been well defined and should be used to classify patients

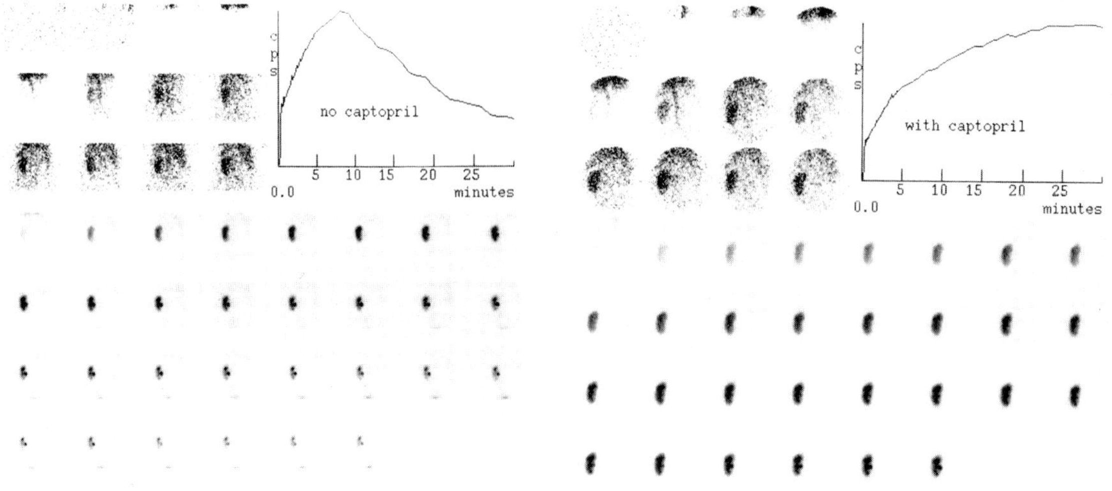

Fig. 5.7a,b. Evaluation of a patient with severe, abrupt-onset hypertension and a single kidney. The baseline ^{99m}Tc-MAG_3 study (no captopril, **a**) shows slightly delayed parenchymal transit but is otherwise normal. The captopril study (25 mg p.o., **b**) discloses severely reduced excretion with worsening of the renographic curve. Note that tracer uptake is not affected by captopril

with high, intermediate and low probability of RVH (Nally et al. 1991). Pitfalls include bilateral RVH, poor global renal function, long-term ACEI therapy and dehydration (Setaro et al. 1991; Mann et al. 1991; Blaufox et al. 1998).

The sensitivity and specificity of ACEI renography have been highly variable, with data ranging between 45% and 100% for sensitivity and between 62% and 100% for specificity. Large studies, however, reported values in the 90% range (Roccatello et al. 1992; Elliot et al. 1993; Fommei et al. 1994). More pessimistic results were recently published in a large series of high-risk hypertensive patients with a sensitivity of 68% and a specificity of 90% (van Jaarsveld et al. 1997). It should be emphasized that the prevalence of the disease has to be considered. Looking critically at the diagnostic performances collected by Taylor et al. (1996) in 1720 patients, the overall sensitivity and specificity were 88.2 and 92.2% respectively. With a prevalence of RVH among the compiled studies of 30%, this leads to a positive predictive value (PPV) of 82.8% (range in individual studies: 46–100%) and a negative predictive value (NPV) of 94.8% (range in individual studies: 81–99%): these results are quite acceptable. On the other hand, if we used these diagnostic performances as a rationale to apply ACEI renography in a general population (prevalence of RVH: 1%) or in a selected hospital-referral population (prevalence of RVH: 10%), the corresponding PPVs would be as low as 10.3% and 55.7%, respectively, with highly confident NPVs of 99.9 and 98.6%, respectively. Although these figures were only generated for illustrative purposes, they indicate that, in a non-selected population, the method is likely to perform adequately as an exclusion test, but would be of little value in the positive diagnosis of functionally significant RAS. This further emphasizes the need for optimal selection of the patients as outlined by Blaufox et al. (1996b). Besides its role in diagnosing RVH, ACEI renography has proven accurate in predicting blood pressure response to revascularization (Fommei et al. 1994; Dondi et al. 1992; Geyskes et al. 1991). Finally, the effect on patient management following ACEI renography has been poorly assessed: Ramsay et al. (1997) concluded from a retrospective study in 95 patients that changes in individual patient management were observed in only 34% of the cases. Outcome studies which more clearly define the place of ACEI renography in the armamentarium of hypertension work-up, particularly on decision making, are therefore needed in order to meet the clinicians' expectations.

In conclusion, ACEI renography has been used successfully over the last 15 years. The methodology is more cost-effective than arteriography (Blaufox et al. 1996b). Although most authors have provided evidence that the test was accurate in selected populations, some rather negative studies indicate the need for standardization of the protocol, including consensus on interpretation criteria, and improved patient selection for clinical applications. Combination of ACEI renography with duplex Doppler sonography may be an appropriate approach before submitting patients to arteriography, as recently suggested by MIRALLES et al. (1997) and KAPLAN-PAVLOVIC and NADJA (1998).

5.4.3 Diuretic Renography and Obstructive Uropathy

Diuresis-augmented renography was first described by RADÓ et al. (1967). In the subsequent years, the method was developed as a simple technique to differentiate between obstructive and non-obstructive dilated upper urinary tracts (O'REILLY et al. 1978; BRITTON et al. 1979). Upper urinary tract obstruction may be due to a variety of causes that can be categorized as intraluminal (e.g., calculi), intramural (e.g., stricture and idiopathic hydronephrosis) and extrinsic (e.g., retroperitoneal fibrosis); in addition, dilatation may be due to lower urinary tract abnormalities such as posterior urethral valves or primary megaureter. Dilatation of the renal pelvis is usually detected by ultrasonography and can be confirmed by intravenous pyelography. These techniques provide little functional information and may not be able to identify obstruction which is characterized by an increased pressure. In acute obstruction, pelvic pressures, which normally range between 4 and 10 cmH_2O, may increase up to 60 cmH_2O (BROWN 1994). This in turn raises tubular pressure, which is followed by a decrease in renal blood flow and reduction in GFR. There is some adaptive elasticity of the pelvis which in some cases reduces the pressure and hence the insult to the tubuli. This protective mechanism is, however, not the rule and at this stage intervention should be considered. The decision depends on the balance between resistance and compliance to flow, urine output and GFR. The first two parameters can be assessed using urodynamic studies as described by WHITAKER (1973, 1976), but these methods are invasive and not widely performed. This is particularly true in children and neonates: in the latter group, idiopathic hydronephrosis is recognized five times more frequently than in the past, due to the development of fetal ultrasonography (BROWN et al. 1987). Since the phenomenon may be transient, all neonates do not need to be operated upon, provided a simple test can assess the degree of obstruction and split renal function.

Many protocols for diuretic renography are described in the literature. The standard conditions are summarized in Table 5.3. In general, the choice of the radiopharmaceutical is not of critical importance and will generally be made between ^{99m}Tc-DTPA, ^{123}I-OIH and ^{99m}Tc-MAG_3. Currently, MAG_3 is preferred and widely used. Its high extraction fraction provides high quality images of both the cortex and collecting system, resulting in sharp curves which are easier to interpret than with DTPA. MAG_3 and to a lesser extent OIH are advisable in case of poor renal function, either in adults or, more generally, in neonates.

Table 5.3. Recommended protocol for diuresis renography

Good hydration (usually oral; in some cases i.v. fluids)
Void bladder completely before starting (indwelling catheter in children)
^{99}Tc-MAG_3 preferred (or ^{123}I-OIH) (^{99}Tc-DTPA adequate if renal function is normal)
Patient usually in supine position (erect position may be useful in selected cases)
Furosemide (40 mg in adults; 0.5–1.0 mg/kg in children)
Injection i.v. 20 min after tracer administration (*F*+20)
In selected cases furosemide injected 15 min before tracer administration (*F–15*)
Bladder voiding after standard scan (per- or postmicturition views)
Advise abundant fluid intake after procedure

Three conditions deserve further comment. First, the degree of hydration should be optimal: this can be achieved by oral hydration in most patients (500 ml water or juice). In young children and when sedation is felt necessary, hydration through an i.v. line is more adequate. Typical flow rates are in the range of 15 ml/kg isotonic saline during the first 30 min, starting 15 min before tracer injection, followed by 200 ml/kg/24 h over the next few hours. The use of hypotonic fluids was proposed by HOWMAN-GILES et al. (1987) as a way to increase the effect of furosemide and to overcome the importance of hydration in avoiding false-positive tests: this technique is known as the *volume expansion diuretic renal scan*. Secondly, the time of administration of furosemide varies between groups. It is usually given as a dose of 40 mg in adults, 0.5 mg/kg in children, and 1 mg/kg in infants (CONWAY 1992). Most publications indicate a time of administration between 20 (known as *F*+20) and 30 min following tracer injection (O'REILLY 1992). However, this may lead to a substantial number of equivocal responses, so an alternative was proposed in which furosemide is injected 15 min before injection (*F*–15) of the radiopharmaceutical (ENGLISH et al. 1987). The rationale for that has been well outlined by BROWN et al. (1992). They showed that after injection of 40 mg furosemide, the increase in urinary flow rates was perceptible after 2 min but maximal at 15 min postinjection. Thus, if maximal diuresis is required throughout the scan, injection of furosemide should take place before administration of the radiopharmaceutical. This method reduces the rate of equivocal results from 15–17% to 3% (O'REILLY 1992; UPSDELL et al. 1988). Nevertheless, the standard *F*+20 seems appropriate in most cases and should be complemented in selected cases by a *F*–15 study (O'REILLY et al. 1996). Thirdly, the role of the bladder in kidney washout should be considered. In all cases, the bladder should be emptied before initiation of the study and a procedure should never be terminated (unless normal) without assessing a potential *bladder effect*. This has been studied by JONES et al. (1990), who noted increased pelvic pressure during bladder filling resulting in a reduced drainage of the pelvicaliceal system, which can cause false-positive results. In children, bladder catheterization is advised (CONWAY 1992). O'REILLY et al. (1996) agues that only children with a high pre-test probability should have a continuous bladder drainage. This is particularly true in case of associated lower urinary tract dilation. An alternative is to perform the test without catheterization and to acquire a postmicturition scan, a procedure that may convert an obstructive to a non-obstructive pattern (GORDON et al. 1988).

Interpretation of a diuretic scan relies both on visual examination of the dynamic images and on inspection of time-activity curves derived for each kidney using the regions of interest (ROI) method (Fig. 5.8). Typical curves were described by O'REILLY (1992). A *type I* curve corresponds to a normal drainage before diuresis: this pattern is not associated with obstruction following diuresis and should be considered as normal. *Type II* curves display a continuous rise or plateau following diuresis. Although this type of curve is usually related to obstruction, unrecognized dehydration, massive dilation and a bladder effect must be excluded. Poor renal function may also be associated with such a pattern and it is well accepted that a single-kidney GFR below 16 ml/min would induce an inadequate diuretic response. In such a patient, the test should be considered inconclusive (O'REILLY et al. 1996). A *type IIIa* curve is characterized by a sharp decline after injection of the diuretic. In this case, dilatation represents stasis and not obstruction (Fig. 5.9). *Type IIIb* is called the equivocal response: in this case, there is some response to furosemide: a drop of less than 50% in 10 min, but not as marked as in type IIIa. In cases with poor renal function, it is unlikely that *F*–15 will improve the accuracy of the test. When the renal function is good and hydration has been well controlled, *F*–15 is useful to confirm the presence of

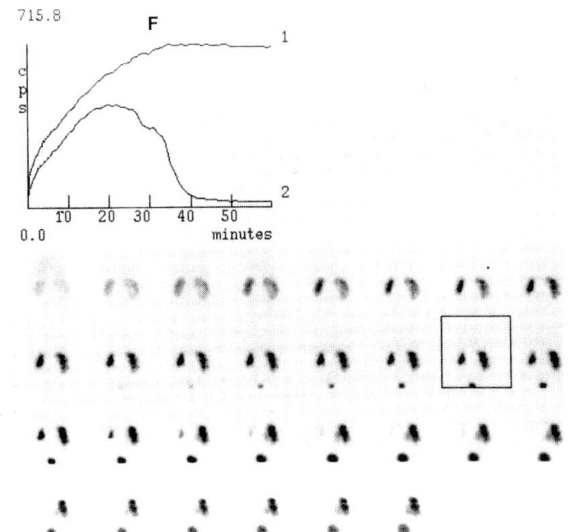

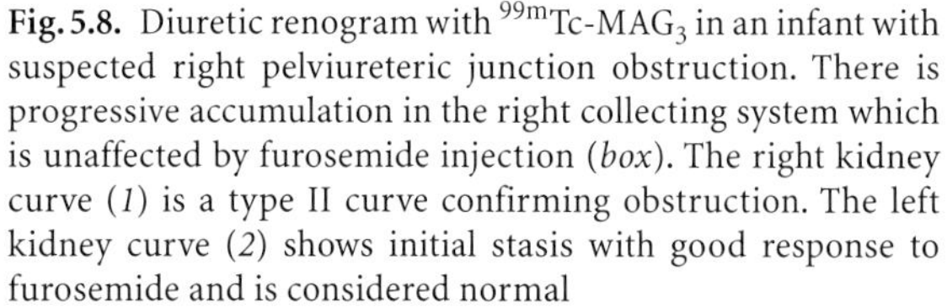

Fig. 5.8. Diuretic renogram with ^{99m}Tc-MAG$_3$ in an infant with suspected right pelviureteric junction obstruction. There is progressive accumulation in the right collecting system which is unaffected by furosemide injection (*box*). The right kidney curve (*1*) is a type II curve confirming obstruction. The left kidney curve (*2*) shows initial stasis with good response to furosemide and is considered normal

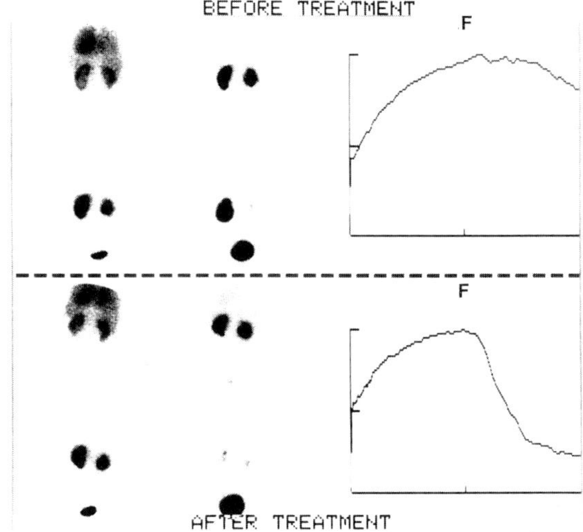

Fig. 5.9. Diuretic renogram with ^{99m}Tc-DTPA in a child with left pelviureteric junction obstruction, before (*top panel*) and after (*bottom panel*) percutaneous pyeloplasty. Note the conversion from a type IIIb (almost type II) curve before intervention to a type IIIa curve thereafter, indicating residual hypotony of the pelvis (*F* time of furosemide injection)

subtotal obstruction. Some authors have proposed evaluating the washout phase using quantitative indices such as $T_{1/2}$ (Kass and Fink-Bennett 1990; Conway 1992). There is general consensus that a $T_{1/2}$ >20 min represents obstruction and that with a $T_{1/2}$ <15 min there is no obstruction. Between 15 and 20 min, the test is considered inconclusive. Alternatively, Kletter and Nurnberger (1989) have proposed the E_{max} or maximal elimination rate. Neither this approach nor the half-time method have proven entirely satisfactory in terms of reproducibility, operator independence and definition of normal and abnormal ranges and hence they have relatively little clinical impact as recently stated by the Consensus Committee on Diuresis Renography (O'Reilly et al. 1996). A fourth pattern was subsequently described and is referred to as the *delayed decompensation* or Homsy's sign (Homsy et al. 1988). In this case, diuretic injection is followed by a transient response which seems decompensated at higher urinary flow rates, i.e., within 15 min of furosemide administration, and most likely represents obstruction – *intermittent hydronephrosis* – which can be confirmed by an *F*–15 study (O'Reilly 1992).

In addition to the excretion pattern, it is important to properly assess the function of the dilated kidney, especially for prenatally detected hydronephrosis. A substantial proportion of babies suspected of having pelviureteric junction obstruction improve spontaneously without treatment (Homsy et al. 1986). Piepsz et al. (1989), therefore, proposed selecting children with an altered single-kidney GFR for immediate surgery. The other children are followed sequentially with a repeat study at 6 months. This approach is more conservative and takes into consideration the maturation potential of renal function.

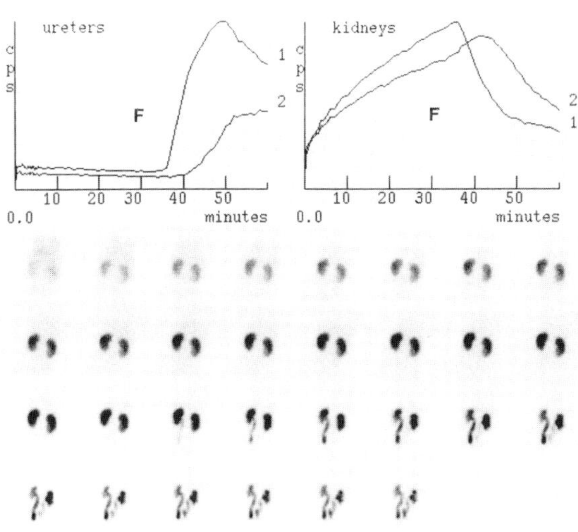

Fig. 5.10. ^{99m}Tc-MAG$_3$ study in a child with primary megaureter, performed with continuous bladder drainage. There is progressive accumulation of the tracer in both ureters after furosemide injection (*F*) and delayed renal washout (*curves, right upper panel*). The ureteric curves (*left upper panel*) are obstructive: type IIa (*curve 2*) and IIc (*curve 1*) according to Jamar et al. (1992)

Finally, little has been published about obstruction of the lower urinary tract. It is important, however, to assess the effect of chronic retention on dilation of the upper urinary tract (George et al. 1983, 1984). The effect of dilated ureters on pelvic washout has been studied and typical ureteral curves, obtained with continuous bladder drainage, were proposed for interpretation of ureter dynamics (Jamar et al. 1992) (Fig. 5.10). Diuretic renography has also been proposed as an alternative to the intravenous pyelogram in the follow-up of posterior urethral valves (Gordon et al. 1987).

In conclusion, the methodology and interpretation of diuresis renography are now well established. Although widely accepted, the validity of this technique for diagnosing obstruction cannot be directly assessed by comparison with a gold standard method. Several outcome studies, both in adults and infants, showed that the function of kidneys with an obstructive pattern did improve after surgery, whereas it remained stable in non-obstructed entities without any intervention (O'Reilly 1989; Upsdell et al. 1992; Piepsz et al. 1989; King et al. 1984). Diuretic renography almost completely replaced the invasive and sophisticated urodynamic studies and has significantly narrowed the spectrum of indications for the intravenous pyelogram.

5.5 Renal Cortical Imaging

Renal cortical scintigraphy was initially used as a morphological imaging tool. The development of ultrasonography and CT along with refinements of intravenous pyelography provided clinicians with excellent anatomical information so that renal scintigraphy, especially with ^{99m}Tc-labeled dimercaptosuccinic acid (DMSA), has evolved to a more functional assessment of the renal parenchyma. Although DMSA scanning can occasionally be useful in assessing congenital abnormalities (e.g., evaluation of a horseshoe kidney) or space-occupying lesions, the major indications now include the diagnosis of urinary tract infection (UTI), renal scarring especially in vesicoureteric reflux (VUR), and measurement of split renal function.

The diagnosis of upper UTI is usually easy in adults, based on clinical signs, elevated erythrocyte sedimentation rate and C-reactive protein, urine analysis and culture. It remains a challenge in children, due to the paucity of the clinical picture. Furthermore, symptoms are rather non-specific, if present, and fever may be the only sign. Prompt diagnosis is necessary because of the potential long-term sequelae. Adequate management of UTI can prevent scarring, which could lead to hypertension, loss of functional cortex and, at the extreme, chronic renal failure (Smellie et al. 1985; Ransley and Risdon 1981). Although the clinical presentation of UTI and VUR may be different, it is impossible to disregard the association between UTI, VUR and scarring. In children, scarring is almost always associated with VUR and was found in 12% of children with primary UTI and in 25% of those with recurrent episodes (Smellie et al. 1981).

The role of DMSA scintigraphy has been well established in identifying potentially reversible defects in acute pyelonephritis and permanent functional damage in scarring (Bingham and Maisey 1978; Merrick et al. 1980; Gordon 1987; Jakobsson et al. 1992). Although a common procedure for almost 20 years, interpretation of DMSA scintigraphy is far from easy. Gacinovic et al. (1996) reported a lack of interobserver consistency though this was not confirmed by two subsequent studies using specific evaluation criteria (Patel et al. 1993; De Sadeleer et al. 1998). The key question remains to determine if a DMSA scan is normal or abnormal. In a recent study by Clarke et al. (1996), images were considered equivocal in 68/496 children. Interestingly, the sensitivity, more precisely the prevalence of abnormalities, of DMSA scanning is relatively low in UTI. This is not due to an intrinsic weakness of the method but to the fact that abnormalities can only be detected when significant damage of the renal cortex has occurred. This was nicely shown in experimental studies in animals where correlation with histopathology was obtained (Majd and Rushton 1992; Parkhouse et al. 1989). Thus, the role of DMSA scintigraphy is not only to help in the diagnosis of UTI but also to assess the functional consequences of UTI on the integrity of the parenchyma.

Normal images demonstrate a fairly uniform distribution in the cortex with centrally located relatively photopenic defects, corresponding to the calices and papillary pyramids (Eggli and Tulchinsky 1993). Activity is not visible in the collecting system except in obstruction (Piepsz et al. 1986). In acute pyelonephritis, three patterns are observed: (1) a focal defect without loss of organ contour, (2) multiple focal defects and diffuse involvement of an entire kidney, and (3) characterized by reduced uptake and often enlargement due to edema (Figs. 5.11, 5.12). In chronic pyelonephritis and scarring, focal retraction(s) of the cortex with loss of organ contour are the most common abnormalities, whereas atrophy of either one or both kidneys is found in 10–20% of the cases (Clarke et al. 1996). Better delineation of the lesions can be obtained using pinhole scintigraphy; some authors have proposed the use of high-resolu-

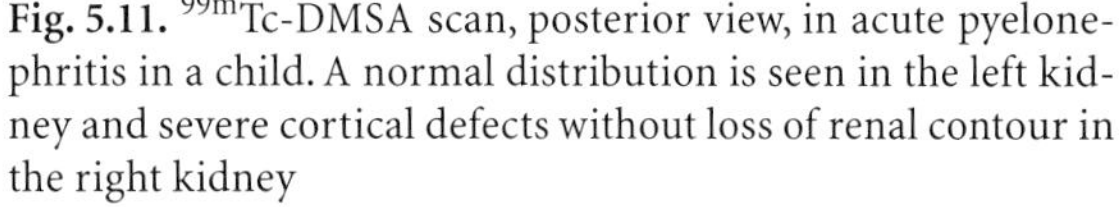

Fig. 5.11. ^{99m}Tc-DMSA scan, posterior view, in acute pyelonephritis in a child. A normal distribution is seen in the left kidney and severe cortical defects without loss of renal contour in the right kidney

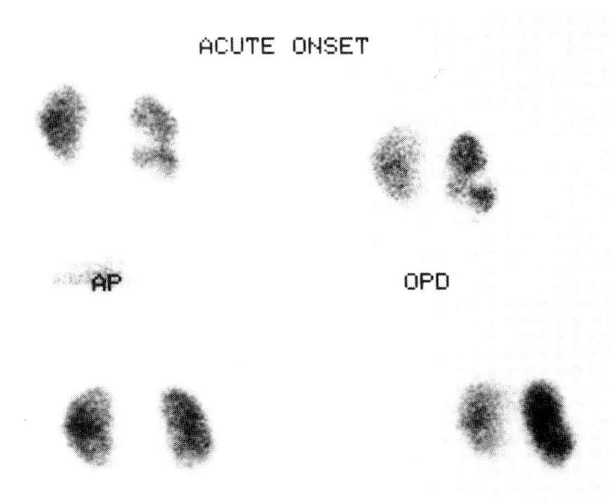

Fig. 5.12. ^{99m}Tc-DMSA study in acute pyelonephritis (*top*) with almost complete resolution of the cortical defects following treatment (*lower panel*) (*AP* posterior view, *OPD* right posterior oblique view)

tion SPECT (Joseph et al. 1990; Tarkington et al. 1990; Yen et al. 1996). Despite experimental evidence that SPECT is more accurate than planar imaging in the diagnosis of acute pyelonephritis (Gilbin et al. 1993), its effect in routine clinical studies appears marginal and is mainly useful for assessing scarring (Williams 1992). Furthermore, a study in normal volunteers demonstrated abnormalities on SPECT images with entirely normal planar images (De Sadeleer et al. 1996): systematic use of SPECT carries the risk of overdiagnosing acute cortical defects or scars.

In clinical practice, DMSA scanning should be performed following UTI, in children younger than 5 years, regardless of the result of ultrasound, to exclude scarring. The decision to proceed with a direct or indirect radionuclide cystogram or a micturating contrast cystogram will depend on the age and gender (Gordon 1990). Finally, it must be emphasized that an abnormal scan at the time of acute infection is not predictive of scarring and some cortical defects may take some time to resolve. Therefore, repeat scanning is required in the follow-up (2–6 months after infection) to identify scarring. The DMSA scan is a better predictor of VUR if performed within 2 months of infection (Jakobsson 1997).

References

Anninga JK, Valdès Olmos RA, de Kraker J et al (1994) Technetium-99 m dimercaptosuccinic acid and ifosfamide tubular dysfunction in children with cancer. Eur J Nucl Med 21:658–662

Bingham JB, Maisey MN (1978) An evaluation of the use of DMSA as a static renal imaging agent. Br J Radiol 51:599–607

Blaufox MD (1991) Procedures of choice in renal nuclear medicine. J Nucl Med 32:1301–1309

Blaufox MD, Aurell M, Bubeck B et al (1996a) Report of the radionuclides in nephrourology committee on renal clearance. J Nucl Med 37:1883–1888

Blaufox MD, Middleton ML, Bongiovanni J et al (1996b) Cost efficacy of the diagnosis and therapy of renovascular hypertension. J Nucl Med 37:171–177

Blaufox MD, Fine EJ, Heller S et al (1998) Prospective study of simultaneous orthoiodohippurate and diethylenetriaminepentaacetic acid captopril renography. The Einstein/Cornell Collaborative Hypertension Group. J Nucl Med 39:522–528

Bourgoignie JJ, Rubbert K, Sfakianakis GN (1994) Angiotensin-converting enzyme-inhibited renography for the diagnostic of ischemic kidneys. Am J Kidney Dis 24:665–673

Britton KE, Nimmon CC, Whitfield HN et al (1979) Obstructive uropathy: successful evaluation with radionuclides. Lancet I:905–907

Bröchner-Mortensen J, Rödbro P (1976) Comparison between total and renal plasma clearance of (51Cr)EDTA. Scand J Clin Lab Invest 36:247–249

Brown SCW (1994) Nuclear medicine in the clinical diagnosis and treatment of obstructive uropathy. In: Murray IPC, Ell PJ (eds) Nuclear medicine in clinical diagnosis and treatment, vol 1. Churchill Livingstone, Edinburgh, pp 271–293

Brown SCW, Upsdell SM, O'Reilly PH (1992) The importance of renal function in the interpretation of diuresis renography. Br J Urol 69:121–125

Brown T, Mandell J, Lebowitz RL (1987) Neonatal hydronephrosis in the era of sonography A. J Roentgenol 148:959–963

Bubeck B (1993) Renal clearance determination with one blood sample: improved accuracy and universal applicability by a new calculation principle. Semin Nucl Med 23:73–86

Carpenter CB (1990) Immunosuppression in organ transplantation. N Engl J Med 322:1224–1226

Chachati A, Meyers A, Godon JP et al (1987) Rapid method for the measurement of differential renal function validation. J Nucl Med 28:829–836

Chantler C, Garnett ES, Parsons V et al (1969) Glomerular filtration rate measurement in man by the single injection method using ^{51}Cr-EDTA. Clin Sci 37:169–180

Clarke SEM, Smellie JM, Prescod N et al (1996) Technetium-99m-DMSA studies in pediatric urinary tract infection. J Nucl Med 37:823–828

Clorius JH, Schmidlin P (1983) The exercise renogram. A new approach documents renal involvement in systemic hypertension. J Nucl Med 24:104–109

Conway JJ (1992) The "well tempered" diuretic renogram: a standard method to examine the asymptomatic neonate with hydronephrosis or hydroureteronephrosis. J Nucl Med 33:2047–2051

De Sadeleer C, Bossuyt A, Goes E et al (1996) Renal technetium-99m-DMSA SPECT in normal volunteers. J Nucl Med 37:1346–1349

De Sadeleer C, Tondeur M, Melis K et al (1998) A Belgian study on the reproducibility in reporting Tc-99 m DMSA planar scintigraphy. Eur J Nucl Med 25:855 (abstract)

Dondi M, Franchi R, Levorato M et al (1989) Evaluation of hypertensive patients by means of captopril enhanced renal scintigraphy with technetium-99 m DTPA. J Nucl Med 30:615–621

Dondi M, Fanti S, De Fabritiis A et al (1992) Prognostic value of captopril renal scintigraphy in renovascular hypertension. J Nucl Med 33:2040–2044

Donker AJM, Van Der Hem GK, Sluiter WJ et al (1977) A radioisotope method for simultaneous determination of the glomerular filtration rate and the effective renal plasma flow. Neth J Med 20:97–103

Dubovsky EV, Russell CD, Erbas B (1995) Radionuclide evaluation of renal transplants. Semin Nucl Med 25:49–59

Eggers PW (1988) Effect of transplantation on the Medicare end-stage renal disease program. N Engl J Med 318:223–229

Eggli DF, Tulchinsky M (1993) Scintigraphic evaluation of pediatric urinary tract infection. Semin Nucl Med 23:199–218

Elliot WJ, Martin WB, Murphy MB (1993) Comparison of two non-invasive screening tests for renovascular hypertension. Arch Intern Med 153:755–764

English PJ, Testa HJ, Lawson RS et al (1987) Modified method of diuresis renography for the assessment of equivocal pelviureteric obstruction. Br J Urol 59:10–14

Erbsloh-Möller B, Dumas A, Roth B et al (1991) Furosemide I-131 hippuran renography after angiotensin-converting enzyme inhibition for the diagnosis of renovascular hypertension. Am J Med 90:23–29

Eshima D, Fritzberg AR, Taylor A (1990) 99m-Tc renal tubular function agents: current status. Semin Nucl Med 20:28–40

Fawdry RM, Gruenewald SM, Collins LT et al (1985) Comparative assessment of techniques for estimation of glomerular filtration rate with 99m-Tc-DTPA. Eur J Nucl Med 11:7–12

Fine EJ (1994) Vascular disorders, with emphasis on hypertension. In: Murray IPC, Ell PJ (eds) Nuclear medicine in clinical diagnosis and treatment, vol 1. Churchill Livingstone, Edinburgh, pp 295–317

Fjeldborg P, Bröchner-Mortensen J (1986) Determination of 51-Cr-EDTA clearance in infants by a single capillary blood sample. Scand J Clin Lab Invest 46:335–340

Fommei E, Ghione S, Hilson AJW et al (1994) Captopril radionuclide test in renovascular hypertension: European multicentric study. In: O'Reilly PH, Taylor A, Nally JV (eds) Radionuclides in nephrourology, vol 1. Field and Wood Medical Periodicals, Blue Bell, PA, pp 33–37

Gacinovic S, Buscombe J, Costa DC et al (1996) Inter-observer agreement in the reporting of ^{DMSA} renal studies. Nucl Med Commun 17:596–602

Gates GF (1982) Glomerular filtration rate: estimation from fractional renal accumulation of 99m-Tc-DTPA (Stannous). AJR 138:565–570

George NJR, O'Reilly PH, Barnard RJ et al (1983) High pressure chronic retention. Br Med J 286:1780–1783

George NJR, O'Reilly PH, Barnard RJ et al (1984) Practical management of patients with dilated upper tracts and chronic retention of urine. Br J Urol 56:9–12

Geyskes GG, de Bruyn AJG (1991) Captopril renography and the effect of percutaneous transluminal angioplasty on blood pressure in 94 patients with renal artery stenosis. Am J Hypertens 4:685S–689S

Giblin JG, O'Connor KP, Fildes RD et al (1993) The diagnosis of acute pyelonephritis in the piglet using single-photon emission computerized tomography dimercaptosuccinic acid scintigraphy: a pathological correlation. J Urol 1150:759–762

Gordon I (1987) Indications for ^{99m}Tc-dimercaptosuccinic acid scan in children. J Urol 137:464–467

Gordon I (1990) Urinary tract infection in paediatrics: the role of diagnostic imaging. Br J Radiol 63:507–511

Gordon I, Ransley PG, Hubbard CS (1987) 99m-Tc DTPA scintigraphy compared with intravenous urography in the follow-up of posterior urethral valves. Br J Urol 60:447–449

Gordon I, Mialdea-Fernandez RM, Peters AM (1988) Pelviureteric junction obstruction. The value of a post-micturition view in 99m-Tc DTPA diuretic renography. Br J Urol 61:409–412

Gordon I, Anderson PJ, Orton M et al (1991) Estimation of technetium-99m-MAG3 renal clearance in children: two gamma camera techniques compared with multiple plasma samples. J Nucl Med 32:1704–1708

Gupta NK, Bomanji JB, Waddington W et al (1995) Technetium-99m-L,L-ethylenedicysteine scintigraphy in patients with renal disorders. Eur J Nucl Med 22:617–624

Ham HR, Piepsz A (1991) Estimation of glomerular filtration rate in infants and in children using a single-plasma sample method. J Nucl Med 32:1294–1297

Hilson AJW (1991) The renal transplant perfusion index: where are we now? Eur J Nucl Med 18:227–228

Hilson AJW, Maisey MN, Brown CB et al (1978) Dynamic renal transplant imaging with Tc-99 m DTPA (Sn) supplemented by a transplant perfusion index in the management of renal transplants. J Nucl Med 19:994–1000

Homsy YL, Williot P, Danais S (1986) Transitional neonatal hydronephrosis: fact or fantasy? J Urol 136:336–340

Homsy YL, Mehta PH, Huot D et al (1988) Intermittent hydronephrosis: a diagnostic challenge. J Urol 140:1222–12226

Howman-Giles R, Uren R, Roy LP et al (1987) Volume expansion diuretic renal scan in urinary tract obstruction. J Nucl Med 28:824–828

Jafri RA, Britton KE, Nimmon CC et al (1988) Technetium-99 m MAG3, a comparison with iodine-123 and iodine-131 orthoiodohippurate, in patients with renal disorders. J Nucl Med 29:147–158

Jakobsson B (1997) Importance of timing when using technetium-99m-dimecaptosuccinic acid scan in urinary tract infection. In: Taylor A, Nally JV, Thomsen H (eds) Radionuclides in nephrourology. Society of Nuclear Medicine, Reston, VA, pp 185–189

Jakobsson B, Nolstedt L, Svensson L et al (1992) Technetium-99m-DMSA scan in the diagnosis of acute pyelonephritis: relation to clinical and radiological findings. Pediatr Nephrol 6:328–334

Jamar F, Piret L, Wese FX et al (1992) Influence of ureteral status on kidney washout during 99m-Tc DTPA diuresis renography in children. J Nucl Med 33:73–78

Jones DA, Lupton EW, George NJR (1990) Effect of bladder filling on upper urodynamics in man. Br J Urol 65:492–496

Joseph DB, Young DW, Jordon SP (1990) Renal cortical scintigraphy and single photon emission computerized tomography (SPECT) in the assessment of renal defects in children. J Urol 144:595–597

Kabasakal L, Atay S, Vural AV et al (1995) Evaluation of ^{99m}Tc-ethylenedicysteine in renal disorders and determination of extraction ratio. J Nucl Med 36:1398–1403

Kaplan-Pavlovic S, Nadja C (1998) Captopril renography and duplex Doppler sonography in the diagnosis of renovascular hypertension. Nephrol Dial Transplant 13:313–317

Kass EJ, Fink-Bennett D (1990) Contemporary techniques for the radioisotopic evaluation of the dilated urinary tract. Urol Clin North Am 17:273–289

King LR, Coughlin PWF, Bloch EC et al (1984) The case for immediate pyeloplasty in the neonate with ureteropelvic junction obstruction. J Urol 132:725–728

Kletter K, Nurnberger N (1989) Diagnostic potential of diuresis renography: limitations by the severity of hydronephrosis and by impairment of renal function. Nucl Med Commun 10:51–61

Kopecky RT, Deaver TF, McAfee JG (1987) Furosemide augments the effects of captopril on nuclear studies in renovascular stenosis. Hypertension 10:181–188

Ladegofed J (1966) Measurements of the renal blood flow in man with the ^{133}Xe washout technique. Scand J Clin Lab Invest 18:299–315

Levey AS, Perrone RD, Madias NE (1988) Serum creatinine and renal function. Annu Rev Med 39:465–490

Levitt BGS, Kogan S, Reda E et al (1988) The dilated urinary tract in children. Br J Urol 61:413–419

Li Y, Lee HB, Blaufox MD (1997) Single-sample methods to measure GFR with technetium-99m-DTPA. J Nucl Med 38:1290–1295

Majd M, Rushton HG (1992) Renal cortical scintigraphy in the diagnosis of acute pyelonephritis. Semin Nucl Med 22:98–111

Majd M, Potter BM, Guzzetta PC et al (1983) Effect of captopril on efficacy of renal scintigraphy in detection of renal artery stenosis. J Nucl Med 24:23 (abstract)

Mann SJ, Pickering TG, Sos TA et al (1991) Captopril renography in the diagnosis of renal artery stenosis; accuracy and limitations. Am J Med 90:30–40

Merrick MV, Uttley WS, Wild SR (1980) The detection of pyelonephritic scarring in children by radioisotopic imaging. Br J Radiol 53:544–556

Meyer G, Piepsz A, Kolinska J et al (1998) Technetium-99 m mercaptoacetyltriglycine clearance values in children with minimal renal disease: can a normal range be determined? Eur J Nucl Med 25:760–765

Miralles M, Covas MI, Martinez-Miralles E et al (1997) Captopril test and renal duplex scanning for the primary screening of renovascular disease. Am J Hypertens 10:1290–1296

Moretti JL, Rapin JR, Saccavini JC et al (1984) 2,3-dimercaptosuccinic-acid chelates. 2. Renal localization. Int J Nucl Med Biol 11:275–279

Müller-Suur R, Müller-Suur C (1989) Glomerular filtration and tubular secretion of MAG-3 in the rat kidney. J Nucl Med 30:1986–1991

Müller-Suur R, Bois-Svensson I, Mesko L (1990) A comparative study of renal scintigraphy and clearance with technetium-99m-MAG3 and iodine-123-hippurate in patients with renal disorders. J Nucl Med 31:1811–1817

Müller-Suur R, Magnusson G, Bois-Svensson I et al (1991) Estimation of technetium 99 m mercaptoacetyltriglycine plasma clearance by use of one single plasma sample. Eur J Nucl Med 18:28–31

Myers BD, Ross J, Newton L et al (1984) Cyclosporine-associated chronic nephropathy. N Engl J Med 311:699–705

Nally JW Jr, Chen C, Fine EJ et al (1991) Diagnostic criteria of renovascular hypertension with captopril renography. Am J Hypertens 4:749S–752S

Nordyke RA, Tubis M, Blahd WH (1960) Use of radioiodinated hippuran for individual kidney function tests. J Lab Clin Med 56:438–445

O'Reilly PH (1989) Functional outcome of pyeloplasty for ureteropelvic junction obstruction: a prospective study in 50 consecutive cases. J Urol 142:273–276

O'Reilly PH (1992) Diuresis renography. recent advances and recommended protocols. Br J Urol 69:113–120

O'Reilly PH, Testa HJ, Lawson RS et al (1978) Diuresis renography in equivocal urinary tract obstruction. Br J Urol 50:76–80

O'Reilly P, Aurell M, Britton K et al (1996) Consensus on diuresis renography for investigating the dilated upper urinary tract. J Nucl Med 37:1872–1876

Parkhouse HF, Godley ML, Cooper J et al (1989) Renal imaging with ^{99}Tc^{m}-labeled DMSA in the detection of acute pyelonephritis: an experimental study in the pig. Nucl Med Commun 10:63–70

Patel K, Charron M, Hoberman A et al (1993) Intra- end interobserver variability in interpretation of DMSA scans using a set of standardized criteria. Pediatr Radiol 23:506–509

Peters AM, Brown J, Crossman D et al (1990) Noninvasive measurement of renal blood flow with technetium-99m-DTPA in the evaluation of patients with suspected renovascular hypertension. J Nucl Med 31:1980–1985

Piepsz A, Ham HR, Roland JH et al (1986) Technetium-99 m DMSA imaging and the obstructed kidney. Clin Nucl Med 11:389–391

Piepsz A, Hall M, Ham R et al (1989) Prospective management of neonates with pelviureteric junction stenosis. Scand J Urol Nephrol 23:31–36

Piepsz A, Gordon I, Hahn K et al (1993) Determination of the technetium-99 m mercaptoacetyltriglycine plasma clearance in children by means of a single blood sample: a multicentre study. Eur J Nucl Med 20:244–248

Piepsz A, Pintelon H, Ham HR (1994) Estimation of normal chromium-51 ethylene diamine tetra-acetic acid clearance in children. Eur J Nucl Med 21:12–16

Piepsz A, Tondeur M, Kinthaert J et al (1996) Reproducibility of technetium-99 m mercaptoacetyltriglycine clearance. Eur J Nucl Med 23:195–198

Prigent A (1993) Diagnosis of renovascular hypertension: the role of captopril renal scintigraphy and related issues. Eur J Nucl Med 20:625–644

Prvulovich EM, Bomanji JB, Waddington WA et al (1997) Clinical evaluation of technetium-99m-L,L-ethylenedicysteine in patients with chronic renal failure. J Nucl Med 38:809–814

Rabito CA, Moore RH, Bougas C et al (1993) Noninvasive, real-time monitoring of renal function: the ambulatory renal monitor. J Nucl Med 34:199–207

Radó JP, Bános C, Takó J (1967) Frusemide renography. Lancet ii:1419–1420

Ramsay D, Belton I, Finlay D (1997) A review of captopril renal scintigraphy and its effect on patient management. Nucl Med Commun 18:631–633

Ransley PG, Risdon RA (1981) Reflux nephropathy: effects of antimicrobial therapy on the evolution of the early pyelonephritic scar. Kidney Int 20:733–742

Roccatello D, Picciotto G, Rabbia C et al (1992) Prospective study of captopril renography in hypertensive patients. Am J Nephrol 12:406–411

Russell CD, Rowell K, Scott JW (1986) Quality control of technetium-99 m DTPA: correlation of analytic tests with in vivo protein binding in man. J Nucl Med 27:560–562

Russell CD, Thorstad BL, Yester MV et al (1988) Quantitation of renal function with technetium-99 m MAG3. J Nucl Med 29:1931–1933

Russell CD, Taylor AT, Dubovsky EV (1996) Measurement of renal function with technetium-99m-MAG3 in children and adults. J Nucl Med 37:588–593

Sapirstein LA, Vidt DG, Mandel MJ et al (1955) Volumes of distribution and clearances of intravenously injected creatinine in the dog. Am J Physiol 181:330–336

Schillig S (1964) Indicator-dilution techniques in the estimation of renal blood flow. Am Heart J 68:675–681

Schreij G, van Es PN, van Kroonenburgh MJPG et al (1996) Baseline and postcaptopril renal blood flow measurements in hypertensives suspected of renal artery stenosis. J Nucl Med 37:1652–1655

Setaro JF, Chen CC, Hoffer PB et al (1991) Captopril renography in the diagnosis of renal artery stenosis and prediction of improvement after revascularization. Am J Hypertens 4:698S–705S

Shattuck LA, Eshima D, Taylor AT et al (1994) Evaluation of the hepatobiliary excretion of ^{99m}Tc-MAG3 and reconstitution factors affecting the radiochemical purity. J Nucl Med 35:349–355

Sherman RA, Blaufox MD (1980) Clinical significance of nonvisualization with ^{131}I-hippuran renal scan. In: Hollenberg NK, Lange S (eds) Radionuclides in nephrology. Thieme, Stuttgart, pp 235–239

Smellie JM, Normand ICS, Katz G (1981) Children with urinary tract infection: a comparison of those with and those without vesicoureteric reflux. Kidney Int 20:717–722

Smellie JM, Ransley PG, Normand ICS et al (1985) Development of new renal scars. A collaborative study. Br Med J 290:1957–1960

Smith HW, Goldring W, Chassis H (1938) The measurement of tubular excretory mass, effective blood flow and filtration rate in the normal human kidney. J Clin Invest 17:263–278

Smith HW, Finkelstein N, Aliminosa L et al (1945) The renal clearances of substituted hippuric acid derivatives and other aromatic acids in dog and man. JCI 24:388–404

Stoffel M, Jamar F, Van Nerom C et al (1994) Evaluation of technetium-99m-L,L-ethylenedicysteine in renal transplant recipients: a comparative study with technetium-99m-mercaptoacetyltriglycine and iodine-125-orthoiodohippurate. J Nucl Med 35:1951–1958

Stoffel M, Jamar F, Van Nerom C et al (1996) Estimation of technetium-99 m L,L-ethylenedicysteine clearance by simplified methods: correlation with effective renal plasma flow. Eur J Nucl Med 23:365–370

Svetkey LP, Himmelstein SI, Dunnick NR et al (1989) Prospective analysis of strategies for diagnosing renovascular hypertension. Hypertension 14:247–257

Taplin GV (1971) Kidney function and disease. In: Blahd WH (ed) Nuclear medicine, 2nd edn. McGraw Hill, New York, NY, pp 382–386

Tarkington MA, Fildes RD, Levin K et al (1990) High resolution single photon emission computerized tomography (SPECT) ^{99m}Technetium-dimercaptosuccinic acid scintigraphy: a state of the art technique. J Urol 144:598–600

Tauxe WH, Dubovsky EV, Kidd TJ et al (1982) New formulas for the calculation of effective renal plasma flow. Eur J Nucl Med 7:51–54

Taylor A, Eshima D, Christian PE et al (1987) Evaluation of Tc-99 m mercaptoacetyltriglycine in patients with impaired renal function. Radiology 162:365–370

Taylor A, Nally J, Aurell M et al (1996) Consensus report on ACE inhibitor renography for detecting renovascular hypertension. J Nucl Med 37:1876–1882

Taylor A, Hansen L, Eshima D et al (1997) Comparison of technetium-99m-LL-Ec isomers in rats and humans. J Nucl Med 38:821–826

Upsdell SM, Leeson SM, Brooman PJC et al (1988) Diuretic-induced urinary flow rates at varying clearances and their relevance to the performance and interpretation of diuresis renography. Br J Urol 61:14–18

Upsdell SM, Testa HJ, Lawson RS (1992) The F-15 diuresis renogram in suspected obstruction of the upper urinary tract. Br J Urol 69:126–131

van Jaarsveld BC, Krijnen P, Derkx FH et al (1997) The place of renal scintigraphy in the diagnosis of renal artery stenosis. Fifteen years of clinical experience. Arch Intern Med 157:1226–1234

Van Nerom CG, Bormans GM, De Roo MJ et al (1993) First experience in healthy volunteers with ^{99m}Tc-L,L-ethylenedicysteine: a new renal imaging agent. Eur J Nucl Med 20:738–746

Verbruggen AM, Nosco DL, Van Nerom CG et al (1992) Technetium-99m-L,L-ethylenedicysteine: a renal imaging agent. I. Labeling and evaluation in animals. J Nucl Med 33:551–557

Vidt DG (1991) The diagnosis of renovascular hypertension: a clinician's viewpoint. Am J Hypertens 4:663S–668S

Visscher CA, de Zeeuw D, Huisman RM (1995) Effect of chronic ACE inhibition on the diagnostic value of renography for renovascular hypertension: a preliminary report. Nephrol Dial Transplant 10:263–265

Walser M, Drew HH, LaFrance ND. (1988) Creatinine measurements often yield false estimates of progression in chronic renal failure. Kidney Int 34:412–418

Whitaker RH (1973) Methods of assessing obstruction in dilated ureters. Br J Urol 45:15–22

Whitaker RH (1976) Equivocal pelviureteric junction obstruction. Br J Urol 47:377–385

Williams ED (1992) Renal single photon computed tomography: should we do it? Semin Nucl Med 22:112–121

Yen T-C, Chen W-P, Chang S-L et al (1996) Technetium-99m-DMSA renal SPECT in diagnosing and monitoring pediatric acute pyelonephritis. J Nucl Med 37:1349–1353

6 Skeletal Scintigraphy

C. Schiepers

Contents

6.1 Introduction 95
6.2 Radio-pharmaceuticals 95
6.2.1 Fluoride 95
6.2.2 Technetium Complexes 96
6.3 Methods 96
6.3.1 Positron Imaging 96
6.3.2 Single-Photon Imaging 96
6.4 Image Interpretation 97
6.5 Selected Clinical Applications 98
6.5.1 Positron Imaging with ^{18}F-Fluoride 98
6.5.2 Oncology 98
6.5.3 Infection and Inflammation 99
6.5.4 Orthopedics 99
6.5.5 Vascular Bone Disorders 101
6.6 Conclusion 101

6.1 Introduction

Bone scintigraphy is one of the common procedures in routine nuclear medicine. The study is relatively simple, no patient preparation is required, and the imaging procedure is well standardized throughout diagnostic imaging departments. Modern equipment has greatly enhanced the ease of operation and permits imaging in planar, tomographic, and whole-body mode.

Bone scintigraphy is an extremely sensitive procedure for evaluating a variety of skeletal disorders, and can also be applied for certain soft tissue evaluations such as calcifications, hematoma, and contusion. The main indications for referral are screening of patients with malignancy, trauma, orthopedic problems, sports injuries, as well as endocrine and rheumatologic disorders.

Bone is a specialized form of connective tissue, with hardness as its characterizing feature. Bone is a dynamic tissue, a metabolically active structure in which osteogenesis and resorption occur continuously, and in which processes can be followed with radioactive tracers. Metabolic rates are affected by disease processes and can be greatly enhanced as in M. Paget, or decreased as in involutional osteoporosis.

Bone scanning has been around for a long time. In 1962 Blau and collaborators introduced ^{18}F-fluoride as a bone-imaging agent. The annihilation radiation of this positron emitter is relatively high and suited for rectilinear scanners. Van Dyke et al. (1965) reported the use of ^{18}F with a gamma camera. Since the advent of positron emission tomography (PET), this radio-pharmaceutical has been revived and allows for true regional quantification of bone blood flow and fluoride influx rate (Schiepers et al. 1990).

A historic breakthrough was the development of ^{99m}Tc-labeled polyphosphate complexes by Subramanian and McAfee (1971). This made bone scanning possible on routine gamma cameras and thus for daily application in the clinic. Gamma cameras have been optimized for ^{99m}Tc, and a high-dose activity can be administered. These developments have led to the present important place of bone scintigraphy in clinical practice.

6.2 Radio-pharmaceuticals

6.2.1 Fluoride

Radioactive fluoride, $^{18}F^-$, is again used in clinical practice since PET systems have become available. The skeletal uptake is high, approximately 70%, and 25% is excreted in the urine by 6 h. The half-life of 109.8 min of $^{18}F^-$ is relatively short but permits transportation and reasonable imaging times. Thus, $^{18}F^-$ forms an excellent tracer to study the fluoride kinetics in the skeleton, and provides a method for absolute quantification of regional blood flow. The small solutes leave the capillaries in bone by passive free diffusion, and traverse through the fluid spaces to reach the osseous tissues. The uptake mechanism

C. Schiepers
Department of Molecular and Medical Pharmacology, UCLA School of Medicine, 10833 Le Conte Avenue, AR-144 CHS, Los Angeles, CA 90095-6942, USA

of fluoride is adsorption in the water shell around newly formed bone crystals, a process of minutes to hours. The exchange with hydroxyl ions of the hydroxyapatite in the bone matrix, i.e., the actual incorporation, takes days and, therefore, cannot be measured accurately with this tracer.

6.2.2 Technetium Complexes

Presently, labeled diphosphonates are the radiopharmaceuticals of choice for skeletal scintigraphy. In order to obtain stable chelated complexes, reducing agents ($SnCl_2$) are needed, which keep technetium in a low valence state so that binding occurs. Generally, the clearance from the vascular compartment is fast, with half-lives of 2–4 min. Peak uptake varies for the different agents but is usually approximately 1 h. The bone-to-background ratio also varies due to the different clearance and uptake rates of other tissues and, therefore, the maximum ratio occurs much later at 4–6 h. Patient convenience is an important factor as well. The combination of contrast, peak uptake, radionuclide decay, and practical issues results in optimal imaging 2–4 h after tracer administration. At this time approximately one third of the administered dose is bound to bone, one third is excreted in the urine, and the remainder is associated with other tissues, approximately 10% of which is bound to blood proteins.

Adverse reactions to the injection of the radiopharmaceutical are virtually non-existent. The reported incidents are usually related to other agents in the kits that are necessary for stabilization, e.g., pH buffers, reducing agents to keep technetium in a low valence state, and/or metabolites.

6.3 Methods

The image acquisition is based on scintillation detection (see Chap. 13). Several geometric configurations have been designed for nuclear imaging equipment. The standard gamma camera has one head, which can be tilted, angled, and moved to image patients in the supine, sitting, or standing position. In addition, whole-body scanning and tomographic imaging is possible. Due to the significantly lower photon flux in nuclear imaging compared with conventional radiography, acquisition duration is prolonged. Presently, gantries with two or three heads are available to shorten the acquisition duration. Varying angles between the camera heads are possible to execute specific protocols and accelerate the acquisition. Systems with detectors over the full 360° are the standard in PET, but not in conventional single-photon imaging. A feature of all tomographic systems in nuclear medicine is the simultaneous acquisition of multiple image planes.

6.3.1 Positron Imaging

The annihilation radiation of ^{18}F is readily detected with a positron camera. The PET systems are optimized for 511 keV and allow correction for attenuation effects. For a more detailed description of this methodology the reader is referred to Chaps. 13 and 14. PET is a tomographic technique that is truly quantitative, i.e., physiologic parameters such as bone blood flow and tracer uptake rate can be determined. A detailed description of the various blood-flow-determination methods with $^{18}F^-$ are in the literature: quantitative with a gamma camera (Charkes 1980), based on whole-body clearance (Wootton et al. 1976, 1981), and with PET (Hawkins et al. 1992).

In general, a transmission scan is necessary to correct for attenuation effects and a dynamic emission scan of 1 h to measure fluoride uptake. The initial framing or sampling rate needs to be high, of the order of 4–6 frames/s, to measure bone blood flow accurately. Arterial blood sampling is recommended to measure the clearance of fluoride from the vascular compartment. However, a large vascular structure in the field of view, e.g., heart, aorta, or major vessel, offers the possibility of measuring the vascular clearance with the PET scanner and sophisticated processing techniques such as factor analysis (Schiepers et al. 1997b, 1998b).

6.3.2 Single-Photon Imaging

The photopeak of 140 keV of ^{99m}Tc is ideal for the sodium iodide detector of a gamma camera, and allows for administration of high doses, e.g., 700–900 MBq of ^{99m}Tc. There is no special patient preparation for a bone scan. After tracer administration, the patient is advised to drink plenty of fluids and to void frequently; thus, excretion of tracer is enhanced and the radiation dose to the bladder minimized. Before scanning, the patient is asked to urinate. Patients need to be instructed about possible contamination because of tracer in the urine. Various protocols are available and imaging can be accomplished in several modes: static, dynamic, or whole body. In addition, tomography can be performed with a dedicated system.

The movement of tracer immediately after the injection can be followed with flow imaging, or radionuclide angiography. Hereafter the tracer disperses in the extracellular space, the so-called second phase or blood-pool phase. After an interval of 2–3 h, the delayed phase of bone scintigraphy is performed; thus, this protocol has been named "three-phase bone imaging." For the flow phase, images of 2- to 4-s duration are acquired for a total time of 60–90 s. According to Fogelman (1993; Ryan and Fogelman 1995) the blood-pool phase needs to be completed within 10 min in order to limit the contribution of bony uptake. The delayed images are usually recorded with high resolution, i.e., pixel size of 3–4 mm.

In the static mode, images are acquired during a "steady state" of the tracer distribution throughout the body. The standard available options of zooming and acquisition of spot views under specific angles, e.g., anterior or posterior oblique, can be attempted if a certain area needs to be inspected in detail. The bladder remains a problem, since urine is being produced continuously during scanning. Most institutions will mount low energy, high-resolution collimators, and preferably ultra-high resolution for tomography, since physicians like high-resolution images. Currently, cameras have a wide field of view, allowing for whole-body scans and spot view that comprise the entire width of the body. This has the advantage that uptake between body parts can be compared directly, in addition to the standard left/right comparison.

Previously, pinhole images were recommended in case high magnification was needed, e.g., evaluation of the caput femoris in osteo-necrosis. With the currently available equipment, this is no longer necessary. Camera sensitivity and resolution have been improved and a zoomed image (1.5 to 4 times) of the area of interest, with a corresponding increase in acquisition time, suffices. It is important to note that the information density is the relevant parameter here. In other words, if the zoom is 2, the imaged area of the object is only a quarter of the original matrix (both x and y dimensions are cut by half). Therefore, the acquisition duration needs to be increased by a factor of 4 in order to maintain the information density, i.e., acquire the same number of counts per pixel.

Whole-body imaging is the routine in most nuclear medicine clinics. The patient is scanned in posterior and anterior views. This can be accomplished by passing the patient through the camera gantry or by moving the detector over the patient on a stationary bed. Special dual-head camera systems have been developed to image both sides in a single pass. This protocol is ideal for screening purposes, e.g., in oncology, and additional spot views of suspicious areas may be acquired later.

Tomographic sections of a certain body part can be reconstructed with single photon emission computed tomography (SPECT). This is available only for the delayed phase, since emission tomography assumes an equilibrium distribution of the radioactivity in the body. Tomography greatly enhances contrast and eliminates superimposed activity by providing three-dimensional images, i.e., in axial, coronal, and sagittal planes. An additional requirement is patient immobility compliance. Whereas PET traditionally has full 360° acquisition, SPECT utilizes a rotating gantry. Currently, single, dual-, and triple-head systems are available. With more camera heads the acquisition can be shortened, greatly enhancing patient convenience and throughput. The best results are obtained with a 360° acquisition, 128×128 matrix for high resolution, 3–6° angular steps, and 20–30 s per view. This results in a 30- to 45-min total acquisition time for a single-head camera, which is tolerable for most patients, but a multi-head system is preferable for a clinically acceptable time.

6.4 Image Interpretation

Knowledge of normal uptake in the skeleton is mandatory. This experience is usually gained through training and interpreting sessions with experts. Fortunately, skeletal scintigraphy is a routine procedure, so that each practicing specialist can easily get acquainted and become proficient. Normal variants, however, can be tricky and many an atlas is devoted to these.

The first step is to check for focal or diffuse abnormalities, i.e., areas of increased and/or decreased uptake. The next step is to compare left and right. In pediatric patients the growth plates are active, which translates into increased uptake. Additional information may be retrieved from the different phases, e.g., increased uptake during the flow phase, indicating hyperemia. Multi-phase imaging is important to differentiate increased uptake in the soft tissues from truly increased bone uptake.

A distinctive feature of bone scintigraphy is its high sensitivity to detect abnormalities such as fractures, infection, degenerative changes, metabolic bone disorders, and metastases, but the test is notoriously nonspecific. Many disease entities present with abnormal uptake on bone scan. However, certain patterns may favor one diagnosis over another. For instance, a linear array of hot spots in the rib cage suggests fractures. Multiple scattered areas of focally increased uptake are highly suspicious for metastatic disease. Slight to moderately increased uptake in a diffuse pattern in joints suggests degenerative changes, especially when it is also seen in neighboring joints. Common pitfalls are: patient rotation obscuring the symmetry; genito-urinary contamination; dental procedures or disease; and radio-pharmaceutical problems.

Clearly, the clinical context is important to determine the possibilities and limit the number of differential diagnoses. Image interpretation was purposely described first, since it is our policy to read the films "blind or blank" to gather all available information. Secondly, the clinical history, signs, and symptoms are added and a final report dictated. This sequence prevents omissions and increases the likelihood that the majority of differential diagnoses are included.

Last, but not least, correlative imaging has to be performed (Pomeranz et al. 1994, Ryan and Fogelman 1995). It is impossible to provide the referring physician with adequate information if the bone scan is not interpreted in conjunction with other image modalities, i.e., conventional radiography, CT, MR, or US. Specialized procedures are usually done after the bone scan, guided by the detected abnormalities. In most cases correlative interpretation of the results of all imaging modalities provides the diagnosis.

6.5 Selected Clinical Applications

6.5.1 Positron Imaging with ^{18}F-Fluoride

Positron emission tomography systems have become more available in the 1990s, making high-resolution imaging and quantitation possible. The quantitative indications are the measurement of local bone blood flow and fluoride influx rate. ^{18}F-fluoride kinetics of vertebrae has been studied in the healthy human male (Schiepers et al. 1990, Hawkins et al. 1992), as well as in metabolic bone disease such as osteoporosis and Paget's disease (Schiepers et al. 1991, 1997a; Ryan and Fogelman 1995). Bone remodeling is closely related to bone blood flow as shown by tetracycline labeling (Reeve et al. 1988); thus, the flow and fluoride influx in bone may be measured non-invasively with PET. One of the applications is the evaluation of bone graft viability (Berding et al. 1995). The applicability of ^{18}F-fluoride PET in clinical practice has been dealt with elsewhere (Schiepers 1993).

An example of a sagittal plane of an upper torso scan with fluoride is shown in Fig. 6.1 with a set of corresponding transverse slices at the levels indicated. Note the exquisite detail and high resolution obtained.

6.5.2 Oncology

Skeletal scintigraphy with technetium complexes is indicated for screening purposes in various cancers, such as prostate and breast. The intent here is to detect

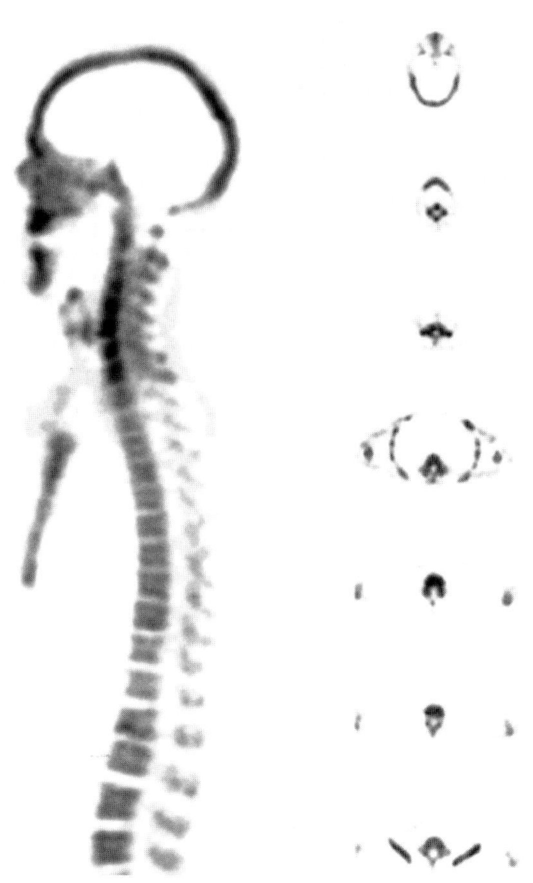

Fig. 6.1. Fluoride positron emission tomography (PET) scan of a 28-year-old man with juvenile osteoporosis. Sagittal plane of the torso of a volumetric data set acquired with a 2D PET system 1 h after administration of 300 MBq of ^{18}F-fluoride. Corresponding axial slices of the head, jaw, neck, thoracic and lumbar spine, and pelvis are given on the *right*. Note the increased uptake in the superior and inferior aspects of thoracic and lumbar vertebrae

occurrence and extent of malignant disease, presenting as hot or sometimes cold spots. The whole-body mode is ideal for surveying the skeleton and is superior to conventional radiography. Since the study is not very specific and in some malignancies the number of false positives exceeds that of true positives, a combination of scintigraphy and radiography is necessary. For the spine, especially vertebrae, MR imaging is recommended to confirm presence of absence of bone metastases. A logical decision tree of imaging modalities may be developed as fits the individual laboratory and/or health system (POMERANZ et al. 1994). In the past decade, referrals for metastasis screening have dropped, since the yield of bone scanning in the early stages of cancer has been shown to be low.

In general, bone metastases reveal increased uptake (BROWN et al. 1993). Since the metastases are usually located in the bone marrow, it is not the metastasis itself that is seen on the bone scan, but the reaction of the bone to the expanding malignant bone marrow. In highly aggressive and fast expanding tumors, therefore, the lesions are cold, since there is not enough time for the bone to respond and the regional bone blood flow may be jeopardized to such extent that the tracer cannot be delivered. Cold lesions have been reported for leiomyosarcoma, ductal breast cancer, and multiple myeloma. The feasibility of whole-body imaging with ^{18}F-fluoride in oncological disorders was reported by HOH et al. (1993). Just as in single-photon bone imaging, there was considerable overlap between uptake in benign and malignant lesions. Given the difference in costs, single-photon imaging with technetium complexes will remain the test of choice for screening of bone metastases.

Of considerable clinical interest is the probability of a solitary lesion on the bone scan to be benign. Widely varying frequencies have been reported: 15–35% in the patient without malignancy, between 40–80% in patients with known malignancy (BROWN et al. 1993). Lesion distribution is sometimes important. In breast cancer, distant metastasis is rare in the absence of lesions in the thorax, i.e., ribs, sternum, and thoracic spine (GOLDFARB et al. 1998).

Primary bone tumors generally show a very high uptake. Bone scintigraphy is indicated to evaluate the extent of disease and screening for metastases. Monitoring of therapy response is no indication since the bone scan remains positive for a long time. ^{201}Tl-chloride or ^{18}F-FDG (fluoro-deoxy-glucose) are better radio-pharmaceuticals for this purpose. Skeletal scintigraphy is useful in diagnosis and screening of osteogenic sarcoma, Ewing's sarcoma, and chondrosarcoma.

An interesting finding is the so-called flare phenomenon, an increasing uptake in lesions and skeleton after initiation of chemotherapy, hemi-body radiation, or high-dose radionuclide therapy. In general, this is related to the response of affected bone to the therapeutic agents and is usually associated with a therapeutic effect.

6.5.3 Infection and Inflammation

In case of osteomyelitis, a three-phase bone scan is performed with increased flow to the affected area in the acute stage. The blood pool is also increased and the delayed images (third phase) show abnormal uptake in the bone, which further increases at 24-h imaging (fourth phase). In case the initial increased uptake decreases in time and appears not to affect the bones, a diagnosis of soft tissue disease, such as cellulitis, may be established. The indication of the bone scan is to demonstrate involvement in the bone. If the test is negative, osteomyelitis is unlikely; if it is positive, further work-up is indicated with an infection survey, i.e., gallium, labeled immunoglobulins, or white blood cells (WBC), which are dealt with in Chap. 7. Alternately, an MR of the affected area may be performed to check for bone marrow edema.

6.5.4 Orthopedics

The bone scan is very sensitive in detecting trauma and, in general, is positive 1–2 days after a traumatic bone event. Fractures show increased uptake up to 1 year in approximately two thirds of cases (COLLIER et al. 1993); therefore, monitoring of therapy is of less value.

Nuclear medicine in sports injuries is an emerging field, a trend that can be expected to continue. Stress fractures in athletes are not infrequent, and routine radiographic evaluation often provides negative or questionable results, especially in the early stages. Stress fractures are most common in the lower extremities, with running the reported cause in most cases. Ultrasound is a possible adjunct to physical examination. Stress fractures occur more frequently in female athletes than in males. A stress fracture is a fatigue fracture, related to repetitive stresses to normal bone (ANDERSON and GREENSPAN 1996). Accurate and timely diagnosis is required to prevent possible costly and disabling complications (REEDER et al.

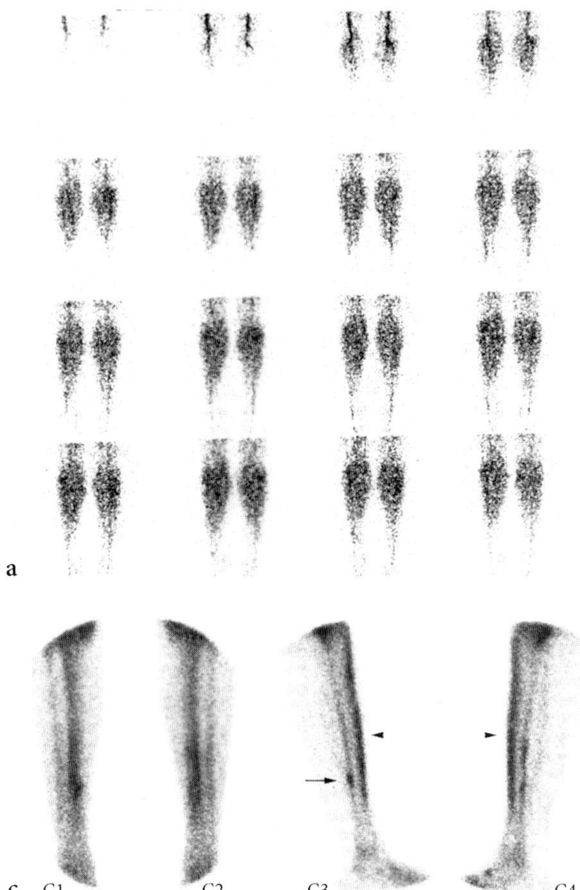

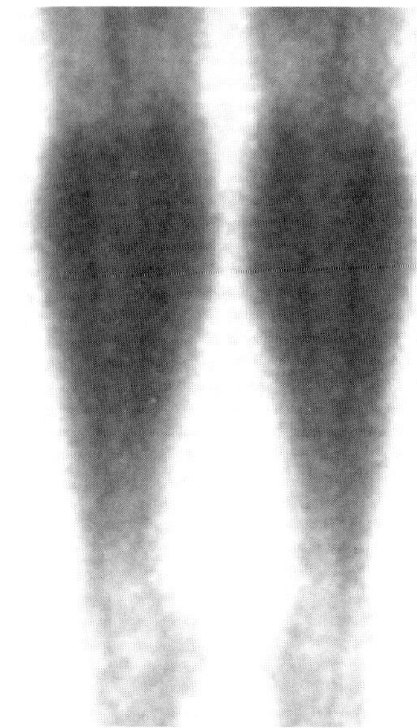

Fig. 6.2a–c. Three-phase bone scan of an 18-year-old woman involved in track and field, who complained of right-sided leg pain. **a** Flow or first phase in the anterior view, 3 s/image, without abnormality or asymmetry. **b** Anterior view of the blood pool or second phase. **c** Delayed or third phase: *C1* anterior right lower leg with focally increased uptake (*arrow*); *C2* anterior left leg; *C3* medial view of the left leg with a stress fracture in the posterior tibia (*arrow*), and shin splints in the anterior tibia (*arrowhead*); *C4* medial view of the right leg with shin splints (*arrowhead*)

1996). Bone scintigraphy is indicated to differentiate stress fractures from shin splints or peri-ostitis. In shin splints there is micro-trauma to the bone, which still has a sufficient reparative ability and healing response, whereas in a stress fracture there is a "critical mass" of injured bone leading to mechanical failure. Since the therapy is so different for these entities, i.e., decreasing but continuing exercise at a lower level in shin splints and "active-rest" plus immobilization in stress fractures, it is important to make the correct diagnosis. In Fig. 6.2 a three-phase bone scan of a young female athlete is shown, having both a shin splint and stress fracture.

A frequent referral for a bone scan is the loosening vs infection of an orthopedic prosthesis. Bone uptake is increased during the first year after prosthesis implantation (hip, knee, shoulder, or elbow implant). The time that the delayed scan is positive is somewhat longer for non-cemented than cemented prostheses, limiting the usefulness of skeletal scintigraphy during the first months after surgery (Rahmy et al. 1994). Increased uptake around the stem and tip usually heralds loosening. The differential diagnosis with infection has to be made by performing an infection survey with ^{67}Ga-citrate or labeled WBC and plain films. If the imaging findings are still inconclusive, addition of a colloid scan may be indicated to assess the presence and location of normal but displaced bone marrow (see Chap. 7).

The SPECT technique has provided new indications for bone scintigraphy. A routine referral is low back pain with normal radiographs. In case of negative planar scintigraphy, tomography needs to be performed to exclude facet syndrome of the spine, occult fracture, spondylolysis, or spondylolisthesis. Tomographic imaging is a real adjunct, because of the increased contrast and resolution and its ability to view the skeleton in 3D (Fig. 6.3). In patients with poorly localized or persistent bone pain, not satisfactorily explained with radiographic imaging, skeletal scintigraphy is helpful. In these situations, planar imaging of the whole body may reveal unsuspected traumatic pathology, and tomographic imaging may disclose small lesions. The SPECT technique is very helpful in delineating the lesion, e.g., in avascular necrosis, Legg-Calve-Perthes disease.

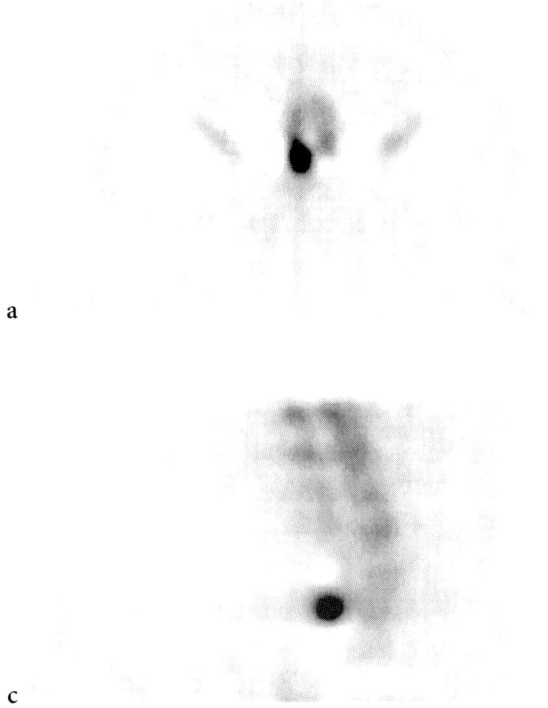

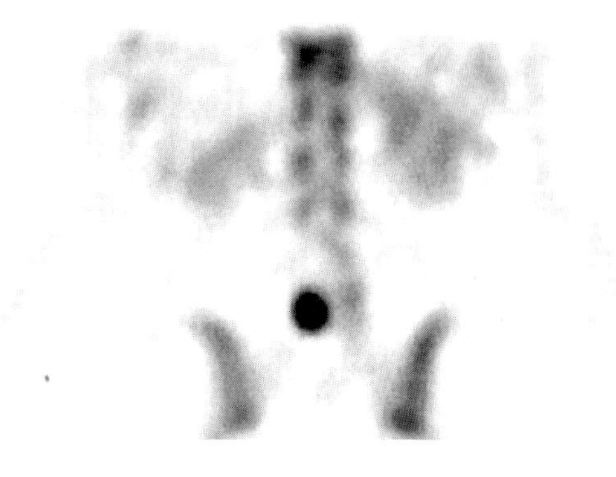

Fig. 6.3. a Transverse, **b** coronal, and **c** sagittal slices of a skeletal single photon emission computed tomography scan of a 39-year-old woman, complaining of low back pain. A focal hot spot is seen in the L5 vertebra, right aspect, consistent with a pars fracture

A role for PET in orthopedic nuclear medicine has yet to be defined. Osteonecrosis has been studied (SCHIEPERS et al. 1998c). In this preliminary study, the healing response of a unilaterally injured femoral head could be predicted. Skeletal flow and fluoride influx rate in the abnormal and normal hips were compared directly, and the relation to final outcome evaluated, i.e., surgical replacement or conservative treatment. A flow ratio of at least 2 between the abnormal and normal femoral head was necessary to predict a successful outcome with a conservative regimen. A minimum flow of 0.04 ml/min per milliliter was measured in a patient, whose affected femoral head healed conservatively. It was concluded that a highly technical procedure, such as PET, appeared feasible in clinical practice, and permitted prediction of outcome depending on regional skeletal flow measurements in vivo.

6.5.5 Vascular Bone Disorders

Reflex sympathetic dystrophy (RSD) is a disorder with a widely variable clinical presentation. The pathophysiology is not completely understood. The syndrome is best described as an exaggerated response to injury due to an abnormal sympathetic reflex. Early and effectively treatment is important; otherwise, the prognosis is guarded, leading to significant disability with lasting socio-economic consequences.

Reflex sympathetic dystrophy is a complex entity which is characterized by increased flow in stage I (3–6 months), and the typical increased peri-articular uptake on the delayed scan. In stage II the flow is decreased. The contribution of scintigraphy in the diagnosis and therapy of upper extremity RSD has been reported previously (SCHIEPERS 1997, SCHIEPERS et al. 1998a), where the utility of dynamic scintigraphy was evaluated. Both the three-phase bone scan and vascular scan were used for diagnosis and staging. Bone scintigraphy was highly accurate in diagnosing RSD, and vascular scintigraphy was best for staging of RSD. Staging by bone and vascular scintigraphy was discordant in 25% of patients. Since the RSD stage determines the type of therapy, a combination of both studies is indicated in the work-up and monitoring of upper extremity RSD.

6.6 Conclusion

Skeletal scintigraphy, both as positron and single-photon imaging, is an extremely sensitive test to evaluate a large spectrum of abnormalities related to the skeleton. The study is non-specific, and other imaging modalities, i.e., plain radiography, CT, MR, and US, are usually necessary to reduce the number of diagnostic possibilities. The addition of sophisticated imaging modalities provides the opportunity of correlative imaging, which will yield the final diagnosis in the vast majority of patients.

For the foreseeable future the place of skeletal scintigraphy will remain the same. Clinical indications for quantitative imaging need to be investigated further. In single-photon imaging, new tracers will be developed with faster uptake and/or clearance from the vascular compartment; thus, the delay of hours between tracer administration and imaging may be shortened, enhancing patient convenience. New equipment may further increase spatial resolution, so that even smaller abnormalities can be detected (see Chap. 13). Development of specialized image reconstruction and processing techniques will produce higher contrast in tomograms and improve image quality (see Chap. 14).

References

Anderson MW, Greenspan A. Stress fractures. Radiology 1996; 199:1–12

Berding G, Burchert W, van den Hoff J, et al. Evaluation of the incorporation of bone grafts used in maxillofacial surgery with [^{18}F]fluoride ion and dynamic positron emission tomography. Eur J Nucl Med, 1995; 22:1133–1140

Blau M, Nagler W, Bender MA. Fluorine-18: A new isotope for bone scanning. J Nucl Med 1962; 3:332–334

Brown ML, Collier BD, Fogelman I. Bone scintigraphy. Part 1: Oncology and infection. J Nucl Med 1993; 34:2236–2240

Charkes ND. Skeletal blood flow: implications for bone scan interpretation. J Nucl Med 1980; 21:91–98

Collier BD, Fogelmann I, Brown ML. Bone scintigraphy. Part 2: Orthopedic bone scanning, J Nucl Med 1993; 34:2241–2246

Fogelmann I, Collier BD, Brown ML. Bone scintigraphy. Part 3: bone scanning in metabolic bone disease. J Nucl Med 1993; 34:2247–2252

Goldfarb CR, Ongseng FO, Finestone H, Szakacs GM, Guelfguat M, Jonas D. Distribution of skeletal metastases in patients with breast carcinoma. J Nucl Med 1998; 39:114P

Hawkins RA, Choi Y, Huang SC, et al. Evaluation of the skeletal kinetics of ^{18}F-fluoride ion with PET. J Nucl Med 1992; 33:633–642

Hoh CK, Hawkins RA, Dahlbom M, et al. Whole body skeletal imaging with [^{18}F]fluoride ion and PET. J Comput Assist Tomogr 1993; 17:34–41

Pomeranz SR, Pretorius HT, Ramsingh PS. Bone scintigraphy and multi-modality imaging in bone neoplasia: strategies for imaging in the new health care climate. Sem Nucl Med 1994; 24:188–207

Rahmy AI, Tonino AJ, Tan WD. Quantitative analysis of technetium-99m-methylene diphosphonate uptake in unilateral hydroxy-apatite-coated total hip prostheses: first year of follow-up. J Nucl Med 1994; 35:1788–1791

Reeder MT, Dick BH, Atkins JK, Pribis AB, Martinez JM. Stress fractures. Current concepts of diagnosis and treatment. Sports Med 1996; 22:198–212

Reeve J, Arlot M, Wootton R, et al. Skeletal blood flow, iliac histomorphometry, and strontium kinetics in osteoporosis: a relationship between blood flow and corrected apposition rate. J Clin Endocrinol Metab 1988; 66:1124–1131

Ryan PJ, Fogelmann I. The bone scan: Where are we now? Sem Nucl Med 1995; 25:76–91

Schiepers C. Skeletal fluoride kinetics of ^{18}F$^-$ and positron emission tomography (PET): in vivo estimation of regional bone blood flow and influx rate in humans in bone circulation and vascularization in normal and pathological conditions. In: Schoutens et al. (eds) Plenum Press, New York, 1993, pp 95–101

Schiepers CWJ, Hawkins RA, Choi Y, et al. Kinetics of bone metabolism assessed with ^{18}F$^-$ and PET. Eur J Nucl Med 1990; 16:450

Schiepers C, Geusens P, Vleugels S, et al. Positron emission tomography (PET) with ^{18}F– to evaluate metabolic rate in bone disorders. J Mineral Bone Res 1991; 6:S243

Schiepers C. Clinical value of dynamic bone and vascular scintigraphy in diagnosing reflex sympathetic dystrophy of the upper limb. In: Cooney WP, Schuind F (eds) Hand clinics, post-traumatic upper extremity RSD. Saunders, Philadelphia, 1997, pp 423–429

Schiepers C, Nuyts J, Bormans G, Dequeker J, Bouillon R, Mortelmans L, Verbruggen A, De Roo M. Fluoride kinetics of the axial skeleton measured in-vivo with positron emission tomography (^{18}F-PET): initial experience in metabolic bone disease. J Nucl Med 1997a; 38:1970–1976

Schiepers C, Wu HM, Nuyts J, Dahlbom M, Hoh CK, Huang SC, Phelps ME. Fluoride PET: Is non-invasive quantitation feasible with factor analysis? J Nucl Med 1997b; 38:93P

Schiepers C, Bormans I, De Roo M. Three-phase bone scan and dynamic vascular scintigraphy in algo-neuro-dystrophy of the upper extremity. Acta Orthop Belg 1998a; 64:322–327

Schiepers C, Hoh CK, Wu HM, Dahlbom M, Phelps ME. Factor analysis for generation of input functions replaces blood sampling in tracer kinetic modeling. J Nucl Med 1998b; 39:206P

Schiepers C, Broos P, Miserez M, Bormans G, De Roo M. Measurement of skeletal flow with positron emission tomography and F-18 fluoride in femoral head osteonecrosis. Arch Orthop Trauma Surg 1998c; 118:131–135

Subramanian G, McAfee JF. A new complex of ^{99m}Tc for skeletal imaging, Radiology 1971; 99:192–198

Van Dyke D, Anger HO, Yano Y, Bozzini C. Bone blood flow shown with ^{18}F and the positron camera. Am J Physiol 1965; 209:65–70

Wootton R, Reeve J, Veall N. The clinical measurement of skeletal blood flow. Clin Sci Mol Med 1976; 50:261–268

Wootton R, Tellez M, Green JR, Reeve J. Skeletal blood flow in Paget's disease of bone. Metab Bone Dis Rel Res 1981; 4:263–270

7 Imaging Infection and Inflammation

W. BECKER

CONTENTS

7.1 Introduction 103
7.7.1 Infection vs Inflammation 103
7.1.2 Clinical Signs and Pathophysiology of Inflammation and Infection 103
7.1.3 Acute Inflammation and Infection 103
7.1.4 Chronic Inflammation and Infection 104
7.1.5 Pathophysiological Aspects of Imaging Infection 104
7.2 Radiopharmaceuticals and Clinical Indications 105
7.2.1 ^{67}Ga-citrate 106
7.2.2 ^{99m}Tc Nanocolloids 107
7.2.3 ^{111}In-Labeled Autologous Leukocytes 108
7.2.4 ^{99m}Tc-HMPAO-Labeled Leukocytes 109
7.2.5 ^{99m}Tc-Labeled Antigranulocyte Antibodies 110
7.2.6 ^{111}In-Labeled HIG 112
7.2.7 ^{99m}Tc-Labeled HIG 113
7.2.8 ^{18}F-FDG 114
7.3 Summary and Recommendations 114
7.4 Future Prospects 116

7.1 Introduction

Nuclear medicine imaging provides information on changes in pathophysiological and pathobiochemical processes in the patient, whereas morphologically based imaging provides information with high resolution on the structural changes which occur in a specific process. Nuclear medicine imaging is available as whole-body imaging in routine clinical practice, whereas computed tomography (CT), magnetic resonance (MR) imaging, and other techniques provide information on one part of the body.

For the localization of an infectious process a nuclear medicine procedure needs high sensitivity in all areas of the body. A typical example is fever of unknown origin. After the localization of an infection or inflammation, further investigations such as CT, MR, biopsy, and culture are necessary. For the differential diagnosis of inflammation or infection, i.e., after a surgical procedure, when the surgeon needs information on whether to reoperate or to administer conservative treatment, infection specific methods are necessary.

W. BECKER
Department of Nuclear Medicine, University of Göttingen, Robert-Koch-Strasse 40, D-37075 Göttingen, Germany

7.1.1 Infection vs Inflammation

The differentiation of infection and inflammation is very important for the clinician in many situations. The clinical symptoms are similar. Infection means contamination with microorganisms. It is very important to keep in mind that there can be infection without inflammation, e.g., in immunosuppressed patients. On the other hand, inflammation can exist without infection when the reaction of tissues is triggered by tissue injury without bacterial contamination. Inflammation can also be triggered by traumatic injury, ischemia, neoplasms, foreign particles, and autoimmune diseases.

7.1.2 Clinical Signs and Pathophysiology of Inflammation and Infection

The clinical signs of inflammation, such as calor, rubor, tumor, and dolor, were described by Celsus (30 B.C.–50 A.D.), together with a reduced function of the infected part of the body (*functio laesa*) by Galen (131–200 A.D.). These clinical signs are based on and are a product of a cascade of different mechanisms.

7.1.3 Acute Inflammation and Infection

Acute inflammation is characterized by hyperemia, increased vascular permeability with exudation of proteins, and migration of leukocytes. Hyperemia and vascular permeability is induced by the release of histamine by mast cells and basophils, and of serotonin by platelets.

These products also induce upregulation of the expression of the adhesion molecule P-selectin and platelet activating factor (PAF) on the endothelial cells. Neutrophils respond to these inflammatory stimuli and adhere to endothelial surfaces, an event mediated by cell-surface glycoproteins (non-specific cross-reacting antigen) and on the epithelial side by adhesion molecules expressed there. Activation of neutrophils makes them more responsive to chemotactic agents. Under the influence of the complement factor C5a and leukotriene B4, the neutrophils then migrate to sites of infection or inflammation. As a consequence, the kinin and plasmin systems get involved. Besides these substances, vasoactive peptides, such as vasoactive intestinal peptide (VIP) and substance P, play a role in the onset of the inflammatory response. Onset of inflammation is also triggered by exogenous mediators including the bacterial chemotactic product formyl-methionyl-leucyl-phenylalanine (fMet-Leu-Phe) and endotoxin, a product of gram-negative bacteria which induces macrophages to secrete cytokines. Neutrophils sense these substances in nanomolar concentrations and migrate toward them with directed movement. This migration of granulocytes out of the circulation is preceded shortly before by increased blood flow and capillary permeability.

Vasodilatation and increased permeability is also induced by prostaglandins. Macrophages secrete interleukin-1 (Il-1) and tumor necrosis factor. Also, E-selectin as an adhesion molecule is upregulated on the endothelial cells. Moreover Il-8, neutrophil-activating peptide-2, platelet factor 4, and other factors are known to play a role in these processes.

7.1.4 Chronic Inflammation and Infection

In chronic inflammation, macrophages, lymphocytes, and plasma cells dominate, whereas hyperemia and vascular permeability are less pronounced. The definition of a chronic inflammation means that inflammation has been present for weeks or months. It may follow a severe acute inflammatory phase if an inflammatory agent persists either because of its resistance to metabolic breakdown or through the inability of the body to clear the microorganisms. The immune response is modulated by various cytokines as well as interleukin-2 and peptides such as somatostatin and substance P.

7.1.5 Pathophysiological Aspects of Imaging Infection

All nuclear medicine procedures use one single step of the infection cascade, i.e., a specific part of the host defense mechanism, to demonstrate all the typical phenomena in infectious disease. Host defense mechanisms may be categorized as non-specific or specific. Non-specific responses protect against a wide range of infectious agents, whereas specific responses are directed against one particular microorganism (Woods et al. 1993).

Specific infection imaging directed against one particular microorganism has been described with a radiolabeled monoclonal antibody against *Pneumocystis carinii*, with a reported sensitivity of 85.7% and a specificity of 86.7% (Goldenberg et al. 1994); however, this approach can only be used in a patient population with a high likelihood of having just one typical infectious agent.

The greatest problem for nuclear medicine imaging of infection is that everything works. This fact is well known to radiologists, who place their contrast agents always in areas of infection or inflammation, because every injected radiopharmaceutical localizes in the area of infection due to hyperemia and increased vascular permeability. The aim of nuclear medicine imaging, on one hand, has to be to find non-specific radiopharmaceuticals, with the best target to background ratio. This means defining particles with an optimal size for leaving the circulation in a large number and small enough to guarantee a rapid excretion. On the other hand, nuclear medicine has to de-

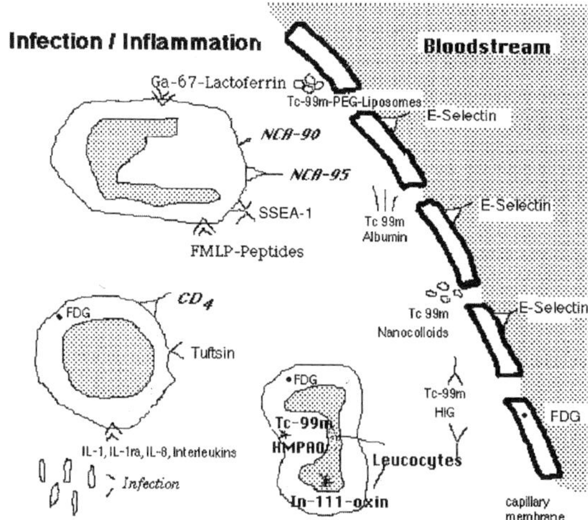

Fig. 7.1. Different radiopharmaceuticals for the detection of intermediate steps in the inflammation cascade, and the pathophysiology of their uptake mechanism

velop highly specific radiopharmaceuticals which target a specific antigen or receptor in the cascade of inflammation or infection (Fig. 7.1).

7.2 Radiopharmaceuticals and Clinical Indications

The available radiopharmaceuticals are discussed in detail herein (see Table 7.1). The commercial availability of different radiopharmaceuticals in various countries and continents is different. In the last section of this chapter, where future prospects are discussed, all of the new developments are mentioned.

The decision to perform a specific infection or inflammation scan always has to be based on the clinical situation; however, biodistribution of the radiopharmaceutical, radiation exposure (Table 7.2), and diagnostic accuracy data from the literature influence this decision. For example, the higher radiation dose of ^{67}Ga citrate or ^{111}In-oxine labeled leukocytes limit their use to special clinical situations; therefore, a sus-

Table 7.1. Routinely available radiopharmaceuticals for imaging infectious diseases. *HIG* human immunoglobulin; *WBC* white blood cells, leukocytes; *HMPAO* hexamethyl propyleneamine oxime

Radiopharmaceutical	Physical characteristics		Uptake mechanism
	Half-life (h)	Energy (keV)	
^{67}Gallium-citrate	78	93, 185, 300, 394	Transferrin receptor binding, lactoferrin receptor binding
^{99m}Tc-nanocolloids	6	140	Non-specific via capillary permeability/ active uptake in activated endothelial cells
^{99m}Tc-HIG	6	140	Non-specific via increased capillary permeability
^{111}In-HIG	67	173, 247	
^{111}In-oxine WBC	67	173, 247	Specific chemotactic activation
^{99m}Tc-HMPAO WBC	6	140	Specific chemotactic activation
^{99m}Tc-labeled granulocyte antibodies	6	140	Increased capillary permeability and specific binding or uptake as antibody-labeled granulocytes

Table 7.2. Estimated radiation dose after injection of various routinely available radiopharmaceuticals to detect infection and inflammation

Radiopharmaceutical	Dose (MBq)	Effective dose equivalent (mSv/dose)	Reference
^{67}Gallium-citrate	220	27	ICRP (1987)
^{99m}Tc-nanocolloids	370	–	–
^{99m}Tc-HIG	370	3	Saptogino et al. (1991)
^{111}In-HIG	75	15	Buijs et al. (1990)
^{111}In-labeled leukocytes	25	15	ICRP (1987)
^{99m}Tc-HMPAO leukocytes	370	6	ICRP (1987)
^{99m}Tc-labeled granulocyte antibodies	370	3.9	Joseph et al. (1988)

Table 7.3. Whole-body distribution of radiopharmaceuticals for imaging infectious lesions (qualitative overview)

Radiopharmaceutical	Liver	Spleen	Kidneys	Bladder	Bowel	Bone marrow	Blood
^{67}Gallium-citrate	Yes	Yes	Yes	Yes	Yes	Yes	No
^{99m}Tc-nanocolloids	Yes	Yes	yes	Yes	No	Yes	No
^{99m}Tc-HIG	Yes	Yes	Yes	Yes	Yes/no	No	Yes
^{111}In-HIG	Yes	Yes	Yes	Yes	Yes/no	Yes	Yes
^{111}In-labeled leukocytes (24 h)	Yes	Yes	No	No	No	Yes	no
^{99m}Tc-HMPAO-labeled leukocytes	Yes	Yes	Yes	Yes	Yes	Yes	no
^{99m}Tc-labeled granulocyte antibodies (24 h)	Yes	Yes	Yes	Yes	No	Yes	no

pected pneumonia is an indication for ^{67}Ga citrate, because other radiopharmaceuticals do not show pneumonia. Also important is the biodistribution of a radiopharmaceutical. If an infection of a transplanted kidney is suspected, we have to use a tracer without renal excretion (Table 7.3), and only ^{111}In-oxine-labeled leukocytes can be considered (Becker 1995).

7.2.1 ^{67}Ga-citrate

7.2.1.1 *Physics and Biodistribution*

^{67}Ga-citrate is a cyclotron-generated radiopharmaceutical with emission of gamma rays over a broad range of 93–388 keV, with dominant energies of 93, 184, 296, and 388 keV. The physical half-life is 78 h.

Physiologically, 10–25% of the nuclide is excreted via the kidneys over the first 24 h, but thereafter the principal route of excretion is the colon. At 48 h after injection approximately 75% of the injected dose remains in the body and is equally distributed among the liver, bone and bone marrow, and soft tissues (Hoffer 1980). This distribution predefines for many organs the indications for imaging. Organs with a high physiological uptake of ^{67}Ga-citrate may be better examined with other radiopharmaceuticals.

7.2.1.2 *Uptake Mechanism*

Leukocytes at the site of inflammation or infection excrete some of their intracellular lactoferrin, which remains localized and bound to macrophages. ^{67}Ga citrate is transported either in ionic form or bound to transferrin, and may leak through the vascular epithelium at the site of infection, where it is then bound to lactoferrin. Another mechanism might be the production, by microorganisms grown in a low iron environment, of siderophores that have a binding affinity for iron as well as for gallium: Because of a lack of freely available iron, ^{67}Ga citrate may be transported directly into the cell in its place.

7.2.1.3 *Clinical Indications*

^{67}Ga-citrate entails high radiation exposure, is not routinely available in the clinic, and has unfavorable physical characteristics for gamma camera imaging. These features, combined with the availability of ^{99m}Tc-labeled radiopharmaceuticals for imaging infections, limit the use of ^{67}Ga citrate to certain indications such as fever of unknown origin, chronic osteomyelitis of the spine, and lung infections, especially in immunocompromised patients.

The diagnosis fever of unknown origin is restricted to patients who have an elevated temperature (>38.8°C) for 2–3 weeks and in whom the cause of fever cannot be ascertained despite intensive investigations (Petersdorf and Beeson 1961). These rigid criteria eliminate obvious bacterial and viral infections, those in whom the diagnosis becomes more obvious with the passage of time and those whose fever is due to a non-infectious cause. However, it does not exclude all patients suffering from an infectious disease who have prolonged fever. In different studies in which a total of 647 patients with fever of unknown origin were examined, the mean percentage with an infectious origin was found to be 32.7% (Petersdorf and Beeson 1961; Shoen and von Ommen 1963; Frayha and Uwaydah 1973; Howard et al. 1977; Larson et al. 1982; Knockaert et al. 1992). It is well known that ^{67}Ga-citrate has a high sensitivity but a low specificity in the diagnosis of infection. This is necessary in fever of unknown origin patients, because a lesion first needs to be detected and then can be diagnosed by other methods such as biopsy. The low specificity also allows the detection of neoplasms or, sometimes, collagen vascular diseases, which subsequently may be further examined using more specific methods.

The results of white blood cell imaging (Palestro et al. 1991), immunoscintigraphy (Reuland et al. 1991; Hotze et al. 1992; Sciuk et al. 1991), and ^{99m}Tc-HIG imaging of infections are not very satisfactory in patients with suspected vertebral osteomyelitis. This is not easy to explain, but it may be that a very high pressure in the disk with chronic infection prevents proteins and granulocytes from migrating to the infection focus during the available imaging time. The data are limited, but ^{67}Ga-citrate may be superior to labeled leukocyte, antibody, and immunoglobulin imaging for vertebral osteomyelitis, although it is less specific and shows tumors as well.

In general, chest radiograph and sputum cultures are easily obtainable and verify most suspected respiratory infections. Radionuclide studies are not of wide importance in this area, because white blood cells, antibodies, and immunoglobulins fail to demonstrate pneumonia with high accuracy. It is within this context that ^{67}Ga-citrate has come to play a role in the diagnosis of AIDS-related respiratory disease.

Lymph node uptake of ^{67}Ga-citrate is a frequent finding in HIV-positive patients and may be identified virtually anywhere in the body (PALESTRO 1994). This is a characteristic finding in patients with *Mycobacterium tuberculosis* and lymphoma. Localized pulmonary uptake is more typical in the setting of bacterial pneumonia, whereas diffuse pulmonary uptake may be caused by *Pneumocystis carinii* pneumonia, *cytomegalovirus* pneumonia, interstitial pneumonia, and pneumonitis (PALESTRO 1994). A negative scan presents strong evidence against an infectious process.

The use of ^{67}Ga-citrate in patients with sarcoidosis is well known. ^{67}Ga-citrate is able to provide staging of the disease activity.

In summary, major indications for ^{67}Ga-citrate are fever of unknown origin, chronic infections, such as tuberculosis and sarcoidosis, chronic spondylodiscitis, and pneumonia.

7.2.2 ^{99m}Tc-Nanocolloids

7.2.2.1 Physics and Biodistribution

The physics of ^{99m}Tc as a generator product is well known, with its physical half-life of 6 h and 140-keV gamma energy. Moreover, it is always available in every nuclear medicine unit and results in a reasonable radiation exposure of the patient.

The biodistribution of ^{99m}Tc-nanocolloids has been studied extensively in the rat model (MCAFEE et al. 1991). The blood activity within the time relevant for imaging decreases from 3.4% (30 min) to 1.8% (1 h) to 0.5% (3 h) of the injected dose; in the liver over the same period it decreases from 72.4 to 68.7 to 52.5%, but for the bone marrow the figures are 14.5, 12.5, and 12.4%, respectively. Consequently, this radiopharmaceutical can also be used for bone marrow imaging. After the active uptake in the reticuloendothelial system, the nanocolloids are lysosomally degraded and 54.5% are renally excreted after 24 h.

7.2.2.2 Uptake Mechanism

Approximately 86% of these particles are 30 nm in diameter or smaller and the remainder are between 30 and 80 mm (DE SCHRIJVER et al. 1987). The passage of these inert particles into the pericapillary spaces and their subsequent accumulation is due to the increased permeability, induced by cytokines, of the capillary basal layer. Unlike macromolecules, the blood clearance is rapid, so that imaging may be completed within 2–4 h. Thereafter, the activity may appear in the gastrointestinal tract, probably from spontaneous oxidation to pertechnetate. The absolute concentration of ^{99m}Tc-nanocolloids is approximately 100 times lower than that of ^{111}In-labeled leukocytes, and the abscess/blood concentration ratios were also lower for ^{99m}Tc-nanocolloids than for other radiopharmaceuticals (MCAFEE et al. 1991). However, in these experimental studies measurements were performed 24 h after injection of the radiopharmaceuticals, which is an improper time for nanocolloids; clinically appropriate times are between 1 and 4 h following injection.

7.2.2.3 Clinical Indications

The main indications for nanocolloids are skeletal and joint infections and inflammations. Soft tissue and especially gastrointestinal infections cannot be diagnosed reliably (WHELLER et al. 1990), which is due perhaps to a slower uptake mechanism in soft tissues and also to a physiological excretion of ^{99m}Tc-degraded particles 4 h after injection.

To date, only a few studies have evaluated ^{99m}Tc-nanocolloids clinically in patients with osteomyelitis (STREULE et al. 1988; VAN DALEN et al. 1989; VORNE et al. 1989; HOTZE et al. 1988). The results indicate values similar to those of ^{111}In-labeled leukocytes, with sensitivities ranging from 87 to 95% and specificities between 77 and 100%. Consequently, some authors have concluded that ^{111}In-labeled leukocytes and ^{99m}Tc-nanocolloids are equivalent (STREULE et al. 1988). Another study (FLIVIK et al. 1988) calculated a sensitivity of 75% with ^{111}In-labeled leukocytes and 94% with ^{99m}Tc-nanocolloids and a specificity of 90 and 84%, respectively. Thus, their diagnostic accuracy was 85 and 87%, respectively. In this study the authors also calculated the sensitivity and specificity when patients with "slightly increased activity" were regarded as being negative. This resulted in a specificity of almost 100%. This "manipulation" or criterion adjustment seems necessary because ^{99m}Tc-nanocolloids are able to leave the circulation wherever the permeability is increased, independent of an infection or non-specific inflammation. The two subtypes of lesions cannot be separated, a fact which is true for most of the other imaging agents as well. The great advantage of these nanocolloids is rapid localization of an infectious process within 30–60 min, after which the study can be terminated.

^{99m}Tc-nanocolloids also work well in rheumatoid arthritis. In a study by LIBERATORE et al. (1992), 79% of all actively inflamed joints had a positive scan with ^{99m}Tc-nanocolloids, whereas 95% of all clinically negative joints had a negative scintigram. In comparing the ^{99m}Tc-nanocolloids to ^{99m}Tc-HIG, they found that the results with both radiopharmaceuticals were in agreement with clinical examinations; only in the initial phase of the disease did ^{99m}Tc-HIG seem to have some advantages.

In summary, the major indications for the nonspecific ^{99m}Tc-nanocolloids are osteomyelitis of the periphery of the skeleton and synovitis.

7.2.3
^{111}In-Labeled Autologous Leukocytes

7.2.3.1
Physics and Biodistribution

^{67}Ga citrate, one of the oldest radiopharmaceuticals for imaging infection, has a poor target-to-background ratio, needs 48- or 72-h images, has bowel excretion, and shows both infection and tumors. A much higher specificity has been demonstrated for ^{111}In-labeled autologous leukocytes (MCAFEE and THAKUR 1976). ^{111}In-, with its physical half-life of 67 h and 173- and 247-keV photopeaks, allows delayed imaging within 24 h and relatively efficient imaging with conventional gamma cameras.

The number of neutrophils that accumulate at sites of inflammation are extremely high: as many as 10% of the circulating neutrophils accumulate in such sites each day (SPECTOR et al. 1967).

Twenty-four hours after reinjection of ^{111}In oxine-labeled cells in dogs, 48.5% of the activity was in the liver, 11% in the spleen, 7.9% in the lungs, and 8.5% in the blood (MCAFEE et al. 1976). This biodistribution, which is similar to that in humans, suggests that the detection of splenic and liver, but also lung abscesses, may be difficult. However, there is no kidney, bladder, or bowel excretion; thus, the whole abdomen is an excellent field for localizing infectious or inflammatory diseases. Also, soft tissue infection in muscles is easily seen.

7.2.3.2
Cell Isolation and Labeling

^{111}In-oxine, ^{111}In-tropolonate, and ^{99m}Tc-hexamethyl propyleneamine oxime (HMPAO) have one common property, their lipophilicity; thus, ^{111}In labels all cell types indiscriminately. For this reason, the leukocytes must first be separated from other blood cells before labeling. In addition, subtypes of cells, such as lymphocytes and monocytes, can be separated and labeled. The labeling technique itself was first described by THAKUR et al (1977) and later, with many modifications, by other authors (BECKER et al. 1986; SAVERYMUTTU et al. 1981). Instead of oxine, other lipophilic agents, such as tropolonate (PETERS et al. 1983) and acetylacetone (SINN and SILVESTER 1979), may be used. Tropolonate-labeled cells especially perform better at early imaging times than oxine-labeled cells, although the difference between the cell kinetics is not uniformly accepted (DATZ 1994).

7.2.3.2.1
UPTAKE MECHANISMS AND PHYSIOLOGY
Neutrophils have a life cycle of 2 weeks (GOLDEN and CLINE 1977). Originating from stem cells in the bone marrow, mature neutrophils are released into the peripheral blood after 6–12 days. There they are distributed into two pools: approximately half of the cells are in the circulating pool and can be removed, whereas the other half are in the marginating pool, temporarily sequestered in capillaries or adhering to the endothelium of larger vessels. The cells can move between the two pools after physical exercise, epinephrine administration, and exposure to bacterial endotoxin. In all conditions, the cells migrate from the marginating to the circulating pool (ATHENS et al. 1961; WEIBLEN et al. 1979). In inflammatory or infectious diseases, the migration of leukocytes via chemotactic stimuli occurs as early as 30–40 min after stimulation of the neutrophils.

7.2.3.2.2
RADIATION EFFECTS
There are two primary sources of radiation to the leukocytes after ^{111}In-leukocyte labeling. The first is external radiation absorbed by the leukocytes during the labeling process itself when the cells are incubated. The second and more important source of radiation is internal, coming from the ^{111}In that is incorporated into the cells. Most of the internally derived dose comes from low-energy Auger electrons (0.6–25.4 keV); these have a range much less than the cell diameter, so that the radiation burden is ex-

tremely high, up to 14.8 Gy (BASSANO et al. 1979). Nevertheless, there is significant evidence that even in mixed-cell populations of leukocytes, labeled with 500 μCi of ^{111}In, the oncogenic risk to the patient is extremely low (THAKUR and MCAFEE 1984).

7.2.3.3
Clinical Indications

Although leukocyte scintigraphy is highly specific for leukocytic infiltration, which can be seen in many different disease entities from infections to tumors (OSWALD et al. 1989), it is not specific for bacterial contamination. Despite the latter fact, ^{111}In-labeled leukocytes have a variety of potential indications due to the high specificity for leukocytic infiltration. Their accuracy has been tested in detail in patients with chronic inflammatory bowel disease (SAVERYMUTTU et al. 1986; BECKER et al. 1986, 1988; FISCHBACH et al. 1991) or other intestinal infections (SAVERYMUTTU et al. 1983), osteomyelitis (MCCARTHY et al. 1988; PRING et al. 1991; PALESTRO et al. 1991), prosthetic valvular heart disease (BECKER et al. 1987; BORST et al. 1993), prosthetic vascular prostheses (VAN ROYEN et al. 1984; BECKER et al. 1987), kidney diseases (BECKER et al. 1986), lung infections (COOK et al. 1984; SAVERYMUTTU et al. 1985), and fever of unknown origin (MACSWEENEY et al. 1990; HAWKER et al. 1985).

Indium-111 is a cyclotron product with a long physical half-life and high radiation burden to the patient. In addition, ^{111}In emits medium energy photons, meaning that the resolution achieved with gamma-camera imaging is suboptimal; therefore, ^{111}In is not favored in clinical practice. Given the possibility of labeling leukocytes with ^{99m}Tc-HMPAO, there are only a few indications for which the use of ^{111}In is mandatory. These indications are related to the biodistribution and excretion of ^{99m}Tc-HMPAO leukocytes, which prevent the diagnosis of infection in the kidneys, the bladder or lower pelvis, and the gallbladder and gut, where 4- and 24-h images are necessary for the differentiation of segmental inflammation from abscess (THAKUR et al. 1977), and ^{99m}Tc-excretion occurs via these organs. For all other indications mentioned previously, ^{111}In-labeled granulocytes may be replaced by ^{99m}Tc-HMPAO-labeled leukocytes.

In summary, the major indications for ^{111}In-oxine-labeled leukocytes are kidney infections (Fig. 7.2), and for quantification of ^{111}In-oxine leukocytes excretion in the bowel in patients with bronchiectasis, or chronic inflammatory bowel disease (PETERS 1994).

7.2.4
^{99m}Tc-HMPAO-Labeled Leukocytes

7.2.4.1
Physics and Biodistribution

The physics of ^{99m}Tc is well known. Its advantages are the energy of 140 keV, the physical half-life of 6 h, availability, and cost. The only reliable and reproducible method is the ^{99m}Tc-HMPAO labeling of leukocytes. The baseline mechanism of ^{99m}Tc-HMPAO labeling is the lipophilicity of HMPAO, which allows the ^{99m}Tc- to enter the cells, which also have to be isolated before labeling.

Whereas ^{111}In is highly stable in all labeled cell types, ^{99m}Tc-HMPAO is not. In vitro we measured an elution of up to 7% of the label per hour out of labeled leukocytes (BECKER et al. 1988). As a consequence of this instability of ^{99m}Tc, bound secondary hydrophilic complexes of HMPAO are excreted via kidney and bladder starting several minutes after reinjection of the labeled cells. Gallbladder visualiza-

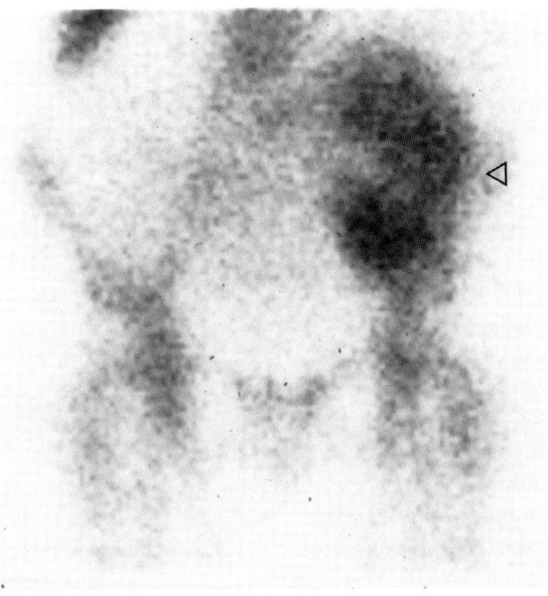

Fig. 7.2. A 49-year-old female with leukocytosis and fever after renal transplantation. ^{111}In-oxine leukocyte scan shows 3.5 h post injection a homogeneous infiltration in the transplanted kidney (*arrowhead*) with a leukocyte uptake index of 2 (normal <0.2) as a sign of transplant infection (proven with biopsy)

tion starts between 2 and 3 h after reinjection and small bowel routinely is seen 3 h after reinjection of the cells. These excretion pathways define the indications for ^{99m}Tc-HMPAO, which are all kinds of infectious diseases other than kidney, bladder and gallbladder infections, inflammatory bowel disease or abscesses with enteric communications, and the differential diagnosis between abscesses and segmental inflammation (BECKER et al. 1988; SAVERYMUTTU et al. 1985). Chronic inflammatory bowel disease is seen 30 min after reinjection of the cells. Thus, the localization of diseased segments can be performed before physiological excretion starts (BECKER et al. 1988).

7.2.4.2
Clinical Indications

Several reports document the superiority of ^{99m}Tc over ^{111}In in the management of inflammatory bowel disease (ARNDT et al. 1991; ALLAN et al. 1993). This is because of its ability to localize disease to specific bowel segments and its ability to identify small bowel disease reliably. The role of labeled white blood cells in chronic inflammatory bowel disease is the localization of diseased bowel segments in highly acute disease with the danger of perforation during endoscopy and in chronic disease with stenosis to localize the total number of diseased segments.

The use of ^{99m}Tc-HMPAO-labeled cells is also indicated for the diagnosis of complications, such as fistulas and abscesses, but only ^{111}In-labeled cells are useful for the quantification of disease activity (PETERS 1994). In the present author's experience, the sensitivity of ^{99m}Tc-HMPAO-labeled leukocytes in patients with osteomyelitis is comparable to that of ^{111}In-labeled leukocytes. Despite its higher resolution, ^{99m}Tc-HMPAO does not seem to be more accurate, because more often imaging of chronic osteomyelitis is necessary in cases in which late scans are required due to the limited granulocyte turnover. In addition, the problem of vertebral osteomyelitis with its usually reduced uptake of cells cannot be solved with ^{99m}Tc-HMPAO-labeled leukocytes. The reason why infection in the vertebrae is more difficult to confirm with labeled leukocytes and antibodies than infection in other areas of the axial skeleton with comparable bone marrow has not been satisfactorily explained. One may hypothesize that the high pressure in one infected vertebra prevents the granulocyte uptake or that the "coldness" of a vertebra is only relative due to the physiological bone marrow in the neighboring vertebral bodies.

Labeled leukocyte scanning has a relatively minor role in the management of patients with intrathoracic disease. Some reports indicate labeled leukocytes to be of use in patients with bronchiectatic lobes before surgery (CURRIE et al. 1987, 1990) and in patients with vasculitis (JONKER et al. 1992).

In patients with fever of unknown origin examination with ^{111}In-labeled leukocytes is probably preferable because of the greater stability in both circulating cells and targeted disease and because of the longer physical half-life; however, this remains to be proven clinically.

In summary, the use of ^{99m}Tc-HMPAO-labeled leukocytes is indicated in chronic inflammatory bowel disease, acute osteomyelitis of the peripheral bone, endocarditis, vascular prosthesis infections, and soft tissue infections.

7.2.5
^{99m}Tc-Labeled Antigranulocyte Antibodies

The advantage of immunoscintigraphy over autologous leukocyte techniques for imaging of infection is the simplicity of its use compared with techniques that require the isolation of autologous white blood cells.

7.2.5.1
Biodistribution

The widely available ^{99m}Tc-labeled antigranulocyte antibodies are directed against the non-specific cross-reacting antigen. The use of such an antibody against granulocytes was first reported by LOCHER et al (1986) with a ^{123}I-NCA-95 immunoglobulin (IgG1); shortly thereafter, JOSEPH et al (1987) reported use of ^{99m}Tc-labeled anti-NCA-95 antibody, which is now the most widely used antibody (Granuloscint, Behring, CIS Bio International, Gif Sur Yvette, France). Recently, we reported the use of a ^{99m}Tc-labeled anti-NCA-90-Fab fragment (BECKER et al. 1994). The antibody targeted epitope is expressed in humans only on granulocytes, promyelocytes, and myelocytes. The affinity constant of the ^{99m}Tc-antigranulocyte antibody (IgG1) BW 250/183 was calculated to be 2×10^9 M, of the Fab-fragment 8×10^8 M. Despite this strong binding capacity, the antibodies do not significantly influence granulocyte-mediated functions (BECKER et al. 1994).

7.2.5.2
Uptake Mechanism

Approximately 10–20% of the injected radiolabeled whole antibody is bound to circulating granulocytes that are functionally normal and may target an infectious area. Approximately 19% of the injected antibody circulates as free immunoglobulin and has the same potential as labeled non-specific human IgG (BECKER et al. 1994). From the fragment even more of the free antibody is available. This often causes problems in routine clinical practice, when inflammatory lesions, due to their increased capillary permeability, are seen, and reliable differentiation of inflammatory non-specific and granulocyte-associated specific uptake in a lesion is not possible. The current hypothesis on the uptake mechanism of radiolabeled monoclonal antigranulocyte whole antibody can be summarized as follows: (a) migration of antibody-labeled circulating granulocytes to the focus due to their undisturbed chemotactic behavior; and (b) non-specific, non-antigen-related uptake of free antibody due to an increased capillary permeability at the focus, with subsequent binding to granulocytes. The resulting image quality with high target-to-background ratios is due to the specific binding of high amounts of the injected antibodies to epitopes in bone marrow and spleen and the consequent low background activity. This rapid endogenous background subtraction allows the detection of small lesions with excellent image quality (BECKER et al. 1994). This low background activity is due to the very rapid binding of the antibody to the bone marrow 55% (4 h), the liver 10% (4 h), and the spleen (6%; BECKER et al. 1994).

7.2.5.3
Clinical Indications

In bone infection the sensitivity of antigranulocyte antibody scintigraphy (BW250/183) in 106 patients was calculated to be 69% for the hips, 79% for the thigh, 85% for the knees, and 100% for the lower leg and ankle (REULAND et al. 1991). The sensitivity decreased from the periphery of the bone to the central parts. This may be due to the physiological uptake of the antibody in the bone-marrow-containing parts of the skeleton, where the normal uptake of the antibody does not allow normal bone marrow to be distinguished from small infectious foci. The overall sensitivity and specificity of the antibody fragment in osteomyelitis was 90 and 84%, respectively, with a

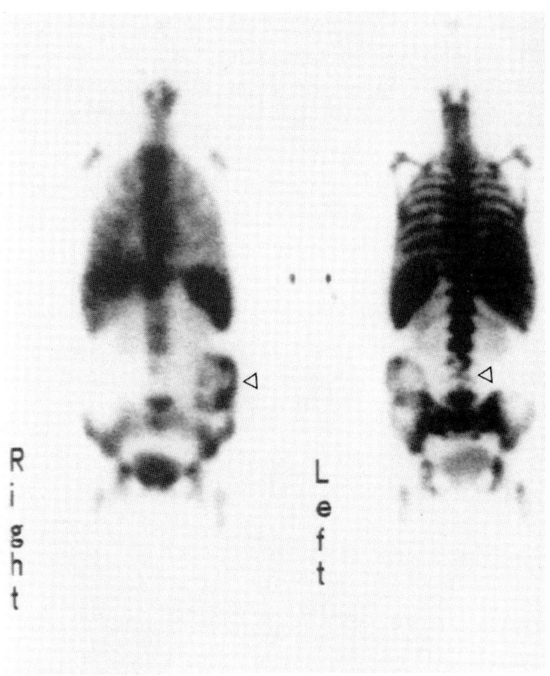

Fig. 7.3. A 63-year-old male with fever of unknown origin with a cold lesion in lumbar spine (*right panel*) as a sign of spondylodiscitis and a hot lesion in the left abdomen (*left panel*) as a sign of soft tissue abscess. Whole-body scan with antibody BW 250/183 4 h post injection

diagnostic accuracy of 87.9%, and was superior to autologous leukocyte scintigraphy (83.9, 76.5, and 81%; BECKER et al. 1996). The worst results were obtained in spondylodiscitis (Fig. 7.3). In 40 patients with spondylodiscitis all lesions showed "cold" patterns (GRATZ et al. 1997). Thus, the disease can be localized, but no differentiation is possible between tumor, fracture, or osteomyelitis. A proposed explanation is increased pressure in the vertebral bodies in case of infection, which prevents labeled white blood cells or antibodies from penetrating.

False-positive uptake can be seen in hematomas, contusions, and aseptic inflammation. Using ^{99m}Tc-BW 250/183 scintigraphy in chronic inflammatory bowel disease, 49% of segments could be detected at 2 h, 55% at 5 h, and 91% at 20 h after injection (BECKER et al. 1990). In another prospective study of chronic inflammatory bowel disease (CIBD), SEGARRA et al (1991) found sensitivity, specificity, and accuracy to be 61, 100, and 78%, respectively, at 4 h, and 79, 92, and 78%, respectively, at 24 h. There is no transport of the activity through the bowel wall, as is known from the use of ^{111}In-labeled white blood cells. The activity increases in the bowel wall over the 24 h following injection. This may be due to an antibody Fc-part interaction with Fc-receptors on granulocytes within the bowel wall (BECKER et al. 1994). The lower sensitivity, in comparison with ^{99m}Tc-HMPAO leukocytes, favors labeled white blood cells (ALMERS et al. 1996).

In vascular graft infection, nuclear medicine procedures are used to determine the extent of the infection following its clinical diagnosis (Fig. 7.4). Immunoscintigraphy with specific anti-granulocyte antibodies offers the best means for the localization of vascular graft infections due to the rapid endogenous background subtraction and low vascular activity.

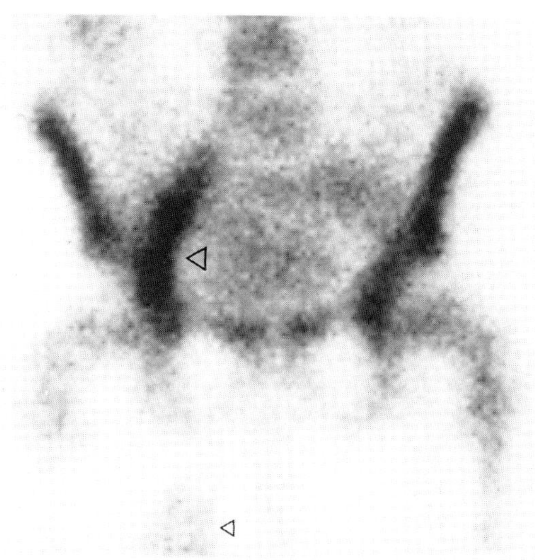

Fig. 7.4. A 61-year-old man with aortobifemoral bypass graft, redness, and swelling of the right inner thigh. The antigranulocyte antibody scan showed at 24 h intensive uptake in the right iliac part of the prosthesis (*top arrowhead*) and a soft tissue uptake (*arrowhead* at lower border of image)

The sensitivity is reported to be 94% and the specificity 85% (CORDES et al. 1991). False-positive results have been observed in perivascular hematoma, especially in late 24-h images; such findings have to be excluded by ultrasonography and CT.

In prosthetic vascular heart disease the combination of immunoscintigraphy with single photon emission computed tomography (SPECT) and echocardiography localizes subacute infective endocarditis with a good sensitivity (MUNZ et al. 1991). In situations where echocardiography and transesophageal echocardiography are inconclusive, 24-h chest SPECT may give additional clinical information.

Use of immunoscintigraphy with antigranulocyte antibodies has not been examined systematically in patients with pneumonia or other infective lung diseases. We found that lung abscesses can be detected well; however, we were not able to detect pneumonia. Our findings concur with another report on false-negative scans in lung abscesses (LIND et al. 1990). Similar findings in AIDS patients demonstrate that extra-abdominal infections can be excluded or shown, whereas opportunistic pneumonia is never shown (PRVULOVICH et al. 1995).

In general, ^{99m}Tc-labeled antibodies are well accepted due to their easy handling and high sensitivity in identifying an infectious focus in the body. However, the scans need careful interpretation in patients in whom the surgeon requires differentiation between postsurgical inflammation and infection, because both situations yield a signal. Although the IgG1 antibodies are widely accepted in routine clinical diagnosis, they induce human anti-mouse antibodies (HAMAs). The production of such antibodies seems to be dose dependent, the frequency ranging from more than 30% in patients receiving repeated injections down to 4.5% in patients with a fixed dose of 125 μg of the antibody. Consequently, we recommend that no more than 250 μg of the antibody be used in order to ensure a low HAMA response rate (BECKER et al. 1994). Technetium-99m antigranulocyte antibodies are known not to induce HAMA; thus, the examinations can easily and safely be performed (BECKER et al. 1994).

7.2.6
^{111}In-Labeled Human Non-Specific Immunoglobulin

In contrast to the aforementioned murine antibodies, ^{111}In-labeled human non-specific immunoglobulin (HIG) preparations have the advantage of absence of a HAMA response. As a spin-off of research on monoclonal antibodies specific for unique antigens on *Pseudomonas aeruginosa* bacteria, RUBIN et al. (1988) discovered serendipitously that the human non-specific polyclonal immunoglobulin G (IgG) in their rat model of infection provided results similar to those for a specific monoclonal antibody. Although there are differences between radiolabeled monoclonal antibodies and polyclonal IgG in terms of origin (murine vs human), specificity, dynamic biodistribution, mechanism of action, etc., there are also many similarities between these radioimmuno-conjugates as agents for detecting infection and inflammation (BUSCOMBE et al. 1993).

7.2.6.1
Biodistribution and Uptake Mechanism

Although the mechanism for accumulation of ^{111}In-HIG, the first labeled immunoglobulin, in inflammatory and infectious foci may not be completely understood, it is obviously related to increased vascular permeability into an expanded extracellular fluid space and to the chemical nature of the radiolabel (CORSTENS et al. 1992). It has been shown that ^{111}In dissociates from HIG in the focus and can be retained, whereas the HIG leaves the abscess (CLAESSENS et al. 1995). This release of ^{111}In provides an explanation for the high ratio between the concentrations of ^{111}In-HIG in the interstitial fluid space of normal muscle and in plasma (JUWEID et al. 1992), and for the high sensitivity of the method especially in the late 48-h scans, when the immunoglobulin in circulation has decreased but the focal ^{111}In uptake is still high.

Physiological uptake of ^{111}In-HIG is observed in liver (17%), spleen (2%), and kidney (6%). Bone marrow uptake is approximately 6% of the injected dose (8%). ^{111}In-HIG clears from the blood pool with a T1/2 alpha of approximately 13 h and a T1/2 beta of approximately 72 h.

7.2.6.2
Clinical Indications

Indium-111 HIG accumulates in various types of pulmonary infection (CORSTENS et al. 1992). Most data are available in immunocompromised patients, in whom ^{111}In-HIG scintigraphy has proved useful in delineating *Pneumocystis carinii* pneumonia (BUSCOMBE et al. 1993). High sensitivity has also been reported in abdominal infection and inflammation (RUBIN et al. 1988).

The majority of patients undergo ^{111}In-HIG scintigraphy for suspected bone and joint infection. The sensitivity and specificity of the method were found to be excellent in a patient population of more than 100 (OYEN et al. 1992). Low-grade *Staphylococcus aureus* infection was missed in only 2 patients. However, ^{111}In-HIG accumulates both in infection and in sterile inflammatory processes such as hematomas, synovitides, and recent fractures, and is not able to distinguish between the two situations. Of special interest are results in patients with a suspected infection of a joint arthroplasty. The reported sensitivity and specificity for infection are 93 and 88%, respectively, whereas for inflammation both are 100% (OYEN et al. 1991; DE KLEIJN et al. 1992). ^{111}In-HIG was also helpful in ruling out or confirming osteomyelitis in the diabetic foot. In vascular graft infection studies, it had a sensitivity of 92% and a specificity of 100% (RUBIN et al. 1988).

The major indication for scintigraphic delineation of infectious foci is fever of unknown origin. Although infection or inflammation is established as the cause of fever in only a minority of patients, scintigraphic delineation of a possible infectious focus is considered for most of the patients. Proven inflammatory processes were missed in only 1 patient with endocarditis and infection of a renal cyst. This method is also helpful in febrile granulocytopenic patients, in whom it may be difficult to isolate enough leukocytes for labeling.

Currently, the chief problem with ^{111}In-HIG is that it is not commercially available and cannot be used in every nuclear medicine unit.

7.2.7
^{99m}Tc-Labeled Human Non-specific Immunoglobulin

Technetium-99m HIG is widely available. Due to the 6-h half-life, images can be obtained at 24 h but not at 48 h.

7.2.7.1
Biodistribution and Uptake Mechanism

In vitro and animal studies have provided some evidence for binding of ^{99m}Tc-HIG to bacteria as a mechanism for scintigraphic detection of infectious foci (OYEN et al. 1992). However, it is difficult to understand how this can play a significant role at sites of infection, because ^{99m}Tc-HIG also accumulates in sterile inflammation. Consequently, the uptake mechanism is probably the same as for ^{111}In-HIG. However, there seems to be retention of ^{99m}Tc in the foci because in a rat model of acute infection there was initially good uptake in the infected area followed by a gradual decrease in after 6 h (OYEN et al. 1992).

The whole-body distribution of ^{99m}Tc-HIG at 4 h p.i. shows 57.7% of the injected activity; the rest has been excreted via the kidneys. Lung uptake is 7.3%, liver uptake 5.1%, splenic uptake 1.3%, kidney uptake 6.5%, estimated bone marrow uptake 22.1%, and gonadal uptake 1% (SAPTOGINO et al. 1991). At 24 h there is still 12.7% of the whole-body activity in the lungs, which is mainly due to the blood-pool activity.

7.2.7.2
Clinical Indications

Twenty-five patients with HIV were studied with both ^{67}Ga citrate and ^{99m}Tc-HIG; poor sensitivity of the latter agent was seen in the chest (BUSCOMBE et al. 1991), which could be explained best by the high physiological blood-pool activity in the lungs. However, the combination of ^{67}Ga citrate and ^{99m}Tc-HIG appeared helpful in differentiating between lymphoma and infection in HIV-positive patients with fever of unknown origin.

In assessing presence or absence of inflammation, a sensitivity of 80% and a specificity of 87% were noted. However, when the extent of intestinal inflammation was evaluated, ^{99m}Tc-HIG appeared to perform poorly, indicating that the technique is of little value in the assessment of patients with proven chronic inflammatory bowel disease. This was studied intensively by SPINELLI et al (1994).

In patients with suspected osteomyelitis the performance of ^{99m}Tc-BW 250/183 was compared with the final diagnosis established by surgery, histology, and bacteriology (SCUIK et al. 1991). In peripherally located osteomyelitis, both agents showed similar and good results. However, in centrally localized osteomyelitis the performance of the two agents was very different because injection of the labeled polyclonal IgG resulted in "hot" lesions, whereas the administration of the monoclonal antibody showed "cold" lesions.

In general, the problem remains the very high vascular uptake during 24 h causing a high background activity, which does not allow diagnosis of low-grade infections.

The use of ^{99m}Tc-HIG for imaging arthritis was first studied in an animal model, which showed that the localization and severity of inflammatory joint diseases can be detected with non-specific IgG (BREEDVELD et al. 1989; BERNA et al. 1992; DE BOIS et al. 1993, 1994). A lot of clinical studies have demonstrated that ^{99m}Tc-HIG is able to distinguish between joints with and without active inflammation in chronic rheumatoid arthritis (DE BOIS et al. 1992), to monitor therapeutic success, to demonstrate septic complications, and to localize other joint infections and inflammation.

7.2.8
^{18}F-FDG Fluoro-2-Deoxy-2 Glucose

^{18}F-FDG has been shown to be a useful tumor-detecting agent (see chap. 10). The mechanism of accumulation of this tracer in malignant tissue is due to the enhanced rate of glucose utilization by neoplastic cells. High ^{18}F-FDG accumulation in abscesses has also been reported (TAHARA et al. 1989; SASAKI et al. 1990).

The accumulation of ^{18}F-FDG is relatively high in macrophages, and in areas where young granulation tissue is formed around tumors demarcating it from the surrounding intact host tissue. The reported uptake of ^{18}F-FDG in abscesses seems to be an active process by phagocytes within the abscess or by granulation tissue surrounding the abscess (KUBOTA et al. 1972, 1980). Interestingly, chemically produced sterile abscesses do not accumulate ^{18}F-FDG (SOM et al. 1980). This may be due to an inflammatory response different from that of infectious agents. It is also known that pneumonia accumulates ^{18}F-FDG intensively, whereas bronchiectasis does not, and ^{11}In-oxine leukocytes behave the other way around (personal communications). Although the ^{18}F-FDG uptake, which is non-specific for infection and inflammation, is not completely understood, some clinical data have been reported. In small numbers of patients with osteomyelitis it was reported that ^{18}F-FDG scanning has a high negative predictive value for excluding osteomyelitis and at least a good positive predictive value for diagnosing osteomyelitis. The major advantage is the high spatial resolution of positron emission tomography (SHNIER et al. 1997). In a comparative study with antigranulocyte antibodies, ^{18}F-FDG and immunoscintigraphy were nearly equivalent in diagnosing chronic osteitis in the peripheral skeleton, whereas in the central skeleton, ^{18}F-FDG seems to be superior (GUHLMANN et al. 1997). A lot of questions still have to be answered, but ^{18}F-FDG proves helpful in fever of unknown origin and in patients where other modalities have problems, such as spondylodiscitis; however, it should be kept in mind that this ^{18}F-FDG method is non-specific for infection (SUGAWARA et al. 1998).

7.3.
Summary and Recommendations

Several radionuclides are available for imaging infection and/or inflammation. They differ in terms of their physical characteristics, biodistribution, need for cell isolation, and radiation exposure. Based on data in the literature regarding all of the advantages and disadvantages of the commercially available radiopharmaceuticals, Table 7.4 shows the present author's conclusions as to appropriate indi-

Table 7.4. Indications for the use of different radiopharmaceuticals in patients with infection and inflammation. *CIBD* chronic inflammatory bowel disease

Indication	*Proposed radiopharmaceutical*
Fever of unknown origin	^{67}Ga-citrate ^{99m}Tc-labeled granulocyte antibodies ^{18}F-FDG
Osteomyelitis Peripheral bone	^{99m}Tc-nanocolloids ^{99m}Tc-labeled granulocyte antibodies ^{99m}Tc-labeled white blood cells
Spine	^{67}Ga-citrate ^{99m}Tc/^{111}In-HIG
Lung infection	^{67}Ga-citrate
Heart valve endocarditis	^{99m}Tc-labeled white blood cells ^{99m}Tc-labeled granulocyte antibodies
Vascular prosthetic infection	^{99m}Tc-labeled white blood cells ^{99m}Tc-labeled granulocyte antibodies
Abdominal infection/inflammation	^{99m}Tc-labeled white blood cells ^{99m}Tc-granulocyte antibodies
Assessment of disease activity in CIBD	^{111}In-labeled white blood cells
Kidney infection/transplant infection	^{111}In-labeled white blood cells
Chronic infection (i.e., tuberculosis, sarcoidosis)	^{67}Ga-citrate

cations for the large variety of available radiopharmaceuticals.

In patients with fever of unknown origin ^{67}Ga citrate has its indications, because ^{67}Ga citrate uptake via lactoferrin and transferrin binding shows infection, pneumonia included, chronic infections (sarcoidosis, tuberculosis), and malignant disease. ^{67}Ga-citrate localizes the disease; other techniques (radiographs, CT, MR) or biopsy provide the underlying process. Easier to use due to availability are ^{99m}Tc-labeled antibodies which also show excellent results (Fig. 7.5). They do not detect pneumonia (which can be excluded clinically and by radiography), sarcoidosis or tuberculosis, but can demonstrate bone marrow pathology. Antibodies may exclude acute infectious disease (MELLER et al. 1998).

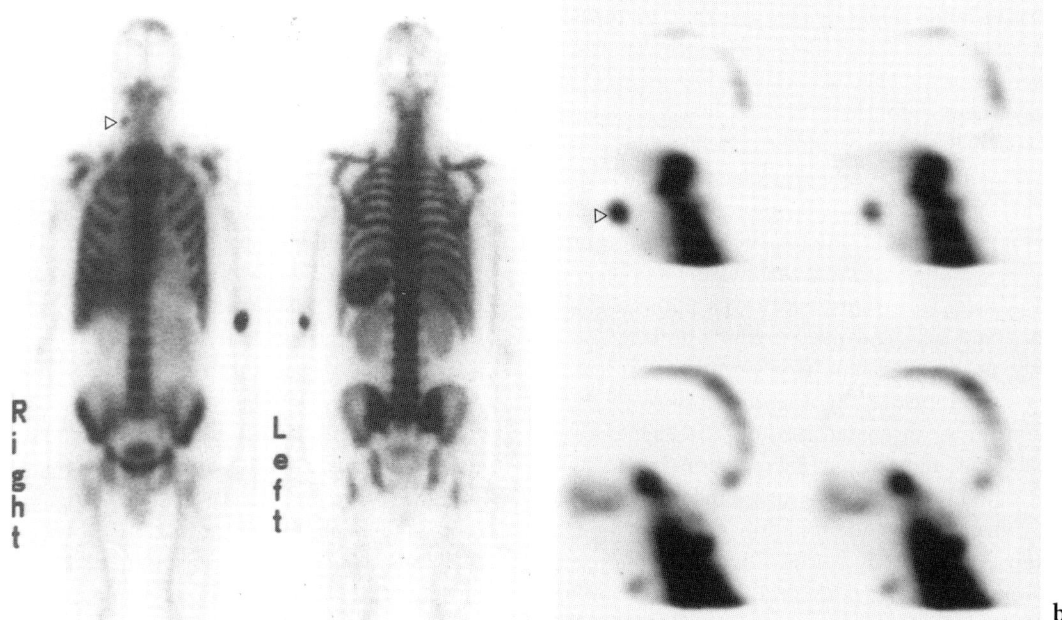

Fig. 7.5. A 57-year-old male with fever and leukocytosis showing tooth granuloma (*arrowhead*) in: **a** whole-body scan and **b** skull single photon emission computed tomography 4.5 h after administration of antigranulocyte antibody BW 250/183

In chronic infections (tuberculosis) or inflammation (sarcoidosis) ^{67}Ga-citrate is obligatory. In osteomyelitis of the peripheral skeleton, ^{99m}Tc-labeled tracers can be used. For the spine, MR should be the method of choice; only ^{67}Ga-citrate gives positive images but does not differentiate between tumors or infections.

In lung infections ^{67}Ga-citrate is the radionuclide of choice, because all other methods fail to show pneumonia.

For the diagnosis of endocarditis, ^{99m}Tc-labeled tracers should be used because of the better resolution and the obligatory SPECT of the chest.

In vascular prostheses ^{99m}Tc-white blood cells or antibodies are best because they have a low vascular background activity.

All tracers other than ^{111}In-leukocytes are excreted via the kidneys; thus, a signal from the kidney yields diagnostic problems. Only ^{111}In-oxine leukocytes have no physiological kidney uptake and make clinical diagnosis easy.

7.4. Future Prospects

The ideal new agent should provide high and early uptake in infections and inflammatory lesions, no accumulation in non-inflamed tissues, low toxicity and radiation dose, and rapid background clearance. The development is targeting smaller peptides. But perhaps even larger molecules are able to fulfill these criteria. Studies on an IgM (925kD) antibody directed against the stage-specific embryonic antigen (SSEA-1) have been published. The reported sensitivities and specificities are 95 and 96%, respectively. Excellent image quality was obtained because of a high target/background ratio due to the very high affinity of the antibody (10–12 M) for the leukocyte antigen (Gratz et al. 1998). Unfortunately, this was accompanied by a higher toxicity, because all patients showed 20 min p.i. a 50% neutropenia, which prevents the antibody at the moment from routine clinical use (Gratz et al. 1998).

None of the discussed methods are able to answer the surgeon's most important question: In a post-surgical patient with clinical signs and symptoms, do they reflect merely inflammation (the normal healing response) or do they herald infection? Whereas inflammation requires conservative treatment only, infection needs further surgical intervention. Nevertheless, the currently available methods do allow some opportunities for differentiation, e.g., if the uptake of a radiopharmaceutical around a knee prosthesis is intensive but homogeneous, it is probably inflammation, whereas if it is more focal, it is likely to represent infection. As a general rule, correct interpretation of scans is feasible when they are considered in conjunction with all available anamnestic and clinical data.

Certain specific steps that have been taken towards the detection of bacterial contamination are worthy of mention. Goldenberg et al (1994) injected ^{99m}Tc-Fab fragments directed against *Pneumocystis carinii* and were able to identify patients infected with microorganisms with a sensitivity of 85.7% and a specificity of 86.7%. It is therefore possible that rapid diagnosis and localization of other infectious lesions may be feasible using organism-specific, radiolabeled monoclonal antibodies. Another approach is the use of labeled antibodies, which may specifically be metabolized by different microorganisms. The best method seems to be the use of a broad-spectrum antibiotic, as has been achieved with the ^{99m}Tc-labeling of a quinolone called "infecton" by Britton et al (1998). These authors found that imaging of infection was possible, but, more interestingly, scans turned positive before white cell scanning showed any uptake. In a multicenter study more than 500 patients were examined with an overall sensitivity of 93%, a specificity of 86%, and an accuracy of 90% (Britton et al. 1998).

Nuclear medicine, with its different approaches, images pathophysiology and pathobiochemistry. The available new techniques, especially within immunology and molecular biology, are yielding new insights into the cascade of infection and inflammation. We now understand that cytokines, especially interleukins, and endothelial cells become activated after a chemotactic signal, and that granulocytes are able to interfere with the expressed molecules, such as E-selectin, before they leave the circulation. The use of ^{111}In-labeled anti-E-selectin fragments is an exciting new method for imaging the expression of E-selectin, an epitope on the vascular surface, which allows specific images to be acquired without the need for an antibody to pass the vessel wall (Keelan et al. 1994).

A new unspecific approach is the use of ^{99m}Tc-pneumoencephalography liposomes, which is, in preliminary studies, as effective as ^{111}In-HIG. Although the uptake mechanism is unspecific, the simple and safe preparation and the ^{99m}Tc-label make this perhaps an attractive agent for imaging infection and inflammation (Dams et al. 1998).

During the past decade, the development of new radiopharmaceuticals has gradually shifted from large proteins with aspecific uptake mechanism via large receptor-specific proteins (e.g., antigranulocyte, anti-E-selectin, and intercellular adhesion molecule antibodies and antibody fragments (BECKER et al. 1994; SIGNORE et al. 1994, 1997; VAN DER LAKEN et al. 1994) to receptor-specific small proteins and peptides, i.e., the mediators of the inflammatory response. The enormous progress in the field of immunology has yielded substantial knowledge about the function and structure of the various mediators of inflammation and their receptors. The mediators became available for applications in synthesis or recombinant DNA techniques. In nuclear medicine, radiolabeled mediators have emerged as a promising class of agents with attractive characteristics for scintigraphic detection of infection and inflammation. Theoretically, the high binding affinity for the receptors, expressed in inflammatory tissue, facilitates retention of these agents in inflammation while their small size permits rapid clearance from blood and other nontarget tissue. For the detection of acute infection and inflammation, rapidly clearing agents targeted to poly-morphoneutrophils are highly preferable. For this application, fMet-Leu-Phe, tuftsin antagonist, Il-1, Il-1ra, Il-8, and PF4 appear to be promising candidates. In contrast, Il-2 octreotide and substance P target specifically to mononuclear cell infiltration and hence are suitable for scintigraphic detection of chronic infection and inflammation.

The promise of these new techniques is the possibility of using peptides in infection. A major problem in the imaging of infection is the fact that nearly every radiopharmaceutical works, because the increased capillary permeability allows radiopharmaceuticals to migrate out of the circulation. For most techniques this yields a high sensitivity but no useful specificity. Small peptides also leave the circulation rapidly, but if they do not specifically bind to their receptor in the focus, they may leave the focus within a given time. The rapid targeting together with rapid clearance from the focus promise to yield high sensitivity and, more importantly, high specificity in the detection of infection. Since the first report of the chemo-attractant properties of small N-formyl peptides (SCHIFFMANN et al. 1972), these compounds have attracted increasing attention (BECKER 1987). The results of FISCHMAN et al (1994) demonstrate the localization of radiolabeled chemotactic peptide analogs at focal sites of infection in experimental models of deep-thigh infection at sufficient concentrations to permit external imaging soon after intravenous administration. Further improvements of such peptide analogs are, however, required before they can be administered to humans. Future aims for peptide imaging of infection are labeling of a small fraction of the available receptor with a high concentration of radioactivity labeling of the peptide with ^{99m}Tc and achievement of a reduced biological activity, e.g., with antagonists or partial agonists (FISCHMAN et al. 1994).

The localization and anatomical delineation of occult sites of infection are frequently important steps in the therapeutic management of critically ill patients. Current imaging procedures, such as computed tomography, ultrasonography, conventional radiography, and magnetic resonance imaging, rely primarily on focal changes in tissue density or composition to define lesions. When an inflammatory process has progressed to tissue necrosis and abscess formation, these modalities can localize the area of involvement. However, early in the course of this process, when the tissue changes associated with necrosis have not yet occurred, lesion localization may be extremely difficult. This is particularly true if normal anatomical landmarks have been obscured by previous surgery of disease. The implantation of prosthetic materials sometimes prevents radiological access and thereby hinders diagnosis. Against this background, and given the available radiopharmaceuticals and future possibilities, one may conclude that nuclear medicine will indeed make an important contribution to the management of the patient with infection (VAN DER LAKEN et al. 1998).

References

Allan RA, Sladen GE, Bassingham S, Lazarus C, Clarke SEM, Fogelman I (1993) Comparison of simultaneous Tc-99m-HMPAO and In-111-oxine labelled white blood cell scan in the assessment of inflammatory bowel disease. Eur J Nucl Med 20: 195–200

Almers S, Granerus G, Franzen L, Strom M (1996) Technetium-99 m scintigraphy: more accurate assessment of ulcerative colitis with exametazime-labelled leukocytes than with antigranulocyte antibodies. Eur J Nucl Med 23: 247–255

Arndt JW, Van der Sluys Veer A, Blok D, Niffioen G, Verspaget HW, Lamers CBHW, Pauwels EKJ (1991) Prospective comparative study of Tc-99m-WBCs and indium-111 granulocytes for the examination of inflammatory bowel disease. J Nucl Med 32: 2029–2034

Athens JW, Haab OP, Raab SO (1961) Leukokinetic studies: the total blood, circulating and marginal granulocyte pools and granulocyte turnover rate in normal subjects. J Clin Invest 40: 989–995

Bassano DA, McAfee JG (1979) Cellular radiation doses of labeled neutrophils and platelets. J Nucl Med 20: 255–259

Becker EJ (1987) The formylpeptide receptor of the neutrophil: a search and conserve operation. Am J Pathol 129: 16–24

Becker W, Bair J, Behr T, Repp R, Streckenbach H, Beck H, Gramatzki M, Winship MJ, Goldenberg DM, Wolf F (1994) Detection of soft-tissue infections and osteomyelitis using a technetium-99 m labeled antigranulocyte monoclonal antibody fragment. J Nucl Med 35: 1436–1443

Becker W, Blair J, Behr T, Repp R, Streckenbach H, Beck H, Gramatzki M, Winship MJ, Goldenberg DM, Wolf F (1994) Detection of soft-tissue infections and osteomyelitis using a technetium-99m-labeled antigranulocyte monoclonal antibody fragment. J Nucl Med 35: 1436–1443

Becker W, Borst U, Maisch B, Epping J, Börner W, Kochsiek K (1987) In-111-labelled granulocytes in inflammatory hear diseases. Eur Heart J 8 [Suppl]: 307–310

Becker W, Düsel W, Berger P, Spiegel W (1987) The In-111-granulocyte scan in prosthetic vascular graft infections: imaging technique and results. Eur J Nucl Med 13: 225–229

Becker W, Fischbach H, Jenett M, Reiners C, Börner W (1986) In-111-oxine labelled white cells in the diagnosis and follow-up of Crohn's disease. Klin Wochenschr 64: 141–148

Becker W, Fischbach W, Reiners C, Börner W (1986) Three-phase white blood cell scan: diagnostic validity in abdominal inflammatory diseases. J Nucl Med, 27: 1109–1115

Becker W, Fischbach W, Weppler M, Mösl B, Jocoby G, Börner W (1988) Radiolabeled granulocytes in inflammatory bowel disease: diagnostic possibilities and clinical indications. Nucl Med Commun 9: 693–701

Becker W, Fleig W, Marienhagen J, Hahn E, Wolf F (1990) Diagnostische Bedeutung der intestinalen Aktivität bei der Immunszintigraphie mit Tc-99m-NCA-95-Antikörpern. Nukl-Med 229: 47–48

Becker W, Goldenberg DM, Wolf F (1994) The use of monoclonal antibodies and antibody fragments in the imaging of infectious lesions. Semin Nucl Med XXIV: 1–13

Becker W, Götz R, Heidbreder W, Börner W (1986) Indium-111 white blood cell scan in the diagnosis of infectious complications in patients undergoing regular dialysis treatment. In: Bischof-Delaloye A, Blaufox MD, eds. Radionuclides in nephrology. Basel: Karger: 191–195

Becker W, Schomann E, Fischbach W, Börner W, Gruner KR (1988) Comparison of Tc-99m-HMPAO and In-111-oxine labelled granulocytes in man: first clinical results. Nucl Med Commun 9: 435–447

Becker W.(1995) The contribution of nuclear medicine to the patient with infection. Eur J Nucl Med 22: 1195–1211

Becker W, Palestro CJ, Winship J, Feld T, Pinsky C.M, Wolf F, Goldenberg D.M, (1996) Rapid imaging of infections with a monoclonal antibody fragment(Leukoscan). Clin Orthop Rel Res 329: 263–272

Berna L, Torres G, Diez C, Estorch M, Martinez-Duncker D, Carrio I (1992) Technetium-99 m human polyclonal immunoglobulin G studies and conventional bone scans to detect active joint inflammation in chronic rheumatoid arthritis. Eur J Nucl Med 19: 173–176

Borst U, Becker W, Maisch B, Börner W, Kochsiek K (1993) Clinical and prognostic effect of a positive granulocyte scan in infective endocarditis. Clin Nucl Med 18: 35–39

Breedveld FC, Kroonenburgh MJPG, Camps JAJ, Feitsma HIJ, Markusse HM, Pauwels EKJ (1989) Imaging of inflammatory arthritis with technetium-99m-labelled IgG. J Nucl Med 30: 2017–2021

Breedveld FC (1992) Tc-99 m human immunoglobulin scintigraphy – a reliable method to detect joint activity in rheumatoid arthritis. J Rheumatol 19: 1371–1376

Britton K, Soroa V, Amaral H, Malamitsi J, Kartamihardja H, Sundram F, Mustafa H, Bhatnagar A, Nair G (1998) Tc-99m-infecton preliminary evaluation in over 500 patients through an IAEA coordinated research programme Eur J Nucl Med 25: 874

Buijs WCAM, Oyen WJG, Claessens RAMJ, Koenders EB, Meeuwis APW, Corstens FHM (1990) Biodistribution and radiation dosimetry of indium-111 labelled immunoglobulin G. Eur J Nucl Med 16: 433

Buscombe JR, Miller RF, Lui D, Ell PJ (1991) Combined Ga-67-citrate and Tc-99 m human immunoglobulin imaging in human immuno deficiency virus-positive patients with fever of unknown origin. Nucl Med Commun 12: 583–592

Buscombe JR, Oyen WJG, Miller RF, Grant A, Claessens RAMJ, Van der Meer J, Corstens FMH, Ell JP, Miller RF (1993) Indium-111 labeled human polyclonal immunoglobulin identifying focal infection in patients positive for human immuno deficiency virus (HIV). J Nucl Med 34: 1621–1625

Calame W, Feitsma HIJ, Ensing GJ, Arndt JW, van Furth R, Pauwels EKJ (1991) Binding of Tc-99m-labelled polyclonal immunoglobulin to bacteria as a mechanism for scintigraphic detection of infection. Eur J Nucl Med 18: 396–400

Claessens RAMJ, Koenders EB, Boerman OC, Oyen, WJG, Borm GF, Van der Meer JWM, Corstens FHM (1995) Dissociation of indium from indium-111-labelled diethylene triamine penta-acetic conjugated non-specific polyclonal human immunoglobulin G in inflammatory foci. Eur J Nucl Med 22: 212–219

Cook PS, Datz EL, Disbro MA, Alazraki NP, Taylor AT (1984) Pulmonary uptake in In-111-leukocyte imaging: clinical significance in patients with suspected occult infection. Radiology 150: 557–561

Cordes M, Hepp W, Langer R, Pannhorst J, Hierholzer J, Felix R (1991) Vascular graft infection: detection by I-123-labeled antigranulocyte antibody (anti-NCA-95) scintigraphy. Nucl Med: 30: 173–177

Corstens FHM, Claessens RAMJ (1992) Imaging inflammation with human polyclonal immunoglobulin: not looked for, but discovered. Eur J Nucl Med 19: 155–158

Corstens FHM, Oyen WJG, Becker WS (1993) Radioimmunoconjugates in the detection of infection and inflammation. Semin Nucl Med XXIII:148–164

Currie DC, Peters AM, Garbett ND, George P, Strickland B, Lavener JP, Cole PJ (1990) In-111-labelled granulocyte scanning to detect inflammation in the lungs of patients with chronic sputum expectoration. Thorax 45: 541–544

Currie DC, Saverymuttu SH, Peters AM, Needham SG, George P, Dhillon DP, Lavender JP, Cole PJ (1987) In-111-labelled granulocyte accumulation in respiratory tract of patients with bronchiectasis. Lancet I: 1335–1339

Dams EThM, Oyen WJG, Boerman O, Laverman P, Beijnen JH, Strom G, van der Meer JWM, Corstens FHM (1998) First clinical evaluation of Tc-99m-PEG liposomes for the detection of infection and inflammation Eur J Nucl Med 25: 897P

Datz FL (1994) In-111-labeled leukocytes for the detection of infection: current status. Semin Nucl Med XXIV: 92–109

De Bois MHW, Arndt JAW, Van der Velde EA, Van der Lubbe PAHM, Westedt ML, Pauwels EKJ,

De Bois MHW, Arndt JW, Tak PP, Kluin PM, Van der Velde EA, Pauwels EKJ, Breedveld FC (1993) Tc-99m-labelled polyclonal human immunoglobulin G scintigraphy before and after intra-articular knee injection of triamcinolone hexacetonide in patients with rheumatoid arthritis. Nucl Med Commun 14: 883–887

De Bois MHW, Arndt JW, Van der Velde EA, Pauwels EKJ, Breedveld FC (1994) Joint scintigraphy for quantification of synovitis with Tc-99m-labelled human immunoglobulin G compared to late phase scintigraphy with Tc-99m-labelled diphosphonate. Br J Rheumatol 33: 67–73

De Kleijn EMHA, Oven WJG, Claessens RAMJ, Corstens FMH, Van der Meer JWM (1992) Scintigraphy with In-111 labeled polyclonal human immunoglobulin G (In-111-IgG) on patients with fever of unknown origin (FUO). Nucl Med Commun 13: 626

De Schrijver M, Streule K, Senekowitsch R, Fridrich R (1987) Scintigraphy of inflammation with nanometer-sized colloid tracers. Nucl Med Commun 8: 895–908

Fischbach W, Becker W (1991) Clinical relevance of activity parameters in Crohn's disease estimated by fecal excretion of In-111-labeled granulocytes. Digestion 50: 149–152

Fischman AJ, Babich JW, Rubin RH (1994) Infection imaging with technetium-99m-labeled chemotactic peptide analogs. Semin Nucl Med XXIV: 154–168

Flivik G, Sloth M, Rydholf U, Herrlin K, Lidgren L (1993) Technetium-99m-nanocolloid scintigraphy in orthopedic infections: a comparison with In-111-labeled leukocytes. J Nucl Med 34: 1646–1650

Frayha R, Uwaydah M (1973) Fever of unknown origin. Lab. Med. J 26: 49

Golden DW, Cline MJ (1977) Production, distribution and fate of granulocytes. In: Williams WJ, Beutler E, Erslev AJ, et al, Eds. Hematology 2nd Ed New York: McGraw Hill. 699–706

Goldenberg DM, Sharkey RM, Udem S, Vagg R, Levine GM, Conte P, Swayne LC, Hansen HJ, Cunnif D, Anton J, Linke MJ, Smulian G, Walzer PD (1994) Immunoscintigraphy of Pneumocytis carinii in AIDS patients. J Nucl Med 35: 1028–1034

Gratz S, Behr T, Hermann A, Dresing K, Tarditi L, Franchesini R, Rhodes B, Stürmer KM, Becker W (1998) Intra-individual comparison of Tc-99 m labelled anti-SSEA-1 antigranulocyte antibody and Tc-99m-HMPAO labelled white blood cells for imaging of infection. Eur J Nucl Med 25: 386–393

Gratz S, Braun HG, Behr TM, Meller J, Hermann A, Conrad M, Rathmann D, Bertagnoli R, Willert HG, Becker W (1997) Photopenia in chronic vertebral osteomyelitis with technetium-99 m antigranulocyte antibody (BW 250/183). J Nucl Med 98: 211–216

Guhlmann CA:, Brecht-Krauss D, Suger G, Moog F, Kotzerke J, Glatting G, Kinzl L, Reske SN (1997) Detecting chronic osteitis with 18F-FDG and immunoscintigraphy using Tc-99 m labeled monoclonal antigranulocyte antibodies. J. Nucl. Med 38: 132P

Hawker RJ, Hall CE, Drole Z, Rhys-Evans PH (1985) Indium-leukocyte imaging in true pyrexia of unknown origin. Eur J Nucl Med 10: 172–174

Hoffer P (1980) Gallium: Mechanisms. J Nucl Med 21: 282–285

Hotze A, Bokisch A, Rüther M, Biersack HJ (1988) Comparison of Tc-99m-HMPAO labelled leukocytes and Tc-99 m nanocolloid in osteomyelitis. Nukl Med 27: 63–65

Hotze A, Briele B, Overbeck B, Knopp J, Grünwald F, Mekkawy MA, von Smekal A, Moeller F, Biersack HJ (1992) Tc-99m-labelled antigranulocyte antibodies in suspected bone infections. J Nucl Med 33: 526–531

Hotze A, Mahlstedt J, Wolf F (1984) Knochenmarkszintigraphie: Methode – Indikationen – Ergebnisse. GIT Verlag Ernst Giebeler

Howard P Jr, Hahn HH, Palmer PL (1977) Fever of unknown origin. A prospective study of 100 patients. Tex Med 73: 56

Jonker N, Peters AM, Carpani de Kaski M, Hodgson HJ, Lavender JP (1992) A retrospective study of granulocytic kinetics in patients with systemic vasculitis. J Nucl Med 33: 491–497

Joseph K, Höffken H, Bosslet K, Schorlemmer HU (1988) In-vivo labelling of granulocytes with Tc-99, anti-NCA monoclonal antibodies from imaging inflammation. Eur J Nucl Med 14: 367–373

Joseph K, Höffken H, Dammann V (1987) In-vivo-Markierung von Granulozyten mit Tc-99m-markierten monoklonalen Antikörpern: erste klinische Ergebnisse. Nuc Compact 18: 223–226

Juweid M, Strauss HW, Yaoita H, Rubin RH, Fischman AJ (1992) Accumulation of immunoglobulin G at focal sites of inflammation. Eur J Nucl Med 19: 159–165

Keelan ETM, Harrison AA, Chapman PT, Binns RM, Peters AM, Haskard DO (1994) Imaging vascular endothelial activation: an approach using radiolabeled monoclonal antibodies against the endothelial cell adhesion molecule E-selectin. J Nucl Med 35: 276–281

Knockaert DC, Vanneste LJ, Vanneste SB (1992) Fever of unknown origin in the 1980 s. An update of the diagnostic spectrum. Arch Intern Med 152: 51

Kubota R, Tamada S, Kubota K, Ishiwata K, Tamahashi N, Ido T (1972–1980) Intratumoral distribution of fluorine-18-fluorrrodeoxyyyglucose in vivo: high accumulation in macrophages and granulation tissue studied by microautoradiography. J Nucl Med 33

Larson EB, Featherstone HJ, Petersdorf RG (1982) Fever of undermined origin: diagnosis and follow-up in 105 patients – 1970–1980. Medicine 61: 269

Liberatore M, Clemente M, Iurilli AP, Zorzin L, Masini M, Di Rocco E, Centi Colella A (1992) Scintigraphic evaluation of disease in rheumatoid arthritis: a comparison of technetium-99 m human non-specific immunoglobulins, leucocytes and albumin nanocolloids. Eur J Nucl Med 19: 853–857

<referenLind P, Langsteger W, Költringer P, Dimai HP, Passl R, Eber O (1990) Immunoscintigraphy of inflammatory process with a technetium-99m-labelled monoclonal antigranulocyte antibody (Mab BW 250/183). J Nucl Med 31: 417–423

Locher JT, Seybold K, Andres RY, Schubiger PA, Mach JP, Buchegger F (1986) Imaging of inflammatory and infectious lesions after injection of radio-iodinated monoclonal antigranulocyte antibodies. Nucl Med Commun 7: 659–670

MacSweeney JE, Peters AM, Lavender JP (1990) Indium labelled leukocyte scanning in pyrexia of unknown origin. Clin Radiol 42: 414–417

McAfee JG, Gagne G, Subramanian G, Schneider RF (1991) The localization of indium-111-leukozytes, gallium-67, polyclonal IgG and other radioactive agents in acute focal inflammatory lesions. J Nucl Med 32: 2126–2131

McAfee JG, Gagne GM, Subramanian G (1980) Distribution of leukocytes labeled with In-111-oxine in dogs with acute inflammatory lesions. J Nucl Med 21: 1059–1068

McAfee JG, Thakur ML (1976) Survey of radioactive agents for in vitro labeling of phagocytic leukocytes. I. Soluble agents. J Nucl Med 17: 480–487

McAfee JG, Thakur ML (1976) Survey of radioactive agents for in vitro labeling of phagocytic leukocytes. II. Particles. J Nucl Med 17: 488–492

McCarthy K, Velchik MG, Alavi A, Mandell GA, Esterhazi JL, Goll S (1988) In-111-labelled white blood cells in the detection of osteomyelitis complicated by a pre-existing condition. J Nucl Med 29: 1015–1021

Meller J, Ivancevic V, Conrad M, Gratz S, Munz DL, Becker W (1998) Clinical value of immunoscintigraphy in patients with fever of unknown origin. J Nucl Med 39; 1248–1253

Munz DL, Morguet AJ, Sandrock D, Heim A, Sold G, Figulla HR, Kreuzer H, Emrich D (1991) Radio-immuno imaging of subacute infective endocarditis using a technetium-99 m monoclonal granulocyte specific antibody. Eur J Nucl Med 18: 977–980

Oswald SG, Norstrand DV, Savory CG, et al (1989) Three phase bone scan and indium white blood cell scintigraphy following porous coated hip arthroplasty: a prospective study of the prosthetic hip. J Nucl Med 30: 1321–1331

Oyen WJG, Claessens RAMJ, van der Meer JMW, Corstens FMH (1992) Biodistribution and kinetics of radiolabeled proteins in rats with focal infection. J Nucl Med 33: 651–656

Oyen WJG, van Horn JR, Claessens RAMJ, Slooff TJJH, Van der Meer WMJ, Corstens FMH (1992) Diagnosis of bone, joint and joint prosthesis infections with indium-111 labelled human immunoglobulin G scintigraphy. Radiology 182: 195–199

Oyen WJG, van Horn JR, Claessens RAMJ, Slooff TJJH, Van der Meer JWM (1991) Diagnosing prosthetic joint infections. J Nucl Med 32: 2195–2196

Palestro CJ, Kim CK, Swyer AJ, Vallabhajosula S, Goldsmith SJ (1991) Radionuclide diagnosis of vertebral osteomyelitis: indium-111-leukocyte and Tc-99 m methylene diphosphonate bone scintigraphy. J Nucl Med 32: 1861–1865

Palestro CJ, Kim DK, Swyer AJ, Vallabhajosula S, Goldsmith S (1991) Radionuclide diagnosis of vertebral osteomyelitis: In-111-leukocyte and Tc-99 m methylene diphosphonate bone scintigraphy. J Nucl Med, 32: 1861–1865

Palestro CJ (1994) The current role of gallium imaging in infection. Semin Nucl Med XXIV: 128–141

Peters AM, Saverymuttu SH, Keshavarzian A, Bell RN, Lavender JP (1983) Imaging of inflammation with In-111-tropolonate labeled leukocytes. J Nucl Med 24: 39–44

Peters AM (1994) The utility of Tc-99m-HMPAO leucocytes for imaging infection. Semin Nucl Med XXIV: 110–127

Petersdorf RG, Beeson PB (1961) Fever of unknown origin: report of 100 cases. Medicine 40: 1–30

Pring DJ, Henderson RG, Keshavarzian A, Rivet AG, Krausz T, Coombs RRH, Lavender JP (1991) Indium granulocyte scanning in painful prosthetic joint. Radiology 179: 645–647

Prvulovich EM, Miller RF, Costa DC, Sevem A, Corbett E, Bomanij J, Becker WS, Ell PJ (1995) Immunoscintigraphy with a Tc-99m-labelled antigranulocyte monoclonal antibody in patients with human immunodeficiency virus infection and AIDS. AIDS 16: 838–845

Radiation dose to patients from radiopharmaceuticals. Technetium labelled white blood cell (leukocytes) (ICRP publication no. 53). Ann ICRP 1987 18: 231–232

Radiation dose to the patients from radiopharmaceuticals (1987). Gallium citrate (ICRP publication no. 53). Ann ICRP 18: 141–143

Radiation dose to the patients from radiopharmaceuticals. Indium labelled white blood cells (leukocytes) (ICRP publication no. 53). Ann ICRP 1987 18: 255–256

Reuland P, Winkler KH, Heuchert T, Ruck P, Müller-Schauenburg W, Weller S, Feine U (1991) Detection of infection in postoperative orthopedic patients with technetium-99m-labeled monoclonal antibodies against granulocytes. J Nucl Med 32: 526–531

Rubin RH, Fischman AJ, Callahan RJ, Khaw BA, Keech F, Ahmed M, Wilkinson R, Strauss HW (1989) In-111 labeled nonspecific immunoglobulin scanning in the detection of focal infection. N Engl J Med 321: 935–940

Rubin RH, Young LS, Hansen P, Nedelman M, Wilkinson R, Nelles MJ, Callahan R, Khaw BA, Strauss HW (1988) Spedific and nonspecific imaging of localized Fisher immunotype. 1. Pseudomas aeruginosa infection with radiolabeled monoclonal antibody, J Nucl Med 29: 651–656

Saptogino A, Becker W, Wolf F (1991) Biokinetics and estimation of dose from Tc-99m-labelled polyclonal human immunoglobulin (HIG). Nucl Med 30: 18–23

Saptogino A, Becker W, Wolf F (1991) Biokinetics and estimation of dose from Tc-99m-labelled polyclonal immunoglobulin (HIG). Nucl Med 30: 18–23

Sasaki M, Ichiya Y, Kuwabara Y (1990) Ring like uptake of 18F-FDG in brain abscesses: a PET study. J. Comput. Assist. Tomogr. 14: 486–487

Saverymuttu SH, Camillieri M, Rees H, Lavender JP, Hodgson HJF, Chadwick VS (1986) Indium-111-granulocyte scanning in the assessment of disease extent and disease activity in inflammatory bowel disease. A comparison with colonoscopy, histology and fecal indium-111 granulocyte excretion. Gastroenterology 90: 1121–1128

Saverymuttu SH, Crofton ME, Peters AM, Lavender JP (1983) Indium-111 tropolonate leukocyte scanning in the detection of intra-abdominal abscesses. Clin Radiol, 34: 593–596

Saverymuttu SH, Peters AM, Chadwick VJ, Hodgson HJ, Lavender JP (1981) Imaging diseased bowel with In-111 labelled white cells. Br J Radiol 54: 707

Saverymuttu SH, Philips G, Peters AM, Lavender JP (1985) Indium-111-analogues leukocyte scanning in lobar pneumonia and lung abscesses. Thorax: 40: 925–930

Saverymuttu, SH, Peters AM, Lavender JP (1985) Clinical importance of enteric communications with abdominal abscesses. Br Med J 290: 23–27

Schiffmann E, Corcoran BA, Wahl SM (1972) Formylmethionyl peptides as chemo-attractants for leukocytes. Proc Natl Acad Sci USA 72: 1059–1062

Sciuk J, Brandau W, Vollet B, Stücker R, Erlemann R, Bartenstein R, Peters PE, Schober O (1991) Comparison of Tc-99 m polyclonal human immunoglobulin and Tc-99m-labeled monoclonal antibodies for imaging chronic osteomyelitis. Eur J Nucl Med 18: 401–407

Sciuk J, Braundau W, Vollet B, Stücker R, Erlemann R, Bartenstein P, Peters PE, Schober O (1991) Comparison of technetium-99 m polyclonal human immunoglobulin and technetium-99 m monoclonal antibodies for imaging chronic osteomyelitis. Eur J Nucl Med 18: 401–407

Segarra I, Roca M, Baliellas C, Vilar L, Ricart Y, Mora J. Puchal R, Martin-Comin J (1991) Granulocyte-specific monoclonal antibody technetium-99 m BW 250/183 and In-111 oxine labelled leukocyte scintigraphy in inflammatory bowel disease. Eur J Nucl Med 18: 715–719

Serafini AN, Garty I, Vargas-Cuba R. Friedman A, Rauh DA, Neptune M, Laundres L, Sfakianakis GN (1991) Clinical evaluation of a scintigraphic method für diagnosing inflammation/infections using indium-111 labeled nonspecific human IgG. J Nucl Med 32: 2227–2232

Shnier D, Bernard F, Alavi A, Garino J, Rhoad R (1997) The role of 18F-FDG -PET in the diagnosis of osteomyelitis. J. Nucl. Med 38: 119P

Shoen RP, van Ommen RA (1963) Fever of obscure origin. Am J Med 34: 486

Signore A, Chianelli M, Ferretti E, Toscano AM, Britton KE, Andreani D, Gale EAM, Pozilli P (1994) A new approach for in vivo detection of insulinitis: activated lymphocyte targeting with I-123-labelled interleukin-2. Eur J Endocrinol 131: 431–437

Signore A, Parman A, Pozilli P, Andreani D, Beverly PCL (1987) Detection of activated lymphocytes in endocrine pancreas of BB/W rats by injection of I-123-interleukin-2: an early sign of type I diabetes. Lancet II: 537–541

Sinn H, Silvester DJ (1979) Simplified cell labelling with In-111 acetyl-acetone. Br J Radiol 52: 758–759

Som P, Atkins HL, Bandooypadhyay D (1980) A fluorinated glucose analog, 18F-FDG, non toxic tracer for rapid tumor detection. J Nucl Med 21: 670–675

Spector WG, Lykke WJ, Willoubhgy PA (1967) A quantitative study of leukocyte emigration in chronic inflammatory granulomata. J Pathol Bacteriol 93: 101–107

Spinelli F, Milella M, Sara R, Busogni F, Possa M, Vigorelli R (1994) The value of Tc-99m-labelled human immunoglobulin scanning in the evaluation of Crohn's disease [abstract]. Eur J Nucl Med 35: 1436–1443

Streule K, de Schrijver M, Friedrich R (1988) Tc-99m-labelled HSA-nanocolloid versus In-111 oxine labeled granulocytes in detecting skeletal septic process. Nucl Med Commun 9: 59–67

Sugawara Y, Braun DK, Kison PV, Russo I.E, Zasadny KR, Wahl R (1998) Rapid detection of human infections with fluorine-18 fluorodeoxyglucose and positron emission tomography: preliminary results. Eur J Nucl Med 25,, 1238–1243

Tahara T, Ichiya Y, Kuwabara Y (1989) High 18F fluorodeoxyglucose uptake in abdominal abscesses: a PET study. J. Comput. Assist. Tomogr. 13: 829–833

Thakur ML, Lavender JP, Arnot RN, Silvester DJ, Segal AW (1977) Indium-111-labeled autologous leukocytes in man. J Nucl Med 18: 1012–1021

Thakur ML, McAfee JG (1984) The significance of chromosomal aberrations in In-111-lymphocytes. J Nucl Med 25: 922–927

Van Dalen H, Stemfort AF, de Jonge-Bok JM, de Schrijver M (1989) Three-phase scintigraphy of Tc-99 m nanocolloid versus Tc-99 m MDP in orthopedics. In: Stuttgart: Schattauer: 474–477

Van der Laken C, Boerman OC, Oyen WJG, Van de Ven M, Van der Meer J, Corstens FHM (1998) Scintigraphic detection of infection and inflammation: new developments with special emphasis on receptor interaction Eur J Nucl Med 25: 535–546

Van der Laken J, Boerman OC, Oyen WJG, Van de Ven MTP, Makarewicz J, Claessens RAMJ, Van der Meer JWM, Corstens FMH (1994) Recombinant human interleukin-1: potential agent to image infectious foci. Eur J Nucl Med 21: 790

Van Royen A, Rövekamp MH, van Dongen RJAM, van der Schoot JB, Hardeman RM (1984) In-111-leukocyte scintigraphy in the diagnosis of vascular graft infection. In: Hardeman MR, Najean Y, eds. Blood cells in nuclear medicine. Part I. cell kinetics and biodistribution. The Hague: Martinus Nijhoff: 341–347

Vorne M, Lantto S, Paakkinen S, Salo S, Soini I (1989) Clinical comparison of Tc-99 m HMPAO labeled leukocytes and Tc-99m-nanocolloid in the detection of inflammation. Acta Radiol 30: 633–637

Weiblen BJ, Forstrom LA, McCullogh J (1979) Kinetics of In-111-labelled granulocytes. J Lab Clin Med 94: 246–255

Wheeler JG, Slack NF, Duncan A, Palmer H, Harvey RF (1990) Tc-99m-nanocolloid in inflammatory bowel disease. Nucl Med Commun 11: 127–133

Woods G, Gutierrez Y, Walker D, Purtilo D, Shanley J (1993) Diagnostic pathology of infectious diseases. Philadelphia: Lea & Febiger

8 Gastrointestinal Nuclear Medicine

J. L. C. Urbain, C. L. Johnson, M. C. Vekemans

Contents

8.1 Esophageal Transit Scintigraphy 123
8.1.1 Introduction 123
8.1.2 Acquisition Procedure 123
8.1.3 Analysis and Quantification 124
8.1.4 Visualization and Interpretation 124
8.1.5 Clinical Applications 125
8.2 Gastric Emptying Scintigraphy 125
8.2.1 Introduction 125
8.2.2 Standard Procedure 125
8.2.2.1 Acquisition 126
8.2.2.2 Visual Assessment and Quantification 126
8.2.2.3 Modeling of Gastric Emptying Curves 127
8.2.2.4 Clinical Applications 127
8.2.3 Compartmental Analysis of the Stomach 127
8.2.4 Dynamic Antral Scintigraphy 127
8.2.4.1 Procedure 127
8.2.4.2 Interpretation and Clinical Significance 128
8.3 Colon Transit Scintigraphy 128
8.3.1 Introduction 128
8.3.2 Acquisition, Analysis, and Quantification 128
8.3.3 Findings and Interpretation 128
8.3.4 Clinical Applications 128
8.3.5 Whole Gut Transit 129
8.4 Gastrointestinal Bleeding Scintigraphy 129
8.4.1 Introduction 129
8.4.2 Acquisition Protocol 130
8.4.3 Findings and Interpretation 130
8.5 Hepatobiliary Scintigraphy 131
8.5.1 Introduction 131
8.5.2 Standard Procedure 131
8.5.3 Challenge Tests 131
8.5.4 Findings and Interpretation 131
8.5.4.1 Baseline Normal Study 131
8.5.4.2 Challenge Test 131
8.5.4.3 Gallbladder Contractility 132
8.5.5 Clinical Significance 132
8.5.5.1 Acute Cholecystitis 132
8.5.5.2 Common Bile Duct Obstruction 132
8.5.5.3 Chronic Cholecystitis 133
8.5.5.4 Gallbladder Dyskinesia 133
8.5.5.5 Sphincter of Oddi Dysfunction 133

J. L. C. Urbain, C.L. Johnson
Department of Diagnostic Imaging, Temple University Hospital, 3401 North Broad Street, Philadelphia, PA 19140, USA
M. C. Vekemans
CHGH, Route de Mons 63, B-7301 Hornu, Belgium

8.1 Esophageal Transit Scintigraphy

8.1.1 Introduction

Esophageal transit scintigraphy is typically performed after a 4- to 6-h fasting period. Medications affecting esophageal motility should be discontinued for at least 24 h. Water is the preferred bolus material because it is homogeneous and does not disperse along the esophagus. Technetium-99 m sulfur colloid is the radiotracer of choice. It is inexpensive, easily prepared, optimally detected by the Anger camera, and neither secreted nor absorbed by the esophageal mucosa. However, in multiple swallow studies, its use is limited by scattered radiation from the stomach.

Typically, a water bolus of 10–20 ml, labeled with 7.5 MBq (200 μCi) of ^{99m}Tc sulfur colloid is given to the patient. Practice swallows with normal water are recommended to educate the patient to swallow the labeled bolus in a single gulp.

8.1.2 Acquisition Procedure

The patient is positioned supine under the camera in order to eliminate the effect of gravity. The upright position is used only to evaluate the effectiveness of medications or surgical procedures. In both instances, the mouth, esophagus, and proximal stomach are visualized in a single field of view.

Anterior imaging is usually performed. The bolus material is administered to the patient with a syringe or a straw, and swallowed in one gulp. In a multiple swallow test, four to six bolus swallows are recommended to decrease the intraindividual variations in esophageal transit time.

In order to adequately assess motility, we acquire a total of 140 dynamic 64×64-pixel images in two steps: 120 images of 0.25 s, followed by 20 images of 30 s each. After the initial bolus swallow, the patient takes "dry swallows" every 30 s to assess the residual activity in the esophagus. In patients with significant stasis delayed images are taken at 15 and 30 min.

8.1.3 Analysis and Quantification

Time-activity curves are generated by drawing regions of interest around the upper, mid, and lower segments of the esophagus (Fig. 8.1). Global esophageal transit is calculated using the following formula:

$$C(t)=100\times[E_{max}-E(t)]/E_{max}. \quad (8.1)$$

In Eq. 8.1, C(t) is the percent esophageal emptying at time (t), E_{max} is the maximal count rate in the esophagus, and E(t) is the esophageal count rate at time (t) (TOLIN et al. 1979). Both global or segmental esophageal transits can be assessed using different parameters, such as the esophageal transit time (ETT), segmental emptying time, global esophageal emptying time, and esophagogastric transit time (TAILLEFER and BEAUCHAMP 1984).

Different methods have been introduced to integrate data obtained from multiple swallows, facilitate the qualitative assessment of radionuclide esophageal transit, and to improve the diagnostic ability of esophageal motor disorders. The technique of condensed images displays in a single image the spatial distribution of the radioactive bolus along the esophageal path (KLEIN 1986). A more recent method integrates the dynamic sequences into a single condensed image to represent average esophageal transit of multiple boluses (TATSCH 1991).

8.1.4 Visualization and Interpretation

Completeness of bolus ingestion, progression through the esophagus, retention in the esophagus, or gastroesophageal reflux are first assessed by cine display of the images. In normal individuals, the esophageal transit time for a liquid bolus is less than 10 s. The condensed picture shows a smooth progression of the bolus along the esophagus, with a physiologic deceleration in its mid portion due to the aortic arch.

8.1.5 Clinical Applications

The role of scintigraphy is to provide a physiological, quantitative, and non-invasive evaluation of suspected esophageal motor disorders, before and after medical or surgical treatment.

Achalasia is characterized by a marked, prolonged, and chaotic retention of the tracer in the distal segment of the esophagus with very little passage into the stomach.

With diffuse esophageal spasm there is a prolonged transit time associated with decreased segmental esophageal emptying, periods of esophageal

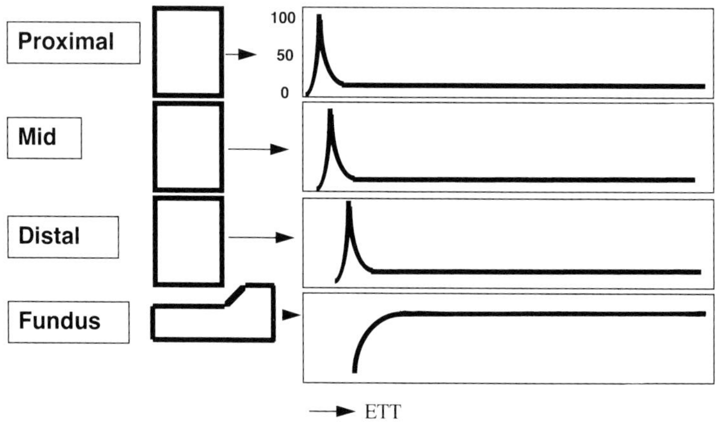

Fig. 8.1. Processing of esophageal transit scintigraphy. Regions of interest are drawn around the upper, middle, and lower third of the esophagus and a time-activity curve is generated for each segment. A curve of fundal activity can also be generated. Esophageal transit time (*ETT*) represents the time required for the bolus to travel from the upper esophageal sphincter to the fundus

retrograde motion, and fragmentation of the tracer. Time–activity curves show multiple peaks of activity in all esophageal segments.

Nutcracker esophagus is characterized by high-amplitude esophageal contractions and shows a prolonged retention of activity in the distal esophagus and a mild distal to mid-level esophageal reflux. However, since the esophageal contractions are peristaltic, scintigraphy can be entirely normal. With non-specific motor disorders the most common finding is a prolonged esophageal transit time with an uncoordinated pattern.

With neuromuscular and connective tissue disorders radionuclide esophageal transit is the only test to assess early involvement of the esophagus by progressive systemic sclerosis and is characterized typically by stagnation of the tracer in the lower two thirds of the esophagus. This retention can be cleared by increasing the pressure in the esophagus either by the upright position or by ingesting a glass of water.

Regarding miscellaneous disorders, radionuclide esophageal transit is the only test which allows for the physiologic quantitative evaluation of esophageal motility before and after surgical treatment for hiatal hernia and reflux and for the assessment of the transposed stomach or colon after esophagectomy.

8.2 Gastric Emptying Scintigraphy

8.2.1 Introduction

Introduced more than 30 years ago, gastric emptying scintigraphy has been significantly refined and optimized over the years. The simultaneous measurement of solid and liquid emptying by scintigraphy is now well established as the gold standard method in evaluation of gastric emptying.

Conventional gastric emptying is a simple procedure that measures the transit of a standardized radiolabeled test meal through the stomach; it requires static imaging at defined time intervals, as well as minimal processing and analysis. Hereafter, we present the technique employed at our institution. Conventional gastric emptying provides little information on gastric physiology and pathophysiology. Over the past 10 years mathematical modeling of the gastric emptying curves, compartmental analysis of the stomach, and more recently, dynamic antral scintigraphy (DAS) have provided new tools in evaluation of the pathophysiology of gastric motors disorders.

8.2.2 Standard Procedure

Gastric emptying is performed after a 12-h overnight fast and discontinuation of any medication likely to interfere with gastric motility. Patients should refrain from smoking since it may delay gastric evacuation. Diabetic patients should be studied early in the morning, after receiving two thirds of their usual insulin dose. There is currently no consensus on the optimal test meal to study gastric emptying. However, radiolabeled eggs, which are readily available, easy to prepare, and consistently labeled are used in most nuclear medicine laboratories. The eggs are mixed with 20–40 MBq (0.5–1.0 mCi) ^{99m}Tc sulfur colloid, cooked till firm in a Teflon-coated pan, and given to the patient as an egg sandwich. To evaluate liquid emptying, water is labeled with 3 MBq (75 μCi) of ^{111}In-DTPA. Ingestion of the test meal should be completed within 10 min.

Imaging is performed preferably with the subject sitting or standing. A ^{57}Co marker placed on the xyphoid process or iliac crest facilitates repositioning of the patient and automated processing.

8.2.2.1 Acquisition

Immediately after the completion of the meal, the patient is positioned in front of the camera fitted with a medium-energy parallel-hole collimator. An initial 1-min image of the stomach is acquired in the 140 keV ±20% technetium window. The patient then ingests the water and a second 1-min image is taken in the technetium window to calculate the downscatter percentage of indium into the technetium window. Simultaneous anterior and posterior static images (dual-head system), or an anterior static image, immediately followed by a posterior view (single head system) of the stomach, are taken in a 64×64 or 128×128 matrix in the technetium and indium windows at regular time intervals up to 50% emptying.

Depth attenuation must be corrected for by calculation of the geometric mean (i.e., the square root of the anterior activity multiplied by the posterior activity) of gastric counts. Counts are then decay and downscatter corrected, and normalized to 100% based on total gastric counts obtained immediately following ingestion of the meal (time t=0). Solid and liquid data are then plotted as percentage retention of food in the stomach over time.

8.2.2.2
Visual Assessment and Quantification

In normal subjects, immediately after meal ingestion, both solid and liquid phases are retained in the proximal stomach. Water distributes then uniformly throughout the stomach and is rapidly emptied into the duodenum. In contrast, solids move progressively from the proximal to the distal stomach where they are ground and slowly emptied into the duodenum (Fig. 8.2).

Measurement of the half-emptying time ($T_{1/2}$), or time required by the stomach to empty 50% of the ingested meal, is the simplest way to assess gastric transit. It is routinely and commonly used for clinical evaluation.

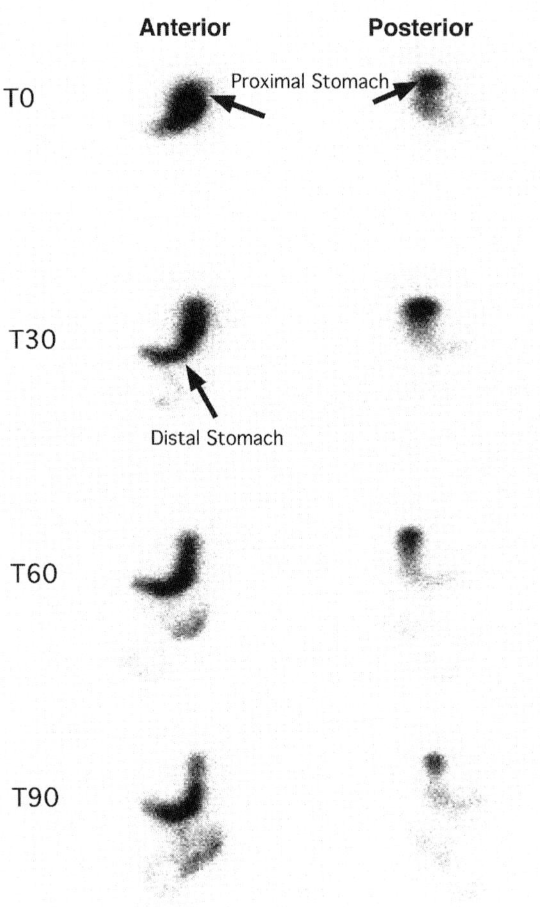

Fig. 8.2. Gastric emptying of solids. Anterior and posterior projections of the stomach are displayed immediately (T_0), 30 min (T_{30}), 60 min (T_{60}), and 90 min (T_{90}) after meal completion. Initially, solid food is stored in the proximal portion of the stomach. Over time, the solid particles move to the distal portion of the stomach for grinding and emptying into the duodenum through the pylorus

8.2.2.3
Modeling of Gastric Emptying Curves

Liquid emptying curves are usually adequately described by the single exponential function:

$$y(t)=e^{-k\times t}. \tag{8.2}$$

In Eq. 8.2, y(t) is the fractional meal retention at time t, and k the emptying rate per minute. $T_{1/2}$ is equal to 0.693/k.

Gastric emptying of solids is sigmoid in shape and characterized by an initial shoulder with little emptying ("lag phase" or T_{lag}), followed by a prolonged linear phase and finally a much slower phase (Fig. 8.3). The lag phase corresponds qualitatively and quantitatively to the redistribution of solid food particles from the fundus to the distal stomach and more specifically to the time to peak activity in the distal stomach (Urbain et al. 1989).

The modified power exponential function adequately fits biphasic solid emptying data:

$$y(t)=[1-(1-e^{-kt})^{ß}]. \tag{8.3}$$

In Eq. 8.3, y(t) is the fractional meal retention at time t, k is the gastric emptying rate in min^{-1} and ß is the extrapolated y-intercept from the terminal portion of the curve. The parameters k and ß are determined

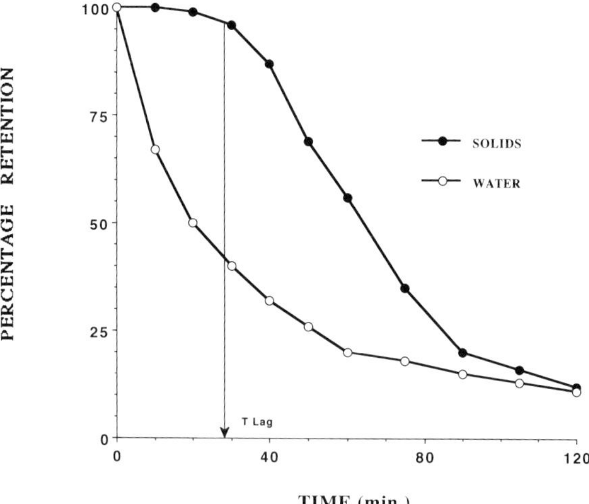

Fig. 8.3. Gastric emptying curves for solids and liquids. A liquid emptying curve follows a mono-exponential pattern. A solid emptying curve is sigmoidal in shape with an initial plateau (lag phase) followed by a linear emptying phase and a late slower portion

by a non-linear least-squares algorithm using the measured fractional retention y(t) and time t as input.

The following physiologic parameters can be derived from the gastric emptying curve: T_{lag} in minutes, i.e., the first part of the curve without emptying where y(t)=y(0), the emptying rate in percent of emptying per minute, and the half emptying time ($T_{1/2}$) in minutes.

8.2.2.4 Clinical Applications

8.2.2.4.1 Diabetes Mellitus

Rapid gastric emptying is observed in the early stages of diabetic autonomic neuropathy (Kong et al. 1996). Delay in solid gastric emptying is very common in symptomatic and asymptomatic long-standing diabetes. This delay is due essentially to a prolonged lag phase while the emptying rate is preserved. Advanced gastroparesis is characterized by a markedly prolonged gastric emptying, with a linear solid emptying curve. A prolonged lag period with a normal $T_{1/2}$ has also been described recently in patients with long-standing disease (Urbain et al. 1993).

Liquid emptying is only abnormal when solid-food emptying is severely impaired (Urbain et al. 1990a).

8.2.2.4.2 Idiopathic Dyspepsia

In functional dyspepsia associated with gastroparesis, there is a prolonged lag phase and slow emptying rate which reflects the retention of food in the distal stomach (Malagelada 1991).

8.2.2.4.3 Gastric Surgery

In patients with partial gastrectomy, such as the Roux-en-Y procedure, there is an initial precipitous emptying followed by a slow evacuation phase resulting in a delay in both solid and liquid emptying. There is no lag phase, and both liquids and solids empty in a similar fashion (Urbain et al. 1990b).

8.2.3 Compartmental Analysis of the Stomach

Scintigraphy, as electrophysiologic and manometric studies, allows characterization of the respective role of the proximal and distal stomach in the gastric emptying process. Distinct regions of interest are drawn over the proximal and distal stomach. Food retention in each compartment is normalized to the total maximum gastric activity at time zero and displayed on time-activity curves. Mathematical compartmental analysis of food distribution in the stomach has just begun to be investigated (Jadali et al. 1994).

In normal subjects total and proximal liquid gastric curves are almost identical because there is no retention of liquid in the distal stomach. In contrast, solids are retained in the stomach by the pylorus and the distal stomach emptying curve for solids takes an asymmetric bell-shape pattern.

In diabetic gastroparesis there is a significant retention of food in the proximal stomach which might correspond to a decrease in fundic motor activity (Urbain et al. 1993).

In contrast, patients with functional dyspepsia with or without gastroparesis display a normal proximal stomach emptying corroborating the normal electromechanical findings (Urbain et al. 1995).

8.2.4 Dynamic Antral Scintigraphy

The most significant development in gastric emptying over the past 5 years has been the introduction of dynamic antral scintigraphy (DAS). This procedure enables characterization of the frequency and amplitude of antral contractions, and correlation between gastric motility and gastric emptying.

8.2.4.1 Procedure

The subject is given a standard solid food test meal labeled with 75 MBq (2 mCi) of ^{99m}Tc sulfur colloid. Static images of the stomach are acquired at regular time intervals; in addition, 1-s anterior dynamic images are acquired for 4 min after each set of static images.

Time–activity curves are generated from proximal, middle, and distal regions of interest in the antrum and then analyzed using the autocorrelation function and a Fourier transform to determine the mean frequency and amplitude of the antral contraction.

8.2.4.2 Interpretation and Clinical Significance

In normal subjects antral contraction frequency and amplitude correlate inversely with the lag phase, emptying rate, and total gastric emptying course, i.e., the greater the antral motility, the faster the gastric emptying (URBAIN et al. 1990c, 1993, 1995).

In diabetic gastroparesis delayed gastric emptying is due to a retention of food in the proximal stomach and a decrease in the amplitude of antral contractions despite a higher frequency (URBAIN et al. 1993).

Patients with functional dyspepsia seem to have a paradoxical increase in the amplitude of antral contractions and gastric emptying delay may be caused by a preponderance of non-expulsive antral contractions and pyloric dysmotility (URBAIN et al. 1995).

8.3 Colon Transit Scintigraphy

8.3.1 Introduction

Patients are asked to discontinue any medications likely to affect colon transit, for at least 3 days before the test. No dietary change is needed. The study should not be performed within a 4-week period following a colonoscopy.

Oral administration of ^{111}In-DTPA is the most commonly used radionuclide to assess colon transit. It is administered either in encapsulated non-digestible capsules (STUBBS et al. 1991), plastic particles (MADSEN and JENSEN 1989), or methylacrylate-coated resin particles that dissolve in the ileocecal region (CAMILLERI et al. 1989). The easiest method consists of the oral administration of 4 MBq (100 μCi) ^{111}In-DTPA in water (SMART et al. 1991).

8.3.2 Acquisition, Analysis, and Quantification

Imaging is performed typically at 6, 24, 48, 72, and 96 h following oral administration of ^{111}In-DTPA. Anterior and posterior images of the abdomen are obtained for 10 min, using a low-field-of-view camera with medium-energy collimator.

Different methods exist to analyze colon transit images. The simplest method consists of determining the percentage of retention in each segment over time and to calculate the time required to clear 50% of the initial radioactivity (MADSEN and JENSEN 1989). Quantitation of residual activity in the different colonic regions at 4 and 24 h provides accurate colon transit information (CAMILLERI and ZINSMEISTER 1992). Colon transit time can also been assessed by the condensed-images technique (NOTGHI et al. 1993).

The geometric mean center (GMC) technique is now widely used to determine the segmental emptying of the anatomic regions of the colon (Fig. 8.4; KREVSKY et al. 1986).

8.3.3 Findings and Interpretation

In normal subjects the ascending colon empties in a linear manner after an initial lag phase suggesting its storage role (PROANO et al. 1990). Periods of no emptying alternating with periods of emptying are observed. A linear progression through the colon is also demonstrated when using the GMC analysis (STUBBS et al. 1991). Solid or liquid tracers produce similar patterns of colon transit (SMART et al. 1991). Significant interstudy variability in transit can be observed. Colon transit is slower and more variable in females than males, but there is no effect of aging (MCLEAN et al. 1992).

In patients with idiopathic constipation, the GMC analysis enables differentiation of colonic inertia from pelvic obstruction of defecation. Colonic inertia is a pancolonic disorder characterized by a very slow transit throughout the entire length of the colon, in patients with significant stasis of radioactivity in the esophagus. In contrast, obstructed defecation is associated with an abnormal retention in the rectosigmoid (KREVSKY et al. 1989a).

8.3.4 Clinical Applications

The most common clinical application of colon transit scintigraphy is the evaluation of patients with idiopathic constipation. It has also been used to demonstrate the prokinetic effect on the colon of drugs such as cisapride or naloxone (KAUFMAN et al. 1988; KREVSKY et al. 1989b).

8.3.5
Whole-Gut Transit

Several methods have been proposed to investigate the entire gastrointestinal tract in a single test. In our institution ^{111}In-DTPA in water is given with a solid meal. The egg sandwich (see above) is labeled with ^{99m}Tc to simultaneously study gastric emptying of solids. In normal subjects water empties from the stomach rapidly (90% within 2 h) and a geometric mean of abdominal counts is obtained at 2–3 h to determine 100% of the administered ^{111}In-DTPA activity. This determination enables generation of terminal ileum filling rates as well as input of bolus into the colon to measure the GMC. Whole-gut transit techniques may be limited in patients with severe gastroparesis, particularly when liquid emptying is markedly delayed.

8.4
Gastrointestinal Bleeding Scintigraphy

8.4.1
Introduction

Over the past 20 years the management of patients with gastrointestinal (GI) bleeding has changed dramatically. The widespread availability of upper and lower GI endoscopy and the progress in interventional radiology and embolization techniques have given nuclear medicine a new role in the diagnostic and therapeutic algorithms of GI bleeding.

In our institution a scan for bleeding is performed in patients with lower GI bleeding to evaluate the importance of the bleeding and, more importantly, to localize the site of bleeding before selective catheterization and embolization or surgery.

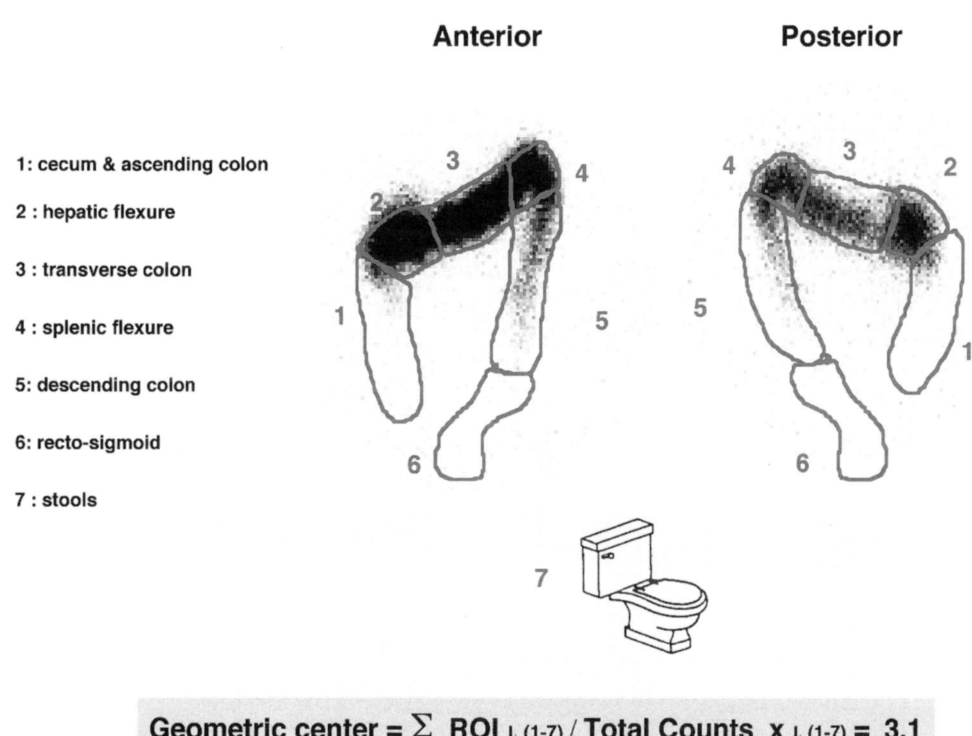

Fig. 8.4. Colon transit geometric center technique. Regions of interest (*ROI*) are generated around the six segments of the colon on the anterior and posterior images to determine the geometric mean of counts in each segment. The counts in ROI 7 are equal to the difference between input activity in the colon and the counts in the entire colon. The weighted numerical value of the geometric center represents the center of the activity as its travels though the colon

Both in vivo and in vitro red cell labeling methods are available for performing GI bleeding studies. In vivo labeling using the injection of stannous ion followed 20–30 min later by ^{99m}Tc-pertechnetate is convenient and easy to perform. However, labeling efficiency is variable and inconsistent varying from 60 to 90%. When present in significant amounts, free pertechnetate is secreted by the gastric mucosa and the kidneys. This may interfere significantly with the ability to detect bleeding in the stomach, proximal small bowel, and/or colon. The in vivo/in vitro technique consists of intravenous administration of the stannous ion, the ^{99m}Tc-pertechnetate labeling of a blood sample collected in a syringe containing an anticoagulant and ^{99m}Tc-pertechnetate, and the reinjection of the labeled sample. The labeling efficiency approaches 95%. The absence of blood manipulation and risk of contamination is a significant advantage of these two techniques. In the in vitro technique a sample of blood is withdrawn from the patient and an anticoagulant and stannous solution are added. Sodium hypochlorite and ACD solution are then added to oxidize the extracellular stannous ion. Technetium-99m pertechnetate is added to the blood sample and diffuses into the red blood cells, where it is reduced and trapped. Labeling efficiency is high and image quality appears superior (Maurer et al. 1998).

8.4.2 Acquisition Protocol

In our institution we acquire sequential sets of 15-min continuous dynamic study with 15-s framing for a total of 60 images in a 128×128-byte matrix. Each 15 min the acquisition is saved at completion. The study is stopped when the bleeding site is identified. If the patient is not bleeding during the initial hour following the administration of the labeled red cells, the study is terminated. Patients are often brought back to the department within the next 24 h for additional imaging if an acute onset of bleeding occurs.

8.4.3 Findings and Interpretation

Bleeding rate detection varies from 0.05 to 0.1 ml/min depending on the efficiency of the labeling procedure and other technical factors (Brown 1995). The cine display of the continuous dynamic set of images allows, most of the time, for the visualization and the precise localization of the bleeding site by tracking down the progression of blood within the bowel (Fig. 8.5). If the patient is bleeding profusely, a quick transfer is organized, either to interventional radiology for selective catheterization and embolization, or to the operating room for surgery.

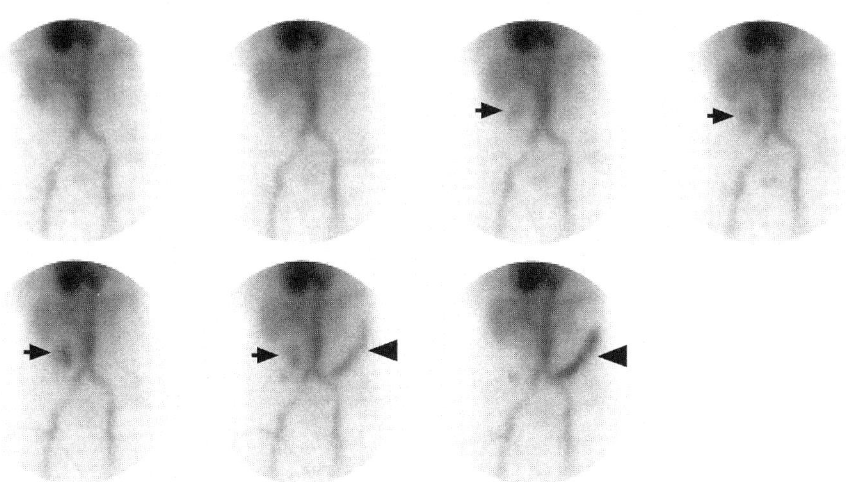

Fig. 8.5. Gastrointestinal bleeding scan. The images are cine displayed on the computer monitor and examined for the site of bleeding and motion of blood within the intestine. Images of this sequence have been reframed for illustration. In this case there is a site of bleeding in the right upper quadrant seen on the third image (*arrow* on the left). Images 6 and 7 show that the blood travels from the right towards the splenic flexure (*arrow* on the right) indicating that the bleeding occurs in the region of the hepatic flexure. Colonoscopy demonstrated that this patient had an angiodysplastic lesion at that level

8.5 Hepatobiliary Scintigraphy

8.5.1 Introduction

Acute cholecystitis resulting from the occlusion of the cystic duct, common bile duct (CBD) obstruction, or biliary leak are the major indications for performing a hepatobiliary scintigraphy. Cholecystagogue-augmented cholescintigraphy is used for the diagnosis of chronic cholecystitis, gallbladder dyskinesia, and sphincter of Oddi dysfunction.

Hepatobiliary scintigraphy is performed after intravenous administration of 175–350 MBq (5–10 mCi) of a ^{99m}Tc-labeled iminodiacetic acid (IDA) derivative such as disofenin (DISIDA) or mebrofenin. Both compounds are first-pass agents and extracted by the hepatocyte by the non-sodium-dependent organic anion transport processes as bilirubin. Eighty five percent of DISIDA and more than 95% of mebrofenin are cleared from the blood pool by the liver, secreted into the bile canaliculi, and transported to the small intestine via the intrahepatic ducts, common hepatic duct, cystic duct, and CBD. When the cystic duct is patent, the gallbladder accumulates a significant amount of the tracer within 1 h.

Patients need to be fasting for 2–5 h prior to the test to enable visualization of the gallbladder. Prolonged fasting and parenteral alimentation may also cause the gallbladder not to fill despite a patent cystic duct due to increased intraluminal pressure and viscous, concentrated bile.

8.5.2 Standard Procedure

The patient is positioned supine and images of the entire abdomen are acquired using a large-field-of-view camera equipped with a low-energy, parallel-hole collimator. An angiographic phase consisting of 60 images of 1 s each in a 128×128 matrix is obtained and is followed by a dynamic study of 59 continuous images of 1 min each.

Right anterior oblique and right lateral projections are then taken for 3 min each to distinguish the gallbladder from activity in the duodenum whenever necessary. Delayed images are acquired up to 6 h post injection if a bile leak is suspected or no activity is seen in the intestines during the 1-h acquisition.

8.5.3 Challenge Tests

If the gallbladder fails to visualize, we administer intravenously 0.02 mg/kg of morphine sulfate and a second lower 110 MBq (3 mCi) dose of tracer if there is not enough activity left in the liver. The acquisition is then continued for another 30 min.

The c-terminal octapeptide portion of cholecystokinin (CCK), Sincalide (Kinevac, Squibb Diagnostics, Princeton, N.J.), is given intravenously at a concentration of 0.02 µg/kg in a baby Baxter of normal serum saline over a period of 30 min to assess the gallbladder ejection fraction and/or the sphincter of Oddi response to CCK.

8.5.4 Findings and Interpretation

8.5.4.1 Baseline Normal Study

Within 15 min of intravenous administration most of the radiopharmaceutical is extracted by the liver and blood pool activity is minimal. The intrahepatic ducts are visualized at approximately 10–15 min. Activity is seen within the CBD at 15–20 min and is quickly followed by passage of the tracer into the intestines. Typically, the gallbladder is visualized between 30 and 60 min and keeps accumulating tracer (Rosenthall 1988).

8.5.4.2 Challenge Test

If the gallbladder fails to visualize within an hour while a fair amount of tracer is seen in the intestines and there is the suspicion of acute cholecystitis, we proceed with intravenous administration of morphine sulfate. Morphine augments the tone of the sphincter of Oddi and increases the intraluminal pressure of the CBD by approximately 50–60% in approximately 85% of patients. If the cystic duct is patent, this increase is sufficient to enable bile flow into the gallbladder. Morphine-augmented cholescintigraphy increases the sensitivity of conventional hepatobiliary scintigraphy in assessing cystic duct patency. A history of drug abuse, an allergy to the drug, pancreatitis, and significant obstruction of the CBD are contraindications to the administration of morphine (Fink-Bennett 1996).

8.5.4.3
Gallbladder Contractility

Cholecystagogues cause the gallbladder to contract, relax the sphincter of Oddi, enhance bowel motility, and cause secretion of bile and pancreatic fluid. In routine practice CCK is administered after maximal filling of the gallbladder and the ejection fraction at 30 min is calculated according to the expression (G_0-G_{30})G_0. In this expression G_0 is the net counts in the gall bladder just before CCK administration and G_{30}, 30 min later. It is usually agreed in the literature that an ejection fraction of 35% or more is a normal response to CCK. The response of the sphincter of Oddi to CCK is usually performed after a conventional baseline study either on a different day or after reinjection of a lower dose of tracer. A paradoxical response is seen when the sphincter of Oddi contracts instead of relaxes. This is witnessed on the scan by a pooling of tracer in the distal CBD. This phenomenon is sometimes referred to as distal CBD "ballooning" (Fig. 8.6).

8.5.5
Clinical Significance

8.5.5.1
Acute Cholecystitis

Increased perfusion to the gallbladder bed, a rim of radiotracer around the gallbladder indicating inflammatory changes of the gallbladder bed, and the non-visualization of the gallbladder, are the stigmata of cystic duct obstruction. The first two signs are very specific but not sensitive. Overall, the sensitivity of cholescintigraphy in detecting acute cholecystitis is greater than 95%. False-positive studies can result from severe chronic cholecystitis, prolonged fasting or a recent meal, or intravenous hyperalimentation. False-negative studies have been described in rare cases of acute acalculous cholecystitis.

8.5.5.2
Common Bile Duct Obstruction

The absence of visualization of the CBD and/or the absence of any activity in the intestines up to 4 h after injection with normal hepatocyte extraction indicates a complete CBD obstruction. The presence of a small

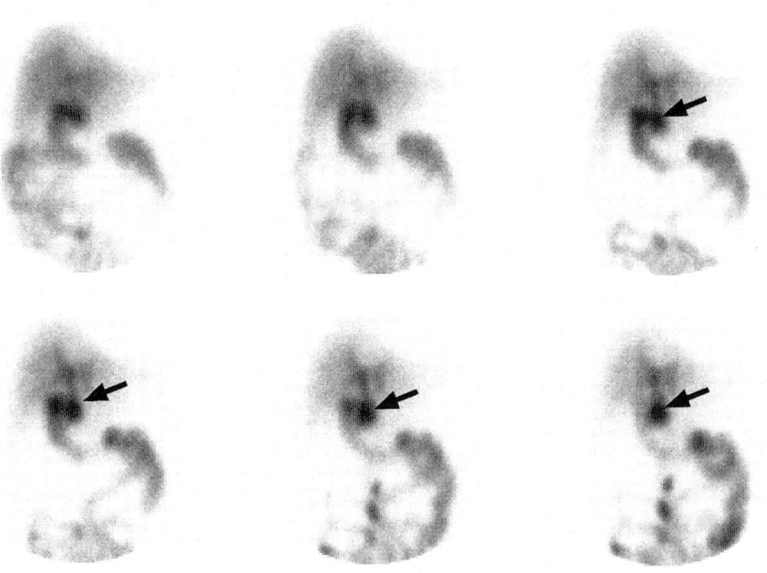

Fig. 8.6. Ballooning of the distal common bile duct (CBD). The paradoxical effect of cholecystokinin (CCK) on the sphincter of Oddi is demonstrated. After a baseline study and injection of a second dose of DISIDA, CCK was infused at a dose of 0.02 µg/kg and images of the liver and abdomen were obtained over a 30-min period. Images were reframed for illustration purposes. After CCK, there is pooling of activity in the distal CBD (*arrow*) indicating a paradoxical response of the sphincter

amount of activity in the intestines at 4 h indicates a high-grade but not complete CBD obstruction. A functional CBD obstruction is represented by a delayed biliary to bowel transit without dilation of the CBD.

8.5.5.3
Chronic Cholecystitis

Delayed gallbladder visualization, i.e., 1–4 h after tracer injection, is considered a positive sign for chronic cholecystitis and often results from increased gallbladder pressure due to sludge.

8.5.5.4
Gallbladder Dyskinesia

The term gallbladder dyskinesia refers to an abnormal response of the gallbladder wall to CCK. It is related to the abnormal or non-homogeneous distribution of CCK receptors or neuromediated contractile receptor cells within the gallbladder wall. These two disorders are characterized by a decreased ejection fraction.

8.5.5.5
Sphincter of Oddi Dysfunction

Sphinter of Oddi dysfunction is characterized by a paradoxical response, i.e., an elevation of the tone of the sphincter triggered by endogenous or intravenous administration of CCK. "Ballooning" (see 8.5.4.3) of the distal CBD is a very specific stigma of this disorder.

References

Brown M (1995) Gastrointestinal bleeding scan. In: Wagner HN Jr (ed) Principles of nuclear medicine, 2nd edn. Saunders, Philadelphia, pp 929–934

Camilleri M, Colemont MJ, Phillips SF, Brown ML, Thomforde GM, Chapman N, Zinsmeister AR (1989) Human gastric emptying and colonic filling of solids characterized by a new method. Am J Physiol 257:G284–G290

Camilleri M, Zinsmeister AR (1992) Towards a relatively inexpensive, non-invasive, accurate test for colonic motility disorders. Gastroenterology 103:36–42

Fink-Bennett D (1996) Hepatobiliary Imaging. In: Gotschalk A, Hoffer PB, Potchen EJ (eds) Diagnostic nuclear medicine, 3rd edn. Williams and Wilkins, Baltimore, pp 759–772

Jadali F, Charkes ND, Urbain JL, Maurer AH (1994) A mathematical model of gastric emptying with a physiological basis. J Nucl Med 35(A684):170

Kaufman PN, Krevsky B, Malmud LS, Maurer AH, Somers MB, Siegel JA, Fischer RS (1988) Role of opiate receptors in the regulation of colonic transit. Gastroenterology 94:1351–1356

Klein HA (1986) Applications of condensed dynamic images. Clin Nucl Med 11:178–182

Kong MF, Macdonald IA, Tattersall RB (1996) Gastric emptying in diabetes. Diabet Med 13:112–119

Krevsky B, Malmud LS, D'Ercole F, Maurer AH, Fisher RS (1986) Colonic transit scintigraphy: a physiologic approach to the quantitative measurements of colonic transit in humans. Gastroenterology 91:1102–1112

Krevsky B, Maurer AH, Fisher RS (1989a) Patterns of colonic transit in chronic idiopathic constipation. Am J Gastroenterol 84:127–132

Krevsky B, Maurer AH, Malmud LS, Fischer RS (1989b) Cisapride accelerates colonic transit in constipated patients with colonic inertia. Am J Gastroenterol 84:882–887

Madsen JL, Jensen M (1989) Gastrointestinal transit of technietium-99m-labeled cellulose fibre and indium-111-labeled plastic particles. JNM 30:402–406

Malagelada JR (1991) Where do we stand on gastric motility? Scand J Gastroenterol 175P [Suppl]:42–51

Maurer AH, Urbain JL, Krevsky B, Knight LC, Revesz G, Brown K (1998) Effects of in vitro versus in vivo red cell labeling on image quality in gastrointestinal bleeding studies. J Nucl Med Technol 26:87–90

McLean RG, Smart RC, Lubowski DZ, King DW, Barbagallo S, Talley NA (1992) Oral colon transit scintigraphy using indium-111-DTPA: variability in healthy subjects. Int J Colorect Dis 7:173–176

Notghi A, Kumar D, Panagamuwa B, Tulley NJ, Hesslewood SR, Harding LK (1993) Measurement of colonic transit time using radionuclide imaging: analysis by condensed images. Nucl Med Commun 14:204–218

Proano M, Camilleri M, Phillips SF, Brown ML, Thomforde GM (1990) Transit of solids through the human colon: regional quantification in the unprepared bowel. Am J Physiol 258:G856–862

Rosenthall L (1988) Hepatobiliary imaging. In: Wagner HN Jr (ed) Diagnostic nuclear medicine, 2nd edn. Williams and Wilkins, Baltimore, pp 582–609

Smart RC, McLean RG, Gaston-Parry D et al (1991) Comparison of oral iodine-131 cellulose and indium-111-DTPA as tracers for colon transit scintigraphy: analysis by colon activity profiles. J Nucl Med 32:1668–1674

Stubbs JB, Valenzuala GA, Stubbs CC, Croft BC, Teates CD, Plankey MW, McCallum RW (1991) A noninvasive scintigraphic assessment of the colonic transit of non-digestible solids in man. J Nucl Med 32:1375–1381

Taillefer R, Beauchamp G (1984) Radionuclide esophagogram. Clin Nucl Med 9:465–483

Tatsch K, Schroettle W, Kirsch CM (1991) Multiple swallow test for the quantitative and qualitative evaluation of esophageal motility disorders. J Nucl Med 32:1365–1370

Tolin RD, Malmud LS, Reillely J, Fisher RS (1979) Esophageal scintigraphy to quantitate esophageal transit (Quantitation of esophageal transit). Gastroenterology 76:1402–1408

Urbain J-LC, Siegel JA, Charkes ND, AH Maurer AH, Fisher RS, Malmud LS (1989) The two-component stomach: effects of meal particle size on fundal and antral emptying. Eur J Nucl Med 15:254–259

Urbain JLC, Vantrappen G, Janssens J, Van Cutsem E, Peeters T, DeRoo M (1990a) Intravenous erythromycin dramatically accelerates gastric emptying in gastroparesis diabeticorum and normals and abolishes the emptying discrimination between solids and liquids. J Nucl Med 31:1490–1493

Urbain JLC, Penninckx F, Siegel JA, Vandenborre PH, VanCutsem E, VanDenMaegdenberg V, DeRoo M (1990b) Effect of proximal vagotomy and Roux-en-Y diversion on gastric emptying kinetics in asymptomatic patients. Clin Nucl Med 15:688–691

Urbain JLC, Van Cutsem E, Siegel JA et al (1990c) Visualization and characterization of gastric contractions using a radionuclide technique. Am J Physiol 259:G1062–G1067

Urbain JLC, Vekemans MC, Bouillon R et al (1993) Characterization of gastric antral motility disturbances in diabetes using the scintigraphic technique. J Nucl Med 34(4):576–581

Urbain JL, Vekemans MC, Parkman H et al (1995) Characterization of gastric antral motility in functional dyspepsia using digital antral scintigraphy. J Nucl Med 36(9):1579–1586

9 Peptide Imaging

I. Virgolini

Contents

9.1 Introduction 135
9.2 Radiolabeled Peptides as Imaging Agents 137
9.2.1 Octreotide-Based Agents 138
9.2.2 ^{111}In-DOTA-Lanreotide 138
9.2.3 ^{99m}Tc-Depreotide 138
9.2.4 ^{99m}Tc-Vapreotide 139
9.2.5 ^{123}I-VIP and Tc-99m-P1666 139
9.3 Scintigraphy with Radiolabeled Peptides 139
9.3.1 Scintigraphy with ^{111}In-DTPA-D-Phe^{1}-Octreotide 139
9.3.2 Scintigraphy with ^{99m}Tc-Depreotide 140
9.3.3 Scintigraphy with ^{123}I VIP 140
9.4 Oncologic Applications 140
9.4.1 Colorectal Cancer 140
9.4.1.1 The Clinical Problem 140
9.4.1.2 ^{123}I VIP Receptor Scintigraphy 140
9.4.1.3 Scintigraphy with Radiolabeled Somatostatin Analogs 142
9.4.2 Pancreatic Cancer 142
9.4.2.1 The Clinical Problem 142
9.4.2.2 ^{123}I-VIP Receptor Scintigraphy 143
9.4.2.3 Scintigraphy with Radiolabeled Somatostatin Analogs 144
9.4.3 Lung Cancer 144
9.4.3.1 The Clinical Problem 144
9.4.3.2 ^{123}I-VIP Receptor Scintigraphy 145
9.4.3.3 Scintigraphy with Radiolabeled Somatostatin Analogs 145
9.4.4 Breast Cancer 146
9.4.4.1 The Clinical Problem 146
9.4.4.2 ^{123}I-VIP Receptor Scintigraphy 147
9.4.4.3 Scintigraphy with Radiolabeled Somatostatin Analogs 147
9.4.5 Neuroendocrine Tumors 148
9.4.5.1 The Clinical Problem 148
9.4.5.2 Carcinoid Tumors 149
9.4.5.3 Insulinomas 150
9.4.5.4 Other Neuroendocrine Tumors 150
9.4.6 Thyroid Cancer 151
9.4.7 Melanomas 151
9.4.8 Lymphomas 152
9.4.9 Other Tumors 152
9.5 Future Aspects 153

I. Virgolini
Department of Internal Medicine, University of Vienna, Währinger Gürtel 18–20, A-1030 Vienna, Austria

9.1 Introduction

Receptors are high-affinity binding proteins that respond to specific ligands with a defined physiological event. Changes in the interaction of a ligand with its receptor have been implemented in a variety of human diseases such as diabetes and hyperlipoproteinemia. Over the past decade, substantial documentation with receptor-mediated imaging has been presented. Radiotracers and nuclear medicine technology are used to detect many types of cancers in their early stages by recognition of tumor-specific properties. However, among thousands of possible candidates, only a few radioligands have entered the clinic and are useful in the daily routine. Over the past three decades, such radioligands have evolved from monoclonal antibodies, which are large proteins, through F(ab')$_2$ and Fab fragments to the smaller "molecular recognition units," and finally to small biologically active (synthetic) peptides. The molecular weight of such peptides is extremely diverse, ranging from small peptides which can be produced by solid phase or solution synthesis to larger polypeptides (>50 residues) which are more efficiently prepared by molecular cloning.

One of the characteristics that can be exploited for imaging is the high-affinity binding of a radiopeptide tracer to receptors expressed on the surface of specific cells. The high level expression of peptide receptors on various tumor cells, as compared with normal tissues or normal peripheral blood cells (Virgolini et al. 1994a; Reubi 1995), has provided the molecular basis for the clinical use of radiolabeled peptides as tumor tracers in nuclear medicine. In fact, receptor scintigraphy using radiolabeled peptide ligands has proven its effectiveness in clinical practice. In particular, somatostatin (SST) and vasoactive intestinal peptide (VIP) analogs have successfully been used for imaging purposes.

Molecular cloning of human SST and VIP receptors (hSSTR, hVIPR) has recently provided new insight into the biology and interaction of SST and VIP.

These receptors are widely distributed throughout the human body and seem to be responsible for the divergent effects observed for SST, VIP, and their analogs. Somatostatin is a 14-amino-acid peptide acting as a neurotransmitter or as a hormone, depending on the site of action and target cell type. Hormonal effects of SST include the suppression of release of growth hormone (GHRF) from the anterior pituitary gland (Brazeau et al. 1973) as well as inhibition of release of other pituitary, pancreatic, and gastrointestinal hormones or secretary proteins (Brazeau et al. 1973; Plewe et al. 1984). In addition, SST inhibits growth and proliferation of various tumor cells (Reichlin 1983). Vasoactive intestinal peptide is a 28-amino-acid neuroendocrine mediator with a broad range of biological activities in various cells and tissues. Initially, VIP was characterized as a vasodilatory substance (Said and Mutt 1970) responsible for the watery diarrhea syndrome in patients with VIP-secreting tumors (Verner and Morrison 1958; Bloom et al. 1973; Said and Faloona 1975). More recent studies have shown that VIP promotes growth and proliferation of both normal and malignant cells (Pincus et al. 1990; Haegerstrand et al. 1989; Virgolini et al. 1994a).

Five different hSSTR (Yamada et al. 1992a,b, 1993; Yasuda et al. 1992; Demchyschyn et al. 1993; Corness et al. 1993; Rohrer et al. 1993; Bell et al. 1995) have been characterized in detail and have been cloned. In several species, VIPR have been characterized and/or cloned (Laburthe and Couvineau 1988; Couvineau and Laburthe 1985; Couvineau et al. 1986, 1990, 1994; Ishihara et al. 1992; Lutz et al. 1993; Sreedharan et al. 1991; Usdin et al. 1994; Ullrich et al. 1998). The human VIPR8 cloned from the small intestinal epithelium (hVIPR; Couvineau et al. 1994) presents a human common VIP/PACAP receptor, similar to the VIPR cloned from human colonic cancer cells (Sreedharan et al. 1991). This receptor has been termed VIPR1, whereas another VIPR (termed VIPR2) has been cloned from animal (Lutz et al. 1993, Inagaki et al. 1994) and human species (Svoboda et al. 1994). VIPR2 is characterized by substantial affinity for helodermin (Robberecht et al. 1989). Also secretin appears to distinguish between these receptors (Adamou et al. 1996). They are members of a distinct subfamily of GTP-binding protein-coupled seven-helix transmembrane spanning receptors, being similar in their amino acid sequences but differing in extracellular amino terminal and intracellular carboxy-terminal domains.

Several efforts have been undertaken to identify hSSTR subtypes expressed by primary human tumors; however, the expression patterns have not been estab-

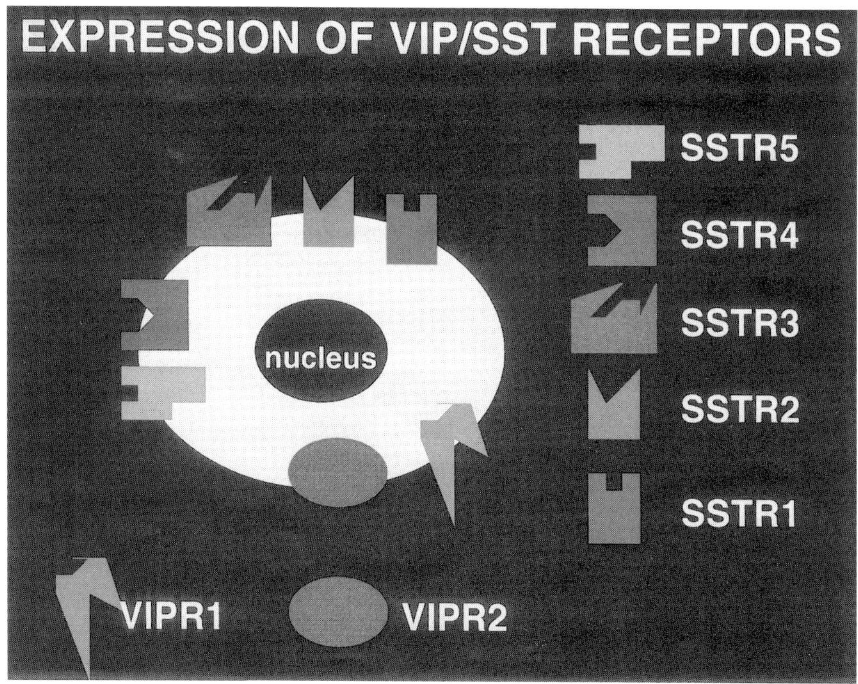

Fig. 9.1. Presentation of somatostatin (*SST*) and vasoactive intestinal peptide (*VIP*) receptor expression in human tumor cells. Five different SST and two different VIP receptors were characterized and cloned

lished in detail (Fig. 9.1). We have reviewed (Virgolini et al. 1997) the results of several attempts to identify hSSTR subtypes in primary human tumors. The patterns of expression of mRNA for hSSTR subtypes and their distributions are different, but often overlapping in various tumors. Using the RT-PCR (reverse transcription polymerase chain reaction) technique, in situ hybridization or Northern blotting, numerous observations suggest that the hSSTR are expressed in various human tumors. However, the expression of hSSTR seems to be very individual and varies from tumor entity to tumor entity. In initial studies only the hSSTR2 was identified frequently in primary human tumors (Reubi et al. 1994). More recently, other hSSTR have been frequently described (Greenman and Melmed 1994a,b; Kubota et al. 1994; Panetta and Patel 1994; Vikic-Topic et al. 1995; Miller et al. 1995; John et al. 1996; Buscail et al. 1996; Janson et al. 1996; Schaer et al. 1997; Laws et al. 1997; Jais et al. 1997; O'Nilsson et al. 1998; Fisher et al. 1998). The data vary from research group to research group, most probably due to the different techniques applied and also to the different tumor entities investigated. We and others have identified the hSSTR3 as another peptide receptor expressed on or in human tumor cells (Pangerl et al. 1997; Schaer et al. 1997). hSSTR3 may be responsible for binding both VIP and SST/octreotide (common binding site), and for the observed cross-competition between these peptides in primary human tumors as well as a variety of human tumor cell lines (Virgolini et al. 1994a, 1996b, 1998a; Peck-Radosavljevic et al. 1998). Contrary to other SSTR subtypes, only the hSSTR3 appears to be over-expressed at a very high level in or on all tumors (Pangerl et al. 1997; Raderer et al. 1998a). In terms of the VIP receptors, the information on subtype receptors in tumor tissues is extremely limited (Jiang et al. 1997).

9.2 Radiolabeled Peptides as Imaging Agents

The SSTR/VIPR imaging agents used for clinical studies are listed in Table 9.1. Some of these radiolabeled agents were also tested for their in vitro binding to hSSTR/hVIPR subtypes expressed on COS7 or CHO cells. Surprisingly, for several of the peptides differences were described in the binding behavior of the parent substance, the labeled and/or unlabeled ligand (Smith-Jones et al. 1998a,b). All these tracers were found to bind to tumor cell lines known to express SSTR as well as to primary human tumors. For most SSTR/VIPR tracers, significantly increased binding to tumor cells as opposed to normal cells was documented.

Native SST exists in two forms (14 or 28 amino acids), but it is readily attacked by aminopeptidases and endopeptidases, and has a short in vivo half-life. Consequently, synthetic SST analogs, which incorporate a Phe-(D)Trp-Lys-Thr (or similar sequence) and which are metabolically stabilized, at both the N- and C-terminals, were developed for clinical applications. Thus far, three commercially available SST analogs, i.e., octreotide (Rosenberg and Brown 1991), lanreotide (Giusti et al. 1997), and vapreotide (Stiefel and Morant 1993), have been shown to be effective in controlling the growth of some human tumors. These SST analogs all have similar binding profiles for four of the five hSSTR subtypes (i.e., a high affinity for hSSTR2 and hSSTR5, moderate affinity for hSSTR3, and very low affinity for hSSTR1), but lanreotide and vapreotide have a moderate affinity for hSSTR4, whereas octreotide has little or no affinity for this hSSTR (Lamberts et al. 1996).

Table 9.1. Overview of imaging agents

Radioligand	Availability	Receptor binding
^{123}I-octreotide	No longer in use	Not available
^{123}I-Tyr^{3}-octreotide	No longer in use	hSSTR2, 5 (3)
^{111}In-DTPA-D-Phe^{1}-octreotide	Mallinckrodt Medical (St. Louis, Mo.)	hSSTR2, 5 (3)
^{111}In-DOTA-lanreotide (MAURITIUS)	University of Vienna	hSST2–5 (1)
^{111}In-DOTA-Tyr^{3}-octreotide	May be prepared in house	hSST2, 5 (3)
^{99m}Tc-depreotide (P829)	Submitted for registration	hSST2, 3, 5
^{99m}Tc-HYNIC-octreotide	May be prepared in house	Not available
^{99m}Tc-vapreotide	May be prepared in house	Not available
^{123}I VIP	University of Vienna	hSSTR3, VIPR1, 2
^{99m}Tc-P1666 (VIP analog)	Phase IIa trial ongoing	Not available
^{99m}Tc-TP 3654 (VIP analog)	Experimental only	Not available

9.2.1 Octreotide-Based Agents

In initial studies ^{123}I-Tyr^3-octreotide was used to demonstrate the feasibility to detect and localize human neuroendocrine tumors (Lamberts et al. 1990; Krenning et al. 1989, 1993; Kvols 1994). However, the labeling with ^{123}I-sodium iodide of high specific activity is expensive and is hardly available worldwide. Furthermore, iodination of peptides requires technology and skills which are usually restricted to larger nuclear medicine institutions. Due to substantial accumulation of ^{123}I-Tyr^3-octreotide in the gut as a result of hepatobiliary clearance of the agent, interpretation of the abdominal images can sometimes be very difficult. Similar high abdominal accumulation was also found with ^{123}I-octreotide (Virgolini et al. 1996a). Some of the aforementioned problems have successfully been overcome by the introduction of ^{111}In-DTPA-D-Phe^1-octreotide which is the first receptor radiopharmaceutical available on the market (OctreoScan, Mallinckrodt Medical, St. Louis, Mo.). In this molecule a DTPA group is coupled to the aNH_2 group of the N-terminal D-Phe residue (Bakker et al. 1991). As opposed to ^{123}I-Tyr^3-octreotide, ^{111}In-DTPA-D-Phe^1-octreotide shows minor accumulation in the liver and is predominantly excreted via the kidneys (Krenning et al. 1992). Therefore, the interpretation of scintigrams of the abdominal region is less affected by intestinal background radioactivity.

Clinical studies with ^{111}In-DTPA-D-Phe^1-octreotide have clearly shown that this receptor radiopharmaceutical is effective in diagnosing and staging tumors and their metastases, due to binding to hSSTR2 (Lamberts et al. 1996; Smith-Jones et al. 1998a,b).

Another analog of octreotide, ^{111}In-DOTA-D-Phe^1-Tyr^3-octreotide, has been prepared showing similar in vivo accumulation as compared with ^{111}In-DTPA-D-Phe^1-octreotide (Krenning et al. 1996, 1997). The purpose of this development was to create a ligand which can be stably labeled with ^{90}Y for receptor-mediated radiotherapy (Otte et al. 1997, 1998). In this molecule the Phe^3 was replaced with Tyr to increase the hydrophilicity of the radiolabeled peptide.

Several efforts have been made to label octreotide with ^{99m}Tc. At our institution, ^{99m}Tc-labeled N-α-(6-hydrazinonicotinoyl)-octreotide (HYNIC-octreotide) did not display sufficiently high binding affinity for SSTR compared with other octreotide analogs (Krois et al. 1996); however, scintigraphic data have demonstrated excellent image quality for a similar HYNIC-octreotide analog in human studies (Bangard et al. 1998).

9.2.2 ^{111}In-DOTA-Lanreotide

^{111}In-DOTA-lanreotide MAURITIUS (Multicenter Analysis of a Universal Receptor Imaging and Treatment Initiative: a European Study) is a novel SST analog which is a conjugate of DOTA coupled directly to the N-terminus of lanreotide (Smith-Jones et al. 1998a,b). The substance can be stably labeled with a variety of radionuclides. ^{111}In-/^{90}Y-DOTA-lanreotide binds with high affinity (dissociation constant K_d 1-12 nM) to numerous primary human tumors such as intestinal adenocarcinomas and breast cancer. ^{111}In-/^{90}Y-DOTA-lanreotide exhibits a similar high binding affinity (K_d 2-11 nM) for the human breast cancer cell lines T47D and ZR75-1, the prostate cancer cell lines PC3 and DU145, the colonic adenocarcinoma cell line HT29, the pancreatic adenocarcinoma cell line PANC1, and the melanoma cell line 518A2. When expressed in COS7 cells, ^{111}In-/^{90}Y-DOTA-lanreotide binds with high affinity to hSSTR2 (K_d≈5 nM), hSSTR3 (K_d 5 nM), hSSTR4 (K_d 3.8 nM), and hSSTR5 (K_d 10 nM), and with lower affinity to hSSTR1 (K_d≈200 nM).

^{111}In-/^{90}Y-DOTA-lanreotide is presently applied at several centers in Europe to prove the concept of receptor-mediated radiotherapy controlled by dosimetry using the same ligand (MAURITIUS).

9.2.3 ^{99m}Tc-Depreotide (P829; Neotect, Amersham-Nycomed, Buckinghamshire, UK)

Although clinical results with ^{111}In- and ^{123}I-labeled peptides have been excellent, extensive efforts have been made in preparing and evaluating peptides labeled with ^{99m}Tc. The SST/VIP peptide analogs are small molecules which target their receptor and clear rapidly from the circulation. Accordingly, radionuclides with short half-lives are the labels of choice. These permit the administration of larger amounts of radioactivity and reduce the radiation dose to the patient. Provided that the energy of the gamma photon emitted is appropriate, this results in a high count rate and high image quality which translates into a high diagnostic efficacy.

In contrast to ^{111}In and ^{123}I, ^{99m}Tc is considered the optimal radionuclide in nuclear medicine, freely available from in-house ^{99}Mo/^{99m}Tc generators, and attempts have been made to label SST/VIP with ^{99m}Tc. Several chelate systems have been used for labeling SST analogs with ^{99m}Tc such as N4-aromatic and N4 aliphatic ligands, N3S ligands, or HYNIC chelators (Maina et al. 1994; Mather and Ellison 1994; Krois et al. 1996; Thakur et al. 1997). None of these methods have proven optimal for in vivo trials with the exception of the N3S system used in the agent P829 (Vallabhajosula et al. 1996). P829 carries a sequence which mimics the binding domain for SST. P829 is synthesized using solid phase peptide synthesis and N-(9-fluorenyl)methoxycarbonyl chemistry. ^{99m}Tc-P829 has been identified as a suitable hSSTR ligand which binds to hSSTR2, 3, and 5 with high affinity (Virgolini et al. 1998a). The cyclic hexapeptide domain of the peptide component of ^{99m}Tc-P829 contains the pharmacophore L-tyrosine-D-tryptophan-L-lysine-L-valine which binds to the SSTR of tumor cells. In fact, ^{99m}Tc-P829 has indicated clinical potential for imaging lung tumors, melanomas, or breast cancers (Virgolini et al. 1998a; Blum et al. 1998; Hustinx et al. 1997; Lastoria et al. 1996).

9.2.4 ^{99m}Tc-Vapreotide (RC-160)

Vapreotide (RC-160, Octastatin) is an SST analog being developed for gastroenterologic, neuroendocrine, and oncologic applications. The peptide binds to hSSTR2 and hSSTR5 with high affinity, and moderately also to hSSTR3 and hSSTR4.

Using CTPA (1,4,8,11-tetraazacyclotetradecane) as a bifunctional agent, RC-160 was labeled with ^{99m}Tc and was evaluated in mice bearing experimental human prostate cancers. In these studies tumor uptake was estimated to be significantly higher compared with other compounds (Thakur et al. 1997). Studies by Guhlke et al. (1997) and Bogatzky et al. (1997) have shown that RC-160 can also be labeled with either ^{131}I, ^{99m}Tc, or ^{188}Re using other chelating systems; however, no clinical data are available presently for humans.

9.2.5 ^{123}I-VIP and ^{99m}Tc-P1666

Vasoactive intestinal peptide (VIP) is a 28-amino-acid neuropeptide with a broad range of biological activities. Vasoactive intestinal peptide receptor scintigraphy uses naturally occurring VIP labeled with ^{123}I in positions 10 and 22 of the amino acids (Virgolini et al. 1994b, 1995).

Although the results obtained thus far suggest ^{123}I VIP to be a promising tumor tracer with the potential to provide additional information to conventional imaging, there are still some shortcomings which hamper widespread clinical use of the compound. Attempts have been made to label VIP with ^{99m}Tc since ^{123}I VIP is difficult and costly to produce.

In developing such a radiopharmaceutical, we have identified P1666 among VIP peptide candidates to be a promising ^{99m}Tc-labeled VIP analog for administration to tumor patients (Shirzad et al. 1998; Lister-James et al. 1998). Other VIP analogs have also been implemented including an ^{18}F-labeled VIP analog (Jagoda et al. 1997) as well as several ^{99m}Tc VIP analogs (Pallela et al. 1998a–c).

9.3 Scintigraphy with Radiolabeled Peptides

9.3.1 Scintigraphy with ^{111}In-DTPA-D-Phe^1-Octreotide

Abundant information exists on the best scanning procedures for OctreoScan (Krenning et al. 1993). In principle, early planar images should be acquired at approximately 4–6 h post injection of 10 µg peptide labeled with approximately 150 MBq (4 mCi) ^{111}In chloride. Late planar images should be acquired at 24 h. Depending on the clinical indication for SSTR scintigraphy, whole-body imaging should be performed in those patients in whom the extent of the disease has to be evaluated. It is very important to use a slow scanning procedure of 6 cm, or less, per minute (Krenning et al.1993). Single photon emission computed tomography (SPECT) should be performed in all patients, preferably at 24 h. In some patients a 48-h acquisition may be necessary to evaluate unclear accumulation in the abdomen. All images should be obtained with a large-field-of-view gamma camera, equipped with a medium-energy parallel-hole collimator. Data from both ^{111}In photon peaks (172 and 245 keV; window width 20%) should be used. For planar imaging a matrix of 128×128 (500 kcounts preset), and for SPECT a 64×64 matrix, should be used (60 projections, 45–60 s per projection). In our institution tomographic reconstruction is performed with a Wiener and ramp filter.

9.3.2 Scintigraphy with ^{99m}Tc-Depreotide

In analyzing early and delayed imaging with ^{99m}Tc-depreotide (Neotect), no appreciable diagnostic difference was reported (Lastoria et al. 1996; Virgolini et al. 1998a; Blum et al. 1998). In general, the image quality was better for the delayed images (i.e., 90 min post injection). We recommend imaging at 15 and 90 min after injection of approximately 50 μg peptide labeled with 740 MBq (20 mCi) ^{99m}Tc-depreotide. Standard planar and SPECT acquisitions should be obtained with a LEAP collimator (see 9.3.1).

9.3.3 Scintigraphy with ^{123}I VIP

Iodine-123 VIP scintigraphy was performed in more than 500 patients at the University of Vienna during the years 1993–1998. In general, the application of ^{123}I VIP is safe; however, blood pressure may drop during the initial minutes after bolus injection. Patients may experience a feeling of "heat" if the tracer is injected too quickly. We recommend early (15–60 min after injection) and delayed (3–6 h after injection) planar images of the abdomen in anterior, posterior, and lateral views. In all patients SPECT imaging should be performed at 2–4 h.

The preferred dose of ^{123}I VIP is 150–200 MBq (2–3 mCi), with 1 μg (300 pmol). The VIP standard planar and SPECT acquisitions should be obtained with a large-field-of-view gamma camera equipped with a low-energy, general-purpose collimator. In clinical routine sequential imaging is not required. Planar images should be acquired in a 128×128 matrix for 500 kcounts. For SPECT imaging, a 64×64 matrix, 60 projections, 30–60 s per projection, are recommended. All patients should receive sodium perchlorate and potassium iodide prior to injection of ^{123}I VIP for thyroid blockade.

9.4 Oncologic Applications

9.4.1 Colorectal Cancer

9.4.1.1 The Clinical Problem

Colorectal cancer is among the leading causes of cancer death worldwide and accounts for approximately 10% of all cancer deaths. It is second to lung cancer in men and to breast cancer in women, and it is estimated that one in 20 persons is affected in Western countries (de Cosse et al. 1994; Boring et al. 1994; Seidman et al. 1985). The only curative therapy is surgical resection, whereas oncologic intervention in patients with advanced, inoperable cancer remains palliative at best (Scheithauer et al. 1993). Because of the strong association between early detection of primary and recurrent tumors or metastases and prognosis, exact determination of the tumor burden is important for the clinical management. Imaging methods available include endoscopy, ultrasound, barium enema, as well as CT and MRI. Although these methods have specific roles in the evaluation of patients with colorectal cancer, none are "optimal," since peritoneal metastasis or small extrahepatic lesions mimicking postoperative scars (Schlag et al. 1989) might escape detection.

Various groups have shown that gastrointestinal adenocarcinomas express high-affinity binding sites for VIP as well as hSSTR3 and other subtypes (Reubi 1995; Virgolini et al. 1994a; Pangerl et al. 1997).

9.4.1.2 ^{123}I VIP Receptor Scintigraphy

In an initial series with ^{123}I-labeled VIP (Virgolini et al. 1994b, 1995) we demonstrated the ability of the tracer to localize even small-sized adenocarcinomas of the gastrointestinal tract along with the safety of the agent. In addition, a higher sensitivity for the peptide tracer was found when compared with an ^{111}In-labeled, commercially available anti-TAG-72.3-antibody (Raderer et al. 1996).

Based on these findings, we have followed 80 consecutive patients in order to determine the diagnostic capability of ^{123}I VIP for visualization of adenocarcinomas of the colon and rectum (Raderer et al. 1998c). Thirteen patients were free of tumor after complete resection of a Dukes' stage C cancer, 8 patients presented with primary and 14 with locally recurrent tumors, but were free of metastases. Ten patients had locally recurrent disease and liver, lung, or lymph node metastases, respectively. Organ metastases (i.e., liver, lung, or lymph nodes) were present in 35 patients. The size of the primary or recurrent tumors varied between 3 and 16 cm, and the size of metastases between 1 and 13 cm. Scan results were evaluated independently by two nuclear medicine physicians in a blinded way, and results were then compared with CT results not older than 4 weeks. Seven of 8 primary (87%) and 21 of 24 (82%) locally relapsing cancers were imaged with ^{123}I VIP (Fig. 9.2). Negative VIP scans were obtained in all 13 patients in whom the cancers had been curatively re-

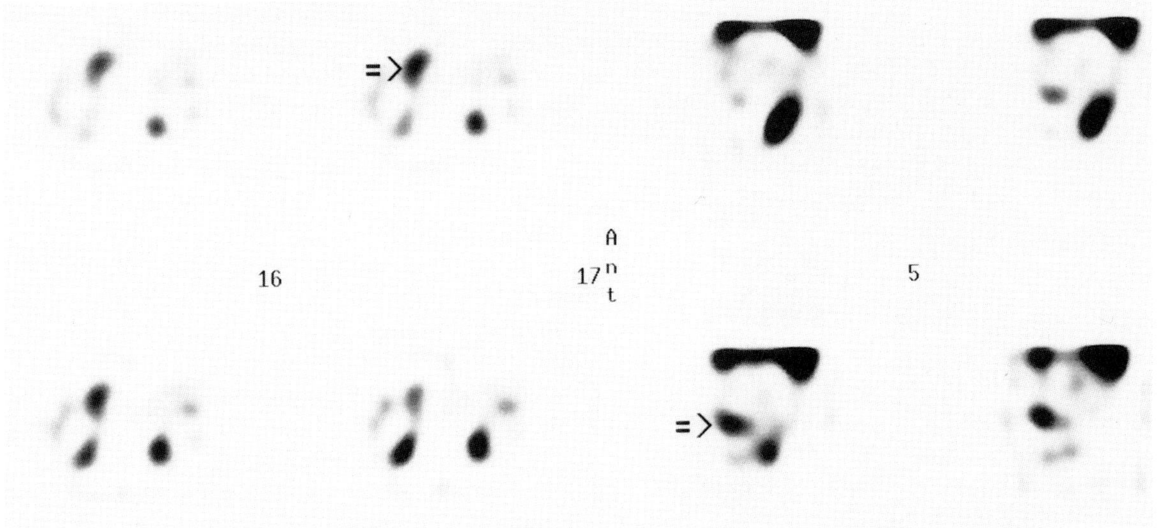

Fig. 9.2. ^{123}I-VIP receptor scintigraphy indicates the primary colorectal tumor (*arrow*) 2 h after injection of 1 µg (150 MBq) radioligand with single photon emission computed tomography (SPECT); four images in left panel *(16, 17)*: transverse reconstruction; four images in right panel *(5)*: sagittal reconstruction

sected. All patients with lymph node metastases showed positive VIP scans (4 of 4), and positive scans were obtained in 25 of 28 (89%) patients with liver metastases and in 2 of 3 cases with lung metastases. In 4 patients with relapsing cancer, the VIP scan indicated the presence of disease before CT, and in 2 patients the diagnosis of scar tissue instead of a local recurrence of rectal cancer as suggested by CT could be established.

Furthermore, our data support in vitro results demonstrating a high expression of VIP receptors in a large percentage of colorectal adenocarcinomas (Reubi 1995; Virgolini et al. 1994a). However, it has to be emphasized that the majority of patients undergoing VIP receptor scanning had not received chemotherapy before injection of the tracer. Virtually nothing is known about the influence of chemotherapeutic agents on receptor expression. Despite the limited number of patients (4 patients with adjuvant treatment and 12 patients with palliative, 5-FU based therapy), a negative impact of cytotoxic agents on scintigraphy cannot be excluded. All patients undergoing adjuvant treatment had negative scans, but also did not develop signs of malignancy in a 3-month follow-up period after scintigraphy. In contrast, 2 patients with locally relapsing cancers and 3 patients with liver lesions had negative scans, whereas the remaining 7 patients with palliative treatment had positive scans. Further investigations to evaluate the influence of treatment on receptor expression are necessary.

Our results add to the accumulating body of evidence that ^{123}I VIP receptor scintigraphy is a highly promising method for imaging and staging of gastrointestinal adenocarcinomas. Apart from the clinical application of peptide-imaging, the over-expression of peptide binding sites offers the potential to apply radiolabeled peptides for targeted tumor therapy. However, despite the capabilities of VIP as an imaging agent, the high lung uptake does not permit the use of the compound labeled with isotopes suitable for therapy. Thus, novel compounds with a different binding profile have been developed at our institution and are currently undergoing clinical testing (Shirzad et al. 1998).

We conclude that ^{123}I VIP offers valuable additional information to conventional radiologic imaging in a broad cohort of patients, including subjects with small cancers or suspected recurrent cancers in scar tissue in the pelvis resulting from initial surgery.

9.4.1.3 Scintigraphy with Radiolabeled Somatostatin Analogs

In several studies we (Virgolini et al. 1994b) and others (Krenning et al. 1993) have found that OctreoScan (Mallinckrodt, Medical, St. Louis, Mo.) is not useful in imaging colorectal adenocarcinomas. This may be explained by the lack of sufficient binding to hSSTR3 or hSSTR4 which both seem to be the major receptors expressed in colonic cancer tissues (Vir-

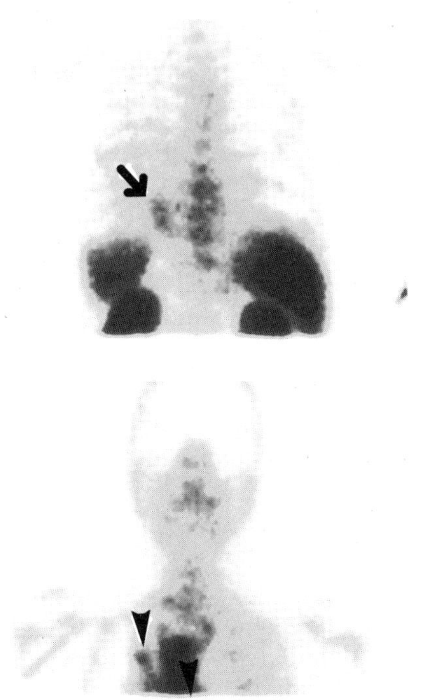

Fig. 9.3. ^{99m}Tc P829 scintigraphy indicates in a patient with rectal adenocarcinoma mediastinal and lung metastases (*arrow*) at 90 min after injection of 50 μg (600 MBq) radioligand. Planar study; *upper panel:* posterior view; *lower panel:* anterior view. At the time of scintigraphy, contrast-enhanced chest CT was negative, lesions were positron on a ^{18}F-FDG positive emission tomography (PET) scan performed 12 weeks later

GOLINI 1997; VIRGOLINI et al. 1997). In contrast, we found significant uptake of ^{99m}Tc-P829 by primary tumors as well as lung metastases from intestinal adenocarcinomas (Fig. 9.3; LEIMER et al. 1998a), underlining our in vitro observations of binding of ^{99m}Tc-P829 to hSSTR3 as well as to a variety of adenocarcinoma cell lines (VIRGOLINI et al. 1998a). In addition, ^{111}In-DOTA-lanreotide which is supposed to bind to the subtype receptors hSSTR3 and hSSTR4, produced positive images in patients with colon cancer (Fig. 9.4; VIRGOLINI et al. 1998c,d).

9.4.2 Pancreatic Cancer

9.4.2.1 The Clinical Problem

Adenocarcinoma of the pancreas is a common cause of cancer death (NATIONAL CANCER INSTITUTE 1991). To date, the only therapeutic measure with curative potential is surgical intervention with total removal of clinically apparent malignant tissue. Despite improvement in terms of perioperative morbidity and mortality, the overall prognosis for patients diagnosed with pancreatic cancer remains poor, since even those individuals undergoing surgical resection have a very high risk of relapse (WARSHAW and FERNANDEZ-DEL CASTILLO 1992; AMERICAN CANCER SOCIETY 1991). More than 80% of all patients die within the first year of diagnosis, and only approximately 3% of patients are still alive after 5 years (AMERICAN CANCER SOCIETY 1991). One of the major obstacles in the treatment of this disease is the fact that pancreatic adenocarcinoma is almost always diagnosed at an advanced stage (KALSER et al. 1985). This is due to the lack of specific symptoms or signs, and lesions smaller than 2 cm may escape detection by conventional radiologic imaging (KELLY and BENJAMIN 1995).

Sonography, endosonography, and CT are the most widely applied methods for diagnosis and staging of pancreatic cancer (VAN DYKE et al. 1985; BALTHAZAR and CHAKO 1990). The most reliable, and thus

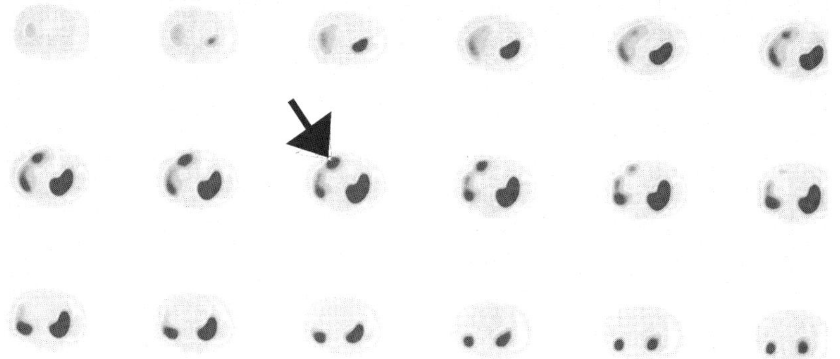

Fig. 9.4. ^{111}In-DOTA-lanreotide scintigraphy in a patient with colon cancer and a single liver metastasis (*arrow*) at 3 h post injection of 150 MBq radioligand. SPECT: transverse reconstruction

most widely applied modality for detection and imaging of pancreatic cancer, remains CT (Van Dyke et al. 1985), whereas MRI still has to prove its advantage over conventional CT (Freeny et al. 1988). Scintigraphic methods, for the time being, continue to be experimental approaches.

9.4.2.2
^{123}I- VIP Receptor Scintigraphy

Pancreatic adenocarcinomas of the gastrointestinal tract have been shown to express abundant numbers of VIP receptors (Virgolini et al. 1994a; Reubi 1995; Jiang et al. 1997). The feasibility and safety of this novel peptide receptor scan has been demonstrated (Virgolini et al. 1994b, 1995) showing the localization of most gastrointestinal adenocarcinomas and liver metastases, including patients suffering from pancreatic adenocarcinoma. As this tumor entity poses a diagnostic challenge, VIP receptor scanning results obtained in a total of 60 consecutive patients with pancreatic adenocarcinomas were evaluated and compared with conventional radiologic imaging methods and surgical exploration results (Fig. 9.5; Raderer et al. 1998a,b). In this series 22 patients presented with organ-confined malignancy (19 at study entry, and 2 developed tumor recurrence during follow-up after initial surgery), whereas 25 patients had distant metastases along with the local malignancy, and 7 patients had liver metastases after resection of the primary lesion (6 upon study entry, 1 case of tumor development during follow-up). In 5 of these patients, abdominal lymph node metastases were present at the time of scanning. Of 10 patients who had undergone potentially curative surgery, 7 remained free of disease during follow-up until death or for at least 6 months. All patients were administered ^{123}I VIP (150–200 MBq, 4–5 mCi); ~1 µg VIP). Primary pancreatic tumors were visualized by ^{123}I VIP in 19 of 21 patients (90%) with disease confined to the pancreas and in 8 of 25 patients (32%) suffering both from locoregional and disease metastatic to the liver. The overall ^{123}I VIP scan sensitivity for primary pancreatic adenocarcinomas was 58% (27 of 46 scans). Liver metastases were detected in 29 of 32 patients (sensitivity 90%) and abdominal lymph node metastases in 4 of 5 patients. In 5 patients the VIP receptor scan indicated the malignant lesion prior to CT. In vitro results confirmed specific binding of ^{123}I VIP to primary pancreatic tumor cells as well as to PANC1 adenocarcinoma cells. We conclude that ^{123}I VIP receptor scanning has additional information to standard diagnostic methods and could influence the decision making process in the treatment of pancreatic cancer. Especially noteworthy are the results obtained in 5 of 60 patients (8.3%) in whom VIP receptor scanning indicated recurrence of disease and/or metastatic liver spread prior to conventional methods. Possible changes in the choice of treatment modalities for pancreatic cancer following VIP receptor scanning suggest a profound impact in terms of quality of life and cost-effectiveness. The diverging results in the two subgroups deserve special emphasis, because our data imply that ^{123}I VIP receptor scintigraphy has the highest diagnostic accuracy in a cohort of patients who usually present a diagnostic problem with conventional radiologic imaging. Thus, ^{123}I VIP receptor scanning may be applied as an additional and complementary method in the evaluation of presurgical patients with suspected cancer of the pancreas.

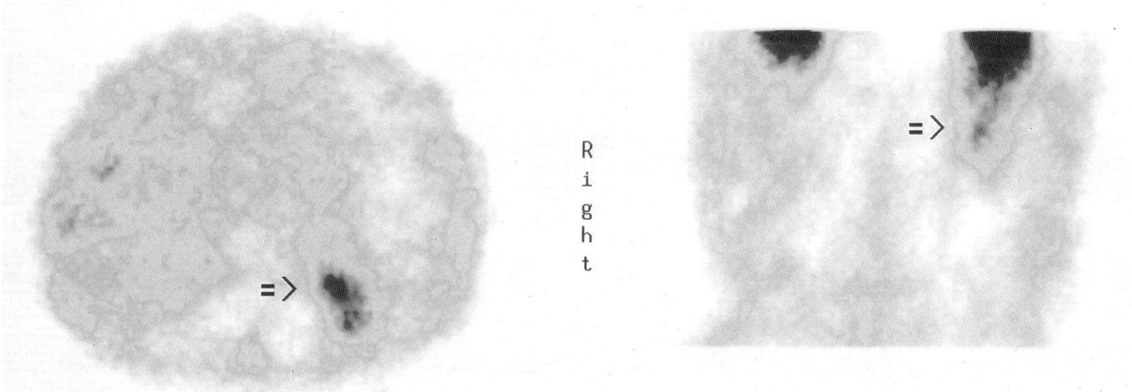

Fig. 9.5. ^{123}I-VIP receptor scintigraphy indicates the recurrent pancreatic tumor (*arrow*) 2 h after injection of 1 µg (150 MBq) radioligand (SPECT; *left panel:* transverse reconstruction; *right panel:* coronal reconstruction)

The diagnostic sensitivity for liver metastases achieved in our study was similar to that reported for conventional radiologic imaging, i.e., sonography or CT (VAN DYKE et al. 1985; FREENY et al. 1988). Iodine-123 VIP is preferentially excreted via the kidneys; thus, it does not concentrate in physiologic liver and biliary tissues, offering the opportunity of visualizing hepatic metastases. The smallest liver lesions imaged in our patients were approximately 1.5 cm with the median size of liver metastases being 3 cm (range 1.5–10 cm). Although the early detection of metastatic disease to the liver may not directly translate into a prolongation of survival, this information nevertheless is important for physicians involved in the management of such patients. There is international consensus that patients with metastatic disease are best spared an operation (WARSHAW and FERNANDEZ-DEL CASTILLO 1992), since extensive surgery does not affect overall survival and bears the risk of increased perioperative mortality and morbidity. The same holds true for the early detection of lymph node metastases, and in this study VIP visualized abdominal lymph node metastases in 4 of 5 patients.

In conclusion, ^{123}I VIP receptor scanning has promising potential for the clinical use in diagnosing and/or staging of pancreatic cancer. As demonstrated in our study, ^{123}I VIP receptor scintigraphy could possibly influence the decision making process in patients with verified or suspected cancer of the pancreas, due to its ability to visualize malignancy even in the absence of conventional radiologic abnormalities. We conclude that scintigraphy with ^{123}I VIP could provide valuable additional information to the available conventional radiologic imaging modalities for staging and early diagnosis of pancreatic cancer. In fact, the high sensitivity especially for small lesions and metastatic deposits might have a profound impact on clinical management of such patients.

9.4.2.3
Scintigraphy with Radiolabeled Somatostatin Analogs

Previously, ^{111}In-DTPA-D-Phe^{1}-octreotide was used for imaging gastrointestinal tumors (KRENNING et al. 1993; VIRGOLINI et al. 1994b). However, whereas VIP scans were positive in a small cohort of patients with pancreatic exocrine tumors, negative imaging results were obtained by labeled octreotide. The most likely explanation for these negative in vivo results is a lack of high-affinity receptors specific for octreotide on pancreatic adenocarcinomas. The VIP receptor scan was also superior to immunoscintigraphy in a study in which a direct comparison of the monoclonal antibody ^{111}In-CYT-103 (OncoScint) with ^{123}I VIP was performed (RADERER et al. 1996). Promising results with the administration of fluorodeoxyglucose (FDG) for positron emission tomography (PET) have been reported (INOKUMA et al. 1995). Forthcoming investigations will have to be performed in order to evaluate the diagnostic value of VIP SPECT and FDG PET in a direct comparison.

Initial imaging results with ^{99m}Tc-P829 (Fig. 9.6; LEIMER et al. 1998a) as well as with ^{111}In-DOTA-lanreotide (VIRGOLINI et al. 1998c,d) have indicated the potential of these tracers to image gastrointestinal adenocarcinomas including pancreatic cancer. This is most probably based on the recognition of different hSSTR subtypes expressed on or in pancreatic tumors (RADERER et al. 1998a,b). For both these SSTR ligands, however, only limited clinical data are available.

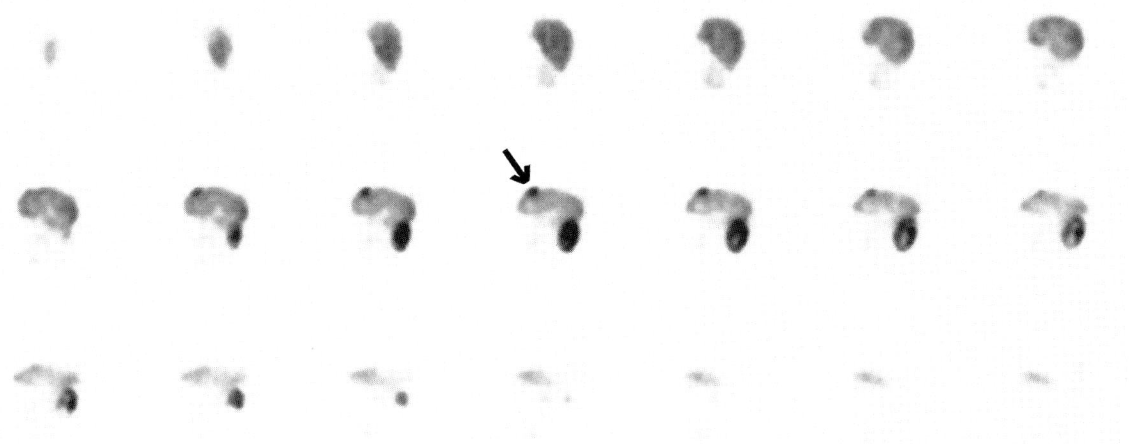

Fig. 9.6. ^{99m}Tc-VIP scintigraphy indicates in a patient with pancreatic adenocarcinoma and a larger liver metastasis (*arrow*) at 90 min post injection of 150 MBq radioligand (SPECT: sagittal reconstruction)

9.4.3
Lung Cancer

9.4.3.1
The Clinical Problem

Lung cancer was the most frequent malignancy in the European Union in 1990 (Black et al. 1997). Also in the United States, lung cancer is the leading cancer site with the highest mortality rate in both men and women, and had a projected mortality of >150,000 deaths in 1997 (Parker et al. 1997). Early detection and treatment may lead to improved survival for some types of lung cancer (Naruke et al. 1997). The best opportunity for cure of lung cancer is surgical excision of the primary tumor and of metastases to regional lymph nodes. If the cancer has spread, then surgery is not an option and other treatment regimes are applied including chemotherapy and external beam radiation, but these measures are rarely curative (Ginsberg et al. 1993). Therefore, an accurate diagnosis with confirmatory cytology or histology and an estimate of the stage of the disease are extremely important.

The major histologic types of lung cancer are squamous cell carcinoma, adenocarcinoma, large cell lung carcinoma (referred to as NSCLC, non-small cell lung cancer) and small cell lung carcinoma (SCLC). In addition, there are other, less common, lung tumors such as carcinoid tumors.

Diagnosis based on histopathology requires bronchoscopy, or open-lung biopsy in order to differentiate benign from malignant lesions before and often after surgical resection or radiation therapy of the primary tumor lesions. Bronchoscopy, including bronchial washings and brushing, has a sensitivity of 65% for malignancy, and transbronchial biopsy increases the sensitivity to 79% for lesions that are accessible (Wang et al. 1988). These invasive procedures have a relatively high incidence of pneumothorax. Beyond the clinical diagnosis conventional imaging techniques are used including chest radiograph, CT, or MRI. These diagnostic methods provide anatomical information and can neither accurately stage the disease when metastases occur without anatomical change nor differentiate between malignant and non-malignant tumors.

Approximately 130,000 new solitary pulmonary nodules (SPNs) are detected each year on chest radiographs performed as part of preoperative evaluations for unrelated surgery or as part of annual physical examinations. In various studies 28–39% of resected SPNs were malignant, accounting for approximately 20% of newly diagnosed lung cancer (Siegelman et al. 1986). Significant progress has been made by the introduction of PET showing overall the highest sensitivity (96%) and specificity (88%) in detecting lung cancer in patients with SPN (Kahn et al. 1991; see Chap. 10).

9.4.3.2
Iodine-123 VIP receptor Scintigraphy

Due to the high physiologic uptake of VIP in the lungs (Virgolini et al. 1995), the visualization of VIPR-positive lung tumors is difficult. Therefore, VIPR scintigraphy does not have application for detecting lung tumors or lung metastases.

9.4.3.3
Scintigraphy with Radiolabeled Somatostatin Analogs

In vitro studies have demonstrated that 50–75% of SCLC have specific high-affinity binding sites for SSTR. Furthermore, SCLC sites have been localized through scintigraphic imaging with the radiolabeled SST analogs ^{123}I-octreotide and ^{111}In-DTPA-D-Phe^{1}-octreotide which bind to tissue expressing hSSTR2 and hSSTR5 (O'Bryne et al. 1994; Kwekkeboom et al. 1991). Controversial reports exist concerning SSTR expression in NSCLC tumors. Whereas some in vitro studies have failed to demonstrate the presence of SSTR in NSCLC (Reubi et al. 1990), SST analog imaging in patients with NSCLC have been successful. Since a tumor may contain numerous different cell types, including neoplastic cells, stroma, inflammatory cells and necrotic tissue, it has been hypothesized that there may be uptake of the radiolabeled SSTR ligand by other cells within the tumor mass, such as lymphocytes, which are known to express SSTR (Sreedharan et al. 1989). O'Bryne et al. (1994) have shown for the first time that NSCLC samples express a single class of specific high-affinity SSTR binding sites. Moreover, we (Virgolini et al. 1998a) identified two classes of specific high-affinity binding sites for ^{99m}Tc-P829 in NSCLC, and the presence of hSSTR was confirmed by mRNA analysis using Northern blot analysis. Thomas et al. (1994) using limiting dilution-PCR (LiD-PCR) found high levels of transcription of SSTR1 in lung tumors, especially in NSCLC. Fujita et al. (1994) showed the expression of SSTR subtype genes at high level in two squamous cell carcinoma cell lines, in which the representative neuroendocrine markers were low.

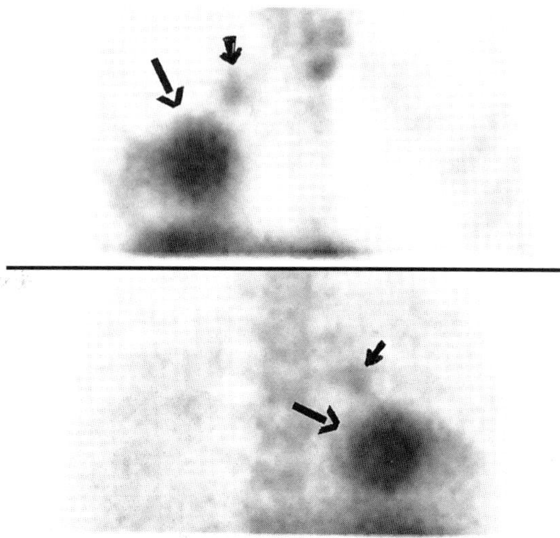

Fig. 9.7. ^{99m}Tc-P829 scintigraphy indicates in a patient with non-small-cell lung carcinoma (NSCLC) the tumor sites at 90 min after injection of 50 μg (600 MBq) radioligand. Planar imaging: anterior (*top panel*) and posterior (*bottom panel*) views. In addition to the large tumor mass (*long arrow*) a small lymph node metastasis was identified above the tumor lesion (*short arrow*) which was not identified on CT but was verified by surgery

The FDG PET technique has been shown to accurately detect SPN with a sensitivity of 98% and a specificity of 69% in a prospective blinded study (Lowe et al. 1998). However, FDG PET is not routinely available and is expensive. Technetium-99m P829 scintigraphy was included into the diagnostic work-up following identification of a suspicious lesion on the chest radiograph or after the CT (Blum et al. 1998). The potential for wider availability and cost-effectiveness of ^{99m}Tc-P829 scintigraphy compared with FDG PET is suggested by kit production and ^{99m}Tc compatibility with existing conventional nuclear medicine detector systems.

The position of ^{99m}Tc-P829 (Fig. 9.7) in the clinical management of patients suspected of having lung cancer might not only be limited to the primary evaluation of the SPN but could be extended to assess post-treatment pulmonary changes. Post-treatment pulmonary changes, such as persistent tumor, scarring, or necrosis, are not adequately characterized by CT or MRI. A tissue biopsy negative for tumor cannot be accepted as definitive because of limitations in accurately sampling regions of viable tumor in the middle of a scar. Suspicious local and distant tumor recurrence can be accurately characterized using whole-body FDG PET (Patz et al. 1994). Whether ^{99m}Tc-P829 would be clinically useful in the secondary management of lung cancer remains to be established.

In initial studies the lanreotide-based ligand MAURITIUS was found to bind to tumors in the lung (Fig. 9.8), as did ^{111}In-DTPA-D-Phe^{1}-octreotide (Kwekkeboom et al. 1991).

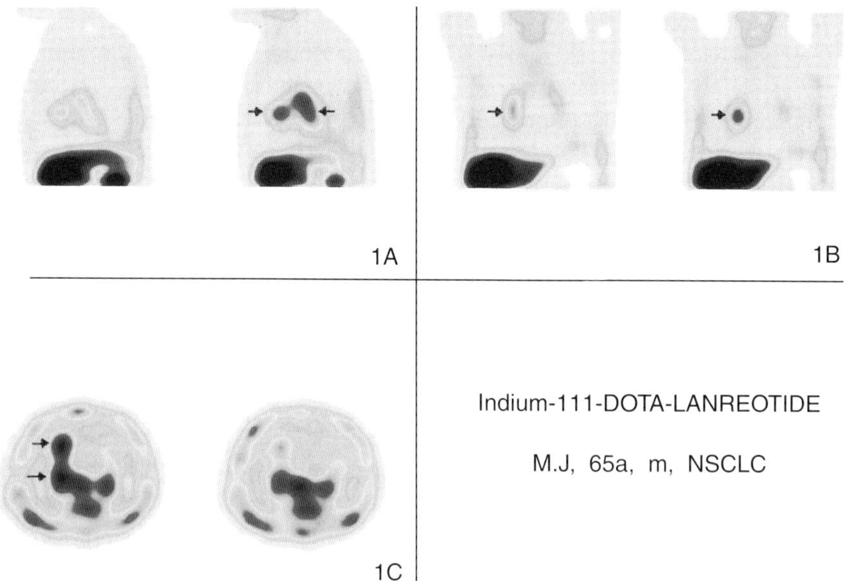

Fig. 9.8. ^{111}In-DOTA-lanreotide scintigraphy indicates in a patient with NSCLC the tumor sites (*arrows*) at 3 h post injection of 150 MBq radioligand. SPECT; *upper panel left* (**1A**): sagittal reconstruction; *upper panel right:* coronal reconstruction (**1B**); *lower panel:* transverse reconstruction (**1C**)

9.4.4
Breast Cancer

9.4.4.1
The Clinical Problem

In women the most common diagnosed cancer was breast cancer (PARKER et al. 1997). The problem with breast cancer is to determine the characteristics and extent of the disease as an aid in planning and monitoring treatment. Which nodes are involved is of importance for prognosis. Several radiopharmaceuticals have been applied in patients with breast cancer, including FDG, sestamibi, tetrofosmin, and receptor tracers (BOMBARDIERI et al. 1997).

The study of breast cancer is complicated by the heterogeneity of the disease. One way of simplifying is to subdivide these tumors into clinically relevant subgroups. There are indications that breast cancer, of which some express the SSTR, can be subdivided this way. It is well recognized that estrogen (ER) and progesterone receptor (PR) expression is associated with prolonged survival time. A retrospective study in 110 patients suggested that the presence of SSTR predict a longer disease-free survival (FOEKENS et al. 1989). In fact, human breast cancers have been shown to express SSTR with high incidence. During the past 10 years this has been demonstrated by several in vitro studies using autoradiography, radioligand binding studies, or Northern blotting. Furthermore, it was documented that the expression of SSTR in breast cancer tissue is significantly higher than in normal breast tissue (VIKIC-TOPIC et al. 1995; SCHAER et al. 1997; VIRGOLINI et al. 1996c; ZIA et al. 1996).

9.4.4.2
^{123}Iodine VIP Receptor Scintigraphy

Whereas ^{123}I VIP has poor sensitivity for localizing ER/PR-positive breast cancer (11%), the sensitivity of VIP in ER/PR-negative breast cancer is approximately 85% (TAUCHER et al. 1996). At several sites (THAKUR et al. 1997; PALLELA et al. 1998a–c) ^{99m}Tc VIP-agonist receptor scintigraphy was used for imaging breast cancer based on the very high expression of VIPR reported in patients with breast cancer (REUBI 1995; VIRGOLINI et al. 1996c; MOODY et al. 1998). No clinical data have been published yet.

9.4.4.3
Scintigraphy with Radiolabeled Somatostatin Analogs

VAN EIJCK et al. (1994) administered ^{111}In-DTPA-D-Phe^1-octreotide to 52 patients with breast cancer and was able to demonstrate the presence of SSTR in 85% of ductal and in 56% of lobular carcinomas. When subdividing the primary tumors according to size, 86% of T2 tumors and 61% of T1 tumors were visualized. Examination of the axillary lymph node status revealed only 4 of 14 histopathologically confirmed metastatic localizations. Higher density in vivo correlated mostly with homogeneous and dense distribution of SSTR at autoradiography, whereas lower dense distribution corresponded with a non-homogeneous and sparse distribution of these receptors in vitro. Moreover, the low density of these receptors seemed to be due to a non-invasive component (mainly ductal carcinoma in situ). Furthermore, a higher sensitivity of SSTR was observed compared with tumor markers such as CA 15-3 and CEA in detecting recurrence in patients with SSTR-positive primary tumors. More recently, VURAL et al. (1997) have shown that ^{111}In-DTPA-D-Phe^1-octreotide was able to detect 16 of 17 histopathologically confirmed breast cancers (15 invasive ductal carcinoma, 1 mucinous adenocarcinoma, 1 intraductal carcinoma) compared with 13 detected by ^{201}Tl. In our series more than 90% of primary human breast tumors were detected using

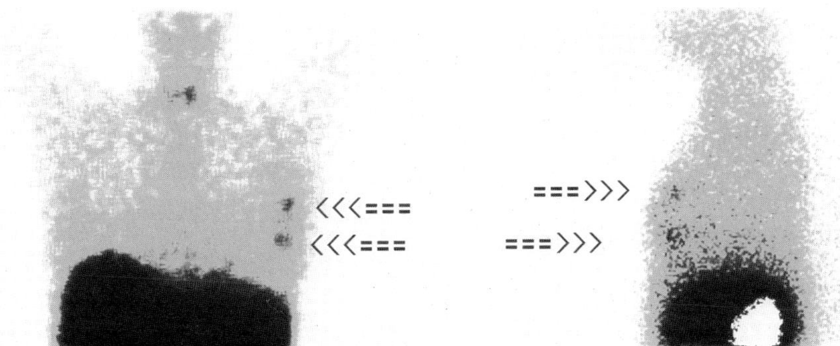

Fig. 9.9. ^{111}In-DTPA-D-Phe^1-octreotide scintigraphy in a patient with breast cancer. The *arrows* indicate two tumor masses in the left breast. Planar images in anterior (*left panel*) and left lateral view (*right panel*)

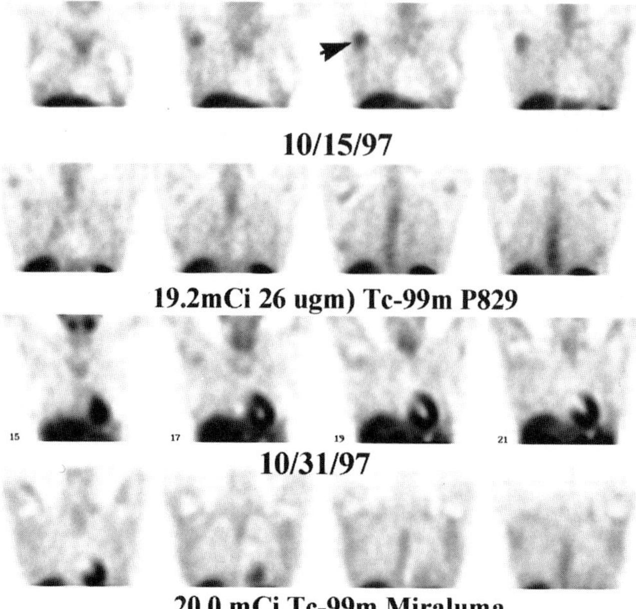

Fig. 9.10. ^{99m}Tc-P829 scintigraphy indicates in a patient with breast cancer (primary tumor resected) axillary lymph node recurrence (*arrow, upper two rows*) 1.5 h after injection of 50 μg (700 MBq) radioligand (SPECT; coronal reconstruction). Scintigraphy with Sestamibi (Miraluma, Dupont Pharma, Billerica, Mass.) showed only faint uptake (*lower two rows*). (Courtesy H. Handmaker)

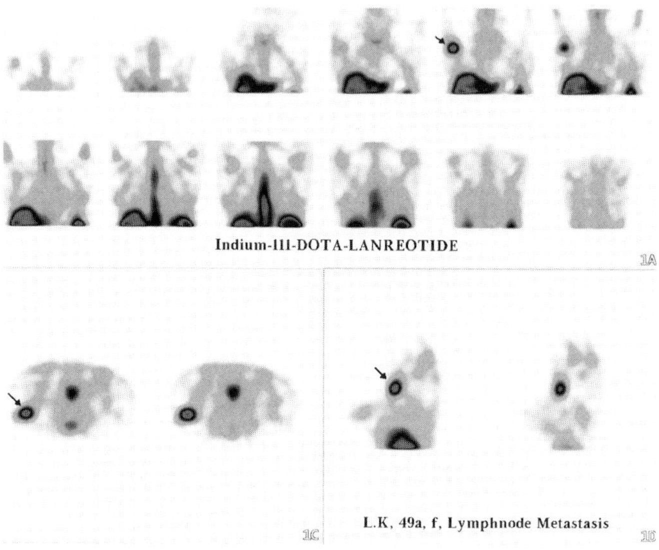

Fig. 9.11. ^{111}In-DOTA-lanreotide scintigraphy in a patient with breast cancer (unknown location of primary). An axillary lymph node metastasis (*arrows*) at 3 h post injection of 150 MBq radioligand is shown (SPECT; *upper two rows:* coronal reconstruction; *lower left panel:* transverse reconstruction; *lower right panel:* sagittal reconstruction)

^{111}In-DTPA-D-Phe^1-octreotide (Fig. 9.9; TAUCHER et al. 1996).

We (VIRGOLINI et al. 1998a) have recently demonstrated the in vivo binding capacity of ^{99m}Tc-P829 in breast cancer patients (Fig. 9.10). This ligand seems to bind with high affinity to hSSTR2 and also to hSSTR 3 and 5. In these studies ^{99m}Tc-P829 performed better than MIBI (H. Handmaker, personal communication). The place of SST therapy in breast cancer has yet to be evaluated. Furthermore, ^{111}In-DOTA-lanreotide may be useful in detecting breast cancer and its metastases (Fig. 9.11).

9.4.5
Neuroendocrine Tumors

9.4.5.1
The Clinical Problem

Neuroendocrine tumors are rare disease entities, often presenting as bizarre diagnostic puzzles (MOERTEL 1987). The fact that these malignancies arise from hormonally active cells explains the wide variety of symptoms encountered in patients with neuroendocrine cancers of various origin. The different manifestations are related to the release of hormones or other biologically active substances produced in excessive amounts, such as insulin, gastrin, VIP, glucagon, or serotonin (KVOLS 1994). Such cancers constitute a group of relatively slow-growing malignancies, which are sometimes diagnosed after years of symptoms in affected patients. This is related to the fact that the amount of hormones secreted does not necessarily correlate with tumor size, whereas small cancers tend to escape clinical detection by conventional radiologic imaging. Thus, the start of successful therapy or symptomatic palliation is often delayed.

9.4.5.2
Carcinoid Tumors

Carcinoid tumors constitute the group with the highest incidence among all cases of neuroendocrine malignancies, predominantly arising in the gastrointestinal tract but also at various other sites (VINIK et al. 1989). According to epidemiologic data, gastrointestinal tract carcinoids occur in 1.5 cases per 100,000 people per year (GODWIN 1975). The onset of symptoms related to excessive serotonin production summarized under the term "carcinoid syndrome" may precede the correct diagnosis and localization of the tumor by years. While long-term symptomatic control of tumor-related symptoms can be achieved in some patients by non-invasive means, the treatment of choice in localized disease remains surgical resection, since it is the only measure with potential cure. On the other hand, the removal of the primary cancer in the absence of symptoms, such as bowel obstruction, does not significantly alter the prognosis in disseminated disease.

In vitro data have demonstrated a high amount of receptors for various hormones and peptides on malignant cells of neuroendocrine origin, including carcinoid tumors (REUBI 1995; REUBI et al. 1989). Among the latter, binding sites for members of the SST family (hSSTR1–5) are frequently found, and their expression has led to therapeutic and diagnostic attempts to specifically target these receptors. The use of OctreoScan (Mallinckrodt-Medical, St. Louis, Mo.) for imaging purposes has been incorporated into the clinical work-up of patients suspected of suffering from neuroendocrine tumors (KRENNING et al. 1993). In our series, which is in line with results reported by KRENNING et al. (1993), primary or recurrent carcinoid tumors could be visualized by means of ^{111}In-DTPA-D-Phe^{1}-octreotide in 95 of 104 patients (91%), whereas metastatic sites were identified in 110 of 116 patients (95%) (Fig. 9.12). In 11 of 21 patients (51%) with suggestive symptoms but without identified lesions by conventional imaging, focal tracer uptake identified the location of the carcinoid tumor. In addition, the presence of metastatic disease was demonstrated in 3 patients after resection. In a direct comparison of 131 patients evaluated with both imaging modalities, ^{111}In-DTPA-D-Phe^{1}-octreotide was found to be superior to ^{123}I VIP, with 35 of 38 (93%) vs 32 of 38 (84%) scans being positive in primary or recurrent tumors, and 58 of 65 (90%) vs 53 of 92 (82%) being positive in patients with metastatic sites, and 7 of 16 (44%) vs 4 of 16 (25%) in patients with symptoms but otherwise negative work-up. Overall, additional lesions not seen by conventional imaging were found in 43 of 158 (41%) vs 25 of 103 (25%) with ^{111}In-DTPA-D-Phe^{1}-octreotide and ^{123}I-VIP, respectively. These results indicate a high sensitivity of both peptide tracers for localizing tumor sites in patients with known or suspected car-

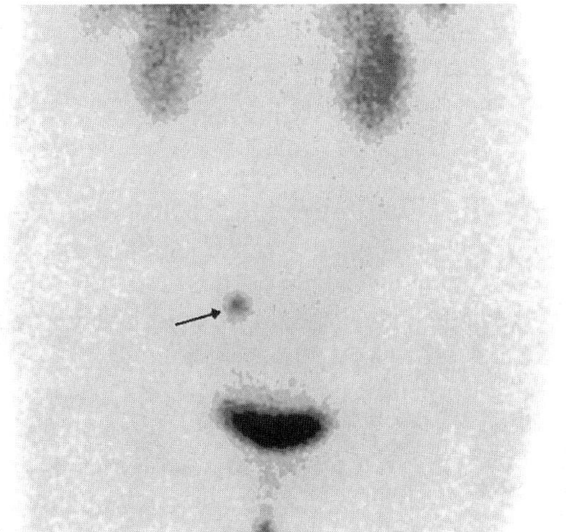

Fig. 9.12. ^{111}In-DTPA-D-Phe^{1}-octreotide scintigraphy in a patient with recurrent carcinoid tumor. Planar anterior view: the *arrow* indicates a single metastatic tumor site in the right ovary at 6 h post injection

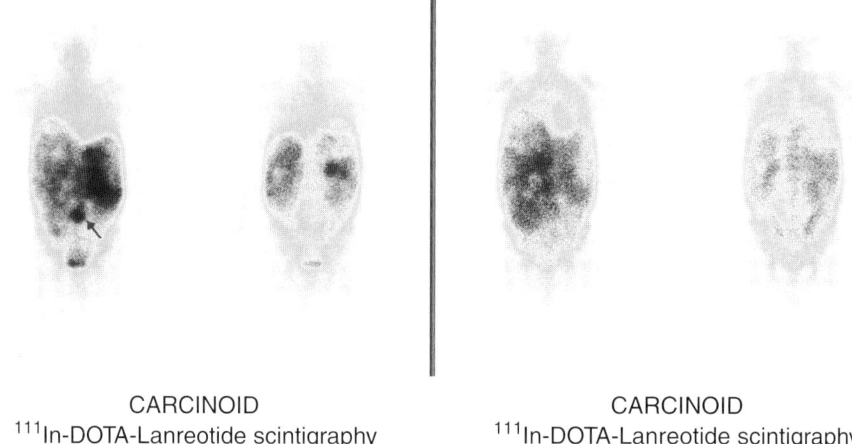

Fig. 9.13. ^{111}In-DOTA-lanreotide scintigraphy indicates in a patient with carcinoid primary an extremely enlarged liver prior to (*left panel*) and after two therapy cycles (*right panel*) with 925 MBq ^{90}Y-DOTA-lanreotide. Planar whole-body study at 3 h post injection

cinoid tumors, with ^{111}In-DTPA-D-Phe^1-octreotide scintigraphy being more sensitive than ^{123}I VIP receptor scanning. Both ^{123}I VIP and ^{111}In-DTPA-D-Phe^1-octreotide had a higher diagnostic yield than conventional imaging, as verified by surgical intervention or long term follow-up. As expected from pharmacokinetic data (Battari et al. 1988; Gespach et al. 1988), one of the shortcomings of ^{123}I VIP is the inability to visualize small pulmonary lesions. In fact, approximately 40% of the tracer is trapped in the lungs a few minutes after administration, supplying a high rate of physiologic background. Thus, small lesions with a low receptor density cannot be distinguished from normal lung uptake. ^{111}In-DTPA-D-Phe^1-octreotide, which is not trapped in the lungs, demonstrated a striking superiority for imaging of lung lesions, whereas less than 50% of pulmonary deposits could be seen on VIP receptor scintigraphy. We conclude that ^{111}In-DTPA-D-Phe^1-octreotide represents the more sensitive method for diagnosis and staging of patients suffering from carcinoid tumors, whereas the combination of both peptide receptor scans does not appear to further enhance diagnostic information.

Our recent data also indicate that ^{111}In-DOTA-lanreotide, similarly to ^{111}In-DTPA-D-Phe^1-octreotide, accumulates in neuroendocrine tumors including carcinoid tumors (Virgolini et al. 1998c,d). Using the ^{90}Y-labeled DOTA-lanreotide compound, receptor-mediated experimental therapy has already been initiated at the University of Vienna (Fig. 9.13; Leimer et al. 1998b).

9.4.5.3 Insulinomas

In reviewing 28 patients with histologically verified insulinomas undergoing ^{123}I VIP as well as ^{111}In-DTPA-D-Phe^1-octreotide scintigraphy, ^{123}I VIP visualized tumor lesions in 15 of 21 patients, whereas ^{111}In-DTPA-D-Phe^1-octreotide visualized tumor lesions in 12 of 28 patients. In 15 patients the two tracers were compared directly: ^{123}I VIP scintigraphy was positive in 12 of 15 patients (80%), whereas ^{111}In-DTPA-D-Phe^1-octreotide scintigraphy was positive in 8 of 15% (60%). In these patients radiologic imaging disclosed primary tumor lesions in 55% only. In vitro experiments indicated predominant expression of hSSTR3 in all insulinoma specimens investigated (Hejna et al. 1998). These results indicate a superior imaging capability for ^{123}I VIP acting as a ligand for hSSTR3, which is probably not sufficiently targeted by ^{111}In-DTPA-D-Phe^1-octreotide (Lamberts et al. 1996).

9.4.5.4 Other Neuroendocrine Tumors

The SSTR scintigraphy using ^{111}In-DTPA-D-Phe^1-octreotide has a high positive predictive value for the vast majority of neuroendocrine tumors (Krenning et al. 1993). ^{111}Indium-DTPA-D-Phe^1-octreotide has earned its place in the diagnostic work-up as well as follow-up of patients with neuroendocrine tumors. These tumors seem to express the hSSTR2 predominantly (Reubi et al. 1994).

Despite positive results in patients with VIPomas (Virgolini et al. 1998b), ^{123}I VIP receptor scintigraphy has no place in the work-up of most other neuroendocrine tumors (Virgolini et al. 1996c). The majority of these tumors have been shown to express hSSTR2 which is not targeted by ^{123}I VIP.

9.4.6 Thyroid Cancer

There is limited information on the expression of hSSTR as well as hVIPR in thyroid cancer, except for medullary thyroid cancer (Kurtaran et al. 1997, 1998; Rainhardt and Moser 1996).

A relatively large number of patients with differentiated metastatic thyroid cancer may present with an ^{131}I-negative whole-body scan. The discovery of neoplastic foci in these patients, even if no ^{131}I-uptake is present, may lead to further treatment, such as surgery or external radiotherapy.

It has been shown that SST and its analogs affect the cell growth of neoplastic thyroid cancer cells through cell surface binding (Ain and Taylor 1994). Furthermore, expression of a specific SSTR on papillary thyroid cancer membranes has been demonstrated (Virgolini et al. 1994b) and initial results have indicated the ability of ^{111}In-DTPA-D-Phe^{1}-octreotide to localize non-medullary thyroid cancer (Tenenbaum et al. 1995; Postema et al. 1996). These results provided the basis for using ^{111}In-DTPA-D-Phe^{1}-octreotide in thyroid cancer patients with a negative ^{131}I-scan: ^{111}In-DTPA-D-Phe^{1}-octreotide scintigraphy was positive in 12 of 16 ^{131}I-scan-negative patients and was positive in 8 of 9 patients with a positive ^{131}I scan (Baudin et al. 1996). A high rate of "false positive" ^{111}In-DTPA-D-Phe^{1}-octreotide imaging was reported for recurrent thyroid carcinoma with negative ^{131}I scans (Garin et al. 1998). Nevertheless, in metastatic thyroid cancer patients SSTR scintigraphy may be helpful in the detection of lesions, and may expand the therapeutic options in these patients. In particular, initial dosimetry with the SST analog ^{111}In-DOTA-lanreotide has indicated a very high tumor dose (up to 50 mGy/MBq) for this type of cancer (Fig. 9.14; Virgolini et al. 1998d).

9.4.7 Melanoma

The sensitivity of the ^{123}I VIP scintigraphy for the detection of melanomas is 70% and is comparable with

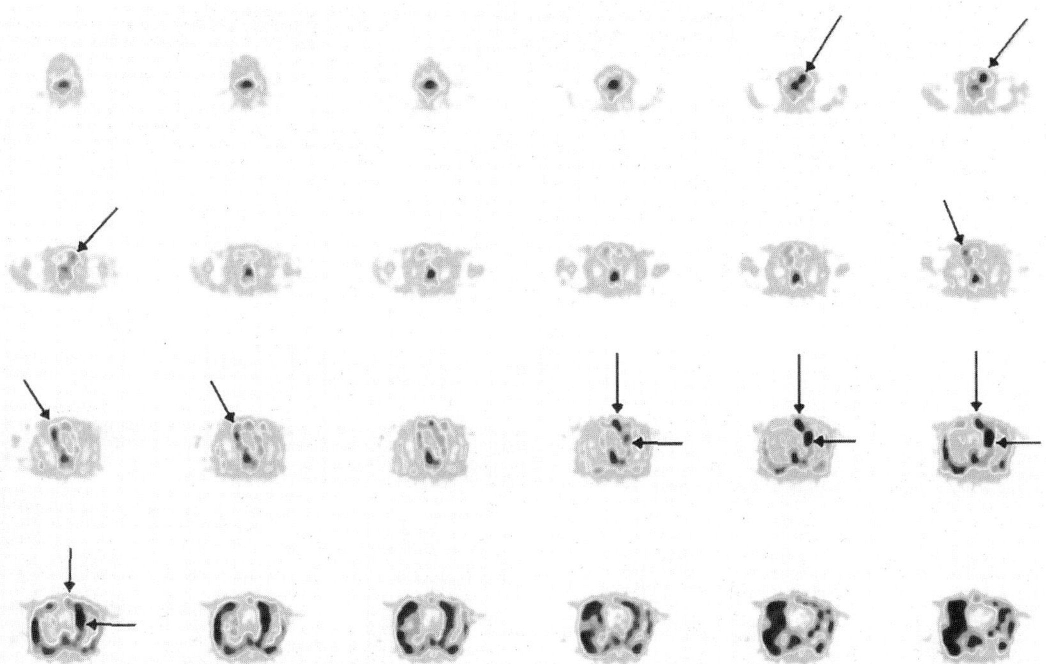

Fig. 9.14. ^{111}In-DOTA-lanreotide scintigraphy in a patient with Hürthle cell carcinoma and an ^{131}I-negative whole-body scan visualizes several tumor sites (*arrows*). Transverse images indicate major tumor lesions in the left neck, mediastinum, and right basal lungs

the sensitivity of ^{111}In-DTPA-D-Phe^1-octreotide scintigraphy (Krenning et al. 1993; Virgolini et al. 1996c). Recently, ^{99m}Tc-P829 was proposed to be a suitable tracer for imaging melanoma sites; however, the results of larger clinical studies remain to be seen (Lastoria et al. 1996).

9.4.8 Lymphoma

The overall sensitivity of the ^{123}I VIP scintigraphy for imaging of lymphomas (Hodgkin's and non-Hodgkin's lymphomas) is reported to be approximately 75% (Virgolini et al. 1996c), whereas the ^{111}In-DTPA-D-Phe^1-octreotide scan sensitivity is somewhat higher (Lugtenburg et al. 1998). The latter authors concluded that in patients with stage-I and stage-IIa supradiaphragmatic Hodgkin's disease SSTR scintigraphy is clearly indicated. We have recently found that tumors in patients with intestinal MALTomas lack the hSSTR3 subtype receptor which may explain why intestinal MALTomas are usually detected with ^{111}In-DOTA-lanreotide but not with ^{111}In-DTPA-D-Phe^1-octreotide.

We have used ^{111}In-DOTA-lanreotide in some patients with Hodgkin's lymphomas showing a high sensitivity (Virgolini et al. 1998c). Also, ^{99m}Tc-P829 has been used successfully to demonstrate lymphoma sites (H. Handmaker, personal communication).

9.4.9 Other Tumors

A variety of other human tumors may express hSSTR or hVIPR, and several peptide tracers have been used to demonstrate these tumors. In over 100 primary human tumors samples as well as over 20 tumor cell lines investigated for hSSTR and hVIPR subtype expression, one of the hSSTR or hVIPR subtypes was found to be expressed (Pangerl et al. 1997). These observations support the notion that the neuroendocrine peptide hormones VIP and SST are important growth regulators. Ideally, the in vivo study should be compared directly with in vitro receptor expression (Fig. 9.15) in order to gain further insights into the complex peptide hormone-receptor interactions.

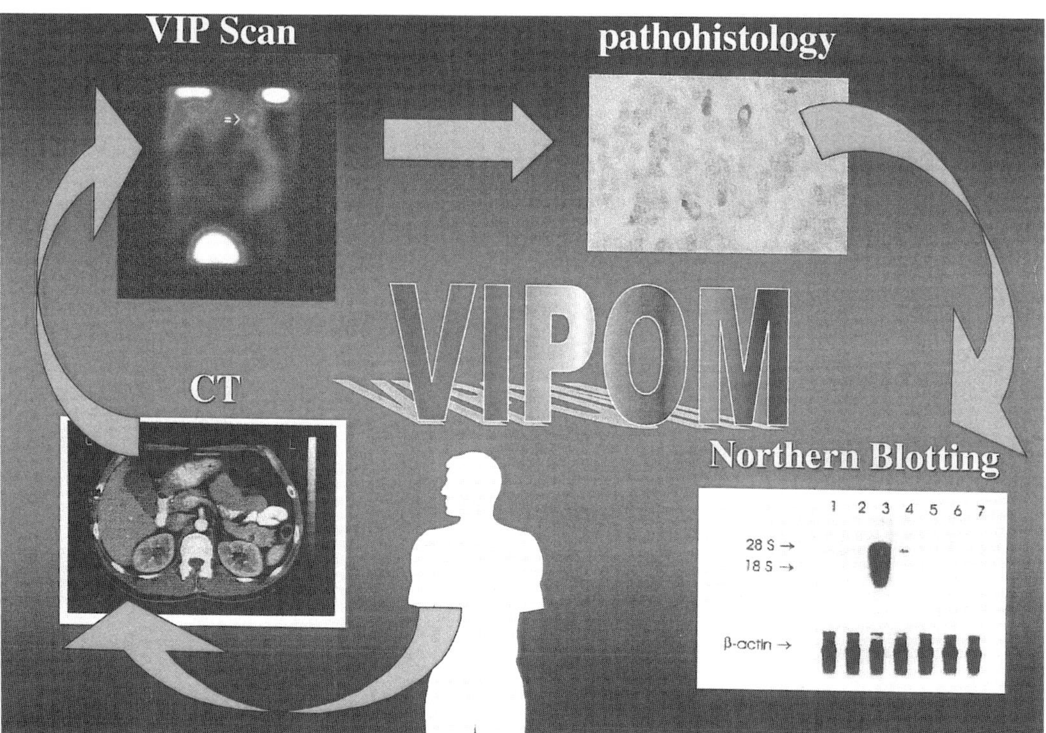

Fig. 9.15. Work-up example. We propose the optimal work-up to gain further insights into the biology and pathophysiology of receptor-ligand interactions on the basis of excellent interactions between a variety of different medical fields, ranging from molecular biology to nuclear medicine and surgery

9.5 Future Aspects

Some peptide tracers have been shown to be effective in both diagnosis and staging of tumors and their metastases. Initial efforts have implemented these peptides to prove the concept of receptor-mediated radiotherapy by using large amounts of the diagnostic compound. Such a therapy has been performed in patients with SSTR2-expressing tumors (Krenning et al. 1994) using large amounts of ^{111}In-DTPA-D-Phe^1-octreotide. However, ^{111}In is not an optimal radionuclide for therapy. We have developed a novel radioligand, termed MAURITIUS (i.e., ^{111}In-/^{90}Y-DOTA-lanreotide). In contrast to ^{111}In-DTPA-D-Phe^1-octreotide, which binds only to hSSTR2 and 5 with high affinity, MAURITIUS is capable of binding to hSSTR2–5 with high affinity and to hSSTR1 with low affinity, both on primary tumor cells as well as a variety of immortalized tumor cells (Smith-Jones et al. 1998a,b; Virgolini et al. 1998a; Leimer et al. 1998b). This makes the peptide a "universal" SSTR subtype recognizing ligand. Especially the high-affinity binding to the SSTR3 is very important since this hSSTR subtype is expressed most often in human tumors. Also, hSSTR3 acts as an acceptor for VIP (Peck-Radoasavljevic et al. 1998). With this concept MAURITIUS is labeled with ^{111}In for diagnostic dosimetry (Virgolini et al. 1998d) and is then used in the ^{90}Y-MAURITIUS version for therapy (Leimer et al. 1998b). Treatment options for patients refractory to standard-dose cytotoxic treatment are limited, and the mostly poor performance status of patients with advanced disease precludes the application of aggressive treatment modalities (e.g., high-dose chemotherapy), which would further impair the quality of life in these patients.

Treatment with "^{90}Y-MAURITIUS" could lead to a significant reduction in analgetic medication, probably sparing patients side effects of higher doses of opiates (constipation, nausea) or non-steroidal anti-inflammatory drugs (gastrointestinal complications). This new therapy could offer palliation and disease control at a reduced cost due to the limited number of administrations. The final peptide therapy strategy in a variety of cancers is most probably cheaper than conventional radiotherapy or prolonged chemotherapy. Overall, receptor-mediated radiotherapy with "^{90}Y-MAURITIUS" might be effective in patients refractory to conventional strategies.

In the past years, fundamental and clinical research on ^{123}I VIP receptor scintigraphy has been extensively pursued. This peptide represents an efficient imaging agent for receptor-positive tumors. Since ^{123}I is not the ideal radionuclide for diagnostic applications, attempts have been made to label VIP and its analogs with ^{99m}Tc, which is available and more cost-effective. ^{99m}Tc-VIP may be superior due to the better imaging quality. Finally, it is postulated that the labeling of VIP or its analog with ß-emitting nuclides would open new therapeutic opportunities to treat receptor-positive tumors. To answer these questions, additional work needs to be done.

Acknowledgements,
This chapter was written with the Experimental Nuclear Medicine Group: A. Kurtaran, M. Leimer, S. Li, T. Pangerl, M. Raderer, T. Traub, and Q. Yang.

References

Adamou A, Aiyar N, Horn van S, Elshourhagy NA (1996) Cloning and functional characterization of human vasoactive intestinal peptide (VIP)-2 receptor. Biochem Biophys Commun 209:383–392

Ain KB, Taylor KD (1994) Somatostatin analogs affect proliferation of human thyroid carcinoma cell lines in vitro. J Clin Endocrinol Metab 78:1097–1102

American Cancer Society (1991) Cancer facts and figures 1991. American Cancer Society, Atlanta

Bakker Wh, Alberts R, Bruns C, Breeman WAP, Hofland LJ, Marbach P, Pless J, Pralet D, Stolz B, Koper JW, Lamberts SWJ, Visser TJ, Krenning EP (1991) [^{111}In-DTPA-D-PHE^1]-octreotide, a potential radiopharmaceutical for imaging of somatostatin receptor-positive tumours: synthesis, radiolabelling and in vitro validation. Life Sci 49:1583–1591

Balthazar EJ, Chako AC (1990) Computed tomography of pancreatic masses. Am J Gastroenterol 85:343–349

Bangard M, Behe M, Bender H, Guhlke S, Risse J, Grünwald F, Mäcke H, Biersack HJ (1998) Technetium-99m-octreotide for the detection of somatostatin receptor positive (SSTR+) tumors: preliminary results. Eur J Nucl Med 25:837

Battari A, Martin JM, Luis J, Pouzol O, Secchi J, Marvaldi J, Pichon J (1988) Solubilization of the vasoactive intestinal peptide receptor from human colonic adenocarcinoma cells. J Biol Chem 263:17685–17689

Baudin E, Schlumberger M, Lumbroso J, Travagli JP, Caillou B, Parmentier C (1996) Octreotide scintigraphy in patients with differentiated thyroid carcinoma: contribution for patients with negative radioiodine scan. J Clin Endocrinol Metab 81:2541–2545

Bell GI, Yasada K, Kong H (1995) Molecular biology of somatostatin receptors. Ciba Found Symp 190:65–88

Black RJ, Bray F, Ferlay J, Parkin DM (1997) Cancer incidence and mortality in the European Union: cancer registry data and estimates of national incidence for 1990. Eur J Cancer 33:1075–1107

Bloom SR, Polak JM, Pearse AGE (1973) Vasoactive intestinal peptide and watery diarrhea syndrome. Lancet ii:14–16

Blum J, Handmaker H, Rinne N (1998) The utility of a somatostatin type receptor binding peptide radiopharmaceutical (P829) in the evaluation of solitary pulmonary nodules. Chest 115:224-232

Bogatzky J, Guhlke S, Bender H, Sartor J, Knapp FF, Biersack HJ (1997) Receptor binding studies with rhenium-RC160, a directly-labeled somatostatin analog, with membranes of the colon cancer cell line HT 29, CHO cells and ovary carcinoma cell line EFO-21. Eur J Nucl Med 24:1059A

Bombardieri E, Crippa F, Maffioli L, Greco M (1997) Nuclear medicine techniques for the study of breast cancer. Eur J Nucl Med 24:809–824

Boring CC, Squires TS, Tong T, Montgomery S (1994) Cancer statistics 1994. CA Cancer J Clin 44:7–26

Brazeau P, Vale W, Burgus R, Ling N, Butcher M, Livier J, Guellemin R (1973) Hypothalamic polypeptide that inhibits the secretion of immunoreactive pituitary growth hormone. Science 119:77–79

Buscail L, Saint-Laurent N, Chastre E, Vaillant JC, Gespach C, Capella G, Kalthoff H, Luis F, Vaysse N, Susini C (1996) Loss of SSTR2 somatostatin receptor gene expression in human pancreatic and colorectal cancer. Cancer Res 54:23–1827

Corness JD, Demchyschyn LL, Seeman P (1993) A human somatostatin receptor (SSTR3), located on chromosome 22, displays preferential affinity for somatostatin-14 like peptides. FEBS 321:279–284

Couvineau A, Laburthe M (1985) The human vasoactive intestinal peptide receptor: molecular identification by covalent cross-linking in colonic epithelium. J Clin Endocrinol Metab 61:50–55

Couvineau A, Amiranoff B, Laburthe M (1986) Solubilization of the liver vasoactive intestinal peptide receptors. J Biol Chem 261:14482–14489

Couvineau A, Voisin T, Guijarro L, Laburthe M (1990) Purification of vasoactive intestinal peptide receptor from porcine liver by a newly designed one-step affinity chromatography. J Biol Chem 265:13386–13390

Couvineau A, Rouyer-Fessard C, Darmoul D, Maoret JJ, Carrero I, Ogier-Denis E Laburthe M (1994) Human intestinal VIP receptor: cloning and functional expression of two cDNA encoding proteins with different N-terminal domains. Biochem Biophys Res Commun 200:769–776

DeCosse JJ, Tsoulias GJ, Jacobson JS (1994) Colorectal cancer: detection, treatment and rehabilitation. CA Cancer J Clin 44:27–42

Demchyschyn LL, Srikant CB, Sunahara RK, Kent G, Seeman P, van Tol HH, Panetta R, Patel YC, Niznik HB (1993) Cloning and expression of a human somatostatin-14-selective receptor variant (somatostatin receptor 4) located on chromosome 20. Mol Pharmacol 43:894–901

Fisher WE, Doran TA, Muscarella II P, Boros LG, Ellison EC, Schirmer WJ (1998) Expression of somatostatin receptor subtype 1–5 genes in human pancreatic cancer. J Natl Cancer Inst 90:322–324

Foekens JA, Portengen H, Putten WLJ (1989) Prognostic value of receptors for insulin-like growth factor 1, somatostatin and epidermal growth factor in human breast cancer. Cancer Res 49:7002–7009

Freeny PC, Marks WM, Ryan JA, Traverso LW (1988) Pancreatic ductal adenocarcinoma: 2 diagnosis and staging with dynamic CT. Radiology 166:125–33

Fujita T, Yamaji Y, Sato M, Murao K, Takhara J (1994) Gene expression of somatostain receptor subtypes, SSTR1 and SSTR2, in human lung cancer cell lines. Life Sci 55:1797–1806

Garin E, Devillers A, Le Cloirec J, Bernard AM, Lescouarché J, Herry JY, Reubi JC, Bourguet P (1998) Use of In-111-pentetreotide somatostatin receptor scintigraphy to detect recurrent thyroid carcinoma in patients without detectable iodine uptake. Eur J Nucl Med 25:687–694

Gespach C, Bawab W, de Cremoux P, Calvo F (1988) Pharmacology, molecular identification and functional characteristics of vasoactive intestinal peptide receptors in human breast cancer. Cancer Res 48:5079–5083

Ginsberg RJ, Kris MG, Armstrong JG (1993) Cancer of the lung. In: De Vita V, Hellman S, Rosenberg SA (eds) Cancer principles and practice of oncology, 4th edn. Lippincott, Philadelphia, pp 673–723

Giusti M, Ciccarelli, Dallabonzana D, Delitala G, Faglia G, Liuzzi A, Gussoni G, Disem GG (1997) Clinical results of long term slow release lanreotide treatment of acromegaly. Eur J Clin Invest 27:277–284

Godwin JD (1975) Carcinoid tumors: an analysis of 2837 cases. Cancer 36:560–569

Greenman Y, Melmed S (1994a) Heterogeneous expression of two somatostatin receptor subtypes in pituitary tumors. J Clin Endocrinol Metab 78:398–403

Greenman Y, Melmed S (1994b) Expression of three somatostatin receptor subtypes in pituitary adenomas: evidence for preferential SSTR5 expression in the mammosomatotroph lineage. J Clin Endocrinol Metab 79:724–729

Guhlke S, Zamora PO, Sartor J, Knapp FF, Rhodes BA, Biersack HJ (1997) Stabilization of rhenium-188 and iodine-131 labeled peptides for radiotherapy. Eur J Nucl Med 24:1059A

Haegerstrand A, Jonzon B, Daalsgard CJ, Dalsgaard CJ, Nilsson J (1989) Vasoactive intestinal polypeptide stimulates cell proliferation and adenylate cyclase activity of cultured human keratinocytes. Proc Natl Acad Sci USA 86:5993–5996

Hejna M, Kurtaran A, Raderer M, Pangerl T, Niederle B, Vorbeck F, Vierhapper H, Angelberger P, Virgolini I (1998) ^{123}I-vasoactive intestinal peptide (VIP) receptor and ^{111}In-DTPA-Phe^{1}-octreotide scanning in patients with insulinoma. Eur J Nucl Med 25:977A

Hustinx R, Paulus P, Foidart J, Bury T, Cataldo D, Rigo P (1997) Efficacy of Tc 99 m P829, a radiolabeled somatostatin analog, in visualising mediastinal spread of non-small cell lung cancer. Eur J Nucl Med 24:959A

Inagaki N, Yoshida H, Mizuta M, Mizuno N, Fujii Y, Gonoi T, Miyazaki JI, Seino S (1994) Cloning and functional characterization of a third pituitary adenylate cyclase-activating polypeptide subtype receptor-expressed in insulin-secreting cells. Proc Natl Acad Sci USA 91:2679–2683

Inokuma T, Tamaki N, Torizuka T, Fujita T, Magata Y, Yonekura Y, Ohshio G, Imamura M, Konishi J (1995) Value of fluorine-18-fluorodeoxyglucose and thallium 201 in the detection of pancreatic cancer. J Nucl Med 36:229–235

Ishihara T, Shigemoto R, Mori K, Takahashi K, Nagata S (1992) Functional expression and tissue distribution of a novel receptor for vasoactive intestinal polypeptide. Neuron 8:811–819

Jagoda E, Aloi L, Seidel J, Lang L, Moody T, Green S, Caraco C, Daube Witherspoon M, Green MV, Eckelman WC (1997) The biodistribution of a F-18 labeled derivate of vasoactive intestinal peptide (dVIP) in a xenograft mouse model of breast cancer. J Nucl Med 38:239A

Jais P, Terris B, Ruszniewski, LeRomancer M, Reyl-Desmars F, Vissuzaine C, Cadiot G, Mignon M, Lewin MGM (1997) Somatostatin receptor subtype gene expression in human endocrine gastroenteropancreatic tumors. Eur J Clin Invest 27:639–644

Janson ET, Gobl A, Kälkner KM, Ölber K (1996) A comparison between the efficacy of somatostatin receptor scintigraphy and that of in situ hybridization of somatostatin receptor subtype 2 messenger RNA to predict therapeutic outcome in carcinoid patients. Cancer Res 56:2561–2565

Jiang S, Kopras E, McMichael M, Bell RH Jr, Ulrich CD (1997) Vasoactive intestinal peptide (VIP) stimulates in vitro growth of VIP-1 receptor-bearing human pancreatic adenocarcinoma derived cells. Cancer Res 57:1475–1480

John M, Meyerhof W, Richter D, Waser B, Schaer JC, Scherübl H, Boese-Landgraf J, Neuhaus P, Ziske C, Mölling K, Riecken EO, Reubi JC, Wiedenmann B (1996) Positive somatostatin receptor scintigraphy correlates with the presence of somatostatin receptor subtype 2. Gut 38:33–39

Kahn A, Herman P, Vorwecki P (1991) Solitary pulmonary nodules: comparison and classification with standard, thin section, and reference phantom CT. Radiology 179:477–481

Kalser MH, Barkin J, MacIntyre JM (1985) Pancreatic cancer: assessment of prognosis by clinical presentation. Cancer 56:397–402

Kelly DM, Benjamin IS (1995) Pancreatic carcinoma. Ann Oncol 6:19–28

Krenning EP, Bakker WH, Breeman WA, Koper JW, Kooij PP, Ausem L, Lamberts JS, Reubi JC, Lamberts SW et al (1989) Localization of endocrine-related tumors with radioiodinated analogue of somatostatin. Lancet 1:242–244

Krenning EP, Bakker WH, Kooij PPM, Breeman WAP, OEI HY, de Jong M, Reubi JC, Visser TJ, Bruns C, Kwekkeboom DJ, Reijs AEM, van Hagen PM, Koper JW, Lamberts SWJ (1992) Somatostatin receptor scintigraphy with [^{111}In-DTPA-D-Phe^{1}]-octreotide in man: metabolism, dosimetry and comparison with [123I-Tyr-3-]-octreotide. J Nucl Med 33:652–658

Krenning EP, Kwekkeboom DJ, Bakker WH, Breeman WA, Kooij PP, Oei Hy, van Hagen M, Postema PT, de Jong M, Reubi JC et al (1993) Somatostatin receptor scintigraphy with (^{111}In-DOTA-d-Phe^{1})- and (^{123}I-Thyt^{3})-octreotide: the Rotterdam experience with more than 1000 patients. Eur J Nucl Med 18:1–16

Krenning EP, Kooij PP, Bakker WH, Breeman WH, Postema PT, Kwekkeboom DJ, Oei HY, Jong M, Visser TJ, Reijs AE (1994) Radiotherapy with a radiolabeled somatostatin analogue, ^{111}In-DTPA-D-Phe^{1}-octreotide. A case history. Ann NY Acad Sci 733:496–504

Krenning EP, Kooij PP, Pauwels S, Breeman WA, Postema PT, Herder de WW, Valkema R, Kwekkeboom DJ (1996) Somatostatin receptor: scintigraphy and radionuclide therapy. Digestion 57:57–61

Krenning EP, Bakker WH, Kwekkeboom DJ, Kooij PPM, van der Pluijm ME, Behe M, Mäcke H (1997) Biodistribution of a new chelated somatostatin analogue, [In-111-DOTA-D-Phe^{1}-Tyr^{3}]-octreotide; comparison with [In-111-DTPA-D-Phe-1]-octreotide in humans. J Nucl Med 38:103A

Krois D, Riedel C, Angelberger P, Kalchberger P, Virgolini I, Lehner H (1996) Synthesis of N-a-(6-hydrazinonicotinoyl)-octreotide: a precursor of a ^{99m}Tc-complex. Liebigs Ann 1463–1469

Kubota A, Yamada Y, Kagimoto S, Kagimoto S, Shimatsu A, Imamura M, Suda K, Imura H, Seino S, Seino Y (1994) Identification of somatostatin receptor subtypes and an implication for the efficacy of somatostatin analogue SMS 201–995 in treatment of human endocrine tumors. J Clin Invest 93:1321–1325

Kurtaran A, Pangerl T, Scheuba C, Schima W, Schober E, Kaserer K, Teleky B, Virgolini I (1997) Vasualization of intestinal splenosis by somatostatin receptor scintigraphy. Am J Gastroenterol 93:1375–1376

Kurtaran A, Scheuba C, Kaserer K, Angelberger P, Niederle B, Virgolini I (1998) Comparison of ^{111}In-DTPA-D-Phe^{1}-octreotide and ^{99m}Tc-(V)-dimercapto-succinic acid scanning in the preoperative localisation of medullary thyroid carcinoma. J Nucl Med 39:1907–1909

Kvols L (1994) Medical oncology considerations in patients with metastatic neuroendocrine tumors. Semin Oncol 21:56–60

Kwekkeboom D, Krenning E, Bakker W (1991) Radioiodinated somatostatin analog scintigraphy in small-cell lung cancer. J Nucl Med 32:1845–1848

Laburthe M, Couvineau A (1988) Molecular analysis of vasoactive intestinal peptid receptors. A comparison with receptors for VIP-related peptides. In: Said S, Mutt V (eds) Vasoactive intestinal peptide and related peptides. N Y Acad Sci 527:296–313

Lamberts SWJ, Bakker WH, Reubi JC, Krenning EP (1990) Somatostatin receptor imaging in the localization of endocrine tumors. N Engl J Med 323:1246–1249

Lamberts SWJ, van der Lely AJ, de Herder WW, Hofland LJ (1996) Drug therapy: octreotide. N Engl J Med 334:246–254

Lastoria S, Muto P, Caracò C, Vergara P, Varrella L, Pezullo F, Ionna F, Mozillo N, Lister-James J, Salvatore M (1996) Somatostatin receptor scintigraphy (SRS) with technetium -99 m labeled synthetic peptides in melanoma. J Nucl Med 37:138A

Laws SAM, Gough AC, Evans AA, Bains MA, Primrose JN (1997) Somatostatin receptor subtype mRNA expression in human colorectal cancer and normal colonic mucosae. Br J Cancer 75:360–366

Leimer M, Kurtaran A, Raderer M, Smith-Jones P, Bischof C, Valencak J, Scima W, Lister-James J, Virgolini I (1998a) In vitro and in vivo binding of ^{99m}Tc-P829 to gastrointestinal adenocarcinomas. Eur J Nucl Med 39:923A

Leimer M, Kurtaran A, Smith-Jones P, Raderer M, Havlik E, Angelberger P, Vorbeck F, Niederele B, Virgolini I (1998b) Response to treatment with 90Y-DOTA-lanreotide of a patient with metastatic gastrinoma. J Nucl Med 39:2090–2094

Lister-James J, Virgolini I, Nelson CA, Pearson DA, Leimer M, Moyer BR, Wilson DM, Dean RT (1998) Tc-99 m 1666: development of a technetium-99m-labeled VIP-receptor imaging agent. J Nucl Med 39:225A

Lowe V, Fletcher J, Gobar L et al (1998) Prospective investigation of positron emission tomography in lung nodules. J Clin Oncol 16:1075–1084

Lugtenburg PJ, Löwenberg B, Eljkemans MJC, Habbema JDF, Lamberts R, Valkema R, Krenning EP (1998) Somatostatin receptor scintigraphy in limited Hodgkin's disease: clinical impact and cost-effectiveness analysis. J Nucl Med 39:39A

Lutz EM, Sheward WJ, West KM, Fink G, Harmar AJ (1993) The VIP2 receptor: molecular characterization of a cDNA encoding a novel receptor for vasoactive intestinal peptide. FEBS Lett 334:3–8

Maina T, Stolz B, Albert R, Bruns C, Koch P, Maecke H (1994) Synthesis, radiochemistry and biological evaluation of a new somatostatin analogue (SDZ 219–387) labeled with technetium-99 m. Eur J Nucl Med 21:437–444

Mather SJ, Ellison D (1994) Technetium-99 m labeled hybrid receptor binding peptides. J Nucl Med Biol 38:480–481

Miller GM, Alexander JM, Bikkal HA, Katzenelson L, Zervas NT, Klibanski A (1995) Somatostatin receptor subtype gene expression in pituitary adenomas. J Clin Endocrinol Metab 80:2974–2979

Moertel CG (1987) Karnovsky memorial lecture: an odyssee in the land of small tumors. J Clin Oncol 5:1503–1522

Moody TW, Leyton J, Unsworth E, John C, Lang L, Eckelman WC (1998) (Arg15, Arg21) VIP: evaluation of biological activity and localization to breast cancer tumors. Peptides 19:585–592

Naruke T, Tsuchiya R, Kondo H, Asamura H, Nakayama H (1997) Implications of staging in lung cancer. Chest 112:242–248

National Cancer Institute (1991) Annual cancer statistics review 1973–1988. Department of Health and Human Services, Bethesda, Md (NIH publication no 91–2789)

O'Byrne K,J, Halmos G, Pinski J, Groot K, Szepeshazi K, Schally AV, Carney DN (1994) Somatostatin receptor expression in lung cancer. Eur J Cancer 30:1682–1687

O'Nilsson L, Kölby L, Wängberg B, Wigander A, Billig H, William-Olsson L, Fjälling M, Forssell-Aronsson E, Ahlman H (1998) Comparative studies on the expression of somatostatin receptor subtypes, outcome of octreotide scintigraphy and response to octreotide treatment in patients with carcinoid tumours. Br J Cancer 77:632–637

Otte A, Jermann E, Behe M, Goetze M, Bucher HC, Roser HW, Heppeler A, Mueller-Brand J, Meacke HR (1997) DOTATOC: a powerful new tool for receptor-mediated radionuclide therapy. Eur J Nucl Med 24:792–795

Otte A, Mueller-Brand J, Dellas S, Nitzsche EU, Herrmann R, Maecke HR (1998) Yittrium-90-labelled somatostatin-analogue for cancer treatment. Lancet 351:417–418

Pallela VR, Chakdar S, Rattan S, Thakur ML (1998a) Tc-99 m labeled VIP receptor agonist: functional and pharmacokinetic studies. J Nucl Med 39:64A

Pallela VR, Reddy MVR, Senadhi VK, Thakur ML (1998b) Synthesis and evaluation of Tc-99m-labeled VIP as potential tumor imaging agents. J Nucl Med 39:226A

Pallela VR, Thakur ML, Chakder S, Rattan S (1998c) Tc-99 m labeled VIP receptor agonist: functional studies. J Nucl Med 40:352–360

Pangerl T, Peck-Radosavljevic M, Kaserer K, Niederle B, Gangl A, Virgolini I (1997) Somatostatin (SST)rand VIP receptor subtype gene expression in human tumors. Eur J Nucl Med 24:995A

Panetta R, Patel YC (1994) Expression of mRNA for all five human somatostatin receptors (hSSTR-1–5) in pituitary tumors. Life Sci 56:333–342

Patz EF, Lowe VJ, Hoffman JM et al (1994) Persistent or recurrent bronchogenic carcinoma: detection with PET and 2-[F-18] fluoro-2-deoxy-D-glucode. Radiology 191:379–382

Parker SL, Tong T, Bolden S, Wingo PA (1997) Cancer statistics 1997. Ca Cancer J Clin 47:5–27

Peck-Radosavljevic M, Yang Q, Leimer M, Bischof C, Virgolini I (1998) Thr somatostatin receptor (sstr) subtype 3 acts as an acceptor of vasoactive intestinal peptide (VIP). Gastroenterology 114:1172A

Plewe G, Beyer J, Krause U, Neufeld M, del Pozo E (1984) Long-acting and selective supression of growth hormon secretion by somatostatin analogue SMS 201–995 in acromegaly. Lancet 6:782–784

Pincus DW, DiCicco-Bloom EM, Black IB (1990) Vasoactive intestinal polypeptide regulates mitosis, differentiation and survival of cultured sympathetic neuroblasts. Nature 343:564–567

Postema PTE, de Herder WW, Reubi JC, Oei HY, Kwekkeboom DJ, Bruining HJ, van Toor H, Hennemann G, Krenning EP (1996) Somatostatin receptor scintigraphy in non-medullary thyroid cancer. Digestion 57:36–37

Raderer M, Becherer A, Kurtaran A, Angelberger P, Li S, Leimer M, Weinländer G, Kornel G, Kletter K, Scheithauer W, Virgolini I (1996) Comparison of iodine-123-vasoactive intestinal peptide receptor scintigraphy and indium-111-CYT-103 immunoscintigraphy. J Nucl Med 37:1480–1487

Raderer M, Pangerl T, Leimer T, Valencak J, Kurtaran A, Hamilton G, Scheithauer W, Virgolini I (1998a) Expression of human somatostatin receptor subtyp 3 in pancreatic cancer in vitro and in vivo. J Nat Cancer Inst 90:1666–1668

Raderer M, Kurtaran A, Yang Q, Susan Meghdadi, Vorbeck Friedrich, Heijn Michael, Angelberger P, Kornek G, Pidlich J, Scheithauer W, Virgolini I (1998b) Iodine-123-vasoactive intestinal peptide receptor scanning in patients with pancreatic cancer. J Nucl Med 39:1570–1575

Raderer M, Kurtaran A, Hejn M, Vorbeck T, Angelberger P, Scheithauer W, Virgolini I (1998c) ^{123}I-labelled vasoactive intestinal peptide receptor scintigraphy in patients with colorectal cancer. Br J Cancer 78:1–5

Rainhardt MJ, Moser E (1996) An update on diagnostic methods in the investigation of disease of the thyroid. Eur J Nucl Med 23:587–594

Reichlin S (1983) Somatostatin. N Engl J Med 309:1556–1563

Reubi JC (1995) In vitro identification of vasoactive peptide receptors in human tumors: implications for tumor imaging. J Nucl Med 36:1846–1853

Reubi JC, Maurer K, von Werder K, Torhorst J, Klijn GM, Lamberts SWJ (1989) Somatostatin receptors in human endocrine tumors. Cancer Res 47:551–558

Reubi JC, Waser B, Sheppard M, Macaulay Y (1990) Somatostatin receptors are present in small-cell but not in non-small primary lung carcinomas: relationship to EGF-receptors. Int J Cancer 45:269–274

Reubi JC, Schaer JC, Waser B, Mengold G (1994) Expression and localization of somatostatin receptor SSTR1, SSTR2 and SSTR3 mRNAs in primary human tumors using in situ hybridization. Cancer Res 54:3455–3459

Robberecht P, de Neef P, Gourlet P, Cauvin A, Coy DH, Christophe J (1989) Pharmacological characterization of the novel helodermin/VIP receptor present in human SUP-T1 lymphoma cell membranes. Regul Pept 26:117–126

Rohrer L, Raulf F, Bruns C, Buetter R, Hofstaedter F, Schüle R (1993) Cloning and characterization of a fourth human somatostatin receptor. Proc Natl Acad Sci USA 90:4196–4200

Rosenberg L, Brown RA (1991) Sandostatin in the management of nonendocrine gastrointestinal and pancreatic disorders: a preliminary study. Cancer J Surg 34:223–229

Said SI, Foloona GR (1975) Elevated plasma and tissue levels of vasoactive intestinal peptide in the watery diarrhea syndrome. N Engl J Med 293:155–158

Said SI, Mutt V (1970) Polypeptide with broad biological activity. Isolation from small intestine. Science 169:1217–1218

Scheithauer W, Rosen H, Kornek GV, Sebesta C, Depisch D (1993) Randomised comparison of combination chemotherapy plus supportive care with supportive care alone in patients with metastatic colorectal cancer. Br Med J 306:752–755

Schaer JC, Waser B, Mengold G, Reubi JC (1997) Somatostatin receptor subtypes sst1, sst2, sst5 expression in human pituitary, gastroentero-pancreatic and mammary tumors: comparison of mRNA analysis with receptor autoradiography. Int J Cancer 70:530–537

Schlag P, Lehner B, Strauss LG, Georgi P, Herfarth C(1989) Scar or recurrent rectal cancer. Positron emission tomography is more helpful for diagnosis than immunoscintigraphy. Arch Surg 124:197–200

Seidman H, Mushnick MH, Gelb SK, Silverberg E (1985) Probability of eventually developing or dying of cancer: United States. CA Cancer J Clin 35:36–56

Shirzad M, Leimer M, Lister-James J, Moyer BR, Angelberger P, Virgolini I (1998) Preclinical characterization of a 99m-technetium labeled vasoactive intestinal peptide (VIP) receptor imaging peptide. Eur J Nucl Med 25:977A

Siegelman S, Khouri N, Leo F, Fishman EK, Braverman RM, Zerhouni EA (1986) Solitary pulmonary nodules: CT assessment. Radiology 160:307–312

Smith-Jones P, Bischof C, Leimer M, Gludovac D, Angelberger P, Pangerl T, Peck-Radosavljevic M, Hamilton G, Kaserer K, Steiner G, Schlagbauer-Wadl H, Mäcke H, Virgolini I (1998a) "MAURITIUS" a novel somatostatin analog for tumor diagnosis and therapy. J Nucl Med 39:223A

Smith-Jones P, Bischof C, Leimer M, Gludovacz D, Angelberger P, Pangerl T, Peck-Radosavljevic M, Steiner G, Virgolini I (1999) "MAURITIUS": a novel tumor diagnostic and therapeutic somatostatin analog. Endocrinology (in press)

Sreedharan SP, Kodama KT, Peterson KE, Goetzl EJ (1989) Distinct subjects of somatostatin receptors on cultured human lymphocytes. J Biol Chem 264:949–952

Sreedharan SP, Robichon A, Peterson KE, Goetzl EJ (1991) Cloning and expression of the human vasoactive intestinal peptide receptor. Proc Natl Acad Sci USA 88:4986–4990

Stiefel F, Morant R (1993) Vapreotide, a new somatostatin analogue in the palliative management of obstructive ileus in advanced cancer. Support Care Cancer 1:57–58

Svoboda M, Tastenoy M, van Rampelsbergh J, de Neef P, Waelbroeck M, Robberecht O (1994) Molecular cloning and functional characterization of a human VIP receptor from sup-T1 lymphoblasts. Biochem Biophys Res Commun 205:1617–1624

Taucher S, Kurtaran A, Leimer M, Angelberger P, Pangerl T, Beck M, Gnant M, Jakesz R, Virgolini I (1996) Validation of VIP and somatostatin receptor scanning in primary breast cancer. Eur J Nucl Med 23:1094A

Tenenbaum F, Lumbroso J, Schlumberger M, Caillou B, Fragu P, Parmentier C (1995) Radiolabeled somatostatin analog scintigraphy in differentiated thyroid carcinoma. J Nucl Med 36:807–810

Thakur ML, Kolan H, Li J, Wiaderkiewicz, Pallela VR, Duggaraju R, Schally AV (1997) Radiolabeled somatostatin analogs in prostate cancer. Nucl Med Biol 24:105–113

Thomas F, Brambrilla E, Friedmann A (1994) Transcription of somatostatin receptor subtype 1 and 2 genes in lung cancer. Lung Cancer 11:111–114

Ullrich CD, Holtmann Martin, Miller LJ (1998) Secretin and vasoactive intestinal peptide receptors: members of a unique family of G protein-coupled receptors. Gastroenterology 114:382.397

Usdin TB, Bonner TI, Mezey E (1994) Two receptors for vasoactive intestinal polypeptide with similar specificity and complementary distributions. Endocrinology 135:2662–2680

Vallabhajosula S, Moyer BR, Lister-James J, McBride BJ, Lipszyc H, Lee H, Bastidas D, Dean RT (1996) Preclinical evaluation of technetium-99m-labeled somatostatin receptor-binding peptides. J Nucl Med 37:1016–1022

van Dyke JA, Stanley RJ, Berland LL (1985) Pancreatic imaging. Ann Intern Med 102:212–7

van Eijck CHJ, Krenning EP, Bootsma A, Oei HY, van Pel R, Lindemans J, Jeekel J, Reubi JC, Lamberts SWJ (1994) Somatostatin-receptor scintigraphy in primary breast cancer. Lancet 343:640–643

Verner JV, Morrison AB (1958) Islet cell tumor and a syndrome of refractory watery diarrhea and hypokalemia. Am J Med 25:374–380

Vikic-Topic S, Raisch KP, Kvols L, Vuk-Pavlovic S (1995) Expression of somatostatin receptor subtypes in breast carcinoma, carcinoid tumors, and renal cell carcinoma. J Clin Endocrinol Metab 80:2974–2979

Vinik AI, McLeod MK, Fig LM, Shapiro B, Lloyd RV, Cho K (1989) Clinical features, diagnosis, and localization of carcinoid tumors and their management. Gastroenterol Clin North Am 18:865–896

Virgolini I (1997) Mack Forster Award Lecture: receptor nuclear medicine: somatostatin receptor scintigraphy for diagnosis and treatment of tumor patients. Eur J Clin Invest 27:793–800

Virgolini I, Yang Q, Li S, Angelberger P, Neuhold N, Niederle B, Scheithauer W, Valent P (1994a) Cross-competition between vasoactive intestinal peptide and somatostatin for binding to tumor cell membrane receptors. Cancer Res 54:690–700

Virgolini I, Raderer M, Kurtaran A, Angelberger P, Banyai S, Yang Q, Li S, Banyai M, Pidlich J, Niederle B, Scheithauer W, Valent P (1994b) Vasoactive intestinal peptide (VIP) receptor imaging for the localisation of intestinal adenocarcinomas and endocrine tumors. N Engl J Med 331:1116–1121

Virgolini I, Kurtaran A, Raderer M, Leimer M, Angelberger P, Havlik E, Li S, Scheithauer W, Niederle B, Valent P, Eichler HG (1995) Vasoactive intestinal peptide receptor scintigraphy. J Nucl Med 36:1732–1739

Virgolini I, Angelberger P, Li S, Yang Q, Kurtaran A, Raderer M, Neuhold N, Kaserer K, Leimer M, Peck-Radosavljevic M, Scheithauer W, Niederle B, Eichler HG, Valent P (1996a) In vitro and in vivo studies of three radiolabelled somatostatin analoges: ^{123}I-octreotide (OCT), ^{123}I-Tyr-3-OCT and ^{111}In-DTPA-D-Phe-1-OCT. Eur J Nucl Med 23:1388–1399

Virgolini I, Pangerl T, Bischof C, Leimer M, Yang Q, Peck-Radosavljevic M, Kaserer K, Niederle B, Angelberger P, Gangl A, Valent P (1996b) Somatostatin (SST) and vasoactive intestinal peptide (VIP) receptor (R) subtype gene expression. Eur J Nucl Med 23:1101A

Virgolini I, Raderer M, Kurtaran A, Angelberger P, Yang Q, Radosavljevic M, Leimer M, Kaserer K, Li S, Kornek G, Hübsch P, Niederle B, Pidlich J, Scheithauer W, Valent P (1996c) ^{123}I-Vasoactive intestinal peptide (VIP) receptor scanning: update of imaging results in patients with adenocarcinomas and endocrine tumors of the gastrointestinal tract. Nucl Med Biol 23:685–692

Virgolini I, Pangerl T, Bischof C, Smith-Jones P, Peck-Radosavljevic M (1997) Somatostatin receptor subtype expression in human tissues: a prediction for diagnosis and treatment of cancer? Eur J Clin Invest 27:645–647

Virgolini I, Leimer M, Hirschmaker H, Lastoria S, Bischof C, Muto P, Pangerl T, Gludovacz D, Peck-Radosavljevic M, Lister-James J, Hamilton G, Kaserer K, Valent P, Dean R (1998a) Somatostatin receptor subtype specificity and in vivo binding of a novel tumor tracer, ^{99m}Tc-P829. Cancer Res 58:1850–1859

Virgolini I, Kurtaran A, Leimer M, Kaserer K, Peck-Radosavljevic M, Angelberger P. Hübsch P, Dvorak M, Valent P, Niederle B (1998b) Location of a VIPoma by iodine-123-vasoactive intestinal peptide scintigraphy. J Nucl Med 39:1575–1579

Virgolini I, Szilvasi I, Angelberger P, Raderer M, Havlik E, Vorbeck F, Bischof C, Leimer M, Dorner G, Kletter K, Niederle B, Scheithauer W, Smith-Jones P (1998c) Indium-111-DOTA-

lanreotide: biodistribution, safety and tumor dose in patients. J Nucl Med 39:1928-1936
Virgolini I, Smith-Jones P, Moncayo R, Kurtaran A, Wenger M, Raderer M, Havlik E, Angelberger P, Szilvaszi I, Zoboli S, Paganelli G, Riccabona G (1998d) 111-In/90-Y-DOTA-lanreotide scintigraphy and therapy: initial clinical results of "Mauritius". Eur J Nucl Med 25:884A
Vural G, ÜnlÜ M, Atasever T, Özur I, Özdemir A, Gökcora N (1997) Comparison of indium-111 octreotide and thallium-201 scintigraphy in patients mammographically suspected of having breast cancer: preliminary results. Eur J Nucl Med 24:312–315
Wang KP, Kelly SJ, Britt JE (1988) Percutaneous needle aspiration biopsy of chest lesions. New instrument and new technique. Chest 9:993–997
Warshaw AL, Fernandez-del Castillo C (1992) Pancreatic carcinoma. N Engl J Med 326:455–65
World Health Organization (1981) Histologic typing of lung cancer, 2nd edn. WHO, Geneva
Yamada Y, Post SR, Wang K, Tager HS, Bell GI, Seino S (1992a) Cloning and functional characterization of a family of human and mouse somatostatin receptors expressed in brain, gastrointestinal tract and kidney. Proc Natl Acad Sci USA 89:251–255
Yamada Y, Reisine S, Law SF, Ihara Y, Kubota A, Kagimoto S, Seino M, Seino Y, Bell I, Seino S (1992b) Somatostatin receptors, an expanding gene family: cloning and functional characterization of human SSTR3, a protein coupled to adenylyl cyclase. Mol Endocrinol 6:2136–2142
Yamada Y, Kagimoto S, Kubota A, Yasuda K, Masuda K, Someya Y, Ihara Y, Li Q, Imura H, Seino S, Seino Y (1993) Cloning, functional expression and pharmacological characterization of a fourth (hSSTR4) and fifth (hSSTR5) human somatostatin receptor subtypes. Biochem Biophys Res Commun 195:844–852
Yasuda K, Res-Domiano S, Breder CA, Law SF, Saper C, Reisine T, Bell GI (1992) Cloning of a novel somatostatin receptor, SST3, coupled to adenylate cyclase. J Biol Chem 267:20422–20428
Zia H, Hida T, Jakowlew S, Birrer M, Gozes Y, Reubi JC, Fridkin M, Gozes I, Moody TW (1996) Breast cancer growth is inhibited by vasoactive intestinal peptide (VIP) hybrid, a synthetic VIP receptor antagonist. Cancer Res 56:3486–3489

10 Clinical Positron Imaging in Oncology

C. Schiepers, C. K. Hoh

Contents

10.1 Introduction 159
10.2 Methods 159
10.2.1 Tracers and Uptake Mechanisms 160
10.2.2 Acquisition 160
10.2.3 Quantification 161
10.2.4 Patient Preparation and Diagnostic Protocol 162
10.3 Objective 162
10.4 Topographical Overview 163
10.4.1 Brain 163
10.4.2 Head and Neck 163
10.4.3 Lung 164
10.4.4 Breast 165
10.4.5 Colorectal 167
10.4.6 Other Gastro-Intestinal Tumors 168
10.4.7 Prostate 169
10.4.8 Other Genito-Urinary Tumors 170
10.4.9 Lymphoma 170
10.4.10 Melanoma 171
10.5 Conclusion 171

10.1 Introduction

The advances in medical imaging technology pose a challenge to both the imaging specialist and the clinician. In this decade a major impact has been made in the field of oncology, where the goals of diagnostic imaging are to: (a) help establish the patients diagnosis; (b) streamline patient management; and (c) enhance the development of accepted treatment protocols.

Improved patient outcome can be expected, if these goals are achieved. Various imaging modalities, such as radiography, computed tomography (CT), magnetic resonance (MR) imaging, ultrasonography (US), and positron emission tomography (PET), are available for this purpose. Positron emission tomography is based on imaging of biochemical processes in vivo, and creates tomographic images similar to other conventional tomographic imaging modalities, i.e., CT and MR. However, PET is unique because it supplies an image representing the metabolic activity of the underlying tissue processes. Positron emission tomography has been in existence since the 1960s, and has slowly gained clinical acceptance.

The basics of PET are beyond the scope of this book. The work by Phelps et al. (1986) is a standard text for the interested reader. Modern instrumentation and image generation is dealt with in Chaps. 13 and 14. Here we focus on the clinical applications of PET and the comparison with conventional radiological techniques, i.e., CT, MR, and US. The place of PET in stratifying patients and in the work-up of clinical problems is discussed. In this respect, it is appropriate to speak of correlative imaging, in which all imaging modalities have their specific contribution, and are not seen as competitive modalities. Diagnostic schemes or algorithms for an efficient diagnostic imaging work-up are presented, if a consensus exists.

A few reports have addressed the cost issue of PET. Generally, algorithms that include a whole-body PET appear cost-effective when compared with a more conventional approach where multiple CT or MR scans of certain body areas are performed. The main advantage of PET in oncology is that with one injection and imaging session the whole body can be imaged in a tomographic mode. Multiple CT scans covering the head, chest, abdomen, and pelvis are likely to be more expensive than a single whole-body PET scan. For the interested reader we refer to articles by Valk et al. (1996) and Gambhir et al. (1996).

10.2 Methods

In order to perform PET imaging there are three essential needs:

1. Injection of a tracer with a positron emitting nuclide (see Chap. 12)

C. Schiepers, C. K. Hoh
Department of Molecular and Medical Pharmacology, UCLA School of Medicine, 10833 Le Conte Avenue, AR-144 CHS, Los Angeles, CA 90095-6942, USA

2. A dedicated camera for detection of the tracer distribution (see Chap. 13)
3. A computer and display with all the necessary hardware and software (see Chap. 14)

10.2.1 Tracers and Uptake Mechanism

A variety of positron emitting tracers are available, which permit the imaging and quantification of physiological parameters such as perfusion, volume distribution, metabolism, or receptor status of normal and abnormal tissues such as tumors. The potential variety of radio-pharmaceuticals which may be developed for PET imaging is unlimited, and this ability will keep PET and nuclear medicine (NM) in the forefront of clinical imaging. As other imaging technologies advance, some NM applications will become obsolete. However, new tracers with better or different biological characteristics will evolve and empower nuclear medicine with a unique adaptive feature in clinical diagnostic imaging.

The most commonly used PET radiopharmaceutical in oncological applications is the glucose analog 2-^{18}F-fluoro-2-deoxy-D-glucose (FDG). The ability to non-invasively image glucose utilization is important, since high rates of glycolysis are found in many malignant tumor cells (Warburg 1931, 1956). Malignant cells also have increased specific membrane glucose transporters and upregulated hexokinase enzymes (Wahl 1997a). This chapter concentrates on the achievements of the 1990s; therefore, we have limited our discussion to the role of FDG as PET radiopharmaceutical in oncology (Conti et al. 1996; Rigo et al. 1996; Brock et al. 1997). The uptake of FDG varies greatly for different tumor types; however, high uptake is usually associated with a high number of viable tumor cells and high expression of glucose transporter 1 (GLUT-1). Lung cancer has among the highest expressions of GLUT-1, and therefore is readily detectable, whereas renal cell cancers show the opposite (Wahl 1997a,b; Brown and Wahl 1993).

Increased FDG uptake is by no means specific for neoplasms. Inflammatory processes also have increased uptake, and false-positive results in the diagnostic setting have been reported for tuberculosis, fungal infections, sarcoidosis, non-specific granulomas, suture granulomas, benign fibrous mesotheliomas, acute post-operative and radiation changes, abscesses, pancreatitis, and fractures. Kubota has studied the uptake of FDG in macrophages and granulation tissues (Kubota et al. 1991, 1992) and has discussed the accumulation of FDG in tumors (Kubota et al. 1993). Higashi et al. (1993a,b) have studied the relation of FDG uptake to proliferation rate and viable cell number after radiation treatment.

10.2.2 Acquisition

Dedicated PET scanners are true volumetric imaging devices with detectors surrounding the full 360° around a patient (see Chap. 13). Modern scanners can simultaneously acquire multiple image planes in a 10- to 15-cm axial span. The PET image acquisitions can be performed in three modes: (a) dynamic; (b) static; and (c) whole body. In the dynamic mode, the image acquisition is initiated at the same time the dose is injected into the patient. The changing blood pool and tissue accumulation of the radiopharmaceutical are recorded in a rapid sequence of image frames. Dynamic acquisition provides a graphical representation of the FDG accumulation in the tissues vs elapsed time which is used in the calculation of in vivo biochemical rate constants. In the static mode of acquisition, an uptake period of 60–90 min is used to allow tracer clearance from the blood pool and sufficient tracer uptake in target tissues. Transverse slices of selected body areas are reconstructed from which coronal and sagittal planes can be extracted and displayed as volumetric data sets. The axial size of the images is determined by the scanner, and larger body areas can be encompassed by joining adjacent bed positions.

The whole-body imaging mode (WBPET) was introduced in the late 1980s by UCLA School of Medicine, and subsequently became the standard for PET imaging in oncology (Dahlbom et al. 1992; Hoh et al. 1993, 1997b). In this mode of scanning, multiple acquisitions are performed sequentially along the length of the patients body, thereby extending the axial field of view to that of the entire body. The intuitive advantage of the whole-body technique is that many cancers are systemic diseases requiring imaging of the entire body. Compared with other whole-body techniques, the PET images are tomographic allowing full three-dimensional review of high-contrast images in the transverse, coronal, and sagittal planes. This is the favorite mode of searching for disease outside the limited primary field of view. In addition, planar (non-tomographic) projections are created, in which the total activity distribution is viewed from different angles around the patient. This data can be displayed as a rotating cine. Although these non-tomographic images have less lesion-to-background contrast, there is no image reconstruction artifact which may obscure tumor foci near bright objects such as the bladder.

As the photons pass through the tissues of the body, varying degrees of attenuation affect the final number which reaches the detectors and can be used for imaging. This attenuation effect can be corrected for by the acquisition of a separate transmission scan, and by calculating the regional attenuation factors. In older PET systems the transmission scan had to be performed before tracer administration. In the newer-generation PET scanners this can be done after tracer injection, thereby allowing the FDG uptake period to be done outside the scanner, enabling higher patient throughput. The transmission scan is also required for dynamic mode acquisitions so that true metabolic activity in units of nanomoles per minute per gram can be calculated. Without attenuation correction, only visual interpretation is possible and quantitative analysis cannot be performed. In general, whole-body images are not corrected for attenuation, since that would increase acquisition times prohibitively. However, new techniques and algorithms are being implemented to overcome this problem (see Chaps. 13, 14). For routine image interpretation, correction for attenuation is not necessary, because the interpreting physician can play with the window settings on the monitor to counteract attenuation effects. Attenuation correction eliminates focal distortions of lesions, but also decreases lesion contrast. No difference in lesion detection was found between corrected and non-attenuation corrected images for a variety of tumors (Bengel et al. 1997).

The spatial resolution of a modern CT or MR system is better than that of a PET system. However, this is not the only determining factor in detecting abnormalities. The difference in metabolic activity of the lesion and its surroundings (target-to-background ratio) or the "contrast resolution" helps determine the presence of disease. Thus, metabolically very active lesions of 5 mm have been detected with FDG PET. Attenuation corrected PET can detect lesions of approximately 1 cm and with the non-attenuation-corrected whole-body PET technique the lower limit is approximately 1.5 cm (Hoh et al. 1997b). This latter difference is due mainly to a difference in image acquisition duration, 10 vs 5 min, respectively.

10.2.3 Quantification

The combination of dynamic imaging and biological tracer detection provides PET the ability to mathematically model in vivo processes. With dynamic imaging, the tissue concentrations of radiotracer can be represented as a function of time. This ability to accurately measure the actual radiotracer distribution in the body enables PET to be similar to autoradiography. A numerical value or index representing the local tracer concentration or accumulation rate in a tumor may provide a new parameter to characterize the unknown tumor or suspicious lesion or to measure a change induced by therapy. A rapid frame acquisition is important in studying the tracer kinetics, since the fast dynamic changes in blood and tissue activity need to be adequately sampled. Currently, no other imaging modality is capable of simultaneously acquiring rapid dynamic tomographic images in a volume of tissue. For a detailed discussion of dynamic imaging and kinetic modeling, the reader is referred to Phelps et al. (1986).

Many clinical studies are analyzed semi-quantitatively by using the standardized uptake value (SUV; Zasadny and Wahl 1993; Hamberg et al. 1994; Kim et al. 1994; Keys 1995), also known as the differential uptake ratio (DUR) or differential absorption ratio (DAR). The SUV is the ratio of the measured radioactivity concentration in a lesion to the estimated body tracer concentration, assuming a uniform distribution throughout the entire body volume. It is generally assumed that tumors achieve a plateau concentration around 1–2 h, at the time of image acquisition. However, many tumor kinetics are not known and tracer uptake may still be increasing at the time of imaging. Therefore, standardization of the SUV is necessary to compare results between institutions. This SUV parameter offers a more objective way of reporting metabolic activity than visual interpretation. Thus far, the SUV technique appears to be satisfactory for clinical purposes, and works very well for some tumors. For other applications, the distinction between benign and malignant lesions is less clear and absolute quantification or an entirely different radiotracer may be required.

Quantification appears especially relevant for monitoring of therapy, i.e., to guide therapy protocols or initiate therapy change. To date, this has not been studied in great detail, and is not discussed here (Wahl 1997a; Hoh et al. 1997b; Brock et al. 1997).

10.2.4 Patient Preparation and Diagnostic Protocol

Patients are studied in a prolonged fasting state to produce low insulin levels and induce low rates of glucose utilization of normal tissues, e.g., the normal muscular tissues including the myocardium. Malignant tissues are less dependent on hormone regulation, and thus have higher contrast when compared with the surrounding normal tissues.

The typical scanning duration of a PET oncology protocol is approximately 1 h. A dose of 250–500 MBq (7–15 mCi) of FDG is the usual adult dose administered intravenously. After an uptake period of 45–75 min, the patient is asked to void and positioned in the scanner. A static scan or whole-body study is acquired as indicated. In general, images are acquired for 6–15 min duration per bed position and reconstructed using available software (see Chap. 14). Modern equipment allows scanning from feet to head, taking advantage of the low bladder uptake after voiding at the beginning of acquisition. After completion of a WBPET, inspection of the images may target a specific body area for an extra limited field of view static acquisition with high count statistics.

Since FDG is filtered but not reabsorbed by the glomerulus, high FDG activity is present in the urinary tract and interventions are sometimes necessary to clear the excreted tracer for better evaluation of the surrounding tissues. This may include administration of diuretics to irrigation of the bladder via a triple-lumen catheter. Several authors have reported high uptake in the bowel, and some propose anti-peristalsis and anti-motility drugs to overcome this problem. However, no consensus consists regarding the interventions necessary in oncological PET protocol. Many institutions utilize mild sedatives for patient comfort during the relatively lengthy acquisition.

10.3 Objective

The unique features of FDG PET in current clinical applications are reviewed to understand its role in relation to other tumor imaging modalities, e.g., in a correlative, corroborative, or complementary mode. The comparison of PET to conventional imaging and, where appropriate, the theoretical advantages of PET in clinical applications are addressed.

In a review by Brock et al. (1997) the viewpoint of the oncologist was used, focusing on grading of tumors and determination of disease extent. Tumor grading generally does not correlate well with FDG uptake. At the moment there is not enough data to propose PET as a prognostic imaging modality in the routine clinical environment. On the other hand, PET appears very well equipped to stage newly detected disease or to signal relapse of disease. If PET discloses unexpected lesions, high-resolution imaging with spiral CT or MR of the suspicious areas is indicated to delineate the structural involvement.

Husband (1995, 1996) has argued that imaging of treated tumors is becoming more important because of the increasing incidence of cancer and scientific progress in imaging and therapy. He distinguished two strategies, imaging for clinical service and for research, and observed two referral patterns: (a) for patients with curable disease and treated according to an established protocol; and (b) imaging employed for individual patient management. The number of patients studied in protocols in which PET has a key function in triage or monitoring is limited. This has lead Price (1997) to question the motives of imaging specialists with respect to diagnostic oncology. In our opinion, PET has matured and reached the level of an imaging modality appropriate for integration into clinical diagnostic algorithms. More emphasis on multi-disciplinary aspects and input from the surgical, medical and radiation oncologist, as well as the imaging specialist, will be of great benefit to the management of cancer patients.

As has been pointed out by Valk (1996), the reference standard in comparing modalities is imperfect, because full validation of findings with biopsy and histology is not feasible. Thus, there are no truly double-blind studies available comparing the performance of whole-body PET to conventional imaging in the majority of cancers. In the typical clinical context, on the other hand, it is not meaningful to evaluate the assumed "separate" contribution of each imaging modality. The purpose of imaging is to supply the diagnosis which will prompt the surgeon or oncologist to watch and observe, or to administer a treatment regimen. In this chapter we discuss the available literature for three diagnostic imaging criteria: (a) diagnosis of presence of neoplasms; (b) initial staging of newly detected disease; and (c) (re)staging of disease, i.e., assess recurrence or relapse after therapy.

This diagnostic imaging scheme implicitly assumes a normal patient work-up with history, physical exam, routine labs, and serum tumor markers, supplemented with standard radiographic imaging, mammography, CT, MR, US, or NM. If there exists a general consensus, the routine sequence of testing is shown.

Hereafter follows a selection of oncological applications in which PET has been shown to have merit. We have chosen the topographical presentation, common in radiology. In addition, we have pooled recent data for the four most common cancers, i.e., lung, breast, colorectal, and prostate (Tables 10.1–10.5).

10.4 Topographical Overview

10.4.1 Brain

The FDG PET technique has been most extensively studied for primary brain neoplasms. This is due mainly to pioneering work of Di Chiro and collaborators (1982, 1987, 1988; Di Chiro 1987). The main applications are in (a) grading of cerebral neoplasms, (b) distinguishing tumor recurrence from radiation necrosis, (c) assessing extent of disease for therapy management, and (d) selecting the optimum site for biopsy. Other investigators have corroborated their results (Doyle et al. 1987; Alavi et al. 1988).

In general, high-grade tumors have high FDG uptake. Similarly, a high FDG uptake is associated with a high-grade tumor and poorer prognosis, although there is considerable overlap. An inherent difficulty concerns the high uptake of normal gray matter. Positron emission tomography has difficulty in detecting low-grade gliomas, because their uptake can be low relative to the normal cortex. For this reason low-grade tumors can be missed by PET; however, correlative imaging, or use of a different tracer, e.g., methionine, tyrosine, or thallium, usually provides the correct diagnosis. On the other hand, high-grade gliomas generally have intense uptake of FDG.

Because of tumor heterogeneity, PET may disclose areas with high metabolic activity, which can be used to guide the optimum site for biopsy (Pirotte et al. 1995). The same principle can be applied in sequential studies, by detecting abnormal foci in a lesion which herald transformation of low-grade to higher-grade gliomas (Delbeke et al. 1995).

Edema is easily diagnosed on CT and MR, but the diagnostic dilemma in distinguishing early recurrence of tumor is well known (Di Chiro et al. 1988; Doyle et al. 1987). Even a metabolic imaging modality as NMR spectroscopy may miss the diagnosis. Metabolic imaging with FDG is helpful in differentiating recurrent tumor from radiation necrosis in lesions demonstrating contrast enhancement on CT or MR. This is only true if the tumor was visible on FDG PET prior to treatment. The differentiation of recurrent tumor vs radiation necrosis is an indication reimbursed by most insurance companies in the United States.

Positron emission tomography with FDG has a clear utility in primary brain tumors, but the data on metastases is limited. A London group claimed in a study of 273 patients that routine screening for cerebral metastasis has a low yield (1.5%) and may not be clinically useful (Larcos and Maisey 1996). For the reasons explained previously, lesions close to the cortex may be difficult to detect.

10.4.2 Head and Neck

This anatomical area is notoriously difficult, due to the small size of anatomic structures and proximity of vessels, nodes, and nerves. Various groups have shown a correlation of high metabolic activity in lesions and poor prognosis. However, the correlation between tumor grade and FDG uptake was not reliable (Lindholm et al. 1993). Haberkorn and coworkers have shown that tumor perfusion did not correlate with proliferation rate. It should be stressed that the number of patients studied is small (Haberkorn et al. 1991a, 1993; Reisser et al. 1993).

Several studies have evaluated the use of PET for accurate staging. An improved diagnostic accuracy for recurrent head and neck cancer of FDG PET over anatomical methods has been demonstrated (Rege et al. 1993a; Jabour et al. 1993; Laubenbacher et al. 1995a; Anzai et al. 1996; Benchaou et al. 1996), whereas other reports show similar numbers for the sensitivity of primaries (>85%) and affected nodes (>80%; Bailet et al. 1992; Wong et al. 1997). The reported specificity for nodal disease is over 90%. Although the accuracy of PET imaging is higher than MR and/or CT, the surgical or radiation treatment of this cancer requires anatomical localization of the abnormal PET foci. Due to the complex anatomy of the head and neck region, the optimal diagnostic modality may be a fusion image showing the abnormal metabolic lesions superimposed onto the anatomical locations.

The proposed diagnostic algorithm, which is reimbursed in California, includes PET for staging of suspected recurrence on CT or MR. Positron emission tomography is used to stratify patients into those who will benefit from surgery and others who will not.

Early on, some studies were performed suggesting that FDG avid thyroid tumors without iodine uptake tended to be more aggressive. Subsequent work has shown that thyroid tumors have FDG uptake which is clearly not specific. Later reports, covering approximately 100 patients, suggested that well-differentiated (low-grade) thyroid cancers are iodine avid and not FDG avid (ADLER and BLOOM 1993; BLOOM et al. 1993; SISSON et al. 1993; FEINE et al. 1996; GRUNWALD et al. 1997). Apparently, both tracers are indicated for the work-up and assessment of recurrence. Thus, the long-awaited method to re-evaluate treated thyroid cancer without interrupting the hormone replacement therapy is not yet available. At present, there is no clinical indication for PET in the work-up of thyroid cancer.

A possible role for PET may be the detection of unknown primaries. In the case of a neck mass and a non-diagnostic FNA, PET may reveal the primary lesion (BRAAMS et al. 1997); however, the data is not sufficient to propose PET as a screening tool.

10.4.3 Lung

The first well-established application of PET in lung cancer was the characterization of solitary pulmonary nodules (size <3 cm) and/or chest masses. Computed tomography cannot reliably distinguish benign from malignant nodules (KUNSTAETTER et al. 1985; CUMMINGS et al. 1986; KEOGAN et al. 1993). The utility of FDG PET in indeterminate lung nodules has been extensively evaluated (Table 10.1) and yields sensitivities over 90% as reported by various institutions (KNIGHT et al. 1996). In general, false-positive lesions can be easily identified through conventional radiography; therefore, FDG PET is best performed after conventional imaging for further lesion characterization. The reproducibility of quantitative measurements is high (MINN et al. 1995). The Institute of Clinical PET (ICP) presented the data of ten participating centers in 1994. The pulmonary task force of the ICP has developed algorithms for solitary pulmonary nodules based on this multi-center study. This investigation has convincingly demonstrated that a reduction in costs can be obtained if PET is included after the conventional work-up and before performing a CT of the chest.

A report on 197 patients in the Duke University series (LOWE et al. 1997; see Table 10.1) revealed a somewhat lower specificity, which the authors contributed to a "verification bias", i.e., the referring physicians no longer chose biopsy to verify "negative" PET studies (Fig. 10.1). A proposed cost-effective diagnostic algorithm for solitary pulmonary nodules consists of chest radiography, followed by an FDG-PET scan, which if positive, then proceeds to a CT-guided biopsy.

The staging of nodes in the mediastinum is very important in stratifying patients for surgery, its relevance being related to the close correspondence between disease involvement and prediction of prognosis. In a meta-analysis study (DALES et al. 1990) it was argued that non-invasive detection of lymph node metastasis must await an approach fundamentally different from the node-size determination. In the prospective NIH sponsored trial of the RDOC (WEBB et al. 1991), both CT and MR imaging had a sensitivity approximately 50% and a somewhat higher specificity approximately 65%. These results are expected since anatomical size of a node may not be directly related to the presence or absence of tumor. For example, in approximately one third of resected nodes between 2 and 4 cm, no tumor cells were detected by histopathology. Similar results on the relative insensitivity of CT have been reported (MCLOUD et al. 1992; DILLEMANS et al. 1994).

Table 10.1. Characterization of solitary pulmonary nodules (*PPV*, positive predictive value; *NPV*, negative predictive value)

First author[a]	Year	No. of patients	PET (%) Sensitivity	Specificity	PPV	NPV
DEWAN	1993	30	95	80	90	89
SCOTT	1994	62	94	80	94	80
DEWAN	1995	76	100	78	93	100
GUPTA	1996	61	93	88	95	82
ICP[b]	1993	237	96	90	–	–
LOWE	1997	197	96	77	86	92

[a] All from the USA
[b] The ICP data are from a multi-center trial in the USA; most of the other data are incorporated in this series

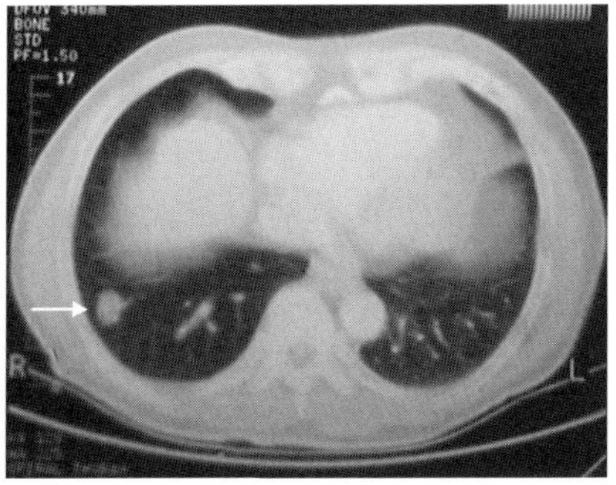

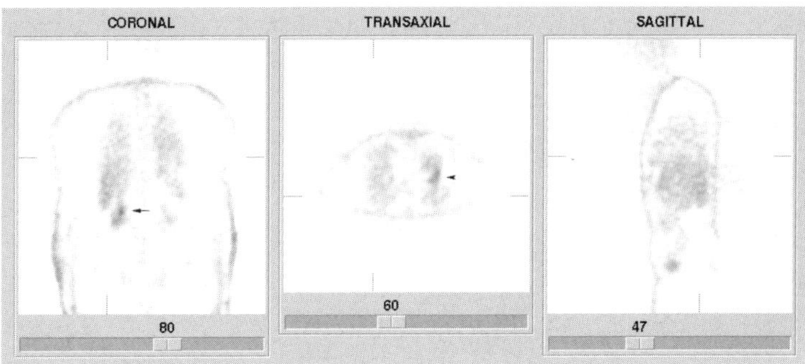

Fig. 10.1. Solitary pulmonary nodule. Transverse CT image shows a nodule in the right lung base (*arrow*). Transverse, coronal, and sagittal positron emission tomography (PET) images do not reveal increased metabolic activity in this area. This 63-year-old white male had a positive skin test, and the lesion was thought to be a tuberculoma. No biopsy was performed and conservative treatment was selected with repeat CT. Note the physiological uptake in the right renal pelvis (*arrow* on coronal image), and myocardium (*arrow* on transaxial image). Cross-sectional CT slice of 8 mm obtained with a PQ 5000 system (Picker, Cleveland, Ohio). The PET slices of 10 mm taken from ECAT ART system (CTI, Knoxville, Tenn.)

Several researchers have established that metabolic imaging with FDG PET is considerably more accurate than CT in staging mediastinal involvement with non-small-cell lung cancer (NSCLC; Table 10.2; Rege et al. 1993b). The available literature reveals for PET a sensitivity of approximately 85% and specificity of 90%, which compares favorably to CT in the same groups of patients with 60 and 80%, respectively. Table 10.2 gives an overview of recently reported series and their origin. The WBPET technique is not only able to evaluate the primary lesion and mediastinum, but especially suited for detection of occult metastases and/or distant lesions (Schiepers 1997).

Gambhir et al. (1996) have performed a study on cost-effectiveness of FDG PET in NSCLC staging and management. By using rigorous decision tree analysis, they were able to show that CT plus PET was theoretically the most economical way to work up primary lung cancer, with a marginal increase in patient life expectancy when compared with staging by CT alone. Frank et al. (1995) have also proposed a decision logic for treatment. Based on the evidence above, it is warranted to conclude that PET has a place in preoperative staging of NSCLC. Figure 10.2 shows an example of initial staging and re-staging after therapy.

The following are considered reimbursable PET indications: (a) characterization of solitary or indeterminate lung nodules as benign or malignant; (b) staging of newly diagnosed lung cancer patients, especially for lymph node involvement.

10.4.4 Breast

A group from Milan reviewed imaging in breast cancer (Bombardieri et al. 1997). They summarized the developments in mammography (MX) which is a very sophisticated imaging technology. Although it is not a three-dimensional volumetric technique, it is widely applied as screening modality of choice for breast cancer. However, in women with dense breasts MX may be non-diagnostic, and it may be difficult to detect tumors in fibrocystic disease. Nuclear medicine techniques may be helpful in providing parameters on vascularity, metabolic activity, and receptor

Table 10.2. Staging of non-small-cell lung cancer

First author	Country	Year	No. of patients	CT Sensitivity %	CT Specificity %	PET Sensitivity %	PET Specificity %
Chin	USA	1995	30	56	86	78	81
Valk	USA	1995	76	63	73	83	94
Sasaki	Japan	1996	29	65	87	76	98
Bury	Belgium	1996	50	72	81	90	86
Guhlmann	Germany	1997	46	50	75	80	100
Steinert	Switzerland	1997	47	57	94	89	99
Vansteenkiste	Belgium	1998	68	75	63	93	95

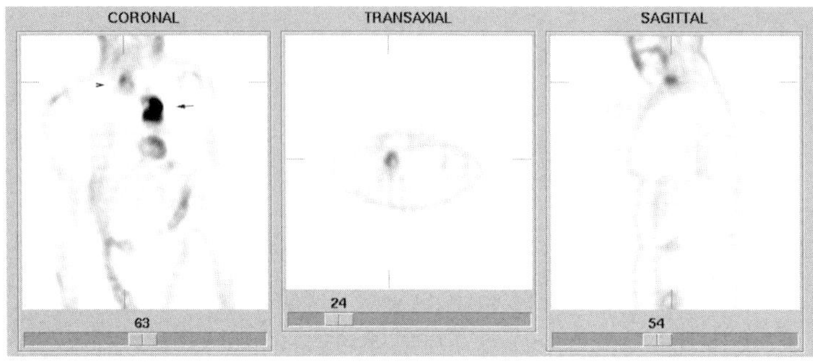

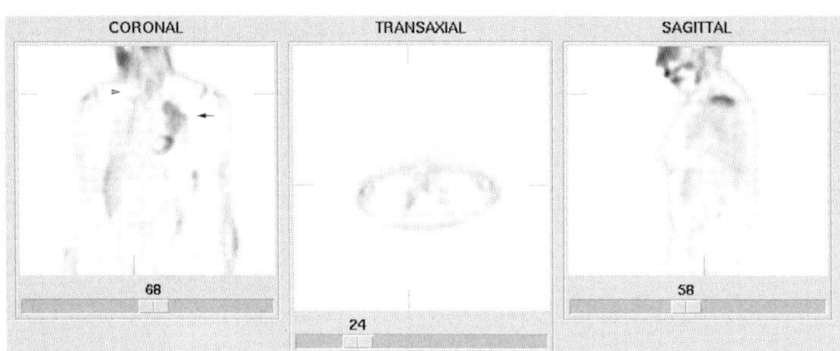

Fig. 10.2. Whole-body PET images in a patient with newly diagnosed non-small-cell lung cancer. *Upper panel:* Large primary tumor in the left upper lobe (*arrow*) and right supra-clavicular node (*arrowhead*). This is advanced disease, clinical stage IIIB, considered unresectable. Note the physiological uptake in the shoulders, myocardium (inferior to the tumor), and mucosa of the bowel. The patient was a 68-year-old Hispanic female who underwent radiation therapy and returned 4 months later. *Lower panel:* The node is no longer seen (*arrowhead*) and the primary tumor has reduced uptake of FDG. Note the different position of shoulders and body rotation relative to the horizontal bed (ECAT 962 PET system)

status. In general, a good sensitivity of PET with FDG has been reported for primary lesions (WAHL et al. 1991; ADLER et al. 1993; NIEWEG et al. 1993). The specificity of PET has not been adequately determined (insufficient studies). Also the weakness of the FDG method concerns the false positives, since both neoplastic and inflammatory lesions have increased uptake (HOH and SCHIEPERS 1999).

Axillary staging is feasible with PET and various studies have shown high specificity (Table 10.3). BOMBARDIERI et al. (1997) have argued that it could replace staging by axillary lymph node dissection. Since the dissection is currently done for prognosis only, the associated morbidity may be avoided in these patients. More studies are needed to confirm the high sensitivity and specificity of axillary staging with FDG PET in stage I–II breast cancer.

In a WBPET study from our institution, 57 patients were imaged with a history of breast cancer and referred for suspicion of recurrence (MOON et al. 1998). Patients were followed for at least 6 months, so that positive or negative diagnoses could be confirmed by biopsy, or follow-up procedures. On a patient-based analysis, the sensitivity and specificity were 93 and 79%, respectively. On a lesion-based analysis, the sensitivity and specificity of WBPET for detecting breast cancer foci was 85 and 79%, respectively. There were six false-negative lesions and 18 false-positive lesions. More extensive metastasis on PET than on CT is shown in Fig. 10.3.

Table 10.3. Breast cancer

First author	Country	Year	No. of patients	PET (%) Sensitivity	Specificity
Primary cancer detection					
AVRIL[a]	Germany	1996	51	92	97
SCHEIDHAUER	Germany	1996	30	90	–
PALMEDO	Germany	1997	20	92	86
Axillary staging					
UTECH	USA	1996	124	100	75
ADLER	USA	1997	52	95	66
CRIPPA	Italy	1998	68	85	91
SMITH	USA	1998	50	90	97

All studies used biopsy or surgery to obtain final diagnosis
[a] Quantitative criterion of SUV>2.5

Table 10.3 represents the literature of adequately sized studies. In short, for screening purposes there is no indication for PET. In primary breast cancer, PET may be helpful in characterizing indeterminate findings on MX. For axillary staging, the data looks very promising but is currently not sufficient to propose PET in the routine staging of newly diagnosed breast cancer patients.

10.4.5 Colorectal

To date, there is no data to support a role for PET in diagnosis of primary colon cancer (Table 10.4). The surgical treatment of recurrent colorectal cancer remains problematic, despite the advancement of MR, spiral CT, intra-operative US, serum tumor markers, or radiolabeled probes (radio-immuno guided surgery, RIGS). Proper selection of patients for secondary surgery with curative intent involves identifying all regional, abdominal, and distant tumor foci. This objective is not easily achieved with non-invasive imaging because of lesion size, occult disease, and lesion characterization problems. Tumor markers, such as CEA, have a low sensitivity to detect recurrence (ca. 60%). The aim of the pre-surgical work-up is to distinguish isolated resectable disease, i.e., local recurrence or solitary liver metastasis, from advanced disease. By correct staging, patients with widespread metastasis may be identified in whom surgery is not an option. This will not only improve the cost–benefit ratio, but also spare the patient extensive surgery with its associated morbidity. The actual selection of patients with recurrent cancer results in 5-year survival rates of only 20–30% after secondary "curative"

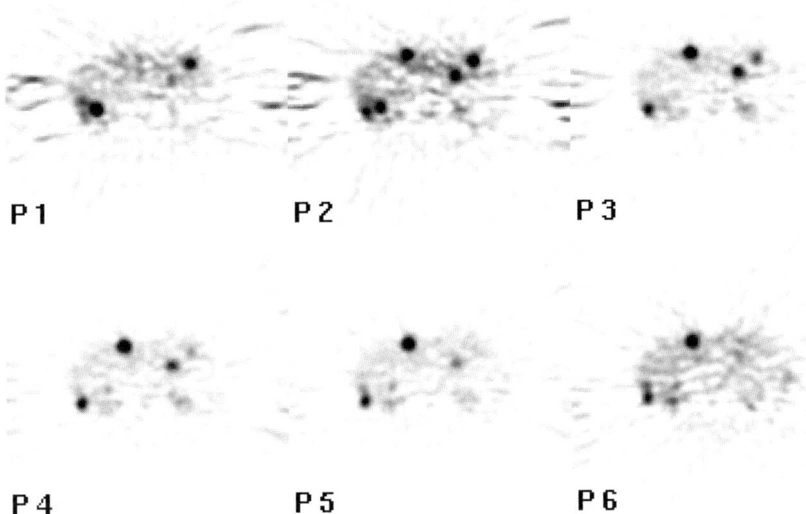

Fig. 10.3. Re-staging of breast cancer. Extensive liver metastasis was found in this 49-year-old white female. A CT exam revealed two metastases in the left liver lobe. Six consecutive slices of 10 mm, *P1–P6*. (ECAT ART PET system)

Table 10.4. Colorectal cancer (*CI* conventional imaging: CT, US, MR)

First author	Country	Year	No. of patients	CI (%) Sensitivity	CI (%) Specificity	PET (%) Sensitivity	PET (%) Specificity
Primary cancer							
Abdel-Nabi	USA	1998	48	37	83	100	43
Recurrent tumor							
Schiepers	Belgium	1995	76	71	88	94	97
Valk	USA	1996	57	68	–	100	–
Delbeke	USA	1997	52	81	–	91	–
Ruhlmann	Germany	1997	59	–	–	100	67
Ogunbiyi	USA	1997	58	68	–	95	–

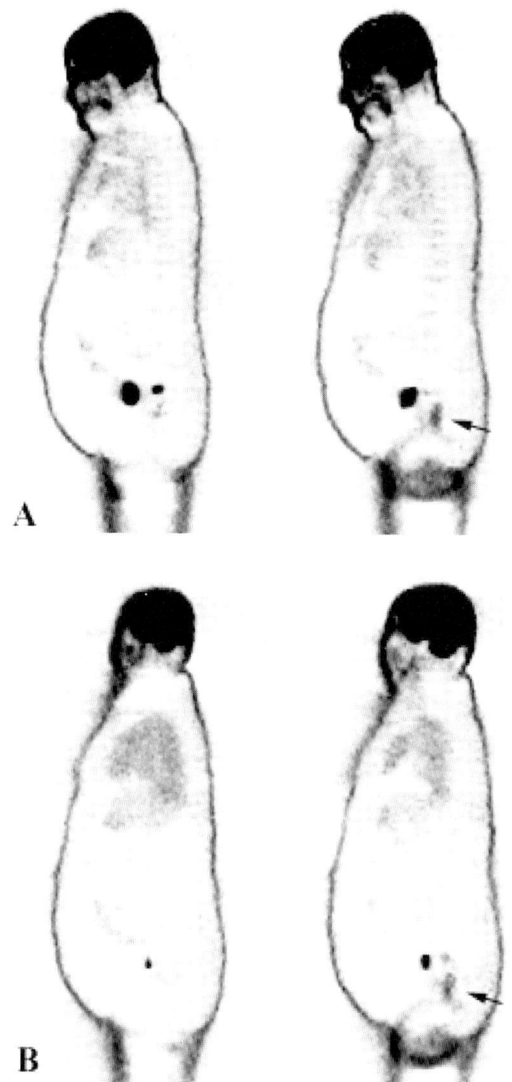

Fig. 10.4A,B. A 70-year-old white male with rectal cancer. cT3N1M0 disease on CT. Sagittal slices **A** before and **B** after radiation therapy. This whole-body PET detected two affected lymph nodes superior of the tumor, which were outside the field of view of 101 mm on the dynamic scan. Note the decrease in metabolic activity of both the tumor (*arrow*) and lymph nodes. Average tumor glucose utilization was 178 nmol/min per milliliter before (**A**) and 72 nmol/min per milliliter after (**B**) radiation therapy. (ECAT 931 PET system)

surgery (Strauss et al. 1989; Haberkorn et al. 1991b; Keogan et al. 1997). Figure 10.4 shows nodal involvement.

Table 10.3 supplies the data on colorectal cancer recurrence. Currently, the largest reported series on comparison of PET to conventional imaging is by Schiepers et al. (1995) with 76 patients. The study was prospective, had surgical confirmation in 63% of patients, and evaluated disease in three "surgical" zones: local pelvic recurrence, hepatic involvement, and distant metastasis. A high accuracy was obtained for PET, 95% for local disease, and 98% for hepatic metastasis. Unexpected advanced disease was diagnosed in 15% of patients. The study by Valk et al. (1996) provided similar results. Delbeke et al. (1997) reported on liver metastasis from colorectal origin. Since all 52 had suspected recurrence on CT, they utilized a lesion-based analysis, which furnished an accuracy of 92% for PET compared with 80% for conventional imaging. The main difference in their protocol with the other two series was the longer image duration of 10 min per bed position and correction for attenuation effects. There were no other reports in the literature with more than 50 patients.

Several reports were published about the impact of PET on patient management, which varied from 28% in the series of Delbeke et al. (1997), 29% in Lai et al. (1996), to 40% in Beets et al. (1994). Presently acknowledged PET indications for colorectal cancer are:

1. Differentiation of a pelvic mass as tumor recurrence vs post-operative fibrosis
2. Assessment of hepatic metastasis
3. Establishment of disease in case of elevated tumor markers and negative conventional imaging
4. Disclosure of occult metastases and (re)staging of disease.

10.4.6 Other Gastro-Intestinal Tumors

Over the past 3 years several papers have been published on the use of FDG PET for the characterization of pancreatic masses with indeterminate CT findings (Inokuma et al. 1995; Ho et al. 1996; Reske et al. 1997). In a study with 73 patients by Stollfuss et al. (1995) the SUV threshold for malignancy was set at 1.5 resulting in both sensitivity and specificity of 93% for lesion detection. Visual interpretation gave a slightly higher sensitivity of 95% but lowered specificity to 90%. With either method for FDG PET interpretation, the results were better than abdominal CT which had a sensitivity and specificity of 80 and 74%, respectively. Similar results were obtained in a previous study by Bares et al. (1994), where PET was compared with abdominal CT, abdominal US, and endoscopic US in 46 patients. Less encouraging results were found when FDG PET was used to differentiate pancreatic carcinoma from mass-forming pancreatitis. The problem of increased FDG uptake in intense inflammatory lesions (e.g., retroperitoneal fibrosis and chronic pancreatitis) requires further studies. False-positive results due to inflammation have occurred in other types of lesions evaluated by PET, emphasizing the non-specific nature of FDG.

If more FDG PET studies in patients with pancreatic masses corroborate these encouraging results, FDG PET may obviate further invasive diagnostic procedures in many patients with benign disease and only patients with abnormal FDG activity will need CT-guided biopsies. At present, there is no consensus on the indications for pancreatic cancer.

10.4.7 Prostate

The results with the common prostate cancer are controversial (Table 10.5). FDG PET helped identify osseous and soft tissue metastases of prostate cancer with a high positive predictive value but had a limited sensitivity (65%) compared with that of routine bone scintigraphy (Shreve et al. 1996). Yeh et al. (1996) also found a low sensitivity (20%) for osseous metastases. It is interesting to note that many of the false-negative lesions on whole-body PET staging of breast carcinoma were also located in the bones (Moon et al. 1998). A reason for this could be that the bone marrow metabolism, which is usually high compared with skeletal FDG metabolism, decreases the contrast with an osseous metastasis (Yao et al. 1995). Laubenbacher et al. (1995b) and Effert et al. (1996) also found that the SUV is relatively low in prostate carcinoma. One observation of Effert et al. (1996) was that in a subgroup of four patients with metastases having SUVs in excess of 5, all had rapid progression of disease and did not respond well to subsequent hormone deprivation or radiation therapy. The relatively low FDG uptake by prostate carcinoma may reflect a characteristic of a slow-growing or indolent neoplasm. However, Shreve et al. (1996) found that an abnormal FDG PET scan had a high positive predictive value of 98% for the presence of tumor.

A study with quantification of FDG activity was performed at our own institution (Hoh et al. 1998). Twelve patients with advanced metastatic disease and on suramin therapy were monitored metabolically with PET and anatomically with CT. In the baseline study, there was a high uptake of FDG in the marker lesions. The relationship of the changes in FDG activity during therapy were less clear. Three patients with clinical partial response to suramin (PSA decreased more than 50%, decreased bone pain, and decreased measurable disease greater than 50%), showed a decrease in FDG activity on follow-up PET scans. In four patients with stable clinical disease, three had decreased tumor FDG activity, but in one patient there was an increase in FDG activity of 40%. In another patient with progressive clinical disease, no change in FDG activity or CT lesion size was noted; however, new lesions were detected both by CT and by whole-body PET. The ability to determine the presence, extent, and metabolic activity of metastatic disease may be important in clinical management decisions concerning hormonal therapy or the institution of experimental therapies. In patients with advanced disease, an abnormal FDG PET has a high positive predictive value for presence of tumor.

From these studies, it appears that imaging the primary tumor in the prostate will be technically challenging due to the relatively low FDG uptake in the tumor in the early stages of disease and due to the intense bladder activity which may obscure the detection of a small tumor focus. Lesions with low FDG uptake will also be a diagnostic challenge to differentiate between an indolent but malignant tumor and a benign or inflammatory lesion. Due to the proximity of the bladder and frequent problems with micturition and retention, significant artifacts may result. Not all of these can be overcome easily. Together with the low uptake in this tumor, it may explain the limited utility of PET in this common cancer, both for primary and recurrent disease.

Table 10.5. Prostate cancer

First author	Country	Year	No. of patients	PET sensitivity (%)
Primary tumor				
Yeh	USA	1996	11	20
Effert	Germany	1996	48	19
Metastasis				
Shreve	USA	1996	34	65

10.4.8 Other Genito-Urinary Tumors

Only a few studies have applied FDG PET to renal cell carcinoma (RCC). In the study by Bachor et al. (1996) 29 patients with solid renal masses were scanned prior to surgery. In 20 of 26 patients, FDG PET scans detected the histologically confirmed RCC and failed in six patients to detect the tumor focus. In 3 patients with benign lesions, false-positive results were obtained. In another 3 patients, FDG PET was able to detect regional lymph node metastases suggesting a role for staging of RCC. Bender et al. (1997) had similar results.

To investigate the reason why some patients with RCC had negative FDG PET scans, the group of Wahl (1997a) compared several biological characteristics. They demonstrated that patients with positive PET scans at the primary tumor site had higher tumor grades and higher GLUT-1 expression than patients with negative PET scans. Since GLUT-1 is the key transporter for FDG, with low expression in RCC, most renal cancers are less well seen. The significance of FDG uptake relative to the prognostic outcomes is unknown. Further clinical and outcome oriented studies may reveal the utility of this imaging technology in RCC (Hoh et al. 1998).

In the few studies reported on patients evaluated for recurrent ovarian carcinoma and confirmed by second look laparotomy, PET had a sensitivity over 90%, whereas CT and US had sensitivities ranging from 33 to 85% (Hubner et al. 1993; Casey et al. 1994). The specificity of PET was 80% and CT 50%. There was a good correlation between PET and histological findings so that patient management will benefit from PET by identifying occult foci that are not apparent on morphological imaging studies (Karlan et al. 1993). More studies are needed to support PET in the clinical work-up of ovarian cancer.

The value of PET imaging for testicular cancers is still under investigation (Stephens et al. 1996; Nuutinen et al. 1997; Reinhardt et al. 1997). For initial staging after orchiectomy, PET may have a role in detecting metastases not seen by conventional imaging, although this has not been proven in the studies completed to date. Following chemotherapy, PET may be able to differentiate viable carcinoma from scar tissue but preliminary findings indicate that it cannot differentiate scar tissue from mature teratoma. Positron emission tomography and for that matter any imaging technology will miss microfoci of viable germ cell tumor. Focal areas of abnormal FDG uptake that are detected within extensive residual radiographic abnormalities may allow a more directed and possibly more limited surgical resection, especially in high-risk patients who have had recurrence following previous medical and surgical treatment. Another application of PET is the patient with a rising tumor marker following chemotherapy and/or retro-peritoneal lymph node dissection, but without evidence of residual mass on conventional imaging. The location of abnormal FDG uptake may be helpful in guiding anatomical imaging, surgical exploration, and tumor resection.

In general, both primary seminomas and malignant teratomas have avid FDG uptake, whereas differentiated teratomas and necrotic or fibrotic tissue have normal uptake. Except for Germany, where it has been incorporated in monitoring therapy, there is at present no consensus on the role of PET in testicular cancer.

10.4.9 Lymphoma

The same diagnostic questions as in lung cancer or colorectal cancer pertain to lymphoma: (a) determine the tumor stage at initial presentation; (b) characterize a residual mass post treatment as scar or tumor; and (c) assess if the tumor has shown a complete relapse after therapy. These questions cannot be appropriately addressed with current anatomical imaging methods (Okada et al. 1991, 1992; Leskinen-Kallio et al. 1991). Moreover, gallium scintigraphy is not sensitive enough in low-grade lymphomas, whereas FDG is (Paul 1987). The accuracy of FDG PET imaging in thoracic–abdominal lymphoma compared with that of CT was studied in 11 patients (Newman et al. 1994). All lesions were detected by PET, and five were missed by CT. No difference was found between low- and intermediate-grade lymphomas. In a study from our institution in 18 patients, both CT and PET detected 33 of 37 lesions, although not all lesions were the same (Hoh et al. 1997a). Staging using WBPET was concordant with conventional staging in 14 of 17 patients, better than conventional staging in 3 and worse in 1 patient. For an analysis of cost-effectiveness, the reader is referred to the original article. Moog et al. (1997) studied 60 consecutive patients and found unexpected lesions with PET, leading to restaging in 4 patients. In another study of 24 patients, PET correctly predicted all patients in complete remission after therapy, and there were no false negatives. These investigators concluded that PET performed for evaluation of

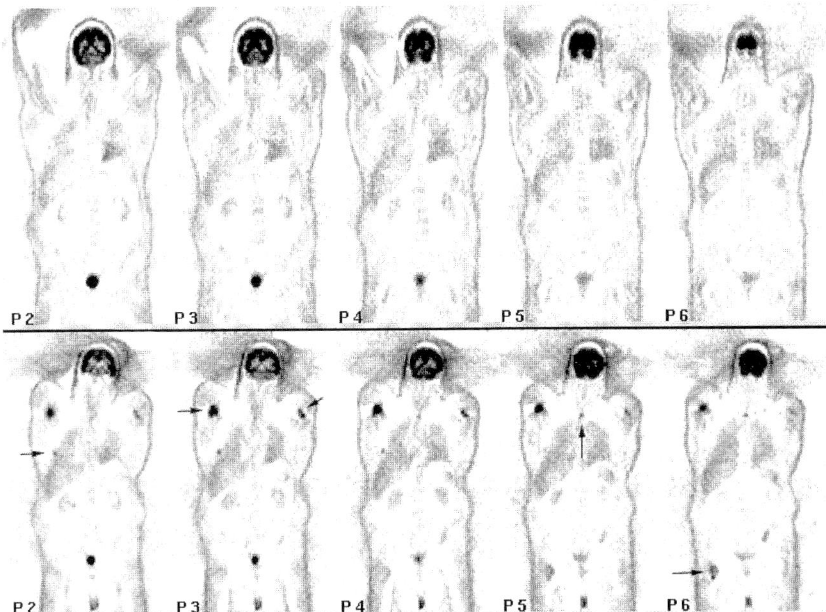

Fig. 10.5. Re-staging of a white male with a history of lymphoma. Contiguous set of five coronal planes (*P2–P6*), slice thickness 1 cm. *Top row* Patient at age 64 years, after chemotherapy and without evidence of metabolically active disease; *bottom row* 2 years later, at age 66 years with abnormal uptake in both shoulders, right more pronounced than left (*arrows* P3). Two small lesions are seen in the thorax, right lateral aspect (*arrow* P2) and in the midline (*arrow* P5). Another area of hyper-metabolism was seen in the right proximal femur (*arrow* P6). Biopsy was performed of the right proximal humerus and right femoral head, and both had involvement with lymphoma (ECAT 961 PET system)

residual mass after treatment of lymphoma has a high predictive value (De Wit et al. 1997). In Fig. 10.5 an example is shown of re-staging after therapy, and the follow-up 2 years later.

It is expected that WBPET will have a significant impact on staging of lymphoma, since biopsy of all lesions is impossible and characterization of abnormalities has shown to be cost-effective in the few studies reported.

10.4.10 Melanoma

In two small studies for staging of metastatic melanoma, PET imaging had an overall accuracy of 100%, detecting all metastatic lesions (intra-abdominal, visceral, and lymph nodes) and correctly predicting all negative lymph node regions (Gritters et al. 1993; Wagner et al. 1997). In a study of 33 patients, Steinert et al. (1995) found a sensitivity of 92%. With blinded reading the specificity was 77%, which could be increased to 100% when clinical information was provided. In a large Australian study of 100 patients, the sensitivity was 93% for detection of metastatic lesions (Damian et al. 1996). Small metastatic foci were seen only on follow-up CT several months later. The sensitivity of the PET technique for detecting small pulmonary lesions was lower than CT, attributed to respiratory motion or prior cancer therapy.

From the studies available, it appears that PET is a sensitive and highly specific test for detecting lymph node metastasis in melanoma. For very small tumor lesions (<5 mm), PET is not as sensitive as CT. Therefore, an algorithm can be proposed for melanoma similar to that of lung and colorectal cancer, in which PET is performed to assess surgical resectability. The clinical indication for a PET study will be exclusion of distant unexpected metastases in a surgically fit patient who has CT evidence of potentially resectable disease.

10.5 Conclusion

The unique imaging capabilities of PET enable physicians to diagnose a disease process in the body and to observe the effect of treatment from a different perspective. The current applications of PET in oncological diagnosis have been in characterizing lesions, differentiating recurrent disease from treatment effects, and staging of cancer. The future developments in medicine may utilize PET not only in diagnostic imaging but also in basic drug development, and in monitoring or evaluating the eligibility of patients for new therapy protocols.

The goal in any staging method is to detect small tumor foci with the highest sensitivity and specificity. Excellent results are obtained for instance with MR of the brain, CT of the neck or liver, and mammography, but the anatomical modalities generally lack specificity. The limiting factor for PET sensitivity will be its resolution, whereas the strength of PET will be in the development of even more specific radiopharmaceuticals for tumor imaging. An inherent difficulty in analyzing and comparing various imaging modalities is that, for ethical reasons, the identified lesions cannot always be confirmed histologically. Therefore other, clinically oriented gold standards will have to be developed to assess the utility of clinical PET in oncology. These include rigorous follow-up of patients to measure progression of disease, disease-free survival, and prognosis. Perhaps the true gold standard may lead to an improved categorization of patients into their correct stages, which is later reflected in an improved patient outcome. The FDG PET technique appears indicated for the evaluation of solitary pulmonary nodules, initial staging of lung cancer, evaluation of recurrence for brain, head, and neck, and colorectal cancer. The FDG PET technique appears very promising for staging and treatment evaluation of melanoma and lymphoma. Its role in staging of breast and ovarian cancer is not clear yet.

The role of clinical imaging a decade from now may be quite different due to the tremendous advances in molecular medicine and genetics. The planning of future cancer therapies may require in vivo tissue specific information which can only be attained through molecular imaging with PET. On the other hand, if there is no effective therapy for a given disease, an imaging procedure which accurately detects that disease process may not be relevant in clinical practice. Scientifically, however, this imaging procedure may play an important role in contributing to the understanding of that disease and assisting in the development of new therapies. In the current and future health care environment, the proper combination of imaging technologies in a well-defined algorithm will provide the most accurate diagnostic information. This, in turn, will achieve the most appropriate clinical management and best patient outcome.

References

Abdel-Nabi H, Doehr RJ, Lamonica M et al. (1998) Staging of primary colorectal carcinomas with Fluorine-18 fluoro-deoxy-glucose Whole body PET:correlation with histo-pathologic and CT findings. Radiology 206:755–760

Adler LP, Bloom AD (1993) Positron emission tomography of thyroid masses. Thyroid 3:195–200

Adler LP, Crowe JP, al-Kaisi NK, Sunshine JL (1993) Evaluation of breast masses and axillary lymph nodes with [18F] 2-deoxy-2-fluoro-D-glucose PET. Radiology 187:743–750

Adler LP, Faulhaber PF, Schnur KC, Al-Kasi NL, Shenk RR (1997) Axillary lymph node metastases: screening with 18F-FDG PET. Radiology 203:323–327

Alavi JB, Alavi A, Chawluk et al. (1988) PET in patients with glioma. Cancer 62:1074–1078

Anzai Y, Carroll WR, Quint DJ, Bradford CR, Minoshima S, Wolf GT, Wahl RL (1996) Recurrence of head and neck cancer after surgery or irradiation: prospective comparison of 2-deoxy-2-[18F]fluoro-D-glucose PET and MR imaging diagnoses. Radiology 200:135–141

Avril N, Dose J, Janicke F et al. (1996) Metabolic characterization of breast tumors with positron emission tomography using F-18 fluorodeoxyglucose. J Clin Oncol 14:1848–1857

Bachor R, Kotzerke J, Gottfried HW et al. (1996) Positron emission tomography in diagnosis of renal cell carcinoma. Urology 35:146–150

Bailet JW, Abemayor E, Jabour BA et al. (1992) Positron emission tomography: a new precise imaging modality for detection of primary head and neck tumors and assessment of cervical adenopathy. Laryngoscope 102:281–288

Bares R, Klever P, Hauptmann S, Hellwig D, Fass J, Cremerius U, Schumpelick V, Mittermayer C, Bull U (1994) F-18 fluorodeoxyglucose PET in vivo evaluation of pancreatic glucose metabolism for detection of pancreatic cancer. Radiology 192:79–86

Beets G, Penninckx F, Schiepers C, Filez L, Mortelmans L, Kerremans R, Aerts R, De Roo M (1994) Clinical value of whole-body positron emission tomography with [18F]fluorodeoxyglucose in recurrent colorectal cancer. Br J Surg 81:1666–1670

Benchaou M, Lehmann W, Slosman DO et al. (1996) The role of FDG-PET in the preoperative assessment of N-staging in head and neck cancer. Acta Otolaryngol 116:332–335

Bender H, Schomburg A, Albers P, Ruhlmann J, Biersack HJ (1997) Possible role of FDG-PET in the evaluation of urologic malignancies. Anticancer Res 17:1655–1660

Bengel FM, Ziegler SI, Avril N et al. (1997) Whole body PET in clinical oncology: comparison between attenuation corrected and uncorrected images. Eur J Nucl Med 24:1091–1098

Bloom AD, Adler LP, Shuck JM (1993) Determination of malignancy of thyroid nodules with positron emission tomography. Surgery 114:728–734

Bombardieri E, Crippa F, Maffioli L, Greco M (1997) Nuclear medicine techniques for the study of breast cancer. Eur J Nucl Med 24:809–824

Braams JW, Pruim J, Kole AC et al. (1997) Detection of unknown primary head and neck tumors by positron emission tomography. Int J Oral Maxillofac Surg 26:112–115

Brock CS, Meikle SR, Price P (1997) Does F-18 fluorodeoxyglucose metabolic imaging of tumours benefit oncology? Eur J Nucl Med 24:691–705

Brown RS, Wahl RL (1993) Overexpression of Glut-1 glucose transporter in human breast cancer. An immunohistochemical study. Cancer 72:2979–2985

Bury T, Dowlati A, Paulus P et al. (1996) Staging of non-small-cell lung cancer by whole-body fluorine-18 deoxyglucose positron emission tomography. Eur J Nucl Med 23:204–206

Casey MJ, Gupta NC, Muths CK (1994) Experience with positron emission tomography (PET) scans in patients with ovarian cancer. Gynecol Oncol 53:331–338

Chin R Jr, Ward R, Keyes JW, Choplin RH, Reed JC, Wallenhaupt S, Hudspeth AS, Haponik EF (1995) Mediastinal staging of non-small-cell lung cancer with positron emission tomography. Am J Respir Crit Care Med 152:2090–2096

Conti PS, Lilien DL, Hawley K, Keppler J, Grafton ST, Bading JR (1996) PET and [18F]-FDG in oncology: a clinical update. Nucl Med Biol 23:717–735

Crippa F, Agresti R, Seregni E et al. (1998) Prospective evaluation of fluorine-18-FDG PET in presurgical staging of the axilla in breast cancer. J Nucl Med 39:4–8

Cummings SR, Lillington GA, Richard RJ (1986) Estimating the probability of malignancy in solitary pulmonary nodules. A Bayesian approach. Am Rev Respir Dis 134:449–452

Dahlbom M, Hoffman EJ, Hoh CK, Schiepers C, Rosenqvist G, Hawkins RA, Phelps ME (1992) Whole-body positron emission tomography. Part I. Methods and performance characteristics. J Nucl Med 33:1191–1199

Dales RE, Stark RM, Raman S (1990) Computed tomography to stage lung cancer: approaching a controversy using meta-analysis. Am Rev Respir Dis 141:1096–1101

Damian DL, Fulham MJ, Thompson E, Thompson JF (1996) Positron emission tomography in the detection and management of metastatic melanoma. Melanoma Res 6:325–329

De Wit M, Bumann D, Beyer W, Herbst K, Clausen M, Hossfeld DK (1997) Whole-body positron emission tomography (PET) for diagnosis of residual mass in patients with lymphoma. Ann Oncol 8:57–60

Delbeke D, Meyerowitz C, Lapidus R et al. (1995) Optimal cut-off levels for 18F-FDG uptake in the differentiation of low-grade from high-grade brain tumors with PET. Radiology 195:47–52

Delbeke D, Vitola J, Sandler MP et al. (1997) Staging recurrent metastatic colorectal carcinoma with PET. J Nucl Med 38:1196–1201

Dewan NA, Gupta NC, Redepenning LS, Phalen JJ, Frick MP (1993) Diagnostic efficacy of PET-FDG imaging in solitary pulmonary nodules. Potential role in evaluation and management. Chest 104:997–1002

Dewan NA, Reeb SD, Gupta NC, Gobar LS, Scott WJ (1995) PET-FDG imaging and transthoracic needle lung aspiration biopsy in evaluation of pulmonary lesions. A comparative risk-benefit analysis. Chest 108:441–446

di Chiro G (1987) Positron emission tomography using [18F]fluorodeoxyglucose in brain tumors: a powerful diagnostic and prognostic tool. Invest Radiol 22:360–371

di Chiro G, de la Paz RL, Brooks RA et al. (1982) Glucose utilization of cerebral gliomas measured by 18F-fluorodeoxyglucose and PET. Neurology 32:1323–1329

di Chiro G, Hatazawa J, Katz DA, Rizzoli HV, De Michele DJ (1987) Glucose utilization by intracranial meningiomas as an index of tumor aggressivity and probability of recurrence: a PET study. Radiology 164:521–526

di Chiro G, Oldfield E, Wright DC et al. (1988) Cerebral necrosis after radiotherapy and/or intra-arterial chemotherapy for brain tumors: PET and neuropathologic studies. AJR 150:189–197

Dillemans B, Deneffe G, Verschakelen J, Decramer M (1994) Value of computed tomography and mediastinoscopy in preoperative evaluation of mediastinal nodes in non-small cell lung cancer. Eur J Cardiothorac Surg 8:37–42

Doyle WK, Budinger TF, Valk PE et al. (1987) Differentiation of cerebral radiation necrosis from tumor recurrence by 18F-FDG and 82Rb PET. J Comput Assist Tomogr 11:563–570

Effert PJ, Bares R, Handt S et al. (1996) Metabolic imaging of untreated prostate cancer by positron emission tomography with [18F]fluorine-labeled deoxy-glucose. J Urol 155:994–998

Feine U, Lietzenmayer R, Hanke JP et al. (1996) Fluorine-18-FDG and iodine-131-iodide uptake in thyroid cancer. J Nucl Med 37:1468–1472

Frank A, Lefkowitz D, Jaeger S et al. (1995) Decision logic for retreatment of asymptomatic lung cancer recurrence based on positron emission tomography findings. Int J Radiat Oncol Biol Phys 32:1495–1512

Gambhir SS, Hoh CK, Phelps ME, Madar I, Maddahi J (1996) Decision tree sensitivity analysis for cost effectiveness of FDG-PET in the staging and management of non-small-cell lung carcinoma. J Nucl Med 37:1428–1436

Gritters LS, Francis IR, Zasadny KR, Wahl RL (1993) Initial assessment of positron emission tomography using 2-fluorine-18-fluoro-2-deoxy-D-glucose in the imaging of malignant melanoma. J Nucl Med 34:1420–1427

Grunwald F, Menzel C, Bender H et al. (1997) Comparison of 18FDG-PET with 131iodine and 99mTc-sestamibi scintigraphy in differentiated thyroid cancer. Thyroid 7:327–335

Guhlmann A, Storck M, Kotzerke J et al. (1997) Lymph node staging in non-small cell lung cancer: evaluation by [18F]FDG positron emission tomography (PET). Thorax 52:438–441

Gupta NC, Maloof J, Gunel E (1996) Probability of malignancy in solitary pulmonary nodules using fluorine-18-FDG and PET. J Nucl Med 37:943–948

Haberkorn U, Strauss LG, Dimitrakopoulou A et al. (1991a) PET studies of fluorodeoxyglucose metabolism in patients with recurrent colorectal tumors receiving radiotherapy. J Nucl Med 32:1485–1490

Haberkorn U, Strauss LG, Reisser C et al. (1991b) Glucose uptake, perfusion, and cell proliferation in head and neck tumors: relation of positron emission tomography to flow cytometry. J Nucl Med 32:1548–1555

Haberkorn U, Strauss LG, Dimitrakopoulou A et al. (1993) Fluorodeoxyglucose imaging of advanced head and neck cancer after chemotherapy. J Nucl Med 34:12–17

Hamberg LM, Hunter GJ, Alpert NM et al. (1994) The dose uptake ratio as an index of glucose metabolism: useful parameter or oversimplification? J Nucl Med 35:1308–1312

Higashi K, Clavo AC, Wahl RL (1993a) Does FDG uptake measure proliferative rate of human cancer cells? In vitro comparison with DNA flow cytometry and tritiated thymidine uptake. J Nucl Med 34:414–419

Higashi K, Clavo AC, Wahl RL (1993b) In vitro assessment of 2-fluoro-2-deoxy-D-glucose, L-methionine and thymidine as agents to monitor the early response of a human adenocarcinoma cell line to radiotherapy. J Nucl Med 34:773–779

Ho CL, Dehdashti F, Griffeth LK, Buse PE, Balfe DM, Siegel BA (1996) FDG-PET evaluation of indeterminate pancreatic masses. J Comput Assist Tomogr 20:363–369

Hoh CK, Schiepers C (1999) ^{18}FDG imaging in breast cancer. Semin Nucl Med 29:49–56

Hoh CK, Hawkins RA, Glaspy JA et al. (1993) Cancer detection with whole-body PET using 2-[18F]fluoro-2-deoxy-D-glucose. J Comput Assist Tomogr 17:582–589

Hoh CK, Glaspy J, Rosen PJ et al. (1997a) Whole body FDG PET imaging for staging of Hodgkin's disease and lymphoma. J Nucl Med 38:343–348

Hoh CK, Schiepers C, Seltzer MA et al. (1997b) PET in oncology: Will it replace the other modalities? Semin Nucl Med 27:94–106

Hoh CK, Seltzer MA, Franklin J et al. (1998) Positron emission tomography (PET) in urologic oncology. J Urol 159:347–356

Hubner KF, McDonald TW, Niethammer JG et al. (1993) Assessment of primary and metastatic ovarian cancer by positron emission tomography (PET) using 2-[18F]deoxyglucose (2-[18F]FDG). Gynecol Oncol 51:197–204

Husband JES (1995) Imaging of treated cancer. Br J Radiol 68:1–12

Husband JE (1996) Monitoring tumour response. Eur Radiol 6:775–785

Inokuma T, Tamaki N, Torizuka T, Magata Y, Fujii M, Yonekura Y, Kajiyama T, Ohshio G, Imamura M, Konishi J (1995) Evaluation of pancreatic tumors with positron emission tomography and F-18 fluorodeoxyglucose: comparison with CT and US. Radiology 195:345–352

Jabour BA, Choi Y, Hoh CK et al. (1993) Extracranial head and neck: PET imaging with 2-[18F]fluoro-2-deoxy-D-glucose and MR imaging correlation. Radiology 186:27–35

Karlan BY, Hawkins R, Hoh C et al. (1993) Whole-body positron emission tomography with 2-[18F]fluoro-2-deoxy-D-glucose can detect recurrent ovarian carcinoma. Gynecol Oncol 51:175–181

Keogan MT, Tung KT, Kaplan DK et al. (1993) The significance of pulmonary nodules detected on CT staging for lung cancer. Clin Radiol 48:94–96

Keogan MT, Lowe VJ, Baker ME, McDermott VG, Lyerly HK, Coleman RE (1997) Local recurrence of rectal cancer: evaluation with F-18 fluorodeoxyglucose PET imaging. Abdom Imaging 22:332–337

Keys JW (1995) SUV: standard uptake or silly useless value? J Nucl Med 36:1836–1839

Kim CK, Gupta NC, Chandramouli B, Alvi A (1994) Standardized uptake values of FDG: body surface area correction is preferable to body weight correction. J Nucl Med 35:164–167

Knight SB, Delbeke D, Stewart JR, Sandler MP (1996) Evaluation of pulmonary lesions with FDG-PET. Comparison of findings in patients with and without a history of prior malignancy. Chest 109:982–988

Kubota K, Ishiwata K, Kubota R et al. (1991) Tracer feasibility for monitoring tumor radiotherapy: a quadruple tracer study with 18F-fluoro-deoxy-glucose or 18F-fluoro-deoxyuridine, L-methyl-[14 C]-methionine, 6-[3H]-thymidine and gallium-67. J Nucl Med 32:2118–2123

Kubota K, Yamada S, Kubota R et al. (1992) Intratumoral distribution of 18F-fluoro-deoxy-glucose in vivo:high accumulation in macrophages and granulation tissues studied by micro-autoradiography. J Nucl Med 33:1972–1980

Kubota K, Kubota R, Yamada Y (1993) FDG accumulation in tumor tissue (editorial). J Nucl Med 34:419–421

Kunstaetter R, Wolkove N, Kreisman H, Cohen C, Frank H (1985) The solitary pulmonary nodule. Decision analysis. Med Decision Making 5:61–75

Laubenbacher C, Saumweber D, Wagner-Manslau C et al. (1995a) Comparison of fluorine-18-fluorodeoxyglucose PET, MRI and endoscopy for staging head and neck squamous-cell carcinomas. J Nucl Med 36:1747–1757

Laubenbacher C, Hofer C, Avril N, Block T, Ziegler S, Herz M, Kruschke C, Hartung R, Schwaiger M (1995b) F-18 FDG PET for differentiation of local recurrent prostate cancer and scar. J Nucl Med 36:198P

Lai DT, Fulham M, Stephen MS, Chu KM, Solomon M, Thompson JF, Sheldon DM, Storey DW (1996) The role of whole-body positron emission tomography with [18F]fluorodeoxyglucose in identifying operable colorectal cancer metastases to the liver. Arch Surg 131:703–707

Larcos G, Maisey MN (1996) FDG-PET screening for cerebral metastases in patients with suspected malignancy. Nucl Med Commun 17:197–198

Leskinen-Kallio S, Ruotsalainen U, Nagren K et al. (1991) Uptake of carbon-11-methionine and fluorodeoxyglucose in non-Hodgkin's lymphoma: a PET study. J Nucl Med 32:1211–1218

Lindholm P, Leskinen-Kallio S, Minn H et al. (1993) Comparison of fluorine-18-fluorodeoxyglucose and carbon-11-methionine in head and neck cancer. J Nucl Med 34:1711–1716

Lowe VJ, Duhaylongsod FG, Patz EF et al. (1997) Pulmonary abnormalities and PET data analysis: a retrospective study. Radiology 202:435–439

McLoud TC, Bourgouin PM, Greenberg RW et al. (1992) Bronchogenic carcinoma: analysis of staging in the mediastinum with CT by correlative lymph node mapping and sampling. Radiology 182:319–323

Minn H, Zasadny KR, Quint LE, Wahl RL (1995) Lung cancer: reproducibility of quantitative measurements for evaluating 2-[F-18]-fluoro-2-deoxy-D-glucose uptake at PET. Radiology 196:167–173

Moog F, Bangerter M, Diederichs CG et al. (1997) Lymphoma: role of whole-body FDG-PET in nodal staging. Radiology 203:795–800

Moon DH, Hoh CK, Silverman DS et al. (1998) Accuracy of whole body FDG PET for the detection of recurrent or metastatic breast carcinoma. J Nucl Med 39:431–435

Newman JS, Francis IR, Kaminski MS, Wahl RL (1994) Imaging of lymphoma with PET with 2-[18F]fluoro-2-deoxy-D-glucose: correlation with CT. Radiology 190:111–116

Nieweg OE, Kim EE, Wong WH et al. (1993) Positron emission tomography with fluorine-18-deoxy-glucose in the detection and staging of breast cancer. Cancer 71:3920–3925

Nuutinen JM, Leskinen S, Elomaa I, Minn H et al. (1997) Detection of residual tumours in postchemotherapy testicular cancer by FDG-PET. Eur J Cancer 33:1234–1241

Ogunbiyi OA, Flanagan FL, Dehdashti F et al. (1997) Detection of recurrent and metastatic colorectal cancer: comparison of positron emission tomography and computed tomography. Ann Surg Oncol 48:613–620

Okada J, Yoshikawa K, Imazeki K et al. (1991) The use of FDG-PET in the detection and management of malignant lymphoma: correlation of uptake with prognosis. J Nucl Med 32:686–691

Okada J, Yoshikawa K, Itami M et al. (1992) Positron emission tomography using fluorine-18-fluorodeoxyglucose in malignant lymphoma: a comparison with proliferative activity. J Nucl Med 33:325–329

Palmedo H, Bender H, Grunwald F et al. (1997) Comparison of fluorine-18 FDG PET and technetium-99 m MIBI scintimammography in the detection of breast tumours. Eur J Nucl Med 24:1138–1145

Paul R (1987) Comparison of fluorine-18-2 fluorodeoxyglucose and gallium 67 citrate imaging for detection of lymphoma. J Nucl Med 28:288–292

Phelps ME, Mazziotta JC, Schelbert HR (eds) (1986) Positron emission tomography and autoradiography: principal applications for the brain and the heart. Raven, New York

Pirotte B, Goldman S, Bidaut LM et al. (1995) Use of PET in stereotactic conditions for brain biopsy. Acta Neurochir (Wien) 134:79–82

Price P (1997) Is there a future for PET in oncology? Eur J Nucl Med 24:587–589

Rege SD, Chaiken L, Hoh CK et al. (1993a) Change induced by radiation therapy in FDG uptake in normal and malignant structures of the head and neck: quantitation with PET. Radiology 189:807–812

Rege SD, Hoh CK, Glaspy JA et al. (1993b) Imaging of pulmonary mass lesions with whole-body positron emission tomography and fluorodeoxyglucose. Cancer 72:82–90

Reinhardt MJ, Muller-Mattheis VG, Gerharz CD et al. (1997) FDG-PET evaluation of retroperitoneal metastases of testicular cancer before and after chemotherapy. J Nucl Med 38:99–101

Reisser C, Haberkorn U, Strauss LG (1993) The relevance of positron emission tomography for the diagnosis and treatment of head and neck tumors. J Otolaryngol 22:231–238

Reske SN, Grillenberger KG, Glatting G et al. (1997) Overexpression of glucose transporter 1 and increased FDG uptake in pancreatic carcinoma. J Nucl Med 38:1344–1348

Rigo P, Paulus P, Kaschten BJ et al. (1996) Oncological applications of positron emission tomography with fluorine-18 fluorodeoxyglucose. Eur J Nucl Med 23:1641–1674

Ruhlmann J, Schomburg A, Bender H et al. (1997) Fluorodeoxyglucose whole-body positron emission tomography in colorectal cancer patients studied in routine daily practice. Dis Colon Rectum z:1195–2004

Sasaki M, Ichiya Y, Kuwabara Y, Akashi Y, Yoshida T, Fukumura T, Murayama S, Ishida T, Sugio K, Masuda K (1996) The usefulness of FDG positron emission tomography for the detection of mediastinal lymph node metastases in patients with non-small cell lung cancer: a comparative study with X-ray computed tomography. Eur J Nucl Med 23:741–747

Scheidhauer K, Scharl A, Pietrzyk U et al. (1996) Qualitative [18F]FDG positron emission tomography in primary breast cancer: clinical relevance and practicability. Eur J Nucl Med 23:618–623

Schiepers C (1997) Role of positron emission tomography in the staging of lung cancer. Lung Cancer 17:S29–S35

Schiepers C, Penninckx F, De Vadder N et al. (1995) Contribution of PET in the diagnosis of recurrent colorectal cancer: comparison with conventional imaging. Eur J Surg Oncol 21:517–522

Scott WJ, Schwabe JL, Gupta NC et al. (1994) PET of lung tumors and mediastinal lymph nodes using FDG. Ann Thorac Surg 58:698–703

Shreve PD, Grossman HB, Gross MD, Wahl RL (1996) Metastatic prostate cancer: initial findings of PET with 2-deoxy-2-[18F]fluoro-D-glucose. Radiology 199:751–756

Sisson JC, Ackermann RJ, Meyer MA, Wahl RL (1993) Uptake of 18-fluoro-2-deoxy-D-glucose by thyroid cancer: implications for diagnosis and therapy. J Clin Endocrinol Metab 77:1090–1094

Smith IC, Ogston KN, Whitford P et al. (1998) Staging of the axilla in breast cancer: accurate in vivo assessment using positron emission tomography with 2-fluorine-18-fluoro-2-deoxy-D-glucose.Ann Surg 228:220–227

Steinert HC, Huch Boni RA, Buck A et al. (1995) Malignant melanoma: staging with whole-body PET and FDG. Radiology 195:705–709

Steinert HC, Hauser M, Allemann F et al. (1997) Non-small cell lung cancer: nodal staging with FDG PET versus CT with correlative lymph node mapping and sampling. Radiology 202:441–446

Stephens AW, Gonin R, Hutchins GD, Einhorn LH (1996) Positron emission tomography evaluation of residual radiographic abnormalities in postchemotherapy germ cell tumor patients. J Clin Oncol 14:1637–1641

Stollfuss JC, Glatting G, Friess H, Kocher F, Berger HG, Reske SN (1995) 2-(fluorine-18)-fluoro-2-deoxy-D-glucose PET in detection of pancreatic cancer: value of quantitative image interpretation. Radiology 195:339–344

Strauss LG, Clorius JH, Schlag P et al. (1989) Recurrence of colorectal tumors: PET evaluation. Radiology 170:329–323

Utech CI, Young CS, Winter PF (1996) Prospective evaluation of fluorine-18 fluorodeoxyglucose positron emission tomography in breast cancer for staging of the axilla related to surgery and immunocytochemistry. Eur J Nucl Med 23:1588–1593

Valk PE (1996) Sense and sensitivity: issues in technology assessment (editorial). J Nucl Med 37:1436–1437

Valk PE, Pounds TR, Hopkins DM et al. (1995) Staging lung cancer by PET imaging. Ann Thorac Surg 60:1573–1581

Valk PE, Pounds TR, Tesar RD, Hopkins DM, Haseman MK (1996) Cost-effectiveness of PET imaging in clinical oncology. Nucl Med Biol 23:737–743

Vansteenkiste JF, Stroobants SG, De Leyn PR et al. (1998) Lymph node staging in non-small-cell lung cancer with FDG-PET scan: a prospective study on 690 lymph node stations from 68 patients. J Clin Oncol 16:2142–2149

Wagner JD, Schauwecker D, Hutchins G, Coleman JJ III (1997) Initial assessment of positron emission tomography for detection of non palpable regional lymphatic metastases in melanoma. J Surg Oncol 64:181–189

Wahl RL, Cody RL, Hutchins G, Mudgett E (1991) Positron emission tomographic scanning of primary and metastatic breast with the radiolabeled glucose analogue 2-deoxy-2[18F]fluoro-D-glucose (letter). N Engl J Med 324:200

Wahl RL (1997a) Clinical oncology update: the emerging role of PET. Part I. Update to: DeVita, Hellman, Rosenberg (eds) Cancer: principles and practice of oncology, vol 11(1). Lippincott-Raven, Philadelphia, pp 1–18

Wahl RL (1997b) Clinical oncology update: the emerging role of PET. Part II. Update to: DeVita, Hellman, Rosenberg (eds) Cancer: principles and practice of oncology, vol 11(2). Lippincott-Raven, Philadelphia, pp 1–24

Warburg O (1931) The metabolism of tumors. Smith, New York, pp 129–169

Warburg O (1956) On the origins of cancer cells. Science 123:309–314

Webb WR, Gatsonis C, Zeerhouni EA et al. (1991) CT and MR imaging in staging non-small cell bronchogenic carcinoma: report of the Radiological Diagnostic Oncology Group. Radiology178:705–713

Wong WL, Chevretton EB, McGurk M et al. (1997) A prospective study of PET-FDG imaging for the assessment of head and neck squamous cell carcinoma. Clin Otolaryngol 22:209–214

Yao WJ, Hoh CK, Hawkins RA et al. (1995) Quantitative PET imaging of bone marrow glucose metabolic response to hematopoietic cytokines. J Nucl Med 36:794–799

Yeh SD, Imbriaco M, Larson SM et al. (1996) Detection of bony metastases of androgen-independent prostate cancer by PET-FDG. Nucl Med Biol 23:693–697

Zasadny KR, Wahl RL (1993) Standardized uptake values of normal tissues at PET with 2-[18F]-fluoro-2-deoxy-D-glucose: variations with body weight and a method for correction. Radiology 189:847–850

11 Pediatric Nuclear Medicine: A Coming of Age

H. R. Nadel, M. E. Stilwell

Contents

11.1 General 177
11.1.1 Patient Preparation 177
11.1.2 Radiation Safety Considerations 177
11.2 *Helicobacter pylori* Infection in Children 178
11.2.1 Diagnostic Tests 180
11.3 Imaging of Inflammatory Bowel Disease 181
11.4 Pediatric Neuronuclear Medicine 183
11.4.1 Scintigraphy in Brain Development 184
11.4.2 Language and Cognition 186
11.4.3 Brain Trauma and Brain Death 187
11.5 Primary Neuro-Psychological Disorders in Childhood 188
11.5.1 Attention Deficit Hyperactivity Disorder 189
11.5.2 Mood Disorders: Depression and Obsessive–Compulsive Disorder 189
11.5.3 Tourette Syndrome 189
11.5.4 Autism 190

11.1 General

Nuclear medicine studies contribute an integral part to the investigation of many disease processes in children. The standard studies of bone, renal, and tumor imaging with scintigraphy are still the backbone of any pediatric nuclear medicine department. Over the past decade we have seen the introduction and increased use of newer scintigraphic approaches in children. This chapter focuses on the use of scintigraphy in children for the assessment of *Helicobacter pylori* infection and inflammatory bowel disease and psychosocial, developmental, and traumatic brain disorders in children.

A discussion of pediatric scintigraphic techniques would not be complete without mention of technical factors required due to the unique needs of imaging pediatric patients who range in age from birth to adulthood. Advances in radiopharmaceutical and instrumentation technology allow greater investigation of physiology as well as anatomy in this diverse group of patients.

11.1.1 Patient Preparation

It is routine in many departments to allow parents and/or siblings to remain in the imaging room to provide a sense of security and safety for the child. The presence of a favorite toy or a prized possession brought with them for the test can also be reassuring. Immobilization needs, which can be an important factor in producing high-quality studies in children, can be broken down by age. For neonates to age 2 years, bundling in a papoose-type holder, sleep deprivation, and feeding the child while on the imaging table are effective immobilization strategies. Videos, music, stories, or distraction techniques, such as bubble blowing, thus ensuring their cooperation, entertain children aged 4–5 years. It is also helpful to have dedicated pediatric nuclear medicine technologists who are secure in their dealings with the various age groups. A simple explanation of the involved procedure tailored to the age of the child will go a long way to gain a child's cooperation; however, some children still require sedation or general anesthesia. In particular, those children who are mentally retarded or have severe attention deficit problems, and often children between the ages of 2 and 4 years, fall into this category. If sedation is necessary, appropriate triage, monitoring, and discharge of the patient are now the standard of care (Weiss 1993; Pintelon et al. 1994). The use of a local anesthetic cream at an intravenous access site is also routine in many laboratories (Sherazi and Gordon 1996; Ljung 1997).

11.1.2 Radiation Safety Considerations

The use of ionizing radiation in the pediatric population is an ongoing issue frequently cited in the pedi-

H. R. Nadel, M. E. Stilwell
Department of Nuclear Medicine, B.C. Children's Hospital, 4480 Oak Street, Vancouver, B.C. V6H 3V4, Canada

atric radiology literature and bears examination by all practitioners. ROEBUCK (1999) examines and re-examines a variety of related issues. He points out rightly that part of the job of the radiologist and/or nuclear medicine physician is to help ensure that the appropriate investigation is performed, and that use of radiation is justifiable. Knowledge of the approximate risk, and more importantly the ability to effectively communicate these to the referring physician and parent, is essential. Nuclear physicians and radiologists alike should be aware of new applications of nuclear medicine tests but remain skeptical (ROEBUCK 1999; BERDON 1999; HALL 1999). Discussions regarding the risks of radiation and what exactly they consist of are frequently misunderstood and misquoted even by the physicians using them. In a letter to the *Lancet*, DIXON and DENDY (1998) posed three valuable questions to be considered before performing a CT scan on a child. These questions can be rephrased for nuclear medicine tests: Can the same or better information be obtained by a method with a lower dose of radiation? Is the utilized technology functioning properly? Is the protocol optimized for the patient? STABIN and GELFAND (1998) have published tables for evaluating absorbed radiation doses for many pediatric nuclear medicine procedures. They used standard MIRD methodology and express absorbed dosimetry in mGy or rad for a body weight adjusted administered activity for each radiopharmaceutical.

11.2 Helicobacter pylori Infection in Children

The battle cry of pediatric medicine is that "children are not just small adults who suffer from small versions of adult diseases." Whereas this is true mainly in pediatric gastrointestinal disease, many entities that we commonly see in adults are seen in children and need to be considered when appropriate. One such entity is *Helicobacter pylori* (*H. pylori*) infection. *H. pylori* infection is endemic worldwide as an asymptomatic infection (NARLA et al. 1999). The recent discovery and growing interest in this gram-negative bacterium as a gut pathogen has had and continues to have significant impact on the management of several gastrointestinal disorders. Peptic ulcer disease and gastritis have been closely linked to *H. pylori* infection, and this infection is implicated in a substantial percentage of cases of acute gastrointestinal bleeding. *H. pylori* has been classified as a type-I carcinogen by the World Health Organization (NARLA et al. 1999). In addition, it has been impugned as a co-factor in other gastrointestinal diseases such as chronic diarrhea, protein-losing enteropathy, and gastric lymphoproliferative disease. CORRADO et al. (1998) studied 90 patients and found a positive association between *H. pylori* infection and food allergy.

H. pylori appears to be acquired early in life with cross-sectional studies suggesting that infection is usually acquired before the age of 5 years, although the time, rate, and modus of colonization are not definitely defined (BUJANOVER et al. 1996). Maternal passive transfer of immunity via IgG antibodies appears to protect infants until approximately 6 months of age when infection of children with *H. pylori* is common in both developed and developing countries (GOLD et al. 1997). There is correlation with socioeconomic and hygiene conditions such as overcrowding and lack of clean running water (DUGGAN et al. 1998; VANDENPLAS and BLECKER 1998). The role of parental infection is not fully understood but is thought to play a role in transmission particularly in infected mothers of young children (ROTHENBACHER et al. 1999). *H. pylori* infection in children is thought to be affected by both the rate of acquisition and loss in different groups based on ethnicity. A study by MALATY et al. (1999) followed 212 children in a biracial community over 12 years from childhood to young adulthood and showed different rates for both acquisition and loss of infection in groups of black children compared with groups of white children. To illustrate, at 7–9 years of age, 19% of children in their population had *H. pylori* infection (40% of black children and 11% of white children). Twelve years later, 22% of the children were positive with the higher prevalence again noted to be present in the black children. GRANSTRÖM et al. (1997) studied a cohort of Swedish children from ages 6 months to 11 years of age measuring both IgG and IgA antibodies to *H. pylori*. They identified that 13.6% (40 of 294) of their children were infected at some time during the study. They noted that at 11 years of age only 3% of the children were seropositive suggesting that spontaneous resolution is common. In a study done in Germany, HORNEMANN et al. (1997) could not find evidence of *H. pylori* infection in infants less than 4 years of age. After age 4 years, the seropositivity increased linearly with age.

H. pylori infection is a well-recognized cause of antral gastritis and a significant factor in peptic ulcer disease in the adult population. In children, peptic ulcer disease does occur, albeit less commonly (STRINGER 1989; HASSALL 1994; HUANG et al. 1999).

Peptic ulcer disease in children is mainly duodenal ulcer disease, and when *H. pylori* is the cause, antral gastritis is also present. *H. pylori* can cause isolated gastritis as well. When *H. pylori* induces antibodies and reacts with them in the gastric mucosa, chronic gastritis may result and it is thought that these mucosal changes play a role in the progression to gastric cancer in adults. IERADI et al. (1998) found that autoreaction of gastric mucosa may be found in *H. pylori* gastritis of childhood. They postulated a role in progression to atrophy and possibly increased risk of late gastric cancer. Numerous properties of the bacteria itself are also suggested as being important, including the presence of the CagA protein and vacA alleles associated with cytotoxin production. *H. pylori* generally falls into one of two groups: a Cag-negative group which does not produce cytotoxin and a Cag-positive which does and is associated with peptic ulcer disease (ÇELIK et al. 1998). ÇELIK et al. (1998) confirmed that the Cag pathogenicity and toxin expression seen in adults is also seen in younger subjects with recurrent abdominal pain. Children and adolescents demonstrate 40% CagA positivity as compared with 80–100% of adults with duodenal ulcer and gastritis. MITCHELL et al. (1999) also found that the presence of CagA is not a marker of specific disease in children. Furthermore, these investigators conclude that children do become persistently infected by *H. pylori* and few carry strains with the virulence properties seen in adults with gastrointestinal pathology. Whether these children should be treated to reduce risk of gastritis and gastric cancer is not clear at this time (ÇELIK et al. 1998). The current view holds that *H. pylori* is spread to children from close person-to-person contact and, because there is familial clustering seen with infection of children, it has been suggested that family treatment may decrease treatment failures due to increased compliance (FALL et al. 1997; ODERDA et al. 1997).

H. pylori is responsible for approximately 80% of duodenal ulcer after other etiologies including Crohn's disease (CD), non-steroidal anti-inflammatory drug ingestion, and Zollinger-Ellison syndrome have been ruled out. In a retrospective review of pediatric gastroscopy carried out in Hong Kong, 88% of patients complaining of dyspepsia had positive histological findings. In this group 25% were positive for *H. pylori* (NG et al. 1997). HEANEY et al. (1998) have suggested that *H. pylori* infection status can be used as a criterion to select patients for gastroscopy when determining management of young dyspeptic patients. In this study 160 "young" patients (<45 years of age) were prospectively recruited when presenting with the complaint of epigastric pain and/or discomfort. Patients who were negative for *H. pylori* using the carbon-13 (^{13}C) urea breath test were reassured that they would likely have a normal gastroscopy. At this point they were given lifestyle advice and symptomatic therapy and then followed at intervals of 6 weeks, 3 months, and 6 months. If they were the same or worse at these intervals, they proceeded to gastroscopy. This management protocol resulted in a 42% reduction in the number of gastroscopy examinations in *H. pylori* patients.

Recurrent abdominal pain is a common presenting complaint in children. There is no substantial evidence to suggest that *H. pylori* has any role in recurrent abdominal pain or so-called non-ulcer dyspepsia in children. WEWER et al. (1998) assessed the IgG seroprevalence of *H. pylori* in children with recurrent abdominal pain compared with healthy children to investigate the presence or absence of related symptoms. IgG antibodies against low molecular weight *H. pylori* were assessed in a total of 438 children and 91 healthy controls. The seroprevalence in children with recurrent abdominal pain was 21%, against 10% in the controls with 46 of 66 of those positive by culture and histology. The presence of *H. pylori* was associated with both parents being born in a country with high prevalence of *H. pylori*, low socioeconomic class, and more pain related to meals but not related to low levels of hemoglobin, leukocytes, thrombocytes, weight, or height. No specific symptomatology was related to *H. pylori* positivity in children. In a case control study of Turkish children by GÜNEL et al. (1998) no association was found between children with *H. pylori* infection, hypergastrinemia, and recurrent abdominal pain. *H. pylori* infection was as high in healthy children as in those with recurrent abdominal pain confirming the findings by GOTTRAND et al. (1997) that normal gastric histology can be associated with infection in children.

The wide interest in this bacterium has spawned many investigations of its relationships, if any, with other gastrointestinal diseases, with inflammatory bowel disease (IBD) being a case in point. The cause or causes of IBD remain incompletely understood with infectious agents including several bacteria and viruses implicated. Since *H. pylori* infection causes changes in both permeability and immunological arrangements in the stomach similar to those seen in the colon in IBD, it is natural to wonder if there is a causal relationship. Currently, there is no epidemiological data to support that conclusion and while, interestingly, there is a low prevalence of *H. pylori* in inflammatory bowel disease, the clinical significance, if any, of *H. pylori* infection against the background of IBD is not yet clear (NARDONE et al. 1998; PARENTE et al. 1997). Permanent colonization of the stomach in pediatric patients with IBD is unusual (KOLHO et al. 1998). In a cross-sectional study with matching of patients with IBD and upper gastrointestinal lesions it is noted that the reduced *H. pylori* infection prevalence is due mainly to decreased frequency of colonization in patients with CD. The prior treatment of patients with sulfasalazine but not 5-aminosalicylic acid, steroids, or immune suppressants is associated with a reduced risk of infection in both patients with ulcerative colitis (UC) and CD. In the group of patients with CD (123 of 216), 10% had gastroduodenal localization of their disease while 15% had *H. pylori* negative gastritis on histological examination (PARENTE et al. 1997).

Celiac disease is a disorder frequently associated with gastritis. In a study performed to assess the prevalence and significance of *H. pylori* infection in children with celiac disease no increase in prevalence or clinical manifestations of *H. pylori* was found (LUZZA et al. 1999). Recurrent abdominal pain was the only symptom that distinguished between *H. pylori* positive and negative children, but this symptom resolved on gluten withdrawal regardless of their *H. pylori* status.

As *H. pylori* is a causal agent for gastritis, the presence of *H. pylori* infection in gastric-body-type mucosa as is seen in Meckel's diverticulum may be pathogenic. HILL and RODE (1998) reported the case of a 25-year-old man who presented with rectal bleeding and a positive Meckel scan. Surgical pathology revealed a diverticulum with gastric-body-type mucosa with active chronic gastritis and positive immunohistochemistry for *H. pylori*. They found only one other case in a retrospective review at their hospital of 21 cases of proven Meckel's diverticulum.

In another line of investigation of gastritis, SALARDI et al. (1999) looked at the prevalence of *H. pylori* in children with type-I diabetes mellitus. Children with diabetes are more susceptible to common acquired bacterial infections and chronic atrophic gastritis if they have longstanding disease. They concluded that, although children with diabetes do not differ from their healthy cohorts in terms of prevalence of *H. pylori* infection in the first few years of disease, they subsequently do have a higher *H. pylori* seroprevalence. They suggest that this could be the cause or one of the causes of chronic atrophic gastritis in children with longstanding diabetes. When BARRIO et al. (1997) looked at a group of children and adolescents with diabetes, they found that 7% (12 of 177) of these patients had gastric parietal cell autoantibodies and 6 of 8 of those who had antral biopsies were found to have *H. pylori* infection leading them to suggest that diabetic children and adolescents should be screened for infection.

In a study looking at the role of *H. pylori* in diminished growth in children, three populations of children were studied including normal, diabetic, and hyposomic children (VAIRA et al. 1998). They looked at the possible role of infection by differing strains of *H. pylori*. As infection with more cytotoxic strains, such as the so-called CagA or VacA strains, lead to more severe gastroduodenal infection, these authors looked for a possible role for these strains in children with decreased growth, but they did not find supportive data.

11.2.1 Diagnostic Tests

When *H. pylori* infection is diagnosed in children and thought to be the cause of the patient's morbidity, a course of double antibiotic therapy is recommended for 4–6 weeks' duration (HASSALL 1994). *H. pylori* infection diagnosis can be achieved using invasive methods, such as endoscopy, to provide tissue samples for rapid urease tests, culture, and histological examination. Noninvasive testing can be performed by blood sampling for IgG antibody tests and urea breath testing using radioactive carbon-14 (^{14}C) or stable ^{13}C. Clinical guidelines for the diagnosis and treatment of *H. pylori* in children currently suggest a fairly limited use in the young age group. Ongoing research into its role in gastrointestinal disease and expanding use of nuclear medicine modalities in children may spur further utilization of these methodologies and knowledge of these for use in children will be valuable.

The noninvasive breath tests are painless and can be performed in children who are old enough to follow simple instruction for ingestion and blowing through a straw. Both ^{13}C and ^{14}C urea breath tests for the diagnosis of *H. pylori* infection can be utilized (CUTLER 1997). Both tests take advantage of the fact that *H. pylori* produces urease which is needed to break down labeled urea. Gastric urease activity can then be measured and used as an indicator of the presence of infection. Both tests rely on the measurement of labeled CO_2 exhaled by the patient after consuming a standard dose of labeled urea.

Urea breath tests have the ability to sample a larger area of the gastric mucosa than individual biopsies. In the ^{13}C breath test the patient is fed a high-carbohydrate, high-protein meal to slow gastric emptying and increase the residence time of ^{13}C-urea in the stomach. ^{13}C-urea is then ingested as a powder that is dissolved in water. Collection of breath samples occurs at baseline and at 30 min. Thirty minutes is the proposed collection time to avoid false-positive results due to urease in the mouth flora. A mass spectrometer is used for the measurement of ^{13}C.

In the ^{14}C-urea breath test the elimination of ^{14}C via exhaled air is measured with a liquid scintillation counting technique. The advantage of ^{14}C over ^{13}C is that smaller concentrations can be detected as radioactive substances are not routinely exhaled. Baseline breath samples are not required; and there is no need to slow gastric emptying. After a 4-h fast, the pediatric patients are given 0.055 MBq dose orally supplied as dissolvable capsules and samples of exhaled air are taken at as early as 10 min after oral administration with cumulative samples taken at 60 min. Caglar et al. (1999) have shown accurate results when comparing a single 10-min sample to 60-min cumulative excretion, thus improving cost-effectiveness and improving patient acceptance. The accepted upper limit of normal for excretion at 10 min is a specific activity of a breath sample corrected for body surface area of 0.3% (Henze et al. 1990; Debongie et al. 1991). An abnormal test result would be a cumulative value of greater than 2% excretion.

In all methodologies the accuracy of the results can be reduced if certain drugs have been taken by the patient. Antimicrobials should be discontinued a minimum of 4 weeks prior to testing; bismuth-containing compounds 1 month prior; proton pump inhibitors and sucralfate or similar compounds at least 1 week prior to the test; histamine (H2) receptor antagonists for 2 days prior; and antacids for 1 day prior. Histological method accuracy is reported to be reduced in the presence of an active or recently bleeding duodenal ulcer (Cutler 1997).

Although there is some controversy as to which of the available methods of diagnosis of *H. pylori* infection in the untreated patient is best, the urea breath test is recognized as the method of choice to confirm *H. pylori* cure (Cutler 1997). Confirmation of eradication of *H. pylori* infection is most accurate when the breath test is performed a minimum of 4 weeks after the completion of therapy.

The ^{14}C-urea breath test is simple, easily performed, and inexpensive. It provides quantitative information regarding the total activity of the *H. pylori* bacterium in the stomach as reflected by urease activity and severity of gastritis and is a sensitive and specific method of confirming its presence in peptic ulcer disease (Henze et al. 1990; Debongie et al. 1991). The test has shown between 95 and 98% reproducibility when repeated after a 1-week interval in a series of children (Steen et al. 1995).

The ^{14}C isotope is radioactive and therefore raises considerations relevant to the use of ionizing radiation in the pediatric population . When ^{14}C-urea is used it is excreted in the breath as $^{14}CO_2$ or in the urine. Biokinetic models have been established to determine dosimetry in the pediatric population (Leide-Svegborn et al. 1999). Approximately 88% of the administered activity is excreted in the urine within 72 h of administration. Approximately 3% is exhaled within 20 days. The bladder wall receives the highest dose of radiation. In children aged 7–14 years this effective absorbed dose measures approximately 0.14–0.36 mGy/MBq. The effective total body dose in children is calculated therefore to be 0.9–2.5 μSv for an administered dose of 0.055 MBq. This is a minimal dose and therefore the use of this examination as a screening test and repeated examinations would be acceptable from a radiation burden standpoint.

11.3 Imaging of Inflammatory Bowel Disease

The demonstration of intra-abdominal sources of infection remains a challenging clinical problem. The front line imaging techniques of ultrasound, CT, and MRI provide structural detail but cannot always differentiate adequately treated residual morphological alterations. A variety of scintigraphic studies can provide physiological information not available through other means. This provides a significant contribution to the clinical problems of whether active infection exists in the abdomen, its location, extent, and response to therapy over time. Whereas gallium has a time-honored place in the visualization of infection, radiopharmaceutical innovations in recent years allow more specific and more sensitive delineation of infectious processes.

The use of radiolabeled autologous white blood cells (WBC) to assess intra-abdominal sites of infection is increasing. Labeled WBC will leave the circulation at sites of infection and migrate into the infected tissues as part of the normal host response. ^{99m}Tc-HMPAO as a practical label for autologous WBC offers high-quality images with favorable dosimetry. ^{111}In-WBC scanning is not used in children because of its unfavorable dosimetry (Gainey et al. 1988). ^{99m}Tc-HMPAO-labeled WBC are proving to be particularly helpful in pediatrics for the assessment of inflammatory bowel disease (CHARRON 1997; BARABINO et al. 1998).

Normal distribution of labeled WBC occurs in the spleen, liver, and red bone marrow (Fig. 11.1), with some faint activity in submandibular glands, kidneys, and bladder. Transient WBC sequestration in the lungs can occur in the first few hours. The gallbladder can be seen in up to 10% of children, but this does not interfere with interpretation. Some activity in normal ascending colon can be seen at 4 h post injection. This activity is usually faint and less intense than iliac crest activity and has a diffuse pattern. This is thought to represent excretion of non-cell bound labeled secondary hydrophilic complexes (CHARRON 1997). Since imaging for the assessment of bowel inflammation is not usually obtained beyond 4 h, this does not decrease specificity.

No bowel preparation is required for this examination, unlike with gallium imaging. The administered dose is adjusted for body weight between a minimum–maximum dose of 185–740 MBq (5–20 mCi). Imaging protocol includes 0.5- to 1-h and 2- to 3-h static images in anterior and posterior projections and SPECT with low-energy high-resolution collimator. Tail on detector views can be used to help distinguish perianal and rectal disease from bladder activity. Upright anterior views of the abdomen can be helpful in separating liver activity from that in transverse colon. All imaging should be performed after the patient has voided. In children suspected of having CD, a view to include anterior chest and mouth can be used to assess for disease in the esophagus (CHARRON 1997). CHARRON et al. (1997) visually grade the inflammatory activity in each segment relative to the iliac crest bone marrow and liver activity: grade 0=no activity; grade 1=less than crest; grade 2=equal to crest; grade 3=greater than crest; grade 4=less than liver; grade 5=equal to liver; grade 6=greater than liver. Abnormal activity in keeping with inflammation appears bowel shaped, does not change configuration on the late scan, and increases in intensity temporally. The SPECT images reviewed in cine mode with maximal intensity can also increase sensitivity for detection of disease, although there may be some reduction in specificity.

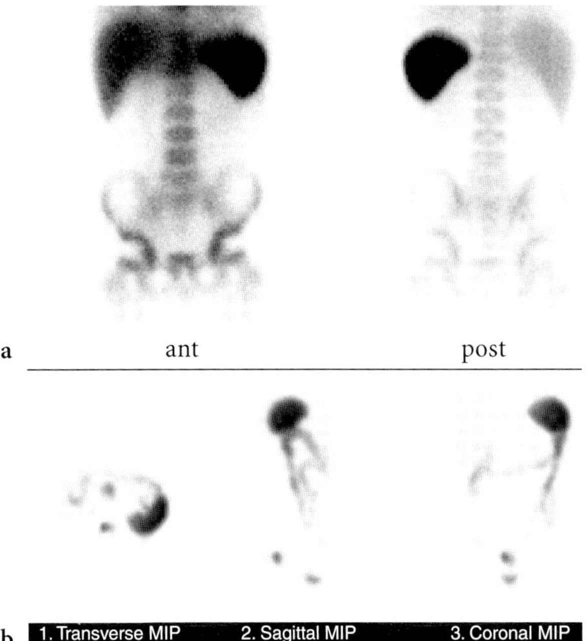

Fig. 11.1**a,b**. **a** Normal distribution of ^{99m}Tc-HMPAO labeled white blood cells in a child. Anterior view of the abdomen and pelvis. Note the prominent activity in the spleen, liver and bone marrow. **b** inflammatory bowel disease (IBD); diffuse involvement of the colon, including proximal ascending colon, transverse colon, splenic flexure, and descending colon to sigmoid colon in a 10 year old girl with Crohn's disease. Note the high uptake in the spleen in all three planes. MIP = maximum intensity projection image, i.e. a volume rendered summation of the maximal counts from the tomographic images, for the transverse, sagittal and coronal planes.

Labeled WBC scintigraphy is particularly helpful for the assessment of small bowel disease. The demonstration of disease distribution influences the selection of therapeutic regimens and has prognostic implications. Labeled-WBC scintigraphy also has the ability to detect extra-intestinal sites of inflammation, such as abscess collections and fistulae (Fig. 11.2). The labeled-WBC scan has also been able to discriminate between continuous and discontinuous disease thereby effectively differentiating UC from CD (CHARRON et al. 1998). In a series of 106 patients with either UC or CD only 6 patients were classified incorrectly. Labeled-WBC scintigraphy allows for accurate assessment of the segmental distribution of disease when correlated with histology and endoscopy (CHARRON et al. 1998). This technique can be particularly helpful in identifying sites of inflammation when technical difficulties preclude this assessment with colonoscopy. Labeled-WBC scintigraphy is less invasive than barium follow-through examination or enteroclysis and is much better tolerated by children. Limitations of labeled-WBC scintigraphy include the inability to assess anatomical detail such as bowel strictures and prestenotic dilations. Fistulae may be difficult to detect. If the abnormal activity is focal, it may be difficult to distinguish large from small bowel due to insufficient anatomical landmarks. In the child who is actively bleeding there may be difficulty in

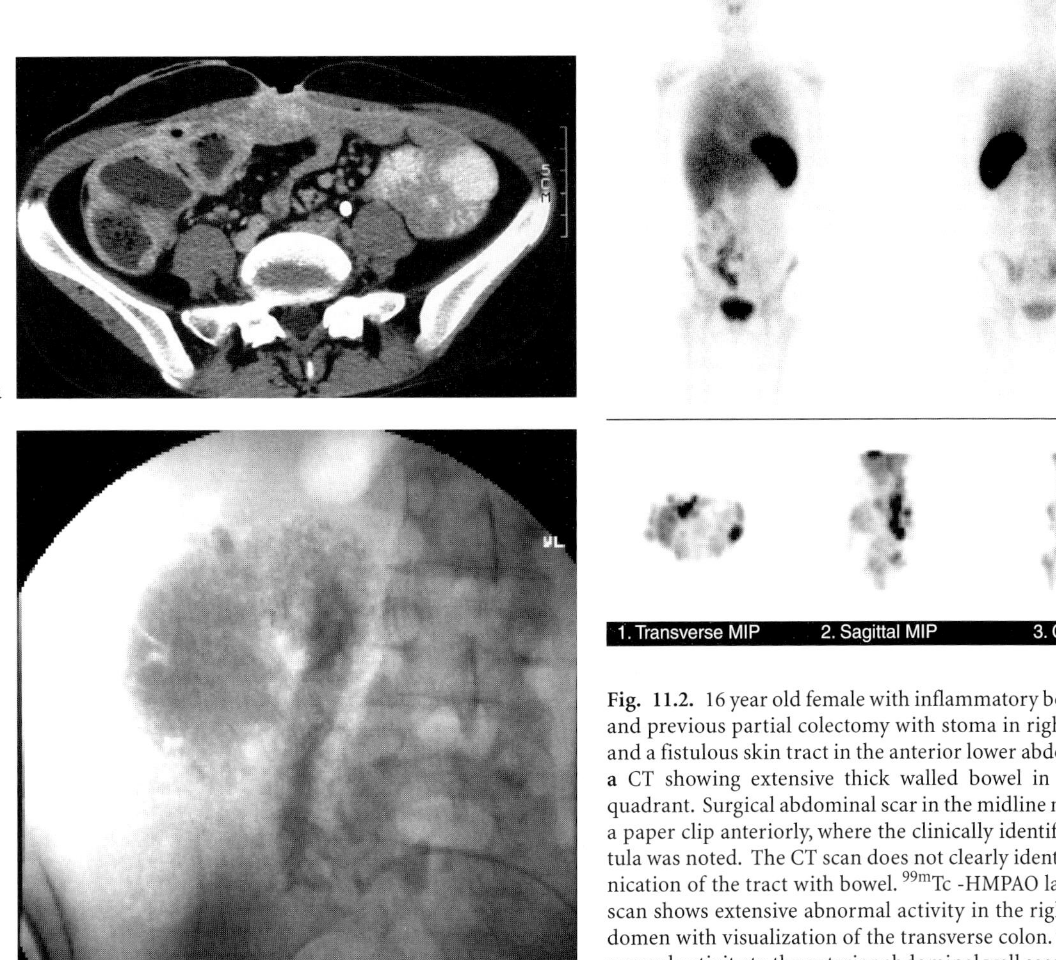

Fig. 11.2. 16 year old female with inflammatory bowel disease and previous partial colectomy with stoma in right iliac fossa and a fistulous skin tract in the anterior lower abdominal wall. **a** CT showing extensive thick walled bowel in right lower quadrant. Surgical abdominal scar in the midline marked with a paper clip anteriorly, where the clinically identified skin fistula was noted. The CT scan does not clearly identify communication of the tract with bowel. ^{99m}Tc -HMPAO labeled-WBC scan shows extensive abnormal activity in the right lower abdomen with visualization of the transverse colon. There is abnormal activity to the anterior abdominal wall seen on the planar views (**b**) and SPECT MIP images (**c**) **d** Fistulogram study showing contrast injected through a catheter placed through the skin fistula filling a connection to the colon in the right iliac fossa. This appearance is consistent with a colocutaneous fistula. MIP = maximum intensity projection image, see Fig. 11-1b

scan interpretation (Charron et al. 1999). Overall accuracy of 93% with 90% sensitivity and 97% specificity has been reported (Charron et al. 1999; Del Rosario et al. 1999). Charron et al. (1999) report a positive predictive value for labeled-WBC scintigraphy of 97%. In the evaluation of 79 control subjects no false-positive results were obtained. Negative predictive value was 93%. The disease distribution can be underestimated in early CD and nonspecific colitis. When there is focal bowel involvement in the region of the cecum, appendicitis as well as involvement of the cecum with IBD must be included in the differential. Although endoscopy and biopsy are still the gold standards, labeled-WBC scintigraphy is helpful in the follow-up of IBD in detecting recurrence, monitor treatment, or plan surgery. This technique can reduce the need for repeated colonoscopies and barium examinations in these children.

11.4 Pediatric Neuronuclear Medicine

Just as there have been advances in the area of brain scintigraphy in adults, so too have there been advances in pediatric neuro-nuclear medicine. The advent of new radiopharmaceuticals for brain imaging has allowed scintigraphy to become a full-fledged member of the multidisciplinary team investigating neurological and psychological illness in the past decade. Cross-sectional imaging with CT and MRI revolutionized the treatment and diagnosis of neurological disease in adults and children; SPECT and PET imaging bring physiological and functional information to vastly improved morphological imaging modalities. This has opened new doors for medical care providers and scientists to study and learn more about neurological disease, neuropsychiatric disorders, brain development, and learning in childhood.

Advances in instrumentation and radiopharmaceuticals have made it easier to perform brain scintigraphy and to obtain more diagnostic information in children. The studies have focused mainly on regional cerebral blood flow, but new research is exploring metabolic and receptor imaging particularly in neuropsychiatric disease. The main indications for pediatric neurological nuclear scintigraphy include seizure disorders, assessment of brain development, evaluation of tumors, and trauma. Knowledge is growing rapidly and expanding our understanding of developmental and neuro-psychological disorders.

While heredity is a large contributor to brain structure and function, we know that development and learning after birth can and will have enormous impact on a child's ultimate motor sensory and intellectual potential and capabilities. When birth or early developmental experiences have a potentially negative impact, parents look anxiously to physicians and allied health personnel for aid. Neuroimaging can be performed to guide intervention, treatment, assessment, or prediction of ultimate outcome (Denays et al. 1990; Kerrigan et al. 1991; O'Tuama and Treves 1993; Kao et al. 1994; Yamada et al. 1995; Lee et al. 1998).

Radiopharmaceuticals used for PET have included ^{18}F-fluorodeoxyglucose (FDG), ^{11}C-L-methionine for tumor imaging, oxygen-^{15}O for cerebral blood flow assessment of intraventricular hemorrhage and infarction, and hypoxic ischemic encephalopathy in infants. SPECT radiopharmaceuticals include ^{99m}Tc-HMPAO and ^{99m}Tc-ECD or less commonly ^{123}I-iodoamphetamine or ^{133}Xe for regional cerebral blood flow assessment. Ligands labeled with ^{123}I or ^{11}C have been used in receptor imaging studies. ^{201}Tl has been used to differentiate recurrent disease from radiation necrosis in children with brain tumors.

Neuroimaging is also used in infants and children to learn about the normal and abnormal development of the brain. Neuroimaging is used more and more in the research and investigations of childhood psychiatric and behavioral disorders, which raises important questions about the value of these tests to children as a group and the individual and group attendant risks. Investigations using ionizing radiation are justified by using the calculation of the so-called risk/benefit ratio of the test. This ratio may not be calculable in the short term and certainly not for a particular child at a particular time in development, assuring that this debate will continue in the future. Ernst (1999) points out correctly that the risk/benefit ratio is essential to the conduct of research and requires the calculation of risks according to the ambiguous definition of "minimal risk." When discussing the risks of exposure to low-level radiation, it is helpful to compare the risk to everyday activities that the child might realistically expect to partake in, such as riding in a car, as well as risks which might be uppermost in the mind of children or their parents such as the risk of developing leukemia or other cancers and the risk of increased chromosomal abnormalities. In another review article assessing health hazards to children of radiation exposure in the context of brain imaging research, the authors conclude that health risks from low-level radiation obtained by radiographic and scintigraphic diagnostic studies are not detectable above random events that occur in everyday life (Ernst et al. 1998).

Brain imaging research has huge potential benefits to society as a whole. Understanding its attendant risks to children is crucial to rational discussion of investigation of neurological and psychological disorders. Members of ethics and grant review boards, as well as individual researchers and practitioners, need to understand the risk of exposure to low-level radiation through research and diagnostic studies. This research needs the participation of both children who are abnormal and those who are normal. It is not unreasonable to assert that normal children will also benefit from further understanding of neurological and psychological dysfunction. PET studies in normal child volunteers have to date recorded very low acceptable radiation exposures (Ernst et al. 1998).

11.4.1 Scintigraphy in Brain Development

Brain development has been extensively studied using PET and FDG. Similarly SPECT radiopharmaceuticals have been used to assess changes in regional cerebral blood flow with brain development in the normal human infant (Chugani et al. 1987; Chiron et al. 1992; Chugani 1998; Kinnala et al. 1996; Schiepers et al. 1997; Rubinstein et al. 1989). Brain development is phylogenetic with developmentally older structures visualized before newer structures. At a gestational age less than 40 weeks, regional cerebral blood flow imaging shows prominent activity seen in the thalami with no parietal or occipital cortical activity and poor if any frontal activity. At 40 weeks or term gestational age, thalamic activity remains prominent. There is increase in activity in the parietal cortex, still low occipital activity and poor frontal activity (Fig. 11.3a). At 44 weeks of gestational age there is a prominent parietal cortex visualized, occipital activity is increasing, the thalami remain prominent, and there is still poor frontal activity. At 2 months of age there is predominance of parietal and occipital cortical activity with still low frontal activity. By 6 months of age there is marked cortical predominance. There is increase in frontal cortex activity but still considerably less than the corresponding parietal and occipital cortical activity (Fig. 11.3b). By 1 year of age all cortical areas show a significant increase in regional cerebral perfusion with either PET or SPECT.

Cerebral glucose metabolism matures through childhood until typical adult activity patterns are seen at approximately age 1 year (Chugani et al. 1987; Chugani and Phelps 1986). Cortical glucose metabolic rate measured with PET shows an increase until age 2–3 years which can exceed adult values. This remains high until 8–10 years of age and declines to normal adult values somewhere between 16–18 years of age. This period of rapidly increasing glucose utilization corresponds to a time of overproduction of nerve terminals and synapses. The plateau phase when glucose utilization remains stable but higher than that of adults represents overconnectivity followed by elimination of the excessive connectivity and corresponding reduction in cerebral glucose utilization to adult levels.

Takahashi et al. (1999) using PET have determined normal values for regional cerebral blood flow (rCBF), regional cerebral metabolic rate for oxygen ($rCRMO_2$), and regional oxygen extraction fraction (rOEF). The children in their series ranged in age from 10 days to 16 years. In the neonatal period the rCBF and $rCRMO_2$ were lowest and increased during early childhood. A temporal sequence of rCBF and $rCRMO_2$ similar to that seen with glucose metabolism and brain SPECT findings was noted, likely reflecting physiological development within anatomical areas of the brain.

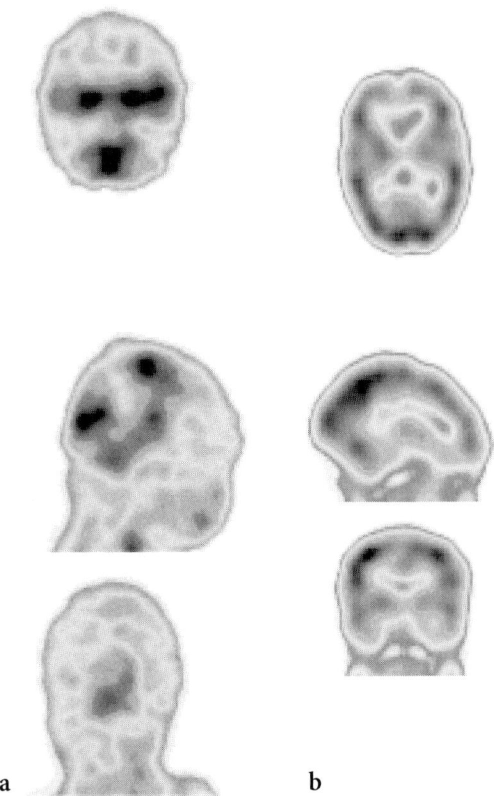

Fig. 11.3. ^{99m}Tc-HMPAO activity pattern in a normal newborn (**a**) and at 6 months of age (**b**). Note the initial lack of frontal activity, prominent brain stem and temporo-parietal perfusion, which increases over the first six months with more uniform cortical activity seen at 6 months.

Chiron et al. (1992) studied 42 neurologically normal children of all ages (2 days to 19 years) with normal CT, EEG at time of study, and normal psychomotor development for 2 years post study using rCBF by SPECT with ^{133}Xe and compared the results to an adult reference group consisting of 32 subjects 19–29 years of age who were free of neuropathology. The mean rCBF was calculated for three age groups and the measurements showed effects of age in all cortical regions and on global blood flow. Global blood flow averaged 50 ml/min per 100 g at birth and increased in all age groups to a maximum at 5 years and decreased to adult levels after 19 years of age. Cortical regions all demonstrated lower perfusion at birth than in adulthood, and all regions peaked at around 5 years of age at levels 70% higher than adult levels. When studied on a relative basis, rCBF was at a lower level at birth than at maturity and increased in the first 2 years of life to plateau during the rest of childhood with less than 10% variation. In addition to refining reference values for large functional areas of the brain, this work reconfirmed the importance of the early years of life in neurological development.

Brain function assessed by regional glucose utilization and PET in the neonate is highest in the thalamic nuclei, brain stem, cerebellar vermis, and sensorimotor cortex which correlates with the dominance of subcortical activity at that age. Early physical examination of an infant elicits the basic reflexes such as rooting and the grasp reflex. As development progresses, the regional utilization of glucose continues to correlate with the development of function in corresponding anatomical regions and these are observed in PET studies in the parietal, temporal, and primary visual cortex, basal ganglia, and cerebellar hemispheres described as encephalization during 2–4 months of age (Chugani 1992).

While work in this area is ongoing, other efforts are aimed at using the neuroimaging techniques of SPECT and PET to attempt to study and, hopefully, predict outcome of neurological insult and catastrophe in the very young. One group of children in whom this would be helpful is the pre-term infant. These infants often have protracted courses in hospitals with superimposed serious illnesses which may conclude in death. Those who survive have often been subject to long periods of artificial ventilation with varying levels of low p_aO_2 and high p_aCO_2, low hematocrit, and low arterial blood pressure, all of which may negatively impact on development and growth. It has been reported that ventilation in neonates is associated with low CBF and specifically with hemorrhage and neurological deficit (Greisen 1986, 1990; Greisen and Pryds 1988; Allan and Volpe 1986; Altman et al. 1993). With respect to intracranial hemorrhage, cranial ultrasound is an effective investigation in the preterm infant for diagnosis and for predicting outcome. Hemorrhage tends to be less damaging to the very young infant than infarction into the periventricular white matter or periventricular leukomalacia. Infants born prior to 30–32 weeks gestational age are at risk due to the thin-walled vessels in those areas and combined factors of decreased cerebrovascular reserve and regulation. Baenziger et al. (1999) studied brain perfusion in these infants in an attempt to elucidate the predictive capacity of CBF measurements in this group. A total of 71 preterm infants (less than 1500 g birth weight and less than 34 weeks gestational age) were studied at three time intervals postnatally: between 2 and 36 h; between 36 and 108 h; and between 108 and 240 h respectively using ^{133}Xe and extracranial cadmium telluride detectors. Corresponding cranial ultrasound was performed. The surviving children were assessed for development at 18 months of age. There was a higher mean CBF and mental or motor development. Other studies in children with cerebral palsy have a spectrum of findings on brain SPECT studies which include absence of cerebral blood flow abnormality to thalamic hypoperfusion, diffuse hemispheric hypoperfusion, focal hypoperfusion in the contralateral hemisphere to an area of motor deficit, and cerebellar areas of hypoperfusion (Denays et al. 1990; Kao et al. 1994; Lee et al. 1998). Pryds et al. (1990) suggest that cerebral hyperperfusion in term asphyxiated infants who lose their ability to autoregulate may be an earlier indicator of cerebral hypoperfusion. There is no definitive pattern identified in children with birth asphyxia which can predict long-term sequelae, but cerebral blood flow imaging studies are helpful in the identification of CBF disturbances.

The brain and skull can be involved in a variety of syndromes or isolated insults in early infancy. Craniosynostosis is one such developmental anomaly. When there is premature fusion of multiple sutures or involvement of only one suture, the result is brain compression which can lead to impaired cognitive development. Surgical correction can include cranial vault remodeling in severe cases and or strip craniectomy. Pre- and post-operative FDG PET studies in a small number of affected children have shown varying regional increases and decreases; however, more consistent postoperative increase in activity has been demonstrated in the posterior occiput in the region where visual development and visual–spatial coordination develops (David et al. 1999).

11.4.2 Language and Cognition

One of the main and best established uses of functional brain imaging is the localization of epileptogenic foci in children in whom surgical treatment is planned. When CT and MRI have ruled out a morphological abnormality, radionuclide perfusion imaging inter- and postictally offers a sensitive method for localization of the seizure activity. The finding of decreased regional perfusion at a focal area and increased perfusion at the same site during a seizure offers a sensitivity of approximately 95%, although this number falls if temporal lobe epilepsy is excluded (Gordon 1996). Nuclear physicians may be unaware that there are substantial considerations for these children regarding language problems and behavioral abnormalities which must be understood to allow the best possible treatment.

There are many language and behavioral manifestations associated with epilepsy and not infrequently these may be epileptic events which are erroneously ascribed to behavioral problems (TUCHMAN 1994). Although the anatomical basis linking seizure disorders to disorders of behavior, such as aggression, depression, and even schizophrenia, have been postulated, this is not yet universally accepted. These areas are fertile fields for functional imaging. The total effects of seizures on the brain are incompletely understood and still debated (DEVINSKY and BEAR 1984; HOLMES 1991; LESSER et al. 1986). In the 1950s LANDAU and KLEFFNER (1957) described a syndrome of acquired aphasia in epilepsy which has been followed by numerous other similar reports, although the exact pathogenesis and neuroanatomical basis for this is unclear. In a study designed to demonstrate the regional cerebral perfusion in Landau-Kleffner syndrome and its correlates with the EEG, O'TUAMA et al. (1992) performed brain SPECT using ^{99m}Tc-HMPAO in five children with this syndrome and in three with other speech difficulties. They found perfusion asymmetry with decreased perfusion in the temporal lobes most marked in the perisylvian cortex. A PET-FDG study performed in three boys with this syndrome showed similar findings, mainly in the temporal lobe distribution. Neither study nor subsequent studies have yet defined the correspondence to EEG abnormalities (MAQUET et al. 1990).

Congenital dysphasia has also been studied using SPECT. This is a clinical diagnosis of exclusion where deafness, mental retardation, speech pathology, and neurological and psychiatric causes have been ruled out. In a study of 14 affected children, SPECT demonstrated decreased activity in the left hemisphere, best localized near Broca's area in 2 patients with expressive aphasia. In 9 of 12 children with both expressive and comprehension problems there were two areas of abnormality best localized to the left temporo-parietal area and the right frontal lobe (DENAYS et al. 1989).

Children suffering from epilepsy have a higher risk of learning and behavioral disorders, which is multi-factorial and can be very complicated to investigate. Many of the important factors are not directly relevant to functional brain imaging; two of interest to nuclear medicine specialists are seizure activity and the location of the epileptogenic focus both of which have significant negative effects on cognition. Specifically, temporal lobe seizures are considered a definite risk factor for cognitive developmental problems and functional brain imaging studies have confirmed this through a suspected negative effect on verbal memory (ALDENKAMP et al. 1990).

11.4.3 Brain Trauma and Brain Death

The determination of brain death relies on unequivocal clinical data indicative of irreversible cessation of brain function, specifically both cortical and brain stem functions. Supportive laboratory studies, most importantly two silent EEG studies separated by various time periods depending on legal jurisdiction, are desirable and often required. In cases of catastrophic injury of a child, the declaration of death can be a highly charged situation for the relatives and physicians involved in the child's care and for physicians involved in harvesting and transplanting organs into other ill children and adults. Not infrequently, an objective test provides comfort for this task. YOUNGER et al. (1989) claim that knowledge of medical and legal criteria for diagnosing death among physicians is surprisingly lacking. It is important that the contribution of nuclear brain scans be available, prompt, and knowledgeable.

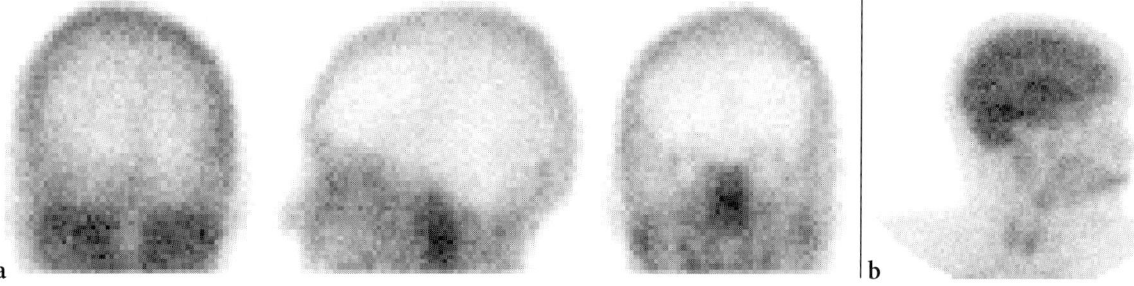

Fig. 11.4. a Brain death. Posterior, left lateral and anterior views obtained with planar scintigraphy. There is absence of normal intracranial activity on these ^{99m}Tc-HMPAO images. **b** Right lateral view of a brain scan showing normal intracranial perfusion after administration of ^{99m}Tc-HMPAO.

Cerebral perfusion studies using tracers, such as ^{99m}Tc-HMPAO or ^{99m}Tc-ECD, are a quick and accurate alternative to traditional gold standard confirmatory four-vessel angiogram examination, to confirm absence of intracranial perfusion and help provide a timely diagnosis of brain death. These radiopharmaceuticals have advantages over the blood-brain barrier agents formerly used in that there is less difficulty in differentiating intra- and extracerebral activity and activity in the dural sinuses is not a potentially confusing picture. Technical aspects of bolus injection and timing of the study are less stringent and assessment of the posterior fossa using the newer ^{99m}Tc-lipophilic perfusion agents is far easier (Fig. 11.4; Laurin et al. 1989; Schiepers et al. 1997).

The absence of perfusion above the tentorium with preservation or persistence of blood flow in the cerebellum and/or brainstem contradicts the diagnosis of brain death, although it has a grave prognosis (Valle et al. 1993). The planar scintigraphy should include a lateral view and SPECT should be performed for the best evaluation of the posterior fossa. A prudent recommendation is to include views of the thyroid bed to confirm radiopharmaceutical quality. Views of the liver and heart also support radiopharmaceutical integrity and an estimation of viability of those organs (Wieler et al. 1993). Imaging can also be done with a portable camera in the ICU setting, if desirable. All patients showing absent brain uptake with these tracers are confirmed as brain dead uniformly in published series. Reported series include mainly adult patients (Larar and Nagel 1992; Wilson et al. 1993; Goodman et al. 1985). The diagnosis of brain death in children can be difficult and adult criteria are not necessarily sufficient or easy to obtain (Holzman et al. 1983). There are several series of pediatric patients which confirm that absence of intracerebral perfusion is a highly reliable aid in diagnosing of brain death (Fig. 11.4). This is particularly useful when the clinical criterion of silent EEG is complicated (Galaske et al. 1988).

Nonfatal head injury ranging from mild to severe has also been studied using lipophilic ^{99m}Tc-labeled brain agents and FDG. Both CT and MRI scans as the front line tools in the diagnosis of head injury can be less sensitive than nuclear medicine studies. Traumatic brain injury abnormalities in regional cerebral blood flow and glucose metabolism can be documented, more extensive, and detected earlier than with CT or MRI (Abu-Judeh et al. 1998). Evidence of ischemic injury is common and can be present in any region of the brain. It is attributed to diffuse or focal axonal shearing in the white matter in the absence of a structural abnormality on CT or MRI scan. Regional hypoperfusion on SPECT can be concordant or discordant with reduced glucose metabolism on PET (Abu-Judeh et al. 1998; Yamaki et al. 1996). When the findings are discordant, it indicates a good prognosis which may be due to vasospasm and edema causing decreased perfusion which is temporary. Most studies demonstrate abnormalities in the temporal frontal or parietal lobes and correlate well with severity of injury generally described by duration, severity of coma, and length of retrograde amnesia (Jacobs et al. 1994; Gordon 1996). An initial negative SPECT examination within 4 weeks of a closed head injury is a robust predictor of full recovery, although a positive scan is of less use prognostically. The role of SPECT and PET brain studies in the clinical and medico-legal work-up and assessment of head injury and its sequelae has not been fully established. Efforts to gain a toe-hold are hampered by lack of knowledge and understanding of the usefulness and applicability by medical practitioners during the acute and chronic phases of head trauma evaluation (van der Kolk 1997). Furthermore, whereas early studies focusing on acute head trauma included patients in the pediatric age group, there are few studies exclusively of children. Studies focusing on the chronic sequelae of brain injury when relationship between the morphological findings may be difficult to confidently relate to the neurological, psychological, or behavioral findings, are also sparse. Goshen et al. (1996) published a series of 28 pediatric patients with chronic sequelae of traumatic brain injury. These patients were referred to the rehabilitation unit of the medical center. They ranged in age from 15 months to 16 years and were assessed using EEG, ^{99m}Tc-HMPAO scintigraphy, CT, and, when available, MRI following substantial head injury (Glasgow coma scale ratings of 3–10). Retrospective analysis showed that cerebral blood flow studies following brain trauma were more sensitive than the anatomical modalities for detection of abnormalities, particularly in the basal ganglia and cerebellum. These authors suggest that brain SPECT may play a role in children who have neurological sequelae in the follow-up of brain trauma.

11.5 Primary Neuro-Psychological Disorders in Childhood

Using the classification of O'Tuama et al. (1999) there are four primary categories of childhood neuro-psychiatric disorders: attention-deficit hyperactivity disorder (ADHD); mood disorders such as depression and obsessive-compulsive disorder (OCD); Tourette syndrome and related disorders; and infantile autism and autistic spectrum disorder. One of the most inspiring uses of functional brain imaging must be the study of neuro-psychological disorders in children. The definition, etiology, diagnosis, and treatment of many of these disorders can be difficult and controversial. Few would dispute the negative outcome on adult life nor deny the often alarming repercussions that many of these disorders have on emotional development and family relationships.

The ability to study cerebral perfusion and metabolism with radionuclides has inspired great hopes for better understanding of psychiatric and developmental disorders in children and adolescents. The hope has been to aid or substantiate the correlation of neuro-psychological deficits or behavioral abnormalities with specific morphological regions and metabolic abnormalities. However, as pointed out by Filipek (1999), behavioral problems in children provide a spectrum of disorders which encompass deficits or derangements in language, cognition, visual-spatial function, and socialization.

11.5.1 Attention Deficit Hyperactivity Disorder

Attention deficit hyperactivity disorder continues to receive enormous attention in the lay media and is a subject of great ongoing study and research. The diagnosis has evolved substantially in recent years in tandem with advances in genetic, cognitive, and pharmacological research among other factors. The American Psychiatric Association includes the following criteria as assessed by reports by parents and teachers: poor impulse control; hyperactivity; poor temper control; and poor attention span. This disorder is relatively common, affecting up to 5–6% of children, and its propensity for boys is well known. The syndrome manifests in adulthood and leads to substantial social problems and alienation. Affected children are generally further classified as predominantly inattentive, predominantly hyperactive, and a combination type. Research using neuroimaging is confounded by frequent overlay of other behavioral disorders, mood, and anxiety disorders, and learning disabilities. Although the exact mechanism for this is not certain, advances in cognitive research in this area consider the main impairment in ADHD to be the inability to inhibit a behavioral response. Multiple models exist in the literature pointing to an arising focus of cognitive and genetic research, and neuroimaging (Tannock 1998).

Neuroimaging, specifically MRI, suggests that developmental abnormality involves the right hemisphere and basal ganglia (Tannock 1998; O'Tuama et al. 1999). Brain SPECT imaging neither confirms nor refutes global changes in cerebral perfusion and currently most convincingly presents hypoperfusion and, therefore, presumably decreased neuronal functioning in the striatal regions (Lou et al. 1989). More recent work using PET has demonstrated decreased glucose metabolism in the pre-frontal cortex (Tannock 1998). Experimental lesions in animals in both the striatal and prefrontal regions may cause hyperactivity (Lou et al. 1989). Although the available studies can be described as embryonic, at best, there is a clear indication that it is appropriate for nuclear brain imaging to join the research in this important disorder.

11.5.2 Mood Disorders: Depression and Obsessive–Compulsive Disorder

One of the most important advances in childhood neuropsychiatric disorders is simply the acknowledgement and understanding that mood and anxiety disorders do occur in young children and should be treated seriously when they exist. Functional brain imaging has shown great promise in the investigation of mood disorders. Decreased perfusion and metabolism has been demonstrated by SPECT and PET in the left prefrontal cortex and limbic areas, most notably in recurrent or chronic depression. In contrast, patients with transient or normal sadness demonstrate increased activity in the same areas when they are asked to recollect sad events (Risch 1997). This supports the theory that this activated circuitry in normals persists when it becomes chronic and ultimately burns out. Functional imaging in depression in adults most frequently demonstrates decreased perfusion in the temporal, frontal, and parietal areas. There is a significant shortage of studies in children in whom depression is now well recognized. Applying adult criteria to children may be completely erroneous as changes in brain activity may fluctuate during the course of an affective illness as well as during normal brain development (Risch 1997; O'Tauma et al. 1999).

The same caution applies to OCD which occurs in adults and children but has mainly been studied in adults. This disorder is not uncommon in children and teenagers and can be debilitating by virtue of intrusive and disturbing obsessive ideation and compulsive behaviors. As in other neuropsychiatric illnesses, a biologic or biochemical basis is suspected, although it is not known where this occurs or what its exact nature is. Functional brain imaging studies suggest involvement of the basal ganglia as well as the orbital–frontal cortex (SWEDO et al. 1989; O'TAUMA et al. 1999).

11.5.3 Tourette Syndrome

Tourette syndrome is a neuropsychiatric disorder that presents with motor and vocal tics most prominently along with frequent associations with ADHD, obsessive-compulsive disorder, and other disturbing behavioral symptoms. Both SPECT and FDG PET studies have demonstrated hypoperfusion in frontal and temporal lobes and basal ganglia regions (LAMPREAVE et al. 1998; SIEG et al. 1993). As in the other conditions discussed herein, the ages of the patients can confound results with changes due to maturity and/or evolution of the disease with or without comorbid features. Data from older age groups should not be assumed to apply to children in general, but they certainly suggest that theory-based studies applied to children may be helpful. As in other disorders the observed hypoperfusion is assumed to be linked to decreased neuronal activity. Improvement observed with neuroleptic treatment may be due to decreased hyperactivity in the dopaminergic system leading to clinical improvement (LAMPREAVE et al. 1998).

11.5.4 Autism

Autism currently referred to as autistic spectrum or pervasive developmental disorders is a wide-ranging gamut of deficits involving verbal and non-verbal behaviors. Pervasive developmental disorders includes autistic disorder, Asperger syndrome, and Rett syndrome among others (O'TAUMA et al. 1999; FILIPEK 1999).

Rett's syndrome is a well-known but rare neurodegenerative disorder which affects very young children, and is only seen in girls. In an effort to better understand the biological basis for this tragic disorder, PET studies have been performed using FDG and D2 receptors agonists, although conclusions are hampered by the small number of subjects. NAIDU et al. (1992) demonstrated decreased activity in the occipital cortex in association with slightly increased activity in the frontal cortex. YOSHIKAWA et al. (1991) studied six patients and suggest that impaired oxidative metabolism exists in Rett syndrome. Using $^{15}O_2$ PET they found that the cerebral metabolic rate of oxygen was decreased in five patients and oxygen extraction fraction in four when compared with three normal controls. Both measures declined with advancing age. The loss of hyperfrontality is also stressed in a study with 13 patients (LAPPALAINEN et al. 1997). SPECT-ECD brain imaging confirms decreased perfusion in the frontal and fronto-parietal cortical areas (BURRONI et al. 1997). These perfusion abnormalities become more marked in the later stages of the disease. In general, the perfusion abnormalities precede abnormal findings on MRI.

Gross brain anatomy in subjects with autism is generally normal and neuroimaging studies are inconsistent or inconclusive. The relationship of cortical migration abnormalities to this spectrum of disorders, if any, is not yet known. MRI studies in high functioning adults with autism, known as Asperger syndrome, have demonstrated abnormalities including polymicrogyria, macrogyria, and schizencephaly without a predilection for a particular region in the brain (FILIPEK 1999; CHAKOS et al. 1998). Findings from neuropathological and neuroimaging studies in groups of patients with autism can be generally summarized as: increased brain volume with patients demonstrating increased head circumference when compared both with normals and patients with other developmental abnormalities; impaired function at the corpus callosum; and impaired frontal lobe function and abnormalities in the areas of the mind where socialization responses and understanding occurs (FILIPEK 1999; DEB and THOMPSON 1998). Data from activation studies would be of potential value in investigating social responses. Data from SPECT and PET studies is only available for a small number of patients with autism many of whom are adults and are further hampered by lack of technical uniformity. Numerous findings are generally not reproduced in other studies (MÜLLER et al. 1999)

Infantile autism is currently described as a developmental disorder for which no specific neurobiological or pathological correlate is defined. SCHIFTER et al. (1994) evaluated retrospectively 13 children with the diagnosis of autism having dysfunctional social interaction skills, decreased or abnormal verbal abilities, and abnormally limited interests and abilities. Unlike other studies, they did not exclude those with significant other abnormalities such as seizure disorders and mental retardation. These children ranging in age from 4.5 to 11 years were studied using FDG PET and CT or MRI, and no common or uniform abnormality was found in the group. The most frequent abnormality found was decreased FDG uptake and for the most part this existed in patients with seizure disorders. The authors feel justified in excluding interictal foci as a cause of this finding due to the multiplicity and multifocal nature of the abnormalities. Furthermore, they conclude that the findings support other work impugning neuronal migration abnormalities, at least in part, as a significant feature. This study illustrates the myriad of technical and logistical difficulties in these and related types of disorders. The sensitivity and specificity of the various imaging studies, although interesting, are far from established but should not discourage ongoing efforts of nuclear physicians to better understand this disease and contribute potential solutions to it.

Functional neuroimaging in childhood disorders continues to be challenging and is complicated by the fact that only pooled data are available, which provides valuable albeit frequently inconsistent information. It is important to understand the large variety of issues to ensure that studies are performed in a manner most likely to enhance and complement ongoing advances in cognitive research, genetics, and therapies. Defining subject groups is difficult and made worse by frequent overlay of more than one disorder. Control groups are often not available in children and subject groups to date are very small. When radionuclide studies are performed, there is variation in scanning techniques, methods of analysis, and activation protocols. None of these factors should discourage informed investigators from further pursuing functional brain imaging research in children.

References

Abu-Judeh HH, Singh M, Masdeu JC, Abdel-Dayem HM (1998) Discordance between FDG uptake and technetium-99m HMPAO brain perfusion in acute traumatic brain injury. J Nucl Med 39:1357–1359

Aldenkamp AP, Alpherts WCJ, Dekker MJA, Overweg J (1990) Neuropsychological aspects of learning disabilities in epilepsy. Epilepsia 31:S9–S20

Allan WC, Volpe JJ (1986) Periventricular-intraventricular hemorrhage. Pediatr Clin North Am 36:47–63

Altman DI, Perlman JM, Volpe JJ, Powers WJ (1993) Cerebral oxygen metabolism in newborns. Pediatrics 92:99–104

Baenziger O, Mueller AM, Morales CG, Jaggi JL, Duc G, von Siebenthal K, Bucher H-U (1999) Cerebral blood flow and neurological outcome in the preterm infant. Eur J Pediatr 158:138–143

Barabino A, Gattorno M, Cabria M, Sormani MP, Occhi M, Villavecchia G, Gandullia P, Buoncompagni A, Castellano E, Picco P (1998) 99mTc-white cell scanning to detect gut inflammation in children with inflammatory bowel diseases or spondyloarthropathies. Clin Exp Rheumatol 16:327–334

Barrio R, Roldán MB, Alonso M, Cantón R, Camerero C (1997) Helicobacter pylori infection with parietal cell antibodies in children and adolescents with insulin dependent diabetes mellitus. J Pediatr Endocrinol Metab 10:511–516

Berdon WE (1999) Editorial comment. Pediatr Radiol 29:721

Bujanover Y, Reif S, Yahav J (1996) *Helicobacter pylori* and peptic disease in the pediatric patient. Pediatr Clin North Am 43:213–234

Burroni L, Aucone AM, Volterrani D, Hayek Y, Bertelli P, Vella A, Zappella M, Vattimo A (1997) Brain perfusion abnormalities in Rett syndrome: a qualitative and quantitative SPET study with 99mTC-ECD. Nucl Med Commun 18:527–534

Caglar M, Belzberg AS, Spruston B, Sexsmith G (1999) Time-optimized carbon-14 breath test for *Helicobacter pylori* contamination of the stomach. Clin Nucl Med 9:674–677

Çelik J, Su B, Tirén U, Finkel Y, Thoresson A, Engstrand L, Sandstedt B, Bernander S, Normark S (1998) Virulence and colonization-associated properties of *Helicobacter pylori* isolated from children and adolescents. J Infect Dis 177:247–252

Chakos MH, Esposito S, Charles C, Lieberman JA (1998) Clinical applications of neuroimaging in psychiatry. MRI Clin North Am 6:155–164

Charron M (1997) Inflammatory bowel disease in pediatric patients. Q J Nucl Med 41:309–320

Charron M, del Rosario JF, Kocoshis S (1998a) Use of technetium-tagged white blood cells in patients with Crohn's disease and ulcerative colitis: is differential diagnosis possible? Pediatr Radiol 28:871–877

Charron M, Fernando del Rosario J, Kocoshis S (1998b) Distribution of acute bowel inflammation determined by technetium-labeled white blood cells in children with inflammatory bowel disease. Inflamm Bowel Dis 4:84–88

Charron M, del Rosario FJ, Kocoshis SA (1999) Pediatric inflammatory bowel disease: assessment with scintigraphy with 99mTc white blood cells. Radiology 212:507–513

Chiron C, Raynaud C, Maziere B, Zilbovicius M, Laflamme L, Masure MC, Dulac O, Bourguignon M, Syrota A (1992) Changes in regional cerebral blood flow during brain maturation in children and adolescents. J Nucl Med 33:696–703

Chugani HT (1992) Functional brain imaging in pediatrics. Pediatr Clin North Am 39:777–799

Chugani HT (1998) A critical period of brain development: studies of cerebral glucose utilization with PET (review). Prev Med 27:184–188

Chugani HT, Phelps ME (1986) Maturational changes in cerebral function in infants determined by [18]FDG positron emission tomography. Science 231:840–843

Chugani HT, Phelps ME, Mazziotta JC (1987) Positron emission tomography study of human brain functional development. Ann Neurol 22:487–497

Corrado G, Luzzi I, Lucarelli S, Frediani T, Pacchiarotti C, Cavaliere M, Rea P, Cardi E (1998) Positive association between *Helicobacter pylori* infection and food allergy in children. Scand J Gastroenterol 33:1135–1139

Cutler AF (1997) Diagnostic tests for *Helicobacter pylori* infection. Gastroenterologist 5:202 212

David LR, Genecov DG, Camastra AA, Wilson JA, Argenta LC (1999) Positron emission tomography studies confirm the need for early surgical intervention in patients with single-suture craniosynostosis. J Craniofac Surg 10:38–42

Deb S, Thompson B (1998) Neuroimaging in autism. Br J Psychiatry 173:299–302

Debongie JC, Pauwels S, Raat A, de Meeus Y, Haot J, Mainguet P (1991) Quantification of Helicobacter pylori infection in gastritis and ulcer disease using a simple and rapid carbon-14-urea breath test. J Nucl Med 32:1192–1198

Del Rosario MA, Fitzgerald JF, Siddiqui AR, Chong SK, Croffie JM, Gupta SK (1999) Clinical applications of technetium Tc 99m hexamethyl propylene amine oxime leukocyte scan in children with inflammatory bowel disease. J Pediatr Gastroenterol Nutr 28:63–70

Denays R, Tondeur M, Foulon M, Verstraeten F, Ham H, Piepsz A, Noel P (1989) Regional brain blood flow in congenital dysphasia: studies with technetium-99m HM-PAO SPECT. J Nucl Med 30:1825–1829

Denays R, Tondeur M, Toppet V, Ham H, Piepsz A, Spehl M, Rubinstein M, Noel P (1990) Cerebral palsy: initial experience with Tc-99m HMPAO SPECT of the brain. Radiology 175:111–116

Devinsky O, Bear D (1984) Varieties of aggressive behavior in temporal lobe epilepsy. Am J. Psychiatry 141:651–656

Dixon AK, Dendy P (1998) How much does radiation dose matter? The Lancet 352:1082–1083

Duggan AE, Usmani I, Neal KR, Logan RF (1998) Appendicectomy, childhood hygiene, *Helicobacter pylori* status, and risk of inflammatory bowel disease: a case control study. Gut 43:494–498

Ernst M (1999) PET in child psychiatry: the risks and benefits of studying normal healthy children. Prog Neuropsychopharmacol Biol Psychiatry 23:561–570

Ernst M, Freed ME, Zametkin AJ (1998) Health hazards of radiation exposure in the context of brain imaging research: special consideration for children. J Nucl Med 39:689–698

Fall CH, Goggin PM, Hawtin P, Fine D, Duggleby S (1997) Growth in infancy, infant feeding, childhood living conditions, and *Helicobacter pylori* infection at age 70. Arch Dis Child 77:310–314

Filipek PA (1999) Neuroimaging in the developmental disorders: the state of the science. J Child Psychol Psychiatry 40:113–128

Gainey MA, Siegel JA, Smergel EM, Jara BJ (1988) Indium-111-labeled white blood cells: dosimetry in children. J Nucl Med 29:689–694

Galaske RG, Schober O, Heyer R (1988) 99mTc-HM-PAO and 123I-amphetamine cerebral scintigraphy: a new, noninvasive method in determination of brain death in children. Eur J Nucl Med 14:446–452

Gold BD, Khanna B, Huang LM, Lee CY, Banatvala N (1997) *Helicobacter pylori* acquisition in infancy after decline of maternal passive immunity. Pediatr Res 41:641–646

Goodman JM, Heck LL, Moore BD (1985) Confirmation of brain death with portable isotope angiography: a review of 204 consecutive cases. Neurosurgery 16:492–497

Gordon I (1996) Cerebral blood flow imaging in paediatrics: a review. Nucl Med Commun 17:1021–1029

Goshen E, Zwas ST, Shahar E, Tadmor R (1996) The role of Tc-99m-HMPAO brain SPET in paediatric traumatic brain injury. Nucl Med Commun 17:418–422

Gottrand F, Cullu F, Turck D, Vincent P, Michaud L, Husson MO, Martin Delasalle E, Farriaux JP (1997) Normal gastric histology in *Helicobacter pylori* -infected children. J Pediatr Gastroenterol Nutr 25:74–78

Granström M, Tindberg Y, Blennow M (1997) Seroepidemiology of *Helicobacter pylori* infection in a cohort of children monitored from 6 months to 11 years of age. J Clin Microbiol 35:468–470

Greisen G (1986) Cerebral blood flow in preterm infants during the first week of life. Acta Paediatr Scand 75:43–51

Greisen G (1990) Cerebral blood flow in mechanically ventilated preterm neonates. Dan Med Bull 2:124–131

Greisen G, Pryds O (1988) Intravenous 133Xe clearance in preterm neonates with respiratory distress. Internal validation of CBF, as a measure of global cerebral blood flow. Scand J Clin Lab Invest 48:673–678

Günel E, Findik D, Caglayan O, Caglayan F, Topgaç Z (1998) *Helicobacter pylori* and hypergastrinemia in children with recurrent abdominal pain. Pediatr Surg Int 14:40–42

Hall E (1999) Commentary. Pediatr Radiol 29:721–722

Hassall E (1994) Clinical practise guidelines for suspected peptic ulcer disease in children. BC Med J 36:538–539

Heaney A, Collins JS, Tham TC, Watson PR, McFarland JR, Bamford KB (1998) A prospective study of the management of the young *Helicobacter pylori* negative dyspeptic patient – can gastroscopies be saved in clinical practice? Eur J Gastroenterol Hepatol 10:953–956

Henze E, Malfertheiner P, Clausen M, Burkhardt H, Adam WE (1990) Validation of a simplified carbon-14-urea breath test for routine use for detecting *Helicobacter pylori* noninvasively. J Nucl Med 31:1940–1944

Hill P, Rode J (1998) *Helicobacter pylori* in ectopic gastric mucosa in Meckel's diverticulum. Pathology 30:7–9

Holmes GL (1991) Do seizures cause brain damage? Epilepsia 32:S14–828

Holzman BH, Curless RG, Sfakianakis GN, Ajmone-Marsan C, Montes JE (1983) Radionuclide cerebral perfusion scintigraphy in determination of brain death in children. Neurology 33:1027–1031

Hornemann F, Nilius M, Malfertheiner P, Bartmann P (1997) Seroprevalence of *Helicobacter pylori* in German infants and children. Helicobacter 2:176–179

Huang FC, Chang MH, Hsu HY, Lee PI, Shun CT (1999) Long-term follow-up of duodenal ulcer in children before and after eradication of *Helicobacter pylori*. J Pediatr Gastroenterol Nutr 28:76–80

Ierardi E, Francavilla R, Balzano T, Negrini R, Francavilla A (1998) Autoantibodies reacting with gastric antigens in *Helicobacter pylori* associated body gastritis of dyspeptic children. Ital J Gastroenterol Hepatol 30:478–480

Jacobs A, Put E, Ingels M, Bossuyt A (1994) Prospective evaluation of technetium-99m HMPAO-SPECT in mild and moderate traumatic brain injury. J Nucl Med 35:942–947

Kao CH, Wang SJ, Yeh SH (1994) The relationship among the quantitative perfusion-defect indices in Tc-99m HMPAO brain SPECT, IQ test, and involved extremities in children with cerebral palsy due to perinatal asphyxia. Clin Nucl Med 19:309–313

Kerrigan JF, Chugani HT, Phelps ME (1991) Regional cerebral glucose metabolism in clinical subtypes of cerebral palsy. Pediatr Neurol 7:415–425

Kinnala A, Suhonen-Polvi H, Aarimaa T, Kero P, Korvenranta H, Ruotsalainen U, Bergman J, Haaparanta M, Solin O, Nuutila P, Wegelius U (1996) Cerebral metabolic rate for glucose during the first six months of life: an FDG positron emission tomography study. Arch Dis Child 74:F153–F157

Kolho KL, Rautelin H, Lindahl H, Savilahti E (1998) *Helicobacter pylori*-positive gastritis in pediatric patients with chronic inflammatory bowel disease. J Pediatr Gastroenterol 27:292–295

Lampreave JL, Molina V, Mardomingo MJ, Bittini A, Dominguez P, Almoguera I, Rubia FJ, Carreras JL (1998) Technetium-99m-HMPAO in Tourette's syndrome on neuroleptic therapy and after withdrawal. J Nucl Med 39:624–628

Landau WM, Kleffner FR (1957) Syndrome of acquired aphasia with convulsive disorder in children. Neurology 7:523–530

Lappalainen R, Liewendahl K, Sainio K et al (1997) Brain perfusion SPECT and EEG findings in Rett syndrome. Acta Neurol Scand 95:44–50

Larar GN, Nagel JS (1992) Technetium-99m-HMPAO cerebral perfusion scintigraphy: considerations for timely brain death declaration. J Nucl Med 33:2209–2213

Laurin NR, Dreidger AA, Hurwitz GA, Mattar AG, Powe JE, Chamberlain MJ, Zabel PL, Pavlovsky WF (1989) Cerebral perfusion imaging with technetium-99m HM-PAO in brain death and severe central nervous system injury. J Nucl Med 30:1627–1635

Lee JD, Kim DI, Ryu YH, Whang GJ, Park CI, Kim DG (1998) Technetium-99m-ECD brain SPECT in cerebral palsy: comparison with MRI. J Nucl Med 39:619–623

Leide-Svegborn S, Stenstrom K, Olofsson M, Mattsson S, Nilsson LE, Nosslin B, Pau K, Johansson L, Erlandsson B, Hellborg R, Skog G (1999) Biokinetics and radiation doses for carbon-14 urea in adults and children undergoing the *Helicobacter pylori* breath test. Eur J Nucl Med 26:573–580

Lesser R, Luders H, Wylie E et al (1986) Mental deterioration in epilepsy. Epilepsia 27:S105–S123

Ljung B (1997) The child in diagnostic nuclear medicine. Eur J Nucl Med 24:683–690

Lou HC, Henriksen L, Bruhn P, Borner H, Bieber Nielsen J (1989) Striatal dysfunction in attention deficit and hyperkinetic disorder. Arch Neurol 46:48–52

Luzza F, Mancuso M, Imeneo M, Mesuraca L, Contaldo A, Giancotti L, La Vecchia AM, Docimo C, Pensabene L, Strisciuglio P, Pallone F, Guandalini S (1999) *Helicobacter pylori* infection in children with celiac disease: prevalence and clinicopathologic features. J Pediatr Gastroenterol Nutr 28:143–146

Malaty HM, Graham DY, Wattigney WA, Srinivasan SR, Osato M, Berenson GS (1999) Natural history of *Helicobacter pylori* infection in childhood:12-year follow-up cohort study in a biracial community. Clin Infect Dis 28:279–282

Maquet P, Hirsch E, Dive D et al (1990) Cerebral glucose utilization during sleep in Landau-Kleffner syndrome: a PET study. Epilepsia 31:778–783

Mitchell HM, Hazell SL, Bohane TD, Hu P, Chen M, Li YY (1999) The prevalence of antibody to CagA in children is not a marker for specific disease. J Pediatr Gastroenterol Nutr 28:71–75

Müller RA, Behen ME, Rothermel RD, Chugani DC, Muzik O, Mangner TJ, Chugani HT (1999) Brain mapping of language and auditory perception in high-functioning autistic adults: a PET study. J Autism Dev Disorders 29:19–31

Naidu S, Wong DF, Kitt C, Wenk G, Moser HW (1992) Positron emission tomography in the Rett syndrome: clinical, biochemical and pathological correlates. Brain Dev 14 [Suppl]:S75–79

Nardone G, Rocco A, Budillon G (1998) Does *Helicobacter pylori* play a role in inflammatory bowel disease? Ital J Gastroenterol Hepatol 30:134–137

Narla LD, Hingsbergen EA, Jones JE (1999) Adult diseases in children. Pediatr Radiol 29:244–254

Ng DK, Liu JH, Ho JC (1997) Paediatric upper gastrointestinal endoscopy: a 2-year review. Chin Med J (Engl) 110:587–589

Oderda G, Ponzetto A, Boero M, Bellis D, Forni M, Vaira D, Ansaldi N (1997) Family treatment of symptomatic children with *Helicobacter pylori* infection. Ital J Gastroenterol Hepatol 29:509–514

O'Tuama LA, Treves ST (1993) Brain single-photon emission computed tomography for behavior disorders in children (review). Semin Nucl Med 23:255–264

O'Tuama LA, Urion DK, Janicek MJ, Treves ST, Bjornson B, Moriarty JM (1992) Regional cerebral perfusion in Landau-Kleffner syndrome and related childhood aphasias. J Nucl Med 33:1758–1765

O'Tuama LA, Dickstein DP, Neeper R, Gascon G (1999) Functional brain imaging in neuropsychiatric disorders of childhood. J Child Neurol 14:207–221

Parente F, Molteni P, Bollani S, Maconi G, Vago L, Duca PG, Rembacken B, Axon AT, Bianchi Porro G (1997) Prevalence of Helicobacter pylori infection and related upper gastrointestinal lesions in patients with inflammatory bowel diseases. A cross-sectional study with matching. Scand J Gastroenterol 32:1140–1146

Pintelon H, Jonckheer MH, Piepsz A (1994) Paediatric nuclear medicine procedures: routine sedation or management of anxiety? Nucl Med Commun 15:664–666

Pryds O, Greisen G, Lou H, Friis-Hansen B (1990) Vasoparalysis associated with brain damage in asphyxiated term infants. J Pediatr 117:119–125

Risch SC (1997) Recent advances in depression research: from stress to molecular biology and brain imaging. J Clin Psychiatry 58:3–6

Roebuck DJ (1999) Risk and benefit in paediatric radiology. Pediatr Radiol 29:637–640

Rothenbacher D, Bode G, Berg G, Knayer U, Gonser T, Adler G, Brenner H (1999) *Helicobacter pylori* among preschool children and their parents: evidence of parent-child transmission. J Infect Dis 179:398–402

Rubinstein M, Denays R, Ham HR, Piepsz A, VanPachterbeke T, Haumont D, Noel P (1989) Functional imaging of brain maturation in humans using iodine-123 iodoamphetamine and SPECT. J Nucl Med 30:1982–1985

Salardi S, Cacciari E, Menegatti M, Landi F, Mazzanti L, Stella FA, Pirazzoli P, Vaira D (1999) *Helicobacter pylori* and type 1 diabetes mellitus in children. J Pediatr Gastroenterol Nutr 28:307–309

Schiepers C, Verbruggen A, Casaer P, De Roo M (1997) Normal brain perfusion pattern of technetium-99m-ethylcysteinate dimer in children. J Nucl Med 38:1115–1120

Schifter T, Hoffman JM, Hatten P, Hanson MW, Coleman E, DeLong GR (1994) Neuroimaging in infantile autism. J Child Neurol 9:155–161

Sherazi Z, Gordon I (1996) Quality of care: identification and quantitation of the process of care among children undergoing nuclear medicine studies. Nucl Med Commun 17:363–366

Sieg KG, Buckingham D, Gaffney GR, Preston DF, Sieg KG (1993) Tc-99m HMPAO SPECT brain imaging of Gilles de la Tourette's syndrome. Clin Nucl Med 18:255

Stabin MG, Gelfand MJ (1998) Dosimetry of pediatric nuclear medicine procedures. Q J Nucl Med 42:93–112

Steen T, Berstad K, Meling T, Berstad A (1995) Reproducibility of the 14 C urea breath test repeated after 1 week. Am J Gastroenterol 90:2103–2105

Stringer DA (1989) Pediatric gastrointestinal imaging. Decker, Philadelphia, Pa

Swedo SE, Schapiro MB, Grady CL, Cheslow DL, Leonard HL, Kumar A, Friedland R, Rapoport SI, Rapoport JL (1989) Cerebral glucose metabolism in childhood-onset obsessive-compulsive disorder. Arch Gen Psychiatry 46:518–523

Takahashi T, Shirane R, Sato S, Yoshimoto T (1999) Developmental changes of cerebral blood flow and oxygen metabolism in children. AJNR Am J Neuroradiol 20:917–922

Tannock R (1998) Attention deficit hyperactivity disorder: advances in cognitive, neurobiological, and genetic research. J Child Psychol Psychiatr 39:65–69

Tuchman RF (1994) Epilepsy, language, and behavior: clinical models in childhood. J Child Neurol 9:95–102

Vaira D, Menegatti M, Salardi S, Ali A, Altomare Stella F, Figura N, Landi F, Holton J, Farinelli S, Cuccaro V, Miglioli M, Cacciari E (1998) *Helicobacter pylori* and diminished growth in children: is it simply a marker of deprivation. Ital J Gastroenterol Hepatol 30:129–133

Valle G, Ciritella P, Bonetti MG, Dicembrino F, Perrone E, Perna GP (1993) Considerations of brain death on a SPECT cerebral perfusion study. Clin Nucl Med 18:953–954

van der Kolk BA (1997) The psychobiology of posttraumatic stress disorder (review). J Clin Psychiatry 58 [Suppl 9]:16–24

Vandenplas Y, Blecker U (1998) *Helicobacter pylori* infection in children. Acta Paediatr 87:1105–1112

Weiss S (1993) Sedation of pediatric patients for nuclear medicine procedures (review). Semin Nucl Med 23:190–198

Wewer V, Andersen LP, Paerregaard A, Gernow AB, Hart Hansen JP, Matzen P, Krasilnikoff PA (1998) The prevalence and related symptomatology of Helicobacter pylori in children with recurrent abdominal pain. Acta Paediatr 87:830-835.

Wieler H, Marohl K, Kaiser KP, Klawki P, Frossler H (1993) Tc-99m HMPAO cerebral scintigraphy. A reliable, noninvasive method for determination of brain death. Clin Nucl Med 18:104–109

Wilson K, Gordon L, Selby JB (1993) The diagnosis of brain death with Tc-99m HMPAO. Clin Nucl Med 18:428–434

Yamada K, Tsuzura S, Matsuda H (1995) Brain MRI and single photon emission computed tomography in severe athetotic cerebral palsy: a comparative study with mental and motor disorders (in Japanese). No To Hattatsu 27:269–275

Yamaki T, Imahori Y, Ohomori Y et al (1996) Cerebral hemodynamics and metabolism of severe diffuse brain injury measured by PET. J Nucl Med 37:1166–1170

Yoshikawa H, Fueki N, Suzuki H, Sakuragawa N, Masaaki I (1991) Cerebral blood flow and oxygen metabolism in Rett syndrome. J Child Neurol 6:237–242

Younger SJ, Landefeld CS, Coulton CJ, Jukialis BW, Leary M (1989) "Brain death" and organ retrieval. A cross-sectional survey.

Basics of Scintigraphic Imaging

12 Radiopharmaceuticals: Recent Developments and Trends

K. Verbeke, A. Verbruggen

Contents

12.1 Production of Radiopharmaceuticals, Quality Control and Availability 197
12.2 Perfusion Agents 198
12.2.1 Myocardial Perfusion Imaging Agents 198
12.2.2 Brain Perfusion Imaging Agents 201
12.2.3 Renal Function Imaging Agents 203
12.2.4 Lung Ventilation Imaging Agents 203
12.3 Metabolism Agents 204
12.3.1 Glucose Metabolism 204
12.3.2 Amino Acid Metabolism 204
12.3.3 Hypoxia Agents 205
12.4 Peptides 207
12.4.1 Somatostatin Receptor Tracers 207
12.4.1.1 ^{111}Indium-Octreotide 207
12.4.1.2 P587 and P829 208
12.4.2 Radioiodinated Vasoactive Intestinal Peptide 208
12.4.3 Peptides for Thrombus Imaging 208
12.5 Receptor Tracers 210
12.5.1 Benzodiazepine Receptor Agents 210
12.5.2 Serotonergic (5-HT) Receptor Tracers 211
12.5.3 Dopaminergic Receptor Tracers 213
12.6 Cell Labeling 214
12.6.1 Red Blood Cell Labeling 214
12.6.2 White Blood Cell Labeling 215

12.1 Production of Radiopharmaceuticals, Quality Control and Availability

Radionuclides used in nuclear medicine are mostly artificial. They are primarily produced in a reactor or cyclotron and supplied by commercial companies to individual nuclear medicine departments and institutions. On the other hand, some radionuclides, in particular short-lived ones, are dispensable at any time due to the availability of appropriate radionuclide generators. By far the most important generator in nuclear medicine is the ^{99}Mo/^{99m}Tc generator, which has led to an almost unlimited availability of ^{99m}Tc. The excellent radiation characteristics of ^{99m}Tc and the commercial availability of efficient labeling kits make this generator the basis of current nuclear medicine clinics.

The very short-lived positron-emitting radionuclides used in clinical positron emission tomography (PET) ^{18}F, ^{11}C, ^{13}N and ^{15}O are only available at or near institutions which have cyclotron facilities and cannot be transported to remote institutions or hospitals due to their rapid decay. Since these facilities are extremely expensive, they are not evenly spread worldwide. Table 12.1 shows the distribution of cyclotron facilities for production of PET radiopharmaceuticals throughout the world. Approximately 80% of all cyclotrons are situated in Europe and the United States. When expressed as number of inhabitants per cyclotron, it can be seen that particularly Belgium and the Scandinavian countries have a high density of cyclotrons.

Numerous PET centers, especially in Germany, the United Kingdom, and the United States, perform clinical imaging but do not have a cyclotron. These sites are usually limited to the use of PET radiotracers labeled with ^{18}F ($t_{1/2}$=110 min), provided by nearby facilities. In the United States a joint venture between CTI and a group of private investors, called P.E.T. Net Pharmaceutical Services, currently operates 13 PET isotope distribution centers: Sacramento (Calif.), Palo Alto (Calif.), Los Angeles (Calif.), Phoenix (Ariz.), Nashville (Tenn.), Tampa (Fla.), Atlanta (Ga.), Chicago (Ill.), Baltimore (Md.), Omaha (Neb.), New York (N.Y.), Royal Oak (Mich.), and Peoria (Ill.). These centers produce and dispense ^{18}F-fluorodeoxy-glucose (FDG) for PET and single photon emission computed tomography (SPECT) imaging facilities in their area.

Incorporation of the cyclotron-produced PET radionuclides into radiopharmaceuticals is performed using dedicated radiochemistry synthesis modules. These units are generally designed as closed systems to minimize radiation exposure, are computer controlled, and are operated automatically. Quality con-

K. Verbeke, A. Verbruggen
Department of Radiopharmacy, UZ Gasthuisberg, Herestraat 49, B-3000 Leuven, Belgium

Table 12.1. Distribution of cyclotron facilities throughout the world

		No. of cyclo-trons	No. of inhab-itants ($\times 10^3$) per cyclotron
Europe[a]	Austria	1	8134
	Belgium	6	1696
	Denmark	2	2667
	Finland	3	1716
	France	3	19,602
	Germany	16	5130
	Italy	3	18,928
	Netherlands	3	15,731
	Norway	1	4420
	Russia	1	146,861
	Spain	2	19,567
	Sweden	3	4443
	Switzerland	3	3630
	United Kingdom	4	19,657
	Total	49	
United States[b]	Arizona	1	
	Arkansas	1	
	California	9	
	Connecticut	1	
	Florida	2	
	Georgia	4	
	Hawaii	1	
	Illinois	3	
	Indiana	1	
	Iowa	1	
	Kansas	1	
	Louisiana	2	
	Maryland	3	
	Massachusetts	1	
	Michigan	4	
	Minnesota	1	
	Missouri	2	
	Nebraska	1	
	New York	13	
	North Carolina	3	
	Ohio	5	
	Pennsylvania	2	
	Tennessee	3	
	Texas	4	
	Utah	1	
	Washington	1	
	West Virginia	1	
	Wisconsin	1	
	Total	73	3703
Other countries[b]	Australia	2	9306
	Canada	3	10,225
	Israel	1	5644
	Japan	20	6297
	Korea	1	46,417
	Saudi Arabia	1	20,786
	Taiwan	1	21,908
	Total	29	

[a] Data from B. Gulyas, Tempus Medical Biology Program, Debrecen University Medical School, Debrecen, Hungary; available at: http://www.neuro.ki.se/neuro/pet/europet.html
[b] Data available at http://www.icppet.org/sitelist.html

trol of the end-products can be performed using radio gas chromatography or radio high-pressure liquid chromatography (HPLC) and should be carried out under the responsibility of a qualified radiopharmacist/radiochemist. Table 12.2 depicts the availability of these synthesis modules from different commercial suppliers. A synthesis unit for production of ^{18}F-FDG can be purchased from each of the companies and also a unit for ^{11}C-CH_3I is readily available. Nuclear Interfaces provides a module which can be used for different nucleophilic substitution reactions with ^{18}F-fluoride using different control programs. In this way, receptor ligands, such as ^{18}F-methylspiperone, ^{18}F-methylbenperidol, ^{18}F-altanserin, as well as ^{18}F-FMISO or ^{18}F-labeled fatty acids, can be synthesized.

12.2 Perfusion Agents

12.2.1 Myocardial Perfusion Imaging Agents

Because of nearly optimal physical properties of the radionuclide, ^{99m}Tc-labeled perfusion agents offer several advantages over ^{201}TlCl for myocardial perfusion imaging. Besides ^{99m}Tc-labeled sestamibi, two other ^{99m}Tc-based perfusion agents have been developed, namely ^{99m}Tc-tetrofosmin (Kelly et al. 1993; Higley et al. 1993) and ^{99m}Tc-furifosmin (Colombo et al. 1992; Rosetti et al. 1992). Each of these agents is a lipophilic mono-ionic cation (Fig. 12.1) and can be prepared in the nuclear medicine department using commercially available freeze-dried kits (Tables 12.3, 12.4).

^{99m}Tc-tetrofosmin is a ^{99m}Tc(V) phosphine dioxo cation which can be prepared by simple addition of ^{99m}Tc generator eluate to the labeling vial. After incubation at room temperature for 15 min, the radiochemical purity (RP) of the labeled product exceeds 95% (Higley et al. 1993). Gluconate, present in the kit, is necessary to keep technetium in a +5 oxidation state after reduction by forming a relatively weak ^{99m}Tc-gluconate intermediary complex. Sulfosalicylic acid presumably accelerates ligand exchange from ^{99m}Tc(V)gluconate to ^{99m}Tc(V)dioxo-tetrofosmin. The radiopharmaceutical can be administered up to 8 h post reconstitution (RP>90%).

^{99m}Tc-furifosmin is a mixed ligand complex comprised of a tetradentate Schiff base ligand (Furomine) and two monodentate phosphine ligands (Trifosmin, TMPP) which are situated in the trans position to

Table 12.2. Availability of synthesis modules for production of positron emission tomography (PET) radiopharmaceuticals

	Nuclear Interfaces (Germany)	Coincid-ence (Belgium)	IBA (Belgium)	CTI (USA)	GE (USA)	EBCO (Canada)
^{18}F-FDG	+	+	+	+	+	+
^{18}F-fluoride nucleophilic substitution	+	–	–	–	–	–
^{18}F-F_2 electrophilic substitution	+	–	–	–	–	–
^{11}C-CH_3I	+	–	+	+	+	+
^{11}C-CO_2	+	–	+	–	–	–
^{13}N-NH_3	+	–	+	–	–	–
^{15}O-H_2O	–	–	+	+	–	+
^{11}C-HCN	–	–	+	+	–	–
$^{11}C^{15}O$	–	–	–	+	–	–

Table 12.3. Properties of the commercially available labeling kits for preparation of ^{99m}Tc-labeled myocardial perfusion imaging agents

Brand name of labeling kit	MIBI Cardiolite	Tetrofosmin Myoview	Furifosmin Technescan Q12
Manufacturer	DuPont Pharma, (Billerica, Mass.)	Amersham-Nycomed (Buckinghamshire, UK)	Mallinckrodt Medical (St. Louis, Mo.)
Chemical name of ligand	2-methoxy-2-isobutyl isonitrile	1,2-bis[bis(2-ethoxyethyl)-phosphino]ethane	1. tris(3-methoxy-1-propyl) phosphine; 2. 1,2-bis-[dihydro-2,2,5,5-tetramethyl-3(2H)-furanone-4-methyleneamino]ethane
Other names	^{99m}Tc-sestamibi (USAN)[a] ^{99m}Tc-hexamibi	–	1. TMPP, trifosmin (USAN) 2. furomine (WHO/INN) furimine (USAN)
Composition of labeling kit	$Cu(MIBI)_4BF_4$ 1.0 mg $SnCl_2$ $2H_2O$ 0.075 mg L-cysteine HCl monohydrate 1.0 mg sodium citrate dihydrate 2.6 mg mannitol 20.0 mg	Tetrofosmin 0.23 mg $SnCl_2$ $2H_2O$ 0.030 mg disodium sulfosalicylate 0.32 mg sodium D-gluconate 1.0 mg sodium hydrogen carbonate 1.8 mg	Trifosmin 1.5 mg furomine 20.0 mg sodium ascorbate 2.0 mg sodium carbonate 1.5 mg g-cyclodextrin 50.0 mg

[a] Other name for the ^{99m}Tc-labeled complex which contains six ligand molecules

Table 12.4. Guidelines for labeling and characteristics of ^{99m}Tc-labeled myocardial perfusion imaging agents. *RT* room temperature

	^{99m}Tc-MIBI	^{99m}Tc-Tetrofosmin	^{99m}Tc-Furifosmin
Oxidation state of ^{99m}Tc	+1	+5	+3
Charge of the complex	+1	+1	+1
Incubation	10 min 100°C	15 min RT	15 min 100°C
Max. activity (GBq)	5.56	8.8	20
Volume (ml)	1–3	4–8	2–3
Eluate restrictions	None	Generator last eluted within 72 h, eluate not older than 6 h	None
pH after reconstitution	5.5	7.5–9.0	9–10
Stability after reconstitution (h)	6	8	8

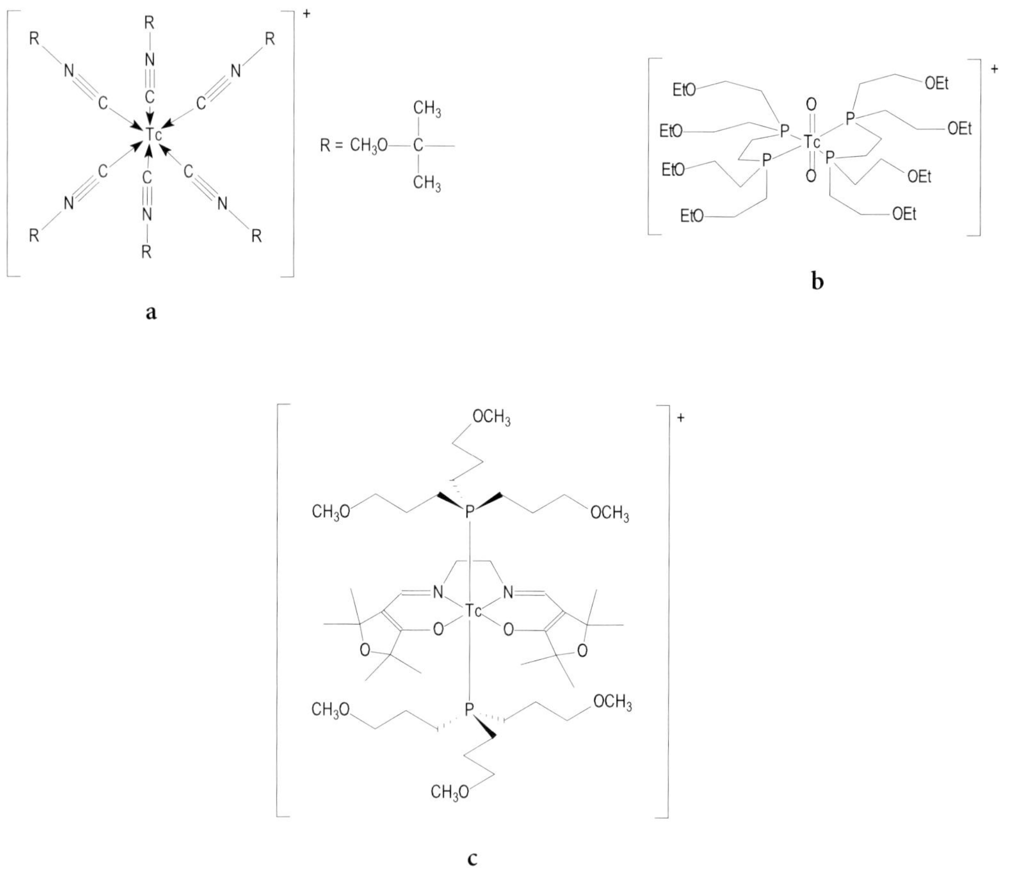

Fig. 12.1a–c. Structures of ^{99m}Tc-labeled myocardial perfusion imaging agents. **a** ^{99m}Tc-MIBI; **b** ^{99m}Tc-tetrofosmin; **c** ^{99m}Tc-furifosmin

each other. Whereas the initial procedure for preparation of ^{99m}Tc-furifosmin involved two steps (forming first the ^{99m}Tc(V) Schiff base intermediate, then reacting with TMPP), a one-vial kit is now available commercially. Labeling is carried out by addition of an appropriate amount of $^{99m}TcO_4^-$ to the kit vial and heating the mixture for 15 min in a boiling-water bath. The phosphine acts both as reductant for pertechnetate and as ligand to bind reduced technetium. For this reason stannous ion is not necessary in the labeling kit to form the ^{99m}Tc complex.

To assess the radiochemical purity of the ^{99m}Tc-labeled agents, simple quality control procedures (thin-layer chromatography or separation on a Sep-Pak cartridge) are proposed by the manufacturers. Using the appropriate stationary and mobile phase (Table 12.5), the amount of ^{99m}Tc complex, $^{99m}TcO_4^-$ and $^{99m}TcO_2$ can easily and rapidly be determined.

Although the images obtained with these new tracer agents are generally similar, there are differences in the myocardial kinetics and body distribution. Unlike ^{201}TlCl, the ^{99m}Tc-labeled perfusion agents accumulate in the myocardium by passive diffusion and are not transported by the Na^+-K^+-ATPase enzymatic pump and the redistribution of ^{99m}Tc-labeled agents is negligible. For each of the tracer agents, myocardial uptake is proportional to blood flow and amounts to approximately 1.0% for ^{99m}Tc-MIBI (Wackers et al. 1989), 1.2% for ^{99m}Tc-tetrofosmin (Higley et al. 1993), and 2.2% for ^{99m}Tc-furifosmin (Rossetti et al. 1994) at rest, and 1.4, 1.1, and 2.4%, respectively during exercise. Heart-to-lung and heart-to-liver ratios of the three ^{99m}Tc-labeled agents are presented in Table 12.6.

Whereas these ^{99m}Tc-labeled agents were originally developed as myocardial perfusion agents, they have been reported to be substrates for P-glycoprotein (Pgp), the product of the human multidrug resistance gene (MDR1), which confers resistance to drugs by transporting cytotoxic agents out of cells (Piwnica-Worms et al. 1993; Ballinger et al. 1996, 1997). As a consequence, they can be used for func-

Table 12.5. Systems proposed by the manufacturer for quality control of ^{99m}Tc-labeled myocardial perfusion imaging agents. *RF* ratio to the front of the chromatogram

	^{99m}Tc-MIBI TLC	^{99m}Tc-Tetrofosmin TLC	^{99m}Tc-Furifosmin Sep-Pak
Stationary phase	Baker-Flex aluminum oxide	Gelman ITLC/SG	Sep-Pak Alumina A cartridges
Mobile phase	Ethanol	Acetone/dichloromethane (35/65)	1. Absolute ethanol (10 ml); 2. 0.9% NaCl (10 ml)
^{99m}Tc-complex	RF=1	RF=0.2–0.8	Elutes in ethanol fraction
$^{99m}TcO_4^-$	RF=0	RF=1	Elutes in 0.9% NaCl fraction
$^{99m}TcO_2$	RF=0	RF=0	Remains on Sep-Pak

Table 12.6. Heart-to-lung and heart-to-liver ratios at rest and during exercise at different time points after injection of ^{99m}Tc-labeled myocardial perfusion imaging agents in humans

		^{99m}Tc-MIBI		^{99m}Tc-Tetrofosmin		^{99m}Tc-Furifosmin	
Time point (min)		Rest	Exercise	Rest	Exercise	Rest	Exercise
15	Heart/lung	–	–	1.9±0.2	1.9±0.3	1.3±0.2	1.5±0.2
	Heart/liver	–	–	0.7±0.1	1.2±0.3	0.6±0.05	0.7±0.1
30	Heart/lung	2.2±0.1	2.3±0.2	2.0±0.4	2.2±0.5	1.5±0.2	1.7±0.2
	Heart/liver	0.5±0.1	1.4±0.2	1.0±0.2	1.4±0.3	0.6±0.3	0.8±0.5
60	Heart/lung	2.4±0.1	2.4±0.2	2.1±0.3	2.1±0.4	1.6±0.5	1.7±0.3
	Heart/liver	0.6±0.1	1.8±0.3	1.3±0.4	1.6±0.4	1.4±0.5	1.6±0.3

tional imaging of multidrug resistance in tumors (see chap. 16).

12.2.2 Brain Perfusion Imaging Agents

Although in recent years no new radiopharmaceuticals for brain perfusion imaging have emerged, considerable efforts have been made in this field to improve technical aspects regarding their preparation and stability and to ascertain and compare the individual value of the established radiopharmaceuticals, namely ^{99m}Tc-d,l-HMPAO and ^{99m}Tc-l,l-ECD (Fig. 12.2; Table 12.7).

^{99m}Tc labeled d,l-HMPAO can be prepared by reconstitution of the commercially available Ceretec kit (Amersham-Nycomed, Buckinghamshire, UK) with generator eluate. However, to ensure adequate radiochemical purity of the resulting ^{99m}Tc preparation, severe restrictions are imposed by the manufacturer on the volume, radioactive concentration, and age of the generator eluate and the total radioactivity added to the kit. Moreover, due to the chemical instability of

Table 12.7. Properties of the commercially available labeling kits for preparation of ^{99m}Tc-labeled brain perfusion imaging agents

	d,l-HMPAO	l,l-ECD
Brand name	Ceretec	Neurolite
Manufacturer	Amersham-Nycomed (Buckinghamshire, UK)	DuPont Pharma (Billerica, Mass.)
Chemical name	[RR,SS]-4,8-diaza-3,6,6,9-tetramethylundecane-2,10-dione bisoxime	N,N'-2-ethylenediylbis-l-cysteine diethyl ester
Other names	Exametazime hexamethyl propylene amine oxime	Bicisate l,l-ethylcysteinate dimer
Composition of labeling kit	Exametazime, 0.5 mg; $SnCl_2$ $2H_2O$, 7.6 µg; NaCl, 4.5 mg	A: ECD 2HCl, 0.9 mg; $SnCl_2$ $2H_2O$, 0.072 mg; Na_2EDTA $2H_2O$, 0.36 mg; mannitol, 24 mg. B: phosphate buffer, pH 7.2–8.0

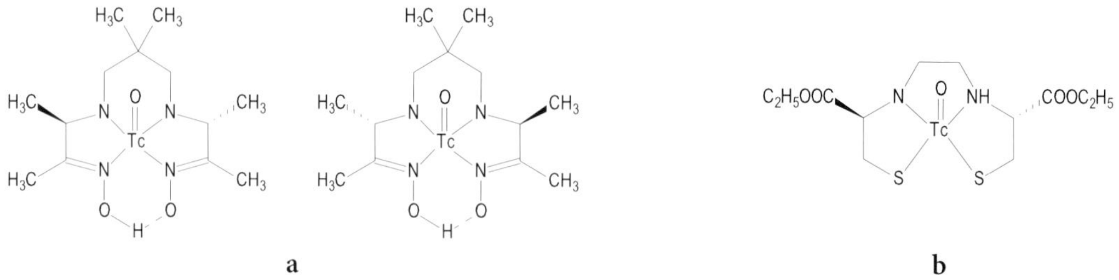

Fig. 12.2a, b. Structures of ^{99m}Tc-labeled brain perfusion imaging agents. **a** ^{99m}Tc-d,l-HMPAO (mixture of d,d (=d) and l,l (=l) isomers), and **b** ^{99m}Tc-l,l-ECD

^{99m}Tc-d,l-HMPAO (conversion of the lipophilic primary complex to a more hydrophilic secondary complex or directly to $^{99m}TcO_4^-$), the preparation should be administered within 30 min after reconstitution. Eluate age and radioactive concentration influence the level of oxidants formed through radiolysis. Due to the low amount of stannous ion (7.6 µg $SnCl_2 \cdot 2H_2O$ at the time of formulation of the kit), only very little amounts of oxidants can be tolerated. In addition, the primary complex is also susceptible to radiolysis (Tubergen et al. 1991) which explains the radioactive concentration restrictions.

To overcome these severe restrictions, several procedures for stabilization of the primary ^{99m}Tc-d,l-HMPAO complex have been reported (Hung et al. 1989; Ballinger and Gulenchyn 1991; Billinghurst et al. 1991; Sampson and Solanki 1991; Anon 1989; Lang et al. 1989), two of which merit special attention. Weisner et al. (1993) described a method for stabilizing 1.11 GBq-^{99m}Tc-d,l-HMPAO preparations by addition of 200 µg cobalt chloride hexahydrate in 2 ml water shortly (within 2 min) after reconstitution of the kit with pertechnetate. In this way, a preparation can be used up to 5 h after reconstitution. Mang'era et al. (1995) studied this method in more detail and found that high-activity preparations (up to 5.55 GBq) can also be stabilized using this method. Radiochemical purity (percent of primary lipophilic complex) exceeds 85% and clinical usefulness for both brain perfusion and white cell labeling is retained up to 6 h after reconstitution. As a consequence, it is possible to prepare a multidose preparation of ^{99m}Tc-d,l-HMPAO.

In the United States the package insert of Ceretec kits (Amersham-Nycomed, Buckinghamshire, UK) prescribes to stabilize the reconstituted ^{99m}Tc-d,l-HMPAO preparation with methylene blue and adjustment of the pH with phosphate buffer. For this purpose a complete labeling set contains the labeling vial with the exametazime ligand plus stannous chloride, a vial of methylene blue injection USP 1% and a vial of 0.003 M monobasic sodium phosphate USP and dibasic sodium phosphate USP in 0.9% sodium chloride injection USP. Up to 2.00 GBq (74 mCi) ^{99m}Tc-pertechnetate may be used for reconstitution of the kit. For brain perfusion imaging, generator eluate less than 30 min old should be used for this stabilizing protocol. For white blood cell labeling, generator eluate less than 2 h old should be used. The final radiopharmaceutical preparation with methylene blue stabilizer may be used up to 4 h after the time of reconstitution.

Unlike ^{99m}Tc-d,l-HMPAO, ^{99m}Tc-l,l-ECD is a chemically stable ^{99m}Tc-complex which can be used up to 8 h after reconstitution of the commercially available Neurolite kit (DuPont Pharma, Billerica, Mass.). In the kit, ECD is supplied in the form of the dihydrochloride for reasons of stability. Because a neutral pH is required to enable efficient labeling, a phosphate buffer of pH 7.2–8.0 is supplied in a separate vial. The standard procedure for preparation of ^{99m}Tc-l,l-ECD, as described by the manufacturer, involves the following manipulations:

1. Add 3.7 GBq generator eluate in 2 ml NaCl 0.9% to vial B (phosphate buffer)
2. Add 3 ml NaCl 0.9% to vial A (containing ECD 2HCl+$SnCl_2 \cdot 2H_2O$ + additives) and mix
3. Within 30 s, add 1 ml of the solution in vial A to vial B and mix
4. Incubate for 30 min

The need for a long incubation period (30 min) is apparently caused by the formation of a weak intermediate complex between reduced ^{99m}Tc and mannitol which slowly converts to ^{99m}Tc-l,l-ECD (Mang'era et al. 1996). In order to shorten the preparation time, alternative procedures for preparation of ^{99m}Tc-l,l-ECD have been evaluated. Hung et al. (1997) found that a 97.4±0.5% radiochemical purity (RCP) could be obtained after an 8-s microwave heating time at 300 W (solution temperature at 69°C) and an average RCP value of 96.4% was maintained throughout the 24-h evaluation period. To prevent the possibility of radioactivity spillage caused by either ejection of the rubber stopper or shattering of the glass vial (HUNG and GIBBONS 1992), an acrylic plastic container should be used or alternatively, incubation in a water bath at 69°C can replace the microwave heating; however, in the latter case, the time gain is more limited.

In the current labeling procedure of Neurolite kits (DuPont Pharma, Billerica, Mass.), 2 of 3 ml of the ligand solution is not used and should be discarded. It has been found (VERBEKE et al. 1997) that such residual portions from vial A of Neurolite kits (DuPont Pharma, Billerica, Mass.) can be efficiently labeled with 3.7 GBq ^{99m}Tc (>95% RCP up to 6 h) after fractionation in 0.5-ml aliquots and storage at -20°C. This requires, of course, the availability of a suitable phosphate buffer, such as the one present in vial B of the Neurolite kit. Although this might be particularly useful and cost-effective for experimental work, such procedures should not be encouraged for patient studies unless applied by or under the supervision of a well-trained radiopharmacist who adheres to strict aseptic techniques and relies on quality control testing of each preparation.

12.2.3 Renal Function Imaging Agents

After it was observed that ^{99m}Tc-l,l-ethylenedicysteine (Fig. 12.3), the di-acid metabolite, of the brain perfusion agent ^{99m}Tc-l,l-ECD, was rapidly and efficiently excreted into the urine (VERBRUGGEN et al. 1990), this agent was further investigated as a possible renal function imaging tracer. Whereas l,l-ECD can easily be labeled with ^{99m}Tc at neutral pH, a pH value of at least 10 and ideally 12 is required for the formation of the ^{99m}Tc-l,l-EC complex (VERBRUGGEN et al. 1992). This is probably due to the amino acid structure of the ligand, and hence, the formation of zwitter ions, by which the amines are ionized up to high pH values. When labeling is performed at high pH, formation of ^{99m}Tc-l,l-EC proceeds immediately with high radiochemical yield (>98%) so that no heating step nor an incubation period is required. Once the desired ^{99m}Tc complex is formed, the preparation may be neutralized and remains stable for at least 8 h.

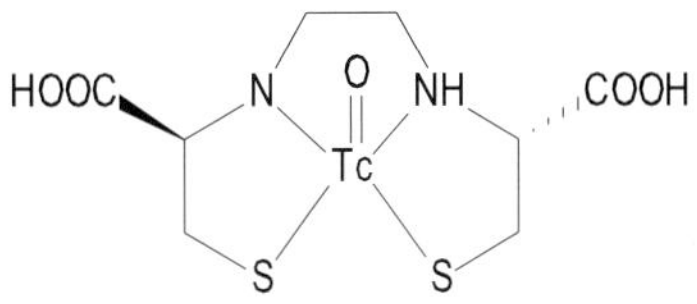

Fig 12.3. Structure of ^{99m}Tc-l,l-EC

After administration, ^{99m}Tc-l,l-EC is excreted into the urine, principally by active tubular transport. As compared with ^{99m}Tc-MAG3, which is generally accepted as the agent of choice for renal function imaging, ^{99m}Tc-l,l-EC exhibits a higher excretion in the urine, a lower renal retention, and a lower excretion from the liver and intestines. The 1-h plasma clearance of ^{99m}Tc-l,l-EC is reproducibly 70–75% of the clearance of Hippuran vs 50–60% in the case of ^{99m}Tc-MAG3 (see Chap. 5, Table 5.1). The high plasma clearance of ^{99m}Tc-l,l-EC is mainly the consequence of the higher distribution volume which is due to the markedly lower plasma protein binding (31±6.8% as compared with 88±5.2% for ^{99m}Tc-MAG3 (VAN NEROM et al. 1993). Labeling kits for the preparation of ^{99m}Tc-l,l-EC are commercially available only in Eastern Europe.

12.2.4 Lung Ventilation Imaging Agents

Radioactive gases with suitable physical characteristics for use as ventilation imaging agents are limited to xenon (^{133}Xe) and krypton (^{81m}Kr). Aqueous aerosols of ^{99m}Tc have been widely developed and refined as replacement for these gases but suffer from practical limitations such as suboptimal particle size and specific activity. BURCH et al. (1984, 1986a,b) developed a technique to produce an ultra-fine dispersion of ^{99m}Tc-labeled carbon particles which can be considered as a pseudogas and is called technegas. After inhalation, technegas is distributed in the lungs in proportion to regional ventilation (LEMB et al. 1993). It does not show central deposition or mucociliary clearance. Technegas is produced using a commercially available generator (Tetley, Carringbah, Australia) by heating a pertechnetate solution with high specific activity (2.6–4.0 GBq/ml) in a crucible of ultrapure (=99.99%) graphite at 2500°C. During this heating step, argon is present (and is consequently inhaled by the patient) to provide a non-reactive, inert shield around the crucible. No evidence has been reported of any compound having been formed with argon under any circumstances.

When technegas is prepared in a mixture of 97% argon and 3% oxygen, a pseudogas "pertechnegas" is formed. Whereas technegas particles remain in the lungs for a long period of time, pertechnegas rapidly disappears with a clearance half-life similar to that of pertechnetate aerosol (TOMINAGA et al. 1995; BURCH and BROWITT 1996; SCALZETTI and GAGNE 1995). Pertechnegas has been reported to be useful for examining the integrity of the alveolar capillary membrane (MONAGHAN et al. 1991) and for identifying individuals having opportunistic infection or other diffuse lung pathology.

The exact size and structure of the ultrafine carbon particles is very difficult to determine. Some authors assume that technegas might consist of small bucky balls (BURCH et al. 1986a; MACKEY et al. 1994) compatible with the buckminsterfullerene model C60 in which ^{99m}Tc atoms are trapped. Most results suggest that technegas and pertechnegas contain ^{99m}Tc-labeled agglomerated graphite particles in the size range of 60–160 nm.

12.3 Metabolism Agents

Metabolic imaging requires endogenous or exogenous radiolabeled substrates which participate in a metabolic pathway. The design of such tracers is based on physiological concepts such as turnover of oxygen, glucose, amino acids, fatty acids, or DNA precursors.

Whereas labeling of candidate tracer agents with ^{11}C can be performed without changing the substrate, labeling with ^{18}F and especially with ^{123}I necessitates chemical changes (F for H, F for OH, alkyl-F for H, I for H, I for OH, I for CH_3) which can alter the physiological properties of the tracer molecule due to steric and electronic effects. For labeling with ^{99m}Tc, the necessity of incorporation of a bifunctional chelating moiety renders it extremely difficult to predict preserved specificity for the metabolic process. As a consequence, examples of metabolic imaging with ^{99m}Tc-labeled tracer agents are scarce (STÖCKLIN 1992).

12.3.1 Glucose Metabolism

2-Fluoro-2-deoxy-D-glucose (^{18}F-FDG; Fig. 12.4), the work horse in clinical PET, is used for the evaluation of glucose metabolism. The energy metabolism of the brain is exclusively based on oxidation of glucose, whereas the heart uses nonesterified fatty acids as primary substrate for energy production and only glucose in the case of low plasma levels of fatty acid. However, after feeding or glucose loading, glucose becomes the primary substrate for the heart (see chap. 3). In addition, certain tumor cells show a higher glucose consumption compared with normal tissues (see chap. 10).

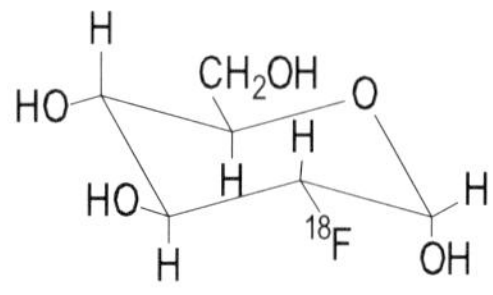

Fig 12.4. Structure of ^{18}F-FDG

In most dedicated cyclotron facilities, ^{18}F-FDG is prepared by a nucleophilic displacement reaction of ^{18}F-fluoride on 1,3,4,6-tetra-O-acetyl-2-O-trifluoromethane-sulfonyl-b-D-mannopyranose followed by hydrolysis of the acetyl esters (HAMACKER et al. 1986).

After administration, FDG is taken up in the cells where it is phosphorylated by hexokinase to FDG-6-phosphate. FDG-6-phosphate is not a substrate for glycolysis and is not further metabolized but remains trapped in the cells for several hours. The blood clearance is triexponential with components having half-lives of 0.2±0.3, 11.6±1.1, and 88±4 min (PHELPS et al. 1978). The brain uptake in dogs is 2–3.5% at 120 min (GALLAGHER et al. 1977), whereas the uptake in the myocardium is approximately 1–4%.

At this moment, no sugar derivative labeled with either ^{123}I or ^{99m}Tc is available as a substitute for ^{18}F-FDG for SPECT.

12.3.2 Amino Acid Metabolism

Radiolabeled amino acids would be important tools for the quantitative assessment of the protein synthesis rate. This would allow diagnosis of various neurological diseases as well as tumor evaluation (diagnosis, tumor grading, and prognosis and therapy monitoring). Radiolabeled amino acids pass the blood-brain barrier and are accumulated in tissues via a specific, large neutral amino acid transport system. ^{11}C-methyl-methionine (Fig. 12.5) is the most widely used labeled amino acid because of ease, reliability and high yield of preparation (BERGER et al. 1979; LANGSTRÖM et al. 1987). However, in the cells, the la-

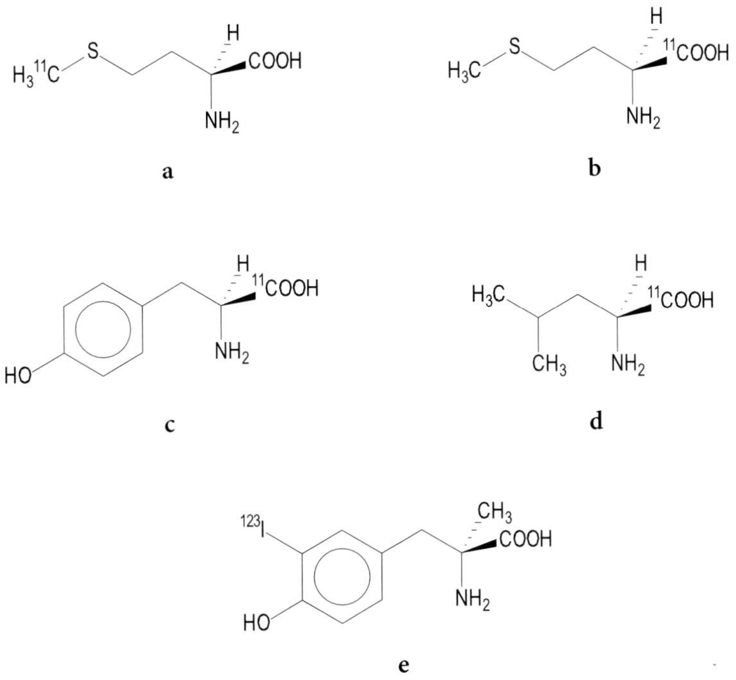

Fig. 12.5a–e. Structures of radiolabeled amino acids. **a** L-^{11}C-methyl-methionine; **b** L-[1-^{11}C]methionine; **c** L-[1-^{11}C]tyrosine; **d** L-[1-^{11}C]leucine; **e** L-[3-^{123}I]iodo-a-methyltyrosine

beled methyl group is transferred to a large number of non-protein acceptor molecules such as lipids and nucleic acids (ISHIWATA et al. 1988). As a consequence, the non-protein metabolism is too complex to allow accurate calculation of the protein synthesis rate.

Alternatively, amino acids such as l-tyrosine, l-methionine, and l-leucine (Fig. 12.5) have been labeled with ^{11}C in the carboxyl position (BOLSTER et al. 1986; KEEN et al. 1989; ISHIWATA et al. 1988). After uptake in the cells, a fraction of the amino acid is incorporated into proteins while the main metabolic route consists of decarboxylation which gives rise to $^{11}CO_2$. Since the formed $^{11}CO_2$ is rapidly eliminated from tissues through blood flow and subsequent ventilation in the lungs, only low levels of ^{11}C-labeled non-protein metabolites are present in the tissues. However, due to in vivo recycling of amino acids coming from protein breakdown (PLANAS et al. 1992), the intracellular amino acid pool is diluted by unlabeled amino acids resulting in a decreased specific activity of the tracer agent. Hence, routine PET measurements of protein synthesis still remain very difficult. Recently, a mathematical model for determination of protein synthesis rate has been developed using ^{11}C-tyrosine on the basis of data obtained from patients with various types of tumors (PAANS et al. 1993; WILLEMSEN et al. 1995; KOLE et al. 1997).

For SPECT studies, l-3-^{123}I-iodo-a-methyltyrosine (^{123}I-IMT) can be considered (KLOSS and LEVEN 1979). There is evidence suggesting that IMT is accumulated in the brain via a specific facilitating l-amino acid transport system. The carrier system for large neutral amino acids which also transports the non-iodinated α-methyltyrosine is likely to be involved (PARDRIDGE 1977). Since IMT is not incorporated into proteins (LANGEN et al. 1990), uptake only reflects amino acid transport (KAWAI et al. 1991; LANGEN et al. 1991). IMT can be prepared by electrophilic substitution via in situ oxidation of ^{123}I-iodide by chloramine-T, hydrogen peroxide, iodogen, or iodate, with radiochemical yields of 70–80%.

12.3.3 Hypoxia Agents

Whereas perfusion agents are often used to identify tissues with reduced flow, and hence, reduced delivery of oxygen, a marker of decreased intracellular oxygen tension would be an effective indicator of tissue that is dysfunctional but still viable (hypoxic tissue). Most hypoxia markers contain a nitroimidazole moiety as the reactive chemical species. Nitroimidazoles are reduced intracellularly in all cells, but in the

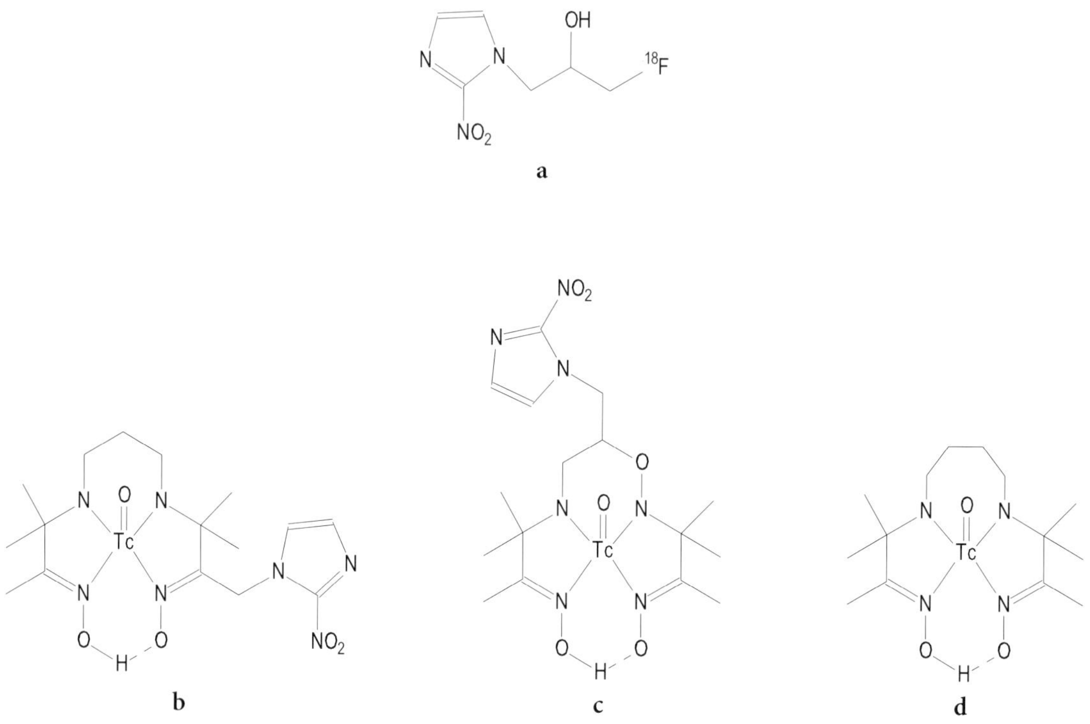

Fig. 12.6a–d. Structures of hypoxia imaging agents. **a** ^{18}F-fluoromisonidazole; **b** BMS181321; **c** BMS194796; **d** ^{99m}Tc-HL91

absence of an adequate supply of oxygen, they undergo further reduction to more reactive products which bind to cell components. In this way, they are trapped in hypoxic tissue (for a review, see NUNN et al. 1995).

Fluoromisonidazole (FMISO; Fig. 12.6) is a fluorinated analog of the chemical radiosensitizer misonidazole and has been radiolabeled with ^{18}F by reaction of [^{18}F]epifluorohydrin with 2-nitroimidazole under basic conditions (GRIERSON et al. 1989).

Although PET imaging with ^{18}F-FMISO has demonstrated the principle of hypoxia imaging, ^{18}F-FMISO is not an ideal tracer agent for this purpose. Since hypoxic tissue usually has decreased perfusion, limiting first-pass delivery of the tracer agent, blood clearance of the tracer agent should be relatively slow. In this way, the tracer is allowed to accumulate in the hypoxic cells and to clear from normoxic tissues, resulting in appropriate target/nontarget ratios. Due to the longer physical half-life and more favorable dosimetry which permits administration of higher doses, a ^{99m}Tc-based hypoxia marker seems to be more convenient than a tracer radiolabeled with a positron emitting isotope.

Several ^{99m}Tc-based compounds have been synthesized and evaluated (LINDER et al. 1993, 1994; NEUMEIER et al. 1990). ^{99m}TcO(PnAO-1-(2-nitroimidazole), called BMS181321, has shown promise as a marker of myocardial and tumor hypoxia in animal models. Labeling of the ligand is achieved by addition of Sn-DTPA to a vial containing the ligand previously reconstituted with an appropriate amount of pertechnetate. After incubation for 10 min at room temperature, the radiochemical purity of the ^{99m}Tc complexes was 90% (LINDER et al. 1994). After intravenous injection, the tracer rapidly distributes throughout the body and is predominantly cleared through the hepatobiliary system (BALLINGER et al. 1996). A “second-generation” ^{99m}Tc-labeled nitroimidazole (BMS194796) has been developed which is more stable, less lipophilic and which clears more rapidly through the liver (STONE et al. 1995). In addition, tumor-to-muscle ratios were similar but tumor-to-blood ratios were significantly higher for BMS194796 than for BMS181321 (MELO et al. 1998).

Investigators at Amersham International developed ^{99m}Tc-HL91 (^{99m}Tc-labeled 4,9-diaza-3,3,10,10-tetramethyldodecan-2,11-dione dioxime, Prognox) which does not contain the bioreductive 2-nitroimidazole moiety (ARCHER et al. 1995). The exact mechanism by which ^{99m}Tc-HL91 is trapped in hypoxic tissue remains to be established. ^{99m}Tc-HL91 can be prepared by simple reconstitution of a freeze-dried labeling kit. After an incubation period of 15 min at room temperature, radiochemical yields exceed 95%

and the preparation remains stable up to 8 h after reconstitution (FUKUCHI et al. 1998). At this moment, phase-II clinical trials are ongoing to estimate the usefulness, safety, and tolerability of ^{99m}Tc-HL91 in patients with suspected recurrent squamous cell carcinomas of the head and neck.

12.4 Peptides

12.4.1 Somatostatin Receptor Tracers

Radiolabeled natural somatostatin cannot be used as a tracer agent for visualization of somatostatin receptors, due to the very short plasma half-life of the peptide (2–4 min); therefore, analogs have been developed which are more stable against the action of peptidases.

12.4.1.1 Indium-111-Octreotide

One somatostatin is octreotide, an octapeptide containing the physiologically active four-amino acid sequence (Phe-D-Trp-Lys-Thr) in a ring form. In order to enable labeling of octreotide with ^{111}In, a diethylenetriaminepentaacetic acid (DTPA) group has been conjugated to the α-NH_2 group of the N-terminal D-Phe residue (BAKKER et al. 1991a). The generic name of this conjugate is pentetreotide (Fig. 12.7). Labeling is performed using the commercially available Octreoscan 111 kit (Mallinckrodt Medical, St. Louis, Mo.) which consists of two vials. ^{111}In-indium chloride (vial A) is added to vial B containing the lyophilized pentetreotide, after which the mixture is incubated for 30 min at room temperature. Labeling yield is higher than 97% and the preparation should be used within 2 h after reconstitution. The pH of the reconstituted product varies between pH 3.5 and 5.0.

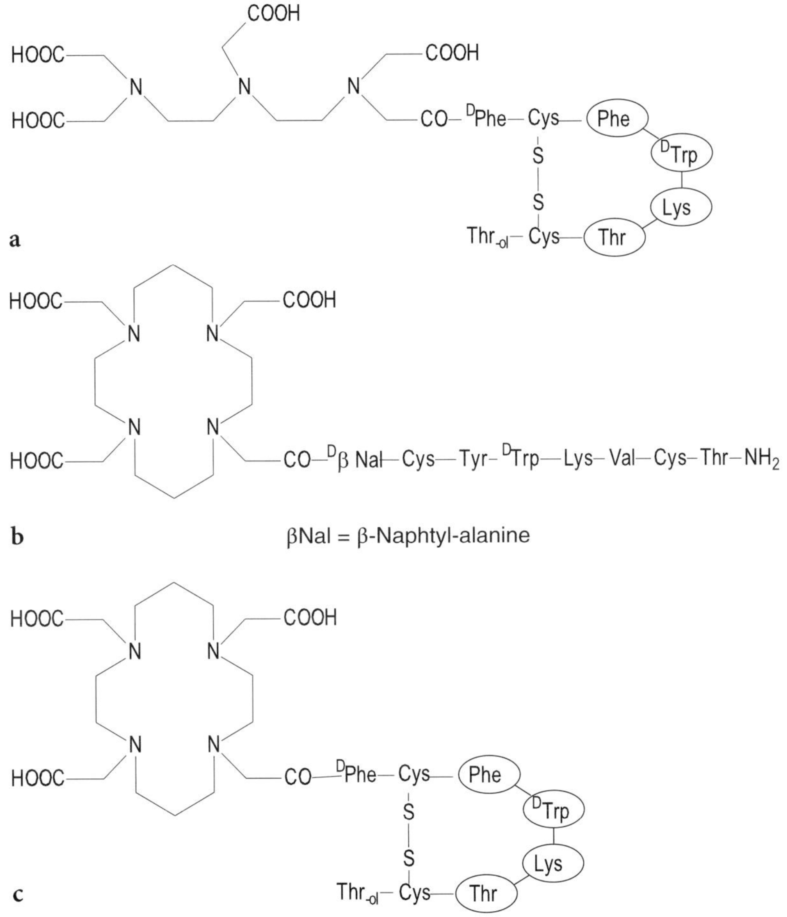

Fig. 12.7a–c. Structures of ligands for somatostatin receptor tracer agents. **a** Pentetreotide; **b** DOTA-lanreotide; **c** DOTA-octreotide

After intravenous administration, ^{111}In-labeled pentetreotide is rapidly cleared from the blood (Krenning et al. 1992). Blood radioactivity decreases within 10 min to 33% of injected dose. Unlike the initially developed ^{123}I-octreotide, which is eliminated to a high degree via the hepatobiliary system (Bakker et al. 1991b), ^{111}In-pentetreotide is excreted mainly into the urine (50% of injected dose after 6 h, 85% after 24 h, and 90% after 48 h). Up to 4 h after injection, radioactivity in plasma and urine is predominantly intact ^{111}In-pentetreotide. The relatively long residence time of ^{111}In-pentetreotide in the kidneys suggests that following glomerular filtration, part of the label is actively reabsorbed into the tubules (Bakker et al. 1991c).

Because pentetreotide only binds with high affinity to the somatostatin receptor subtype SSTR2, with moderate affinity to SSTR3 and SSTR5 and not to SSTR1 and SSTR4, research has continued to develop other somatostatin analogs, which have a high affinity for the other receptor subtypes. Lanreotide is an octapeptide which binds to SSTR2 through SSTR5 with high affinity and to SSTR1 with low affinity. This peptide is modified with DOTA (Fig. 12.7) and labeled with ^{111}In in a similar way as octreotide. The high-affinity binding of lanreotide to SSTR3 and SSTR4 enables visualization of certain tumors, such as intestinal adenocarcinomas, which are not visualized by ^{111}In-pentetreotide scintigraphy (Virgolini et al. 1998).

12.4.1.2
P587 and P829

Despite the encouraging results obtained with ^{111}In-labeled somatostatin analogs, a ^{99m}Tc-labeled SSTR-binding tracer agent is highly desirable for routine nuclear medicine procedures, because ^{99m}Tc is less expensive than ^{111}In. Also, ^{99m}Tc provides a higher photon flux per unit of absorbed radiation dose and better-quality images.

Diatide Inc. (Londonderry, New Hampshire) has developed numerous synthetic high-affinity SSTR-binding peptides, designed for labeling with ^{99m}Tc. From these peptides, ^{99m}Tc-P587 and ^{99m}Tc-P829 (Fig. 12.8) were selected to enter clinical trials. These are peptides designed in a cyclic configuration which is not susceptible to reductive cleavage, in order to avoid the incompatibility of having a disulfide in a molecule that is to be radiolabeled with ^{99m}Tc in reducing conditions. In the peptides a sequence is incorporated to provide a donor atom set which allows stable complexation of ^{99m}Tc (Vallabhajosula et al. 1996). Labeling is performed by ligand exchange from ^{99m}Tc-glucoheptonate. Since the labeling sequence is in fact a diamide monoamine monothiolate chelator (P829) and a triamide thiolate chelator (P587), heat needs to be applied (15 min at 100°C) to promote subtraction of the amide protons and afford stable ^{99m}Tc complexes. In this way, labeling yields >90% can be obtained.

12.4.2
Radioiodinated Vasoactive Intestinal Peptide

The observation that various tumors express significantly higher amounts of radioiodinated vasoactive intestinal peptide (VIP) receptors as compared to normal peripheral blood cells or tissues, provides the basis for the clinical use of radiolabeled VIP (Virgolini et al. 1994a).

Synthetic VIP, a 28-amino acid peptide of the glucagon-secretin family (Fig. 12.9), is labeled with ^{123}I on one of the tyrosine residues using a modified iodogen method (Virgolini et al. 1995). To obtain a high specific activity (>500 TBq/mmol), ^{123}I VIP is purified by HPLC. ^{123}I-VIP can thus be administered as an intravenous bolus injection without causing serious side effects, except for a transient drop in blood pressure. After administration, ^{123}I VIP is rapidly cleared from the circulation (calculated half-life is approximately 1 min) and accumulated to a high degree in the lungs, whereas no substantial uptake is observed in liver, spleen, or normal gastrointestinal tissues. Radioactivity is mainly eliminated via the urine. This tissue distribution is very favorable for detection of gastrointestinal tumors and constitutes a distinct advantage of this agent over other iodinated peptides which are excreted through the hepatobiliary system (Lamberts et al. 1990).

Because of the observed cross-competition of VIP and octreotide for binding to certain primary tumors (Virgolini et al. 1994b), it has been hypothesized that there could be a receptor which can bind both peptides. Recently, SSTR3 has been identified as a common binding site for octreotide and VIP (Peck-Radosavljevic et al. 1998).

12.4.3
Peptides for Thrombus Imaging

Platelet activation and deposition, the initial events of active thrombus formation, involve expression of the GPIIb/IIIa receptor, which recognizes proteins

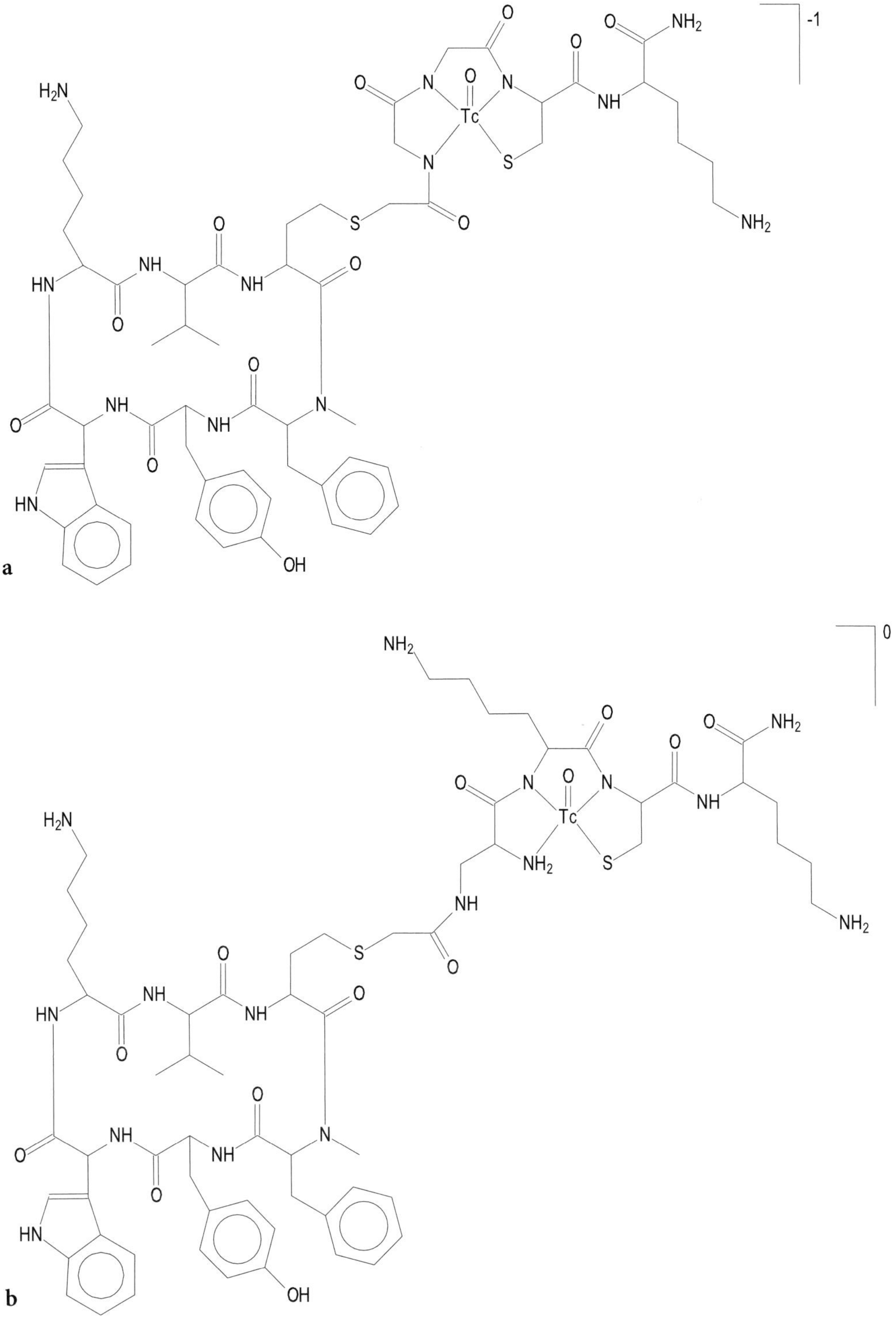

Fig. 12.8a, b. Structures of ^{99m}Tc-labeled somatostatin receptor tracer agents. **a** P547 and **b** P829

H-His-Ser-Aso-Ala-Val-Phe-Thr-Ara-Lvs-Gln-Met-Ala-Val-Lvs-Lvs-Tvr-Leu-Asn-Ser-Ile-Leu-Asn-NH_2

Fig. 12.9. Amino acid sequence of vasoactive intestinal peptide

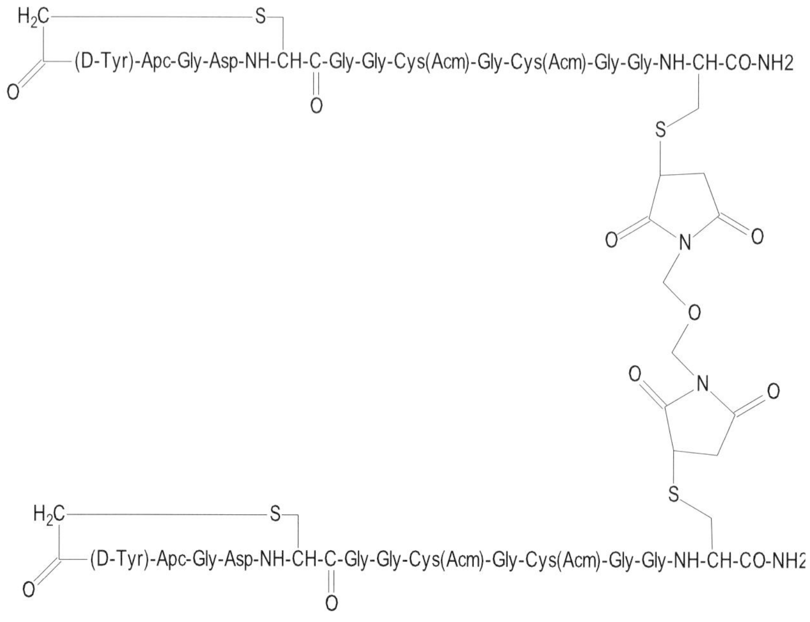

Fig. 12.10. Structure of the thrombus imaging peptide bibapcitide

and peptides bearing the Arg-Gly-Asp (RGD) tripeptide sequence.

LISTER-JAMES and co-workers (1996; PEARSON et al. 1996) at Diatide Inc. developed a ^{99m}Tc-labeled GPIIb/IIIa receptor antagonist for scintigraphic detection of deep venous thrombosis. P280 (now called bibapcitide) is a small oligopeptide that consists of two identical, linked, cyclic 13-amino acid monomers (Fig. 12.10). Each monomer (called apcitide) contains a (S-aminopropyl)cysteine-Gly-Asp tripeptide sequence which mimics the RGD sequence and a Cys(Acm)-Gly-Cys(Acm) tripeptide sequence, which forms after deprotection an N_2S_2 diamidedithiol-type chelator for ^{99m}Tc labeling. Because of the presence of protecting groups (acetamidomethyl, Acm) on the two thiol groups of the diamidedithiol and the presence of two amide protons, ^{99m}Tc labeling of P280 requires heating at 100°C for 15 min. At this time bibapcitide is split and a ^{99m}Tc-apcitide complex is formed. Recently, ^{99m}Tc-apcitide has been approved by the FDA and a kit for the preparation of ^{99m}Tc-apcitide has become available commercially (AcuTect, Diatide, Londonderry, N.H.). Each vial contains besides 100 µg bibapcitide, 89 µg $SnCl_2 \cdot 2H_2O$ for reduction of ^{99m}Tc-pertechnetate, and 75 mg sodium glucoheptonate which forms an intermediary ^{99m}Tc-glucoheptonate complex which exchanges for apcitide upon heating. After administration, ^{99m}Tc-apcitide exhibits a fast plasma clearance and predominantly renal excretion which is favorable for rapid delineation of thrombi.

12.5 Receptor Tracers

Scintigraphic imaging and especially PET are powerful non-invasive techniques that use suitable radioligands to image receptors and binding sites at low (nM) concentrations. In this way, the relationship between changes in receptor or binding-site concentration and the progress of certain diseases can be elucidated. In current research, interest has been shown mainly in peptide receptor tracer agents (which have been discussed separately) and neuroreceptor radioligands.

12.5.1 Benzodiazepine Receptor Agents

Central benzodiazepine receptors have been studied in relation to diseases such as epilepsy (SAVIC et al. 1988), hepatic encephalopathy (SAMSON et al. 1987), Alzheimer's disease (YAMASAKI et al. 1986), Huntington's disease (HANTRAYE et al. 1984), and chronic alcoholism (LITTON et al. 1991).

Whereas diazepam and flunitrazepam were the first classical benzodiazepines to be labeled with ^{11}C in the N-methyl group (MAZIÈRE et al. 1980), [N-methyl-^{11}C]flumazenil and its iodinated analogue ^{123}I-iomazenil (Fig. 12.11) are currently the radioligands of choice for studies of central benzodi-

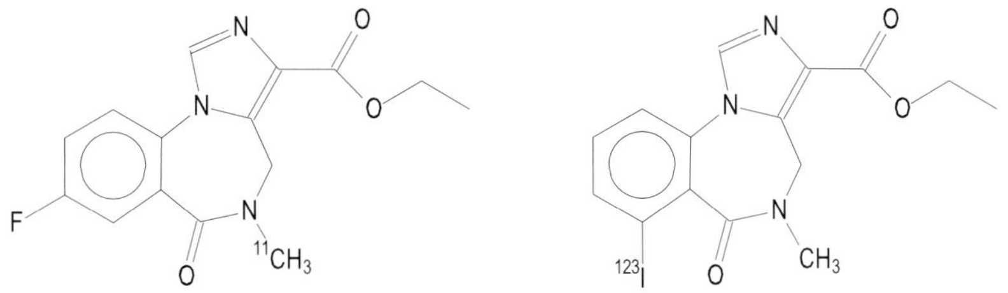

Fig. 12.11. Structures of the benzodiazepine receptor agents **a** [N-methyl-^{11}C]flumazenil and **b** ^{123}I-iomazenil

azepine receptors with PET and SPECT, respectively. They are benzodiazepine antagonists with high affinity for the receptor, whereas they lack major intrinsic pharmacological effects.

Radiosynthesis of [N-methyl-^{11}C]flumazenil involves N-methylation of N-*des*-methyl-flumazenil with NCA [^{11}C]iodomethane. Several conditions have been reported for routine labeling of flumazenil with ^{11}C whereby radiochemical yields ranging from 70 to 88% were obtained in 1–10 min (Mazière et al. 1984; Ehrin et al. 1984; Suzuki et al. 1985; Halldin et al. 1988; Jewett et al. 1991). Specific activity is usually approximately 37 TBq (1000 Ci)/mmol at the end of radiosynthesis.

^{123}I-iomazenil is prepared with high specific activity, i.e., >185 TBq (5000 Ci)/mmol, by oxidative radioiodination of the tributylstannyl precursor (Beer et al. 1990).

After administration, the initial uptake of ^{11}C-flumazenil and ^{123}I-iomazenil in the brain is similar to the rCBF seen with ^{99m}Tc-HMPAO (Yamamoto et al. 1983; Bartenstein et al. 1991). Within 30 min post injection, unbound tracer agent is almost completely cleared from the brain and the distribution of both radioligands closely resembles the known biodistribution of benzodiazepine receptors. As compared with ^{11}C-flumazenil, ^{123}I-iomazenil has a tenfold higher affinity for the neuronal-type benzodiazepine receptor and a slower brain wash-out (Johnson et al. 1990).

12.5.2 Serotonergic (5-HT) Receptor Tracers

The in vivo investigation of brain serotonergic (5-HT) receptors has been pursued for several years. There is evidence suggesting a role for the 5-HT system, in particular 5-HT_2 receptors in the regulation of a wide range of central mechanisms (Cowen 1991). Abnormalities in 5-HT_2 receptors have been proposed in several neuropsychiatric conditions including major depression, Alzheimer-type dementia, drug abuse, and schizophrenia.

A great number of ligands have been prepared and evaluated for probing the 5-HT receptors. At this moment ^{18}F-setoperone (Mazière et al. 1988) and ^{18}F-altanserin (Lemaire et al. 1991) are the only radioligands used for PET studies of 5-HT_2 receptors (Fig. 12.12). Both can be obtained by a direct one-pot nucleophilic substitution of the nitro-precursor by n.c.a. ^{18}F-fluoride. The binding affinity values for different neurotransmitter receptor sites have been reported by Leysen (1989; Table 12.8). In rats the frontal cortex-to-striatum ratio, which is a good index for ligand specificity (5-HT_2/D_2), reached 2.56 at 1 h post injection for ^{18}F-altanserin, whereas this ratio did not exceed 1.18 for ^{18}F-setoperone; hence, ^{18}F-altanserin appeared more selective for binding to 5-HT2 receptors than ^{18}F-setoperone.

For SPECT, ^{123}I-5-I-R91150 ([^{123}I]-4-amino-N-[1-[3-(4-fluorophenoxy)-propyl]-4-methyl-4-piperidinyl]-5-iodo-2-methoxybenzamide) has been synthesized by Mertens et al. (1994) by electrophilic

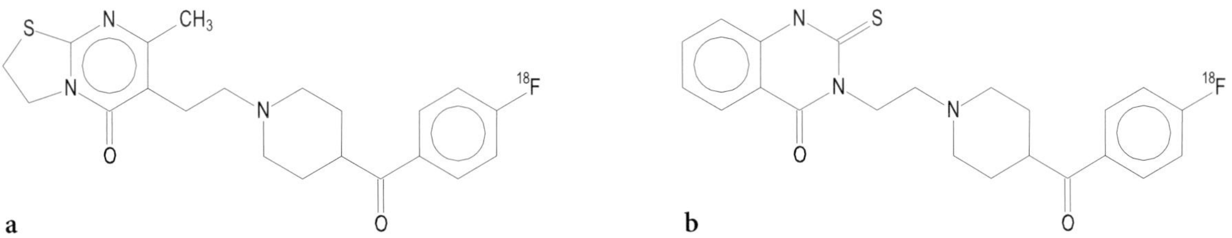

Fig. 12.12. Structures of the 5-HT_2 receptor tracers **a** ^{18}F-setoperone and **b** ^{18}F-altanserin

Table 12.8. Binding affinity values (K_i, nM) of setoperone and altanserin for different neurotransmitter receptor sites

	5-HT_2 [^{3}H]ketanserin	D_2 [^{3}H]haloperidol	a_1 [^{3}H]WB-4101
Setoperone	0.37	25	13
Altanserin	0.13	62	4.55

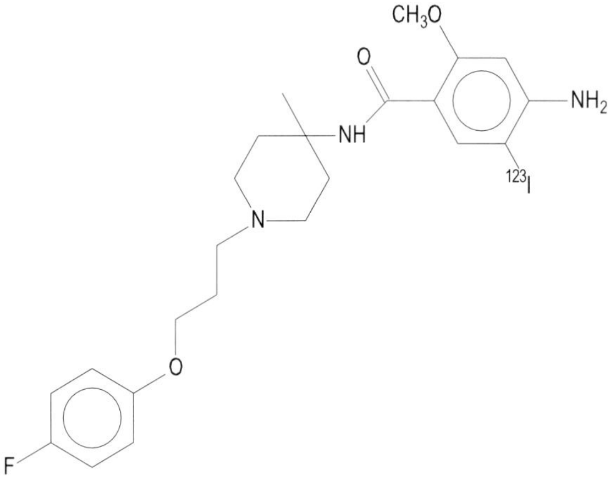

Fig. 12.13. Structure of the 5-HT_2 receptor tracer ^{123}I-5-I-R91150

substitution on the 5-position of the methoxybenzamide group of R91150 (Fig. 12.13). It is a 5-HT_2 antagonist with high affinity and selectivity for the 5-HT_{2A} receptor (the main subtype of 5-HT_2 receptors in the brain). The in vitro binding constant (Ki) for 5-HT_2 receptors is 0.2 nM, whereas the selectivity to other neurotransmitter receptors (5-HTx, α_1, α_2, D_1, and D_2) is at least a factor of 50 (Terriere et al. 1995). Preliminary results with this tracer agent have been reported (Busatto et al. 1997), and this radioligand might be very useful for in vivo 5-HT_{2A} receptor mapping, especially since SPECT is cheaper and more available than PET.

Receptors of the 5-HT_1 family (5-HT_{1A} and 5-HT_{1D}) are distributed among several cortical and subcortical structures where they mediate neuronal hyperpolarization and inhibit the release of neurotransmitters (Hoyer et al. 1994). A selective ligand with high potency, high selectivity, and pure antagonistic action of 5-HT_{1A} receptors is WAY-100635 (Fig. 12.14). The ligand can be radiolabeled with ^{11}C in the O-methyl as well as in the carbonyl position. In primates it was found that the descyclohexane carbonyl analogue [O-methyl-^{11}C]WAY-100634 is a major radiolabeled metabolite of [O-methyl-^{11}C]WAY-100635 (Osman et al. 1996). WAY-100634 is known to have a high affinity for 5-HT_{1A} receptors and α1-adrenoreceptors, suggesting that this radioactive metabolite contributes to brain radioactivity in human PET studies (Osman et al. 1996). Therefore, WAY-100635 is now being labeled in the carbonyl position (Pike et al. 1996) to avoid formation of radioactive WAY-100634 or any other pharmacologically active metabolite.

[Carbonyl-^{11}C]WAY-1003635 is prepared by reaction of cyclohexane[carbonyl-^{11}C]chloride with WAY-100634 and is obtained in a 30–50% decay-corrected radiochemical yield from trapped ^{11}C-carbon dioxide in 20 min from end of bombardment (EOB). After semi-preparative reversed phase HPLC, radiochemical purity exceeds 99% (Pike et al. 1995).

Within 60 min after administration, the ratio of radioactivity uptake in the receptor-rich medial temporal cortex to that in the cerebellum reaches a value

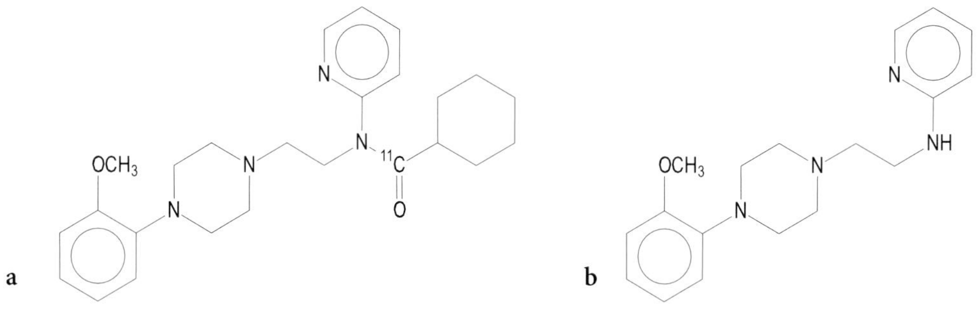

Fig. 12.14. Structure of the 5-HT_1 receptor tracer [carbonyl-^{11}C]WAY-100635 (**a**) and (**b**) its metabolite WAY-100634

of 25, indicating the very low non-specific binding of this radioligand. Plasma analysis showed rapid metabolism but only to very polar radioactive compounds (most probably ^{11}C-cyclohexanecarboxylic acid and derivatives) which are not expected to enter the brain nor to be pharmacologically active.

12.5.3 Dopaminergic Receptor Tracers

The brain dopaminergic system lies in a well-defined region in the striatum and localization is relatively easy; hence, a large number of ligands for the dopaminergic system, and in particular the D_2 receptors, have been studied. The most prominent reversible and highly selective D_2 receptor ligands are the benzamides of the salicylamide type such as raclopride and eticlopride (Fig. 12.15); the latter has a 30-fold higher affinity for the D_2-receptor than raclopride (Halldin et al. 1991; Mazière et al. 1992). For both ligands the (S)-enantiomer is the most potent form (Högberg et al. 1991). They can be radiolabeled with ^{11}C by O-methylation of the desmethyl-precursor with ^{11}C-methyl iodide. In the case of eticlopride, two different O-methylated products are obtained (Fig. 12.15) which have to be separated by HPLC. Alternatively, eticlopride can be labeled in the N-ethyl position as well. The ^{18}F labeled analogs have also been prepared but show generally inferior binding properties.

The favorable results obtained with these PET tracers stimulated the design of a ^{123}I-labeled analog for SPECT, namely (S)-N-[(1-ethyl-2-pyrrolidinyl)]methyl-2-hydroxy-3-iodo-6-methoxybenzamide (^{123}I-IBZM; Fig. 12.16; Kung et al. 1988). It can be prepared with high yield and high specific activity by oxidative iodination of the enantiomerically pure BZM precursor with n.c.a. ^{123}I-iodide via in situ formation of peracetic acid (Bobeldijk et al. 1990). Biodistribution studies have demonstrated that the agent is concentrated in the basal ganglia, although some non-specific binding was noted in cerebral cortex and cerebellum (Kung et al. 1990). If receptor occupancy or blockade is being quantified, it is necessary to correct for this non-specific binding.

Dopamine reuptake sites can be visualized using radioligands which bind to the dopamine transporter, a protein which plays an important role in the inactivation and recycling of dopamine released into the synaptic cleft. Measurement of the decrease in the dopamine transporters may be a useful indicator of dopamine neuronal loss in Parkinson's and other neurodegenerative diseases (Kaufman and Madras 1991). Beta-carbomethoxy-3b-(4-iodophenyl)tropane (β-CIT; Fig. 12.17) is a more potent analog of the cocaine congener in the inhibition of dopamine uptake (Boja et al. 1990) and has been radiolabeled with ^{123}I for use in SPECT imaging (Carroll et al. 1991). Alternatively, ^{11}C-β-CIT can be used for PET imaging (Laihinen et al. 1995). In addition, the N-fluoroethyl (β-CIT-FE) and N-fluoropropyl analogue (β-CIT-FP) have

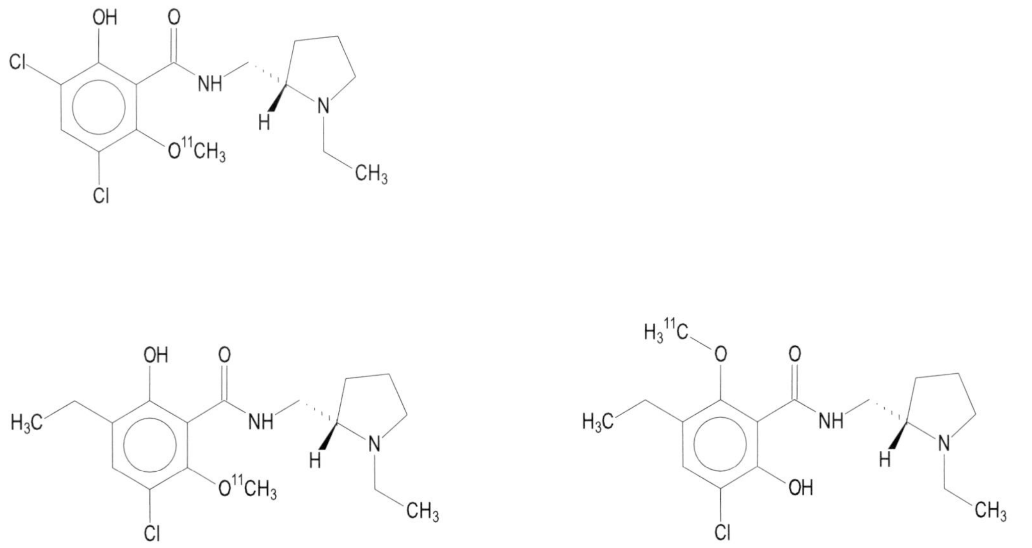

Fig. 12.15. Structures of the dopaminergic tracer agents **a** (S)-[O-methyl-^{11}C]raclopride, **b** (S)-[2-O-methyl-^{11}C]eticlopride, and **c** (S)-[6-O-methyl-^{11}C]eticlopride

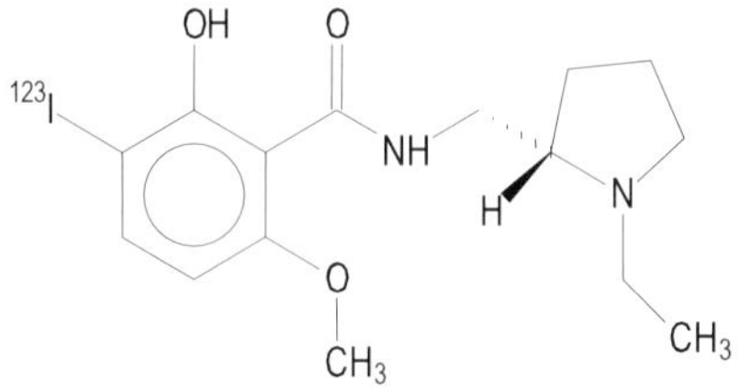

Fig. 12.16. Structure of the dopaminergic tracer agent ^{123}I-IBZM

been synthesized and radiolabeled with the relatively long-lived radionuclides ^{123}I and ^{76}Br. Due to the high proportion of homology between the dopamine transporter (DAT), the serotonin transporter and the norepinephrine transporter, these ligands are not selective for DAT (Amara and Kuhar 1993). Table 12.9 shows the K_i values of β-CIT, β-CIT-FE, β-CIT-FP and cocaine to inhibit the uptake of [^{3}H]dopamine, [^{3}H]serotonin and [^{3}H]1-norepinephrine (Okada et al. 1998).

Recently, Meegalla et al. (1997) synthesized a tropane derivative, TRODAT-1, designed for labeling with ^{99m}Tc, by conjugation of a N_2S_2 diaminedithiol-type chelator with tropane at the 2β-position (Fig. 12.18). Labeling of the conjugate by ligand exchange from ^{99m}Tc-glucoheptonate yields a neutral, lipophilic ^{99m}Tc-TRODAT-1 complex in high yield (RP>93%). The in vitro binding of the dopamine transporter was assessed using the surrogate Re-complex, Re-TRODAT-1, and a K_i value of 14 nM was obtained (Kung et al. 1997). As compared with iodinated receptor ligands, the ratio of specific to non-specific binding of ^{99m}Tc-TRODAT-1 appears to be lower than that of ^{123}I-β-CIT (1.66 vs 7). Nevertheless, animal studies and a preliminary study in normal humans (Kung et al. 1996) indicate that ^{99m}Tc-TRODAT-1 is a useful SPECT-imaging agent for localization of dopamine transporters.

12.6 Cell Labeling

12.6.1 Red Blood Cell Labeling

Several studies comparing the biological behavior of ^{99m}Tc red blood cells (^{99m}Tc RBCs) labeled via the in vitro, in vivo, or modified in vivo method all revealed higher heart-to-background ratios and better subjective images with in-vitro-labeled RBCs (Hamilton and Alderson 1977; Hegge et al. 1978). A labeling kit for in vitro labeling of RBCs with ^{99m}Tc in whole blood was originally developed at Brookhaven National Laboratory (Srivastava et al. 1983) and is since a few years commercially available under the brand name Ultra-Tag.

Each kit consists of three separate non-radioactive components with the following constituents:

1. Labeling vial: $SnCl_2.2H_2O$, 105 µg (50 µg stannous ion minimum); sodium citrate; $2H_2O$, 3.67 mg; dextrose, 5.50 mg; pH prior to lyophilization, 7.1–7.2

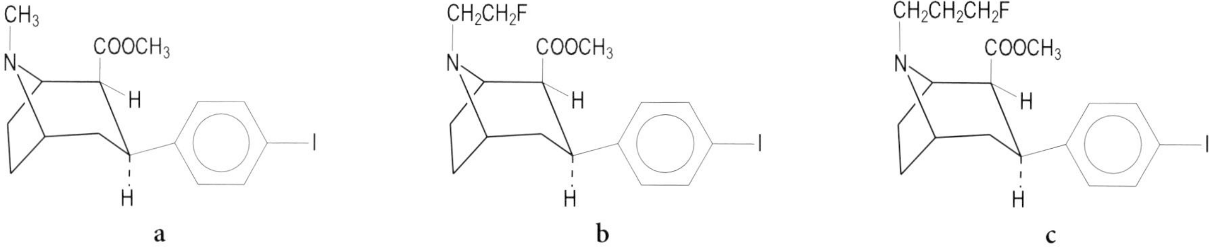

Fig. 12.17. Structures of the dopamine reuptake tracer agents **a** β-CIT and its analogs **b** β-CIT-FE and **c** β-CIT-FP

Table 12.9. Ki values for inhibition of [^{3}H]dopamine, [^{3}H]serotonin, and [^{3}H]1-norepinephrine uptake

	Dopamine transporter (45 nM) [^{3}H]dopamine	Serotonin transporter (20 nM) [^{3}H]serotonin	1-Norepinephrine transporter (50 nM) [^{3}H]1-norepinephrine
β-CIT	6.34±1.68	29.17±6.40	32.77±13.41
β-CIT-FE	90.88±4.92	132.73±31.90	130.45±49.18
β-CIT-FP	27.97±7.36	113.39±63.77	70.42±15.37

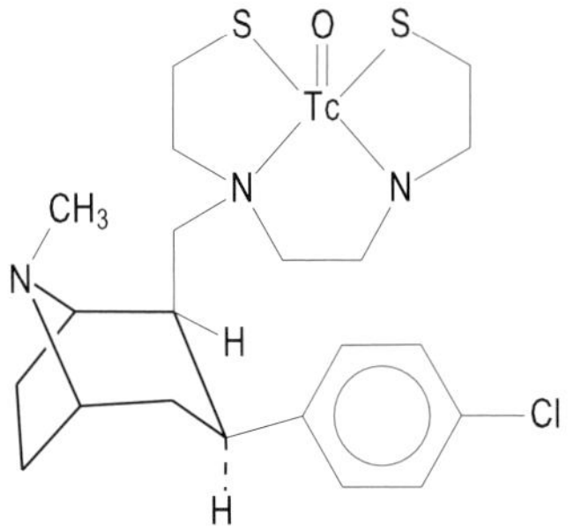

Fig. 12.18. Structure of the ^{99m}Tc-labeled dopamine reuptake tracer agent TRODAT-1

2. Syringe I (to be protected from light): sodium hypochlorite, 0.6 mg; water for injection, 0.6 ml; pH 11–13
3. Syringe II: citric acid; H_2O, 8.7 mg; sodium citrate; $2H_2O$, 32.5 mg; dextrose, 12.0 mg; water for injection, 1.0 ml; pH 4.5–5.5

Red blood cell labeling is started by addition of 1–3 ml of autologous whole blood, anticoagulated with heparin or anticoagulant citrate dextrose solution (ACD) to the labeling vial. In this vial the citrate complexes stannous ion and the dextrose is present to sustain red cell metabolism, which improves RBC viability. After an incubation period of 5 min, during which a portion of the stannous ion in the reaction vial diffuses across the RBC membrane and is bound intracellularly, the hypochlorite solution of syringe I is added to the vial to oxidize the extracellular stannous ion. To render the extracellular tin more readily available for oxidation by hypochlorite, the solution in syringe II is added. Finally, a pertechnetate solution (0.5–3 ml, 370–3700 MBq ^{99m}Tc) is added and the vial is incubated with occasional gentle mixing for 20 min.

An RBC labeling efficiency of 95% is typically obtained using this in vitro labeling procedure. As the yield can decrease in the presence of excessive amounts of the long-lived daughter nuclide ^{99}Tc, the use of fresh (<24 h in growth time) generator eluate is recommended.

12.6.2 White Blood Cell Labeling

Radiolabeled autologous white cells offer the most widely accepted method for imaging infection and inflammation. Methods for labeling can be classified depending on the choice of the radionuclide (^{111}In or ^{99m}Tc) and the choice of the cell preparation (pure granulocytes or mixed white cell populations).

Both mixed leukocytes and pure granulocytes have been labeled with ^{111}In. Although pure granulocytes offer the advantage of theoretically better sensitivity and specificity and avoid the risk of malignant transformations of lymphocytes, mixed leukocytes are more practical for routine use because they can be prepared easier and faster while having a comparative sensitivity in acute infections (Schauwecker et al. 1988). Hydroxyquinoline (oxine) was the first established and mostly used lipophilic chelating agent to transport ^{111}In into the cell (McAfee and Thakur 1976).

Because of the favorable physical characteristics of ^{99m}Tc, many attempts have been made to label leukocytes. The first approaches to label leukocytes with ^{99m}Tc implied phagocytic engulfment of technetium-labeled colloid (Schroth et al. 1981; Pullman et al. 1986). However, this technique has not been established worldwide, because by deliberately inducing the cells to phagocytose, they become activated prior to injection (McAfee et al. 1984). Successful labeling of leukocytes with ^{99m}Tc was achieved in 1986 when ^{99m}Tc-HMPAO was used, like ^{111}In-oxine, as a neutral lipophilic chelate capable of penetrating blood cells (Peters et al. 1986; Roddie et al. 1988). Since ^{99m}Tc-HMPAO is relatively selectively taken up by granulocytes in mixed cell populations and elutes more rapidly from lymphocytes and monocytes than from granulocytes, labeling can be performed in a mixed white cell population which avoids the need for complex and lengthy cell purification (Frier 1994).

Leukocytes can be labeled with either ^{111}In or ^{99m}Tc by a variety of accepted procedures (Datz 1993, 1994; Thakur et al. 1977; Danpure et al. 1988; Dewanjee 1990; Mortelmans et al. 1989).

A major concern when preparing radiolabeled cells is the effect of the labeling procedure on granulocyte viability and function. In vitro tests examining chemotaxis, superoxide generation in response to activation, and morphological changes can be used to assess granulocyte function; however, these tests cannot discriminate between cell damage and activation, since the techniques themselves often activate the granulocytes.

The most sensitive and practical means of quality control of radiolabeled granulocytes are based on their in vivo distribution following injection. When radiolabeled granulocytes are damaged or activated, they are sequestrated in the lung microvasculature by a mechanism which is poorly understood. As a consequence, dynamic imaging over the lungs is a useful test. Alternatively, the radiolabeled granulocyte recovery, defined as the fraction of injected labeled granulocytes that are circulating in blood, can be determined. Normal recovery factors at 45 min p.i. are approximately 35%, whereas these values fall to less than 5% when the cells are severely activated or damaged (Peters 1994). These tests need not be performed with every preparation but are useful when setting up a white cell labeling procedure.

The normal biodistribution of ^{99m}Tc-leukocytes is not fully identical to that of ^{111}In-labeled leukocytes. Whereas ^{111}In-leukocyte distribution at 18–24 h is primarily confined to the reticuloendothelial system of liver, spleen, bone marrow, and major blood vessels (Seabold et al. 1997), a non-specific bowel activity appears from approximately 3–4 h after administration of ^{99m}Tc-labeled white cells. This is due to elution of secondary hydrophilic ^{99m}Tc-HMPAO species which are excreted in the gut via biliary excretion and in the urine (Peters et al. 1988). As a consequence, imaging of inflammatory bowel disease (IBD) and intra-abdominal abscesses using ^{99m}Tc-labeled leukocytes needs to be performed within 2 h of injection.

References

Amara SG, Kuhar MJ (1993) Neurotransmitter transporters: recent progress. Annu Rev Neurosci 16:73–93

Anon (1989) In vitro stabilization of technetium-99 m exametazime (HM-PAO). Res Discl 305:666

Archer CM, Edwards B, Kelly JD et al. (1995) Technetium labeled agents for imaging tissue hypoxia in vivo. In: Nicolini M, Bandoli G, Mazzi U (eds) Technetium and rhenium in chemistry and nuclear medicine 4. SGEditoriali, Padova, pp 535–539

Bakker WH, Brunss AC, Breeman WAP et al. (1991a) [^{111}In-DTPA-D-Phe^{1}]-octreotide, a potential radiopharmaceutical for imaging of somatostatin receptor-positive tumors: synthesis, radiolabeling and in vitro validation. Life Sci 49:1583–1591

Bakker WH, Krenning EP, Breeman WAP et al. (1991b) In vivo use of radioiodinated somastatin analogue: dynamics, metabolism and binding to somatostatin receptor positive tumors in man. J Nucl Med 32:1184–1189

Bakker WH, Krenning EP, Reubi JC et al. (1991c) In vivo application of [^{111}In- DTPA-D-Phe^{1}]-octreotide for detection of somatostatin receptor-positive tumors in rats. Life Sci 49:1593–1601

Ballinger JR, Gulenchyn K (1991) Alternative formulations for technetium-99 m HMPAO. Int J Appl Radiat Isotop 42:315–316

Ballinger JR, Banneman J, Boxen I et al. (1996) Technetium-99m-tetrofosmin as a substrate for P-glycoprotein: in vitro studies in multidrug-resistant breast tumor cells. J Nucl Med 37:1578–1582

Ballinger JR, Muzzammil T, Moore MJ (1997) Technetium-99m-furifosmin as an agent for functional imaging of multidrug resistance in tumors. J Nucl Med 38:1915–1919

Bartenstein P, Ludolph A, Schober O et al. (1991) Benzodiazepine receptors and cerebral blood flow in partial epilepsy. Eur J Nucl Med 18:111–118

Beer HF, Blauenstein PA, Hasler PH et al. (1990) In vitro and in vivo evaluation of iodine-123-Ro 16-0154: a new imaging agent for SPECT investigations of benzodiazepine receptors. J Nucl Med 31:1007–1014

Berger G, Mazière M, Comar D (1979) Automated synthesis of ^{11}C-labeled radiopharmaceuticals: imipramine, chlorpromazine, nicotine, methionine. Int J Appl Radiat Isot 30:393–399

Billinghurst MW, Abrams DN, Lawson MS (1991) Stabilization of [^{99m}Tc]HMPAO-1. Ethanolic preparation. Int J Appl Radiat Isotop 42:607–612

Bobeldijk M, Verhoeff NPLG, Vekemans JAJM et al. (1990) A simple and high-yield synthesis of (S)-BZM, (R)-BZM and (S)-IBZM for the preparation of (S)-^{123}I-IBZM. J Labeled Compds Radiopharm 28:1247–1256

Boja JW, Carroll FI, Rahman MA et al. (1990) New, potent cocaine analogs: ligand binding and transport studies in rat striatum. Eur J Pharmacol 184:329–332

Bolster JM, Vaalburg W, Paans AM, van Dijk TH, Elsinga PH, Zijlstra JB, Piers DA, Mulder NH, Woldring MG, Wynberg H (1986) Carbon-11 labelled tyrosine to study tumor metabolism by positron emission tomography (PET). Eur J Nucl Med 12:321–324

Burch WM, Browitt RJ (1996) The transition from technegas to pertechnegas. J Nucl Med 37:1917–1918

Burch WM, Tetley IJ, Gras JL (1984) Technetium-99 m 'Pseudogas' for diagnostic studies in the lung. Clin Phys Physiol Meas 5:79–85

Burch WM, Sullivan PJ, Lomas FE et al. (1986a) Lung ventilation studies with technetium-99 m pseudogas. J Nucl Med 27:842–846

Burch WM, Sullivan PJ, McLaren CJ (1986b) Technegas – a new ventilation agent for lung scanning. Nucl Med Commun 7:865–871

Busatto GF, Pilowsky LS, Costa DC et al. (1997) Initial evaluation of ^{123}I-5-I-R91150, a selective 5-HT$_{2A}$ ligand for single-photon emission tomography, in healthy human subjects. Eur J Nucl Med 24:119–124

Carroll FI, Rahman MA, Abraham P et al. (1991) [^{123}I]3b-(4-iodophenyl)tropan-2b-carboxylic acid methyl ester (RTI-55), a unique cocaine receptor ligand for imaging the dopamine and serotonin transporters in vivo. Med Chem Res 1:289–294

Colombo F, Marmion M, Deutsch K et al. (1992) A new ^{99m}Tc radiotracer named Q-12: a myocardial perfusion agent with optimized imaging properties. J Nucl Biol Med 36:114

Cowen P (1991) Serotonin receptor subtypes: implications for psychopharmacology. Br J Psychiatry 159 [Suppl 12]:7–14

Danpure HJ, Osman S, Carroll MJ (1988) Development of a clinical protocol for radiolabeling of mixed leukocytes with ^{99m}Tc-hexamethylpropyleneamine oxime. Nucl Med Commun 9:465–475

Datz FL (1993) The current status of radionuclide infection imaging. In: Freeman LM (ed) Nuclear medicine annual. Raven, New York

Datz FL (1994) Indium-111-labeled laukocytes for the detection of infection: current status. Semin Nucl Med 24:92–109

Dewanjee MK (1990) The chemistry of Tc-99m-labeled radiopharmaceuticals. Semin Nucl Med 20:5–27

Ehrin E, Johnström P, Stone-Elander S et al. (1984) Preparation and preliminary positron emission tomography studies of ^{11}C-Ro 15-1788, a selective benzodiazepine antagonist. Acta Pharm Suec 21:183–188

Frier M (1994) Leucocyte radiolabeling techniques: practical aspects. Scand J Gastroenterol 29 [Suppl]:32–35

Fukuchi K, Kusuoka H, Yutani K et al. (1998) Assessment of reperfused myocardium using a new ischaemia-avid imaging agent, technetium-99 m HL91: comparison with myocardial glucose uptake. Eur J Nucl Med 25:361–366

Gallagher BM, Ansari A, Atkins H, Casella V, Christman DR, Fowler JS, Ido T, MacGregor RR, Som P, Wan CN, Wolf AP, Kuhl DE, Reivich M (1977) Radiopharmaceuticals XXVII. 18F-labeled 2-deoxy-2-fluoro-d-glucose as a radiopharmaceutical for measuring regional myocardial glucose metabolism in vivo: tissue distribution and imaging studies in animals. J Nucl Med 18:990-996

Grierson IR, Link JM, Mathis CA et al. (1989) A radiosynthesis of fluorine-18 fluoromisonidazole. J Nucl Med 30:343–350

Halldin C, Stone-Elander S, Thorell J-O et al. (1988)^{11}C-labeling of Ro 15–1788 in two different positions, and also ^{11}C-labeling of its main metabolite Ro 15–3890 for PET studies of benzodiazepine receptors. Appl Radiat Isot 39:993–997

Halldin C, Farde L, Högberg T et al. (1991) A comparative PET-study of five carbon-11 or fluorine-18 labeled salicylamides. Preparation and in vitro dopamine D-2 receptor binding. Nucl Med Biol 18:871–881

Hamacker K, Coenen HH, Stöcklin G (1986) Efficient stereospecific synthesis of no-carrier-added 2-[18F]-fluoro-2-deoxy-D-glucose using aminopolyether supported nucleophilic substitution. J Nucl Med 27:235–238

Hamilton RG, Alderson PO (1977) A comparative evaluation of techniques for rapid and efficient in vivo labeling of red cells with [^{99m}Tc]pertechnetate. J Nucl Med 18:1010–1013

Hantraye P, Kaijima M, Prenant C et al. (1984) Central type benzodiazepine binding sites: a positron emission tomography study in the baboon's brain. Neurosci Lett 48:115–120

Hegge FN, Hamilton GW, Larson SM et al. (1978) Cardiac chamber imaging: a comparison of red blood cells, labeled with Tc-99 m in vitro and in vivo. J Nucl Med 19:129–134

Higley B, Smith FW, Smith T et al. (1993) Technetium-99m-1,2 bis[bis(2-ethoxyethyl)phosphino]ethane: human biodistribution, dosimetry and safety of a new myocardial perfusion imaging agent. J Nucl Med 34:30–38

Högberg T, Ström P, de Paulis T et al. (1991) Potential antipsychotic agents. 9. Synthesis and stereoselective dopamine D-2 receptor blockade of a potent class of substituted (R)-N-((1-benzyl-2-pyrrolidinyl)methyl)benzamides. Relation to other side chain congeners. J Med Chem 34:948–955

Hoyer D, Clarke D, Fozard J et al. (1994) International union of pharmacology classification of receptors for 5-hydroxytrypamine. Pharmacol Rev 46:157–203

Hung JC, Gibbons RJ (1992) Breakage of technetium-99m-sestamibi vial with the use of a microwave oven. J Nucl Med 33:176–178

Hung JC, Volkert WA, Holmes RA (1989) Stabilization of technetium-99m-d,l-hexamethylpropyleneamine oxime (^{99m}Tc-d,l-HM-PAO) using gentisic acid. Nucl Med Biol 16:675–680

Hung JC, Chowdhury S, Redfern MG et al. (1997) Rapid preparation method for technetium-99m-bicisate. Eur J Nucl Med 24:655–659

Ishiwata K, Vaalburg W, Elsinga PH et al. (1988) Comparison of l-[1-^{11}C]methionine and l-methyl-[^{11}C]methionine for measurement of in vivo protein synthesis rate with PET. J Nucl Med 29:1419–1427

Jewett DM, Magner TJ, Watkins GL (1991) Captive solvent methods for fast, simple carbon-11 radioalkylations. In: Emran AM (ed) New trends in radiopharmaceutical synthesis, quality assurance and regulatory control. Plenum, New York

Johnson EW, Woods SW, Zoghbi SS et al. (1990) Receptor binding characterization of the benzodiazepine radioligand ^{125}I-Ro 16–0154: potential probe for SPECT brain imaging. Life Sci 47:1535–1546

Kaufman MJ, Madras BK (1991) Severe depletion of cocaine recognition sites associated with the dopamine transporter in Parkinson's diseased striatum. Synapse 49:43–49

Kawai K, FujibayashiY, Saji H et al. (1991) A strategy for the study of cerebral amino acid transport using iodine-123 labeled amino acid radiophamaceutical: 3-iodo-alpha-methyl-l-tyrosine. J Nucl Med 32:819–824

Kelly JD, Foster AM, Higley B et al. (1993) Technetium-99m-tetrofosmin a new radiopharmaceutical for myocardial perfusion imaging. J Nucl Med 34:222–227

Keen M, Kelly E, Nobbs P, MacDermot J (1989) A selective binding site for 3H-NECA that is not an adenosine A2 receptor. Biochem Pharmacol 38:3827–3833

Kloss G, Leven M (1979) Accumulation of radioiodinated tyrosine derivatives in adrenal medulla and in melanomas. Eur J Nucl Med 4:179–186

Kole AC, Pruim J, Nieweg OE et al. (1997) PET with L-[1-carbon-11]-tyrosine to visualize tumors and measure protein synthesis rates. J Nucl Med 38:191–195

Krenning EP, Bakker WH, Kooij PPM et al. (1992) Somatostatin receptor scintigraphy with indium-111-DTPA-D-Phe-1-octreotide in man: metabolism, dosimetry and comparison with iodine-123-Tyr-3-octreotide. J Nucl Med 33:652–658

Kung HF, Guoy Z, Billings D (1988) Preparation and biodistribution of [^{123}I]IBZM: a potential CNS D_2 dopamine receptor imaging agent. Nucl Med Biol 15:195–201

Kung HF, Alavi A, Chang W et al. (1990) In vivo SPECT imaging of CNS D-2 dopamine receptors: initial studies with iodine-123-IBZM in humans. J Nucl Med 31:573–579

Kung HF, Kim H-J, Kung M-P et al. (1996) Imaging of dopamine transporters in humans with technetium-99 m TRODAT-1. Eur J Nucl Med 23:1527–1530

Kung M-P, Stevenson DA, Plössi K et al. (1997) [^{99m}Tc]TRODAT-1: a novel technetium-99 m complex as a dopamine transporter imaging agent. Eur J Nucl Med 24:372–380

Laihinen AO, Rinne JO, Nägren K et al. (1995) PET studies on brain monoamine transporters with carbon-11-b-CIT in Parkinson's disease. J Nucl Med 36:1263–1267

Lamberts SWJ, Bakker WH, Reubi JC et al. (1990) Somatostatin receptor imaging in the localization of endocrine tumors. N Engl J Med 323:1246–1249

Lang J, Barbarics E, Lazar J et al. (1989) Effects of labeling conditions and formulation of kit on in vitro stability of 99mTc-d,l-HM-PAO. Eur J Nucl Med 15:424

Langen K-J, Coenen HH, Roosen N et al. (1990) SPECT studies of brain tumors wirh L-3-[^{123}I]iodo-a-methyl tyrosine: comparison with PET, ^{124}IMT and first clinical results. J Nucl Med 31:281–286

Langen K-J, Roosen N, Coenen HH et al. (1991) Brain and brain tumor uptake of L-3-[^{123}I]iodo-a-methyl tyrosine: competition with natural L-amino acids. J Nucl Med 32:1225–1228

Langström B, Antoni G, Gullberg P et al. (1987) Synthesis of L- and D-[methyl-11 C]methionine. J Nucl Med 28:1037–1040

Lemaire C, Cantineau R, Guillaume M et al. (1991) Fluorine-18-altanserin: a radioligand for the study of serotonin receptors with PET: radiolabeling and in vivo biologic behavior in rats. J Nucl Med 32:2266–2272

Lemb M, Oei TH, Eifert H et al. (1993) Technegas: a study of particle structure, size and distribution. Eur J Nucl Med 20:576–579

Leysen JE (1989) Use of 5-HT receptor agonists and antagonists for the characterization of their respective receptor sites. In: Boulton AB, Baker BG, Jurio AV (eds) Drugs as tools in neurotransmitter research. Neuromethods, vol 12. Humana, Clifton, pp 299–349

Linder KE, Chan YW, Cyr JE et al. (1993) Synthesis, characterization and in vitro evaluation of nitroimidazole-BATO complexes: new technetium compounds designed for imaging hypoxic tissue. Bioconj Chem 4:326–333

Linder KE, Chan YW, Cyr JE et al. (1994) ^{99m}TcO(PnAO-1-2-nitroimidazole)[BMS181321], a new technetium-containing nitroimidazole complex for imaging hypoxia: synthesis, characterization and xanthine oxidase-catalyzed reduction. J Med Chem 37:9–17

Lister-James J, Knight LC, Mauer AH et al. (1996) Thrombus imaging with a technetium-99m-labeled activated platelet receptor-binding peptide. J Nucl Med 37:775–781

Litton J, Farde L, Neiman J et al. (1991) Positron emission tomography of benzodiazepine receptor binding in alcoholics – equilibrium quantification. J Cereb Blood Flow Metab 11 [Suppl]:617

Mackey DW, Jackson P, Baker RJ et al. (1994) The observation of fullerenes in a Technegas lung ventilation unit. Nucl Med Commun 15:430–434

Mang'era KO, Vanbilloen HP, Schiepers CW et al. (1995) Stabilisation of high-activity ^{99m}Tc-d,l-HMPAO preparations with cobalt chloride and their biological behaviour. Eur J Nucl Med 22:1163–1172

Mang'era KO, Vanbilloen HP, Bellande E et al. (1996) Influence of a ^{99m}TcN core on the biological and physicochemical behavior of ^{99m}Tc complexes of l,l-EC and l,l-ECD. Nucl Med Biol 23:987–993

Mazière M, Godot JM, Berger G et al. (1980) High specific activity carbon-11 labeling of benzodiazepines: diazepam and flunitrazepam. J Radioanal Chem 56:229–235

Mazière M, Hantraye P, Prenant C et al. (1984) Synthesis of ethyl 8-fluoro-5,6-dihydro-5-[^{11}C]methyl-6-oxo-4H-imidazo[1,5-a][1,4]benzodiazepine-3-carboxylate (Ro 15.1788-^{11}C): a specific radioligand for the in vivo study of central benzodiazepine receptor of rat kidney mitochondria. Neuroscience 15:642

Mazière B, Crouzel C, Venet M et al. (1988) Synthesis, affinity and specificity of ^{18}F-setoperone, a potential ligand for in-vivo imaging of cortical serotonin receptors. Nucl Med Biol 15:463–468

Mazière B, Coenen HH, Halldin C et al. (1992) PET radioligands for dopamine receptors and re-uptake sites: chemistry and biochemistry. Nucl Med Biol 19:497–512

McAfee JG, Thakur ML (1976) Survey of radioactive agents for in vitro labeling of phagocytic leukocytes. I. Soluble agents. J Nucl Med 17:480–487

McAfee JG, Subramanian JG, Gagne G (1984) Techniques of leucocyte harvesting and labeling: problems and perspectives. Semin Nucl Med 14:83–106

Meegalla SK, Plössi K, Kung M-P et al. (1997) Synthesis and characterization of Tc-99 m labeled tropanes as dopamine tansporter imaging agents. J Med Chem 40:9–17

Melo T, Duncan J, Ballinger JR et al. (1998) BMS194796, a second-generation Tc-99m-labeled 2-nitroimidazole for imaging hypoxia in tumours. J Nucl Med 39:219P

Mertens J, Terriere D, Sipido V et al. (1994) Radiosynthesis of a new radioiodinated ligand for serotonin-5HT2-receptors, a promising tracer for g-emission tomography. J Labeled Comp Radiopharm 34:795–806

Monaghan P, Provan I, Murray C (1991) An improved radionuclide technique for the detection of altered pulmonary permeability. J Nucl Med 32:1945–1949

Mortelmans L, Malbrain S, Stuyck J et al. (1989) In vitro and in vivo evaluation of granulocyte labeling with (^{99m}Tc)d,l-HMPAO. J Nucl Med 30:2022–2028

Neumeier R, Kramp W, Macke H (1990) Chelating agents for forming complexes with radioactive isotopes, metal complexes thereof and use thereof in diagnosis and therapy. Eur Patent Appl 0417870 A2

Nunn A, Linder K, Strauss HW (1995) Nitroimidazoles and imaging hypoxia. Eur J Nucl Med 22:265–280

Okada T, Fujita M, Shimada S et al. (1998) Assessment of affinities of beta-CIT, beta-CIT-FE, and beta-CIT-FP for monoamine transporters permanently expressed in cell lines. Nucl Med Biol 25:53–58

Osman S, Lundkvist C, Pike V et al. (1996) Characterization of the radioactive metabolites of the 5-HT$_{1A}$ receptor radioligand [O-methyl-^{11}C]WAY-100635 in monkey and human plasma by HPLC-comparison of the behaviour of an identified radioactive metabolite with parent radioligand in monkey using PET. Nucl Med Biol 23:627–634

Paans AMJ, Elsinga PH, Vaalburg W (1993) Carbon-11-labeled tyrosine as a probe for modelling the protein synthesis rate. In: Mazoyer BM, Heiss WD, Comar D (eds) PET studies on amino acid metabolism and protein synthesis. Dordrecht, Kluwer, pp 161–174

Pardridge WM (1977) Kinetics of competitive inhibition of neutral amino acid transport across the blood-brain barrier. J Neurochem 28:103–108

Pearson DA, Lister-James J, McBride WJ et al. (1996) Thrombus imaging using technetium-99 m labeled high potency GPI-Ib/IIIa receptor antagonists. Chemistry and initial biological studies. J Med Chem 39:1372–1382

Peck-Radosavljevic M, Yang Q, Leimer M et al. (1998) The somatostatine receptor subtype 3 (SSTR) acts as a VIP-receptor. Gastroenterology 114:1172

Peters AM (1994) Quality control of radiolabeled white cells. In: Martin-Comin J, Thakur ML, Piera C, Roca M, Lomena F (eds) Radiolabeled blood elements. Recent advances in techniques and applications. Plenum, New York, pp 29–32

Peters AM, Danpure HJ, Osman S et al. (1986) Preliminary clinical experience with ^{99m}Tc-HMPAO for labeling leucocytes and imaging inflammation. Lancet 2:946–949

Peters AM, Roddie ME, Danpure HJ et al. (1988) Tc-99 m HM-PAO labeled leucocytes: a comparison with In-111-tropolonate labeled granulocytes. Nucl Med Commun 9:449–463

Phelps ME, Hoffman EJ, Selin C, Huang SC, Robinson G, MacDonald N, Shelbert H, Kuhl DE (1978) Investigation of [18F]-2-fluoro-2-deoxyglucose for the measure of myocardial glucose metabolism. J Nucl Med 19:1311–1319

Pike VW, McCarron J, Hume SP et al. (1995) Preclinical development of a radioligand for studies of central 5-HT$_{1A}$ receptors in vivo –[^{11}C]WAY-100635. Med Chem Res 5:208–227

Pike VW, McCarron J, Lamertsmaa A et al. (1996) Exquisite delineation of 5-HT$_{1A}$ receptors in human brain with PET and [carbonyl-^{11}C]WAY-100635. Eur J Pharmacol 301:R5–R7

Piwnica-Worms D, Chiu ML, Budding M et al. (1993) Functional imaging of multidrug-resistant P-glycoprotein with an organo-technetium complex. Cancer Res 53:977–984

Planas AM, Prenant C, Mazoyer BM et al. (1992) Regional cerebral L-[^{14}C-methyl]methionine incorporation into proteins: evidence for methionine recycling in the rat brain. J Cereb Blood Flow Metab 12:603–612

Pullman W, Hanna R, Sullivan P et al. (1986) Tc-99 m autologous phagocyte scanning: a new imaging technique for inflammatory bowel disease. Br Med J 293:171–174

Roddie ME, Peters HM, Danpure HJ et al. (1988) Imaging inflammation with Tc-99 m hexamethyl propyleneamineoxime (HMPAO) labeled leucocytes. Radiology 166:767–772

Rossetti C, Paganelli G, Vanoli G et al. (1992) Biodistribution in humans and preliminary clinical evaluation of a new tracer with optimized properties for myocardial perfusion imaging: [^{99m}Tc]Q12. J Nucl Biol Med 36 [Suppl]:29–31

Rossetti C, Vanoli G, Paganelli G et al. (1994) Human biodistribution, dosimetry and clinical use of technetium(III)-99m-Q12. J Nucl Med 35:1571–1580

Sampson CB, Solanki C (1991) Stabilisation of Tc-99m-exametazine using ethanol and storage at low temperature. Eur J Nucl Med 18:532

Samson Y, Bernuau J, Pappata S et al. (1987) Cerebral uptake of benzodiazepine measured by positron emission tomography in hepatic encephalopathy. N Engl J Med 316:414–415

Savic I, Roland P, Sedvall G et al. (1988) In vivo demonstration of reduced benzodiazepine receptor binding in human epileptic foci. Lancet 16:863–866

Scalzetti EM, Gagne GM (1995) The transition from technegas to pertechnegas. J Nucl Med 36:267–269

Schauwecker DS, Burt RW, Park HM et al. (1988) Comparison of purified indium-111 granulocytes and indium-111 mixed leukocytes for imaging of infections. J Nucl Med 29:23–25

Schroth HJ, Oberhausen E, Berberich R (1981) Cell labeling with colloidal substances in whole blood. Eur J Nucl Med 6:469–472

Seabold JE, Forstrom LA, Schauwecker DS et al. (1997) Procedure guideline for indium-111-leukocyte scintigraphy for suspected infection/inflammation. J Nucl Med 38:997–1001

Srivastava SC, Babich JB, Richards P (1983) A new kit method for the selective labeling of erythrocytes in whole blood with technetium-99 m. J Nucl Med 24:128P

Stone CK, Mulnix T, Nickles RJ et al. (1995) Comparison of the myocardial and hepatic uptake of two technetium-labeled nitroimidazoles after regional ischemia and reperfusion using a dual-isotope technique. J Nucl Med 36:138P

Stöcklin G (1992) Tracers for metabolic imaging of brain and heart. Radiochemistry and radiopharmacology. Eur J Nucl Med 19:527–551

Suzuki K, Inoue O, Hashimoto K et al. (1985) Computer-controlled large scale production of high specific activity[11 C]Ro 15–1788 for PET studies of benzodiazepine receptors. Int J Appl Radiat Isot 36:971–976

Terriere D, Janssen PMF, Gommeren W et al. (1995) Evaluation of radioiodo-4-amino-N-[1-[3-(4-fluorophenoxy)-propyl]-4-methyl-4-piperidinyl]-5-iodo-2-methoxybenzamide as a potential 5HT2 receptor tracer for SPE(C)T. Nucl Med Biol 22:1005–1010

Thakur ML Lavender JP, Arnot RN et al. (1977) Indium-111-labeled autologous leukocytes in man. J Nucl Med 18:1014–1019

Tominaga S, Shimada T, Kawakami K (1995) Physicochemical characterization and lung clearance of pertechnegas. Kaku Ikagu 32:563–567

Tubergen K, Corlija M, Volkert WA et al. (1991) Sensitivity of technetium-99m-d,l-HMPAO to radiolysis in aqueous solutions. J Nucl Med 32:111–115

Vallabhajosula S, Moyer BR, Lister-James J et al. (1996) Preclinical evaluation of technetium-99m-labeled somatostatin receptor-binding peptides. J Nucl Med 37:1016–1022

Van Nerom CG, Bormans GM, De Roo MJ et al. (1993) First experience in healthy volunteers with technetium-99 m l,l-ethylenedicysteine, a new renal imaging agent. Eur J Nucl Med 20:738–746

Verbeke K, Boonen C, Verbruggen A (1997) Usefulness of residual fractions of L,L-ethylcysteinate dimer (NeuroliteÒ) for the preparation of ^{99m}Tc-L,L-ethylcysteinate dimer. Nucl Med Commun 18:535–539

Verbruggen A, Bormans G, Van Nerom C et al. (1990) Isolation of the mono-ester mono-acid derivatives of ^{99m}Tc-ECD and their metabolites in mice. In: Nicolini M, Bandoli G, Mazzi U (eds) Technetium and rhenium in chemistry and nuclear medicine 3. Cortina International, Verona / Raven, New York, pp 445–452

Verbruggen AM, Nosco DL, Van Nerom CG et al. (1992) Technetium-99m-l,l-ethylenedicysteine: a renal imaging agent. I. Labeling and evaluation in animals. J Nucl Med 33:551–557

Virgolini I, Raderer M, Kurtaran A et al. (1994a) Vasoactive intestinal peptide-receptor imaging for the localization of intestinal adenocarcinomas and endocrine tumors. N Engl J Med 331:1116–1121

Virgolini I, Yang Q, Li S et al. (1994b) Cross-competition between vasoactive intestinal peptide and somatostatin for binding to tumor cell membrane receptors. Cancer Res 54:690–700

Virgolini I, Kurtaran A, Raderer M et al. (1995) Vasoactive intestinal peptide receptor scintigraphy. J Nucl Med 36:1732–1739

Virgolini I, Szilvasi I, Kurtaran A et al. (1998) Indium-111-DOTA-Lanreotide: biodistribution, safety and radiation absorbed dose in tumor patients. J Nucl Med 39:1928–1936

Wackers FJT, Berman DS, Maddahi J et al. (1989) Technetium-99 m hexakis 2-methoxyisobutyl isonitrile: human biodistribution, dosimetry, safety and preliminary comparison to thallium-201 for myocardial perfusion imaging. J Nucl Med 30:301–311

Weisner PS, Bower GR, Dollimore LA et al. (1993) A method for stabilising technetium-99 m exametazime prepared from a commercial kit. Eur J Nucl Med 20:661–666

Willemsen ATM, van Waarde A, Paans AMJ et al. (1995) In vivo protein synthesis rate determination with L-[1-^{11}C]-tyrosine and positron emission tomography: methods, metabolism, modeling and results in patients with primary or recurrent brain tumors. J Nucl Med 36:411–419

Yamamoto YL, Meyer E, Menon D et al. (1983) Regional cerebral blood measurement and dynamic positron emission tomography. In: Heiss WD, Phelps ME (eds) Positron emission tomography of the brain. Springer, Berlin Heidelberg New York, pp 78–84

Yamasaki T, Inoue O, Shinotoh H et al. (1986) Benzodiazepine study in the elderly using PET and clinical application of a new tracer, C-11-a-methyl-N-methyl benzylamine. In: Kitane K (ed) Liver and aging, liver and brain. Elsevier, Amsterdam, pp 265–276

13 Instrumentation and Data Acquisition

S. I. Ziegler

Contents

13.1 Detectors and Imaging Systems 221
13.1.1 Principles of Scintillation Detectors 221
13.1.2 From Single-Head, Multi-Head and Ring Geometry to Hybrid Systems 222
13.2 Requirements of Imaging Systems 228
13.2.1 Fundamentals of Clinical Imaging Protocols and Technical Factors 228
13.2.2 Acquisition Parameters and Procedural Factors 229
13.2.2.1 Sampling Requirements 229
13.2.2.2 Whole-Body Acquisition 230
13.2.2.3 Attenuation Correction 230
13.2.3 Quality Control 231
13.3 Is There a Future for Dedicated Systems? 233

13.1 Detectors and Imaging Systems

Nuclear medical images are formed by the detection of gamma-rays, X-rays or annihilation quanta (in the case of positron imaging). The camera detects the density of gamma rays per unit area, their energy and their direction of flight. If single photon emitters are used the direction of flight has to be determined by geometric collimation. In contrast, coincidence detection uses the unique feature of positron annihilation which results in two high-energy gamma rays simultaneously emitted back-to-back. The detection of both gamma rays within a very short time window defines the line of response in space and thus the direction of flight. Scintigraphic instrumentation consists of scintillation crystals to convert gamma-ray energy into visible light, suitable light sensors, readout electronics and image processing units.

S. I. Ziegler
Nuklearmedizinische Klinik und Poliklinik, Klinikum rechts der Isar der TU München, Ismaninger Strasse 22, D-81675 Munich, Germany

13.1.1 Principles of Scintillation Detectors

Scintillators emit light after a gamma ray has deposited its energy in the crystal. The wavelength (UV, visible), the intensity and time distribution of the scintillation light are properties of the scintillating material. There are organic (plastic) and inorganic scintillators, each having some unique advantages or disadvantages for the detection of either charged particles or gamma- and X-rays. All clinical nuclear medicine cameras are built with inorganic scintillators because of their high detection efficiency for X-rays and gamma rays.

The search for new scintillation crystals which are suitable for nuclear medicine imaging is guided by the following requirements: the higher the density of the material and the higher the atomic number, the better is the detection efficiency for gamma rays. More scintillation light emitted in a shorter period of time allows the detection of events in short time intervals. Although there are numerous scintillation crystals available, NaI(Tl) (thallium activated sodium iodide) remains the crystal of choice for single photon detection with energies of 70–360 keV. This is mainly because of its high light output, reasonable decay time and inexpensive production in large quantities. One disadvantage of NaI(Tl) is that it is a hygroscopic material and needs to be sealed in airtight containers.

For efficient detection of high-energy gamma rays in positron imaging, requirements are even more stringent: if coincidence detection is used, detection efficiency is most important, since the total efficiency is the product of the individual detector sensitivities. High density and atomic number are essential for detection of photons at 511 keV. The specific necessity of fast timing in coincidence measurements can be met by short decay times of scintillation light.

Although the energy resolution of a gamma camera is determined by the whole system, the light yield of the scintillation crystal is an important determinant. Better image contrast can be reached if the se-

Table 13.1. Characteristics of scintillation crystals which are used in nuclear medicine. *NaI* thallium-activated sodium iodide; *BGO* bismuth germanate; *YSO* cerium-activated yttrium oxy-orthosilicate; *LSO* cerium activated lutetium oxy-orthosilicate

	NaI:Tl	BGO	YSO:Ce	LSO:Ce
Light yield (% of NaI)	100	15	120	75
Wavelength (nm)	410	480	420	420
Light decay time (ns)	230	300	70	40
Attenuation length for 140 keV (mm)	4.2	0.8	7.7	1.0
Attenuation length for 511 keV (mm)	30	11	26	12

lection of accepted energy is improved. An energy resolution of less than 10% allows the choice of a narrow window with less loss in unscattered radiation (Kojima et al. 1993). Good energy resolution can be achieved with crystals of high light output. Additionally, luminous crystals provide improved event localization in a continuous detector.

Although the very first positron tomographs consisted of NaI(Tl) scintillation detectors, the most commonly used scintillator in positron emission tomography is bismuth germanate (BGO), which has high detection efficiency for annihilation quanta (Table 13.1). However, BGO has a low light yield and long light decay time, prohibiting short coincidence windows and high count rate capability. More recently, new scintillation materials became available specifically for coincidence detection. The most promising scintillator is cerium activated lutetium oxy-orthosilicate (LSO; Melcher and Schweitzer 1992). It has a similar detection efficiency as BGO, but a higher light yield and shorter light decay time. A high-resolution positron tomograph with this fast, luminous scintillation material is being constructed for brain research (Casey et al. 1997; Schmand et al. 1998a,b), and once large quantities of LSO can routinely be produced, it will substitute BGO most likely in clinical positron tomographs. These devices will perform at much higher count rates and will be less affected by random events in 3D mode (see below) since short coincidence windows can be implemented.

The light which is emitted by the scintillation crystal is detected by sensors coupled to the crystal. The coupling is achieved through a light pipe or directly on the entrance window of the light sensor. Photomultiplier tubes (PMT) are the light sensors which are in routine use. The photo-sensitive cathode of the PMT converts the impinging light into electrons, which are multiplied in the dynode structure of the PMT and read out as a pulse whose amplitude is proportional to the amount of light (Fig. 13.1). Semiconductor sensors may offer the advantage of very compact detector modules but are not yet implemented in commercial systems. First results in research imaging devices show their potential for the detection of signals from luminous, fast scintillators (Schmelz et al. 1995; Lecomte et al. 1996; Levin et al. 1997). In combination with PMTs, they offer novel designs for high-resolution detector modules (Huber et al. 1997).

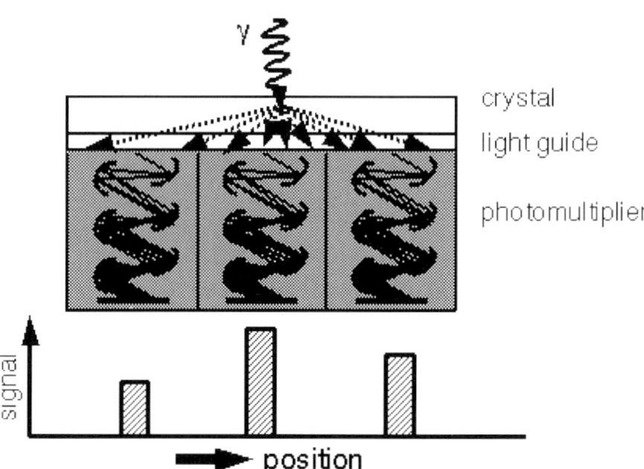

Fig. 13.1. Principle of the gamma camera. An incoming photon (γ) causes scintillations in the crystal which are guided to and amplified by photo multipliers. The position of the incoming photon is calculated from the signal intensity of the photomultiplier tubes

Direct detection of gamma rays in semiconductor material such as cadmium-zinc-telluride (CdZnTe) has become more realistic since the production process and signal processing have been improved (Butler et al. 1998; Kipper et al. 1998). Future investigations will show if these devices will find widespread application in clinical systems.

13.1.2 From Single-Head, Multi-Head and Ring Geometry to Hybrid Systems

Most nuclear medicine imaging is performed using a scintillation camera either in static or in dynamic acquisition mode. It consists of a single large area (typical 40×50 cm^2) NaI(Tl) scintillation crystal, which is read out by photomultiplier tubes (Fig. 13.1). A crystal of only 9.5 mm thickness has a detection efficiency of 90% for 140 keV gamma rays. Light sharing among the PMTs and centroid calculation of the light distribution is exploited for event localization on the detector head according to the scheme first proposed by Anger (1958). The technological improvements of this device which is in routine use since the 1960s, include higher spatial resolution, better uniformity and much higher count rate performance. Introduction of individual PMT-signal digitization resulted in new and better possibilities for the correction of system imperfections. In general, the Anger camera is optimized for imaging ^{99m}Tc-labeled compounds; thus performance is usually best for the detection of gamma rays of 140 keV.

Since the emission of gamma-rays from the patient is isotropic, collimation is needed to restrict data to gamma rays of certain, predefined directions. Most commonly used are parallel-hole collimators made of lead with very small holes separated by septa. The thickness and length of the septa are chosen such that for a given energy the gamma rays with inadequate direction are absorbed (Fig. 13.2). Obviously this leads to thicker septa for higher-energy gamma rays. Collimator design always is a compromise between spatial resolution and sensitivity: reducing the size of the holes or using longer septa improves spatial resolution but reduces sensitivity at the same time. This fact is the most important tradeoff in the imaging process using Anger cameras. The spatial resolution of a parallel-hole collimator decreases linearly with increasing distance between object and collimator (Fig. 13.2), whereas sensitivity stays approximately constant.

For transaxial tomography (single photon emission computed tomography, SPECT), the camera is rotated around the patient, acquiring multiple views from different angles. The transverse activity distribution is calculated from these projections using adequate reconstruction techniques (see chap. 14). The SPECT systems with two or three camera heads (Fig. 13.3) were developed to increase detection efficiency. Thus, for the same number of counts in the image, total scan duration can be reduced or higher-resolution collimators can be used.

Positron emission tomography (PET) utilizes the unique feature of two high-energy gamma rays emitted back-to-back after positron annihilation (Fig. 13.4). Detector pairs count all events which occur in both of them within a very short time interval (10–20 ns). From data along these lines of response, the distribution of radioactivity can be reconstructed by similar mathematical methods as are used in SPECT. The measured counts are the sum of true coincidences, belonging to a single positron decay, random events, which occur if two uncorrelated gamma rays are accidentally detected in a detector pair, and

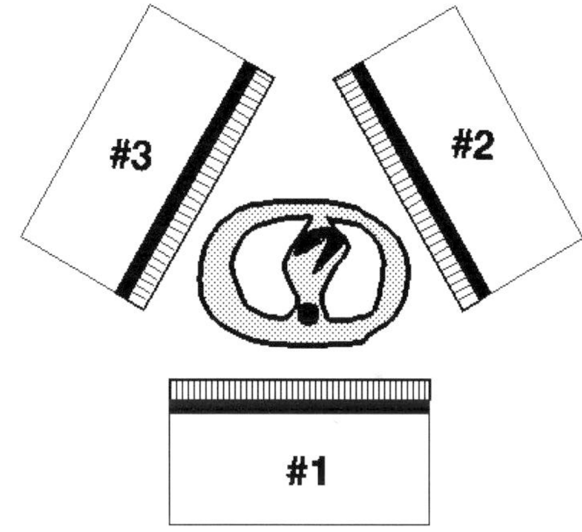

Fig. 13.3. Geometry of a triple-head SPECT system

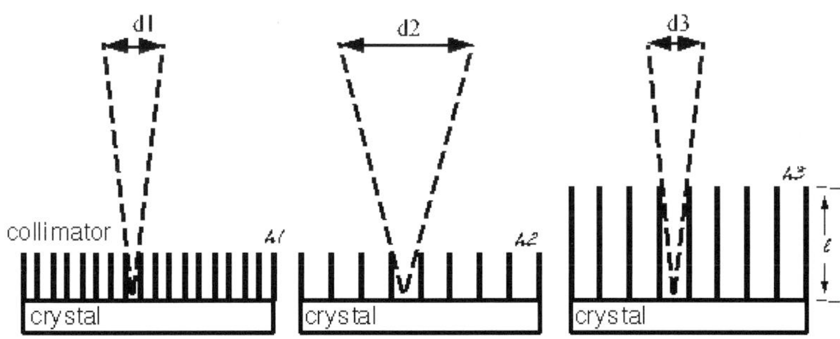

Fig. 13.2. Geometrical design of lead collimators defines the spatial resolution which can be achieved with a gamma camera. Septa length (l), thickness and hole width (h_1, h_2, h_3) define the blur in the image, represented by the visual field angle of the collimator (d_1, d_2, d_3). Spatial resolution degrades rapidly for larger distances

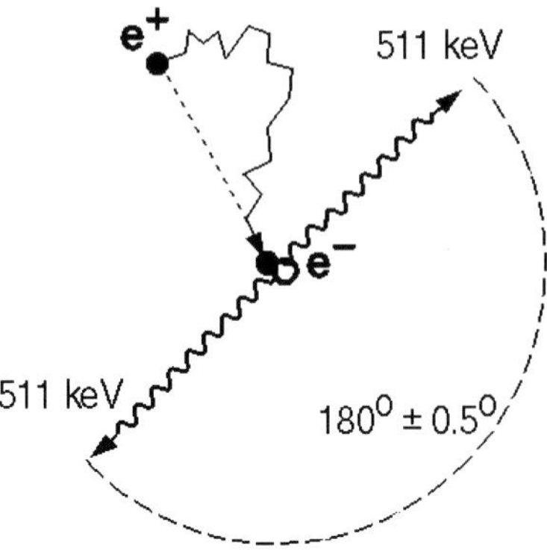

Fig. 13.4. Positron annihilation. Two high-energy gamma rays are emitted back-to-back, which can be used for "electronic collimation"

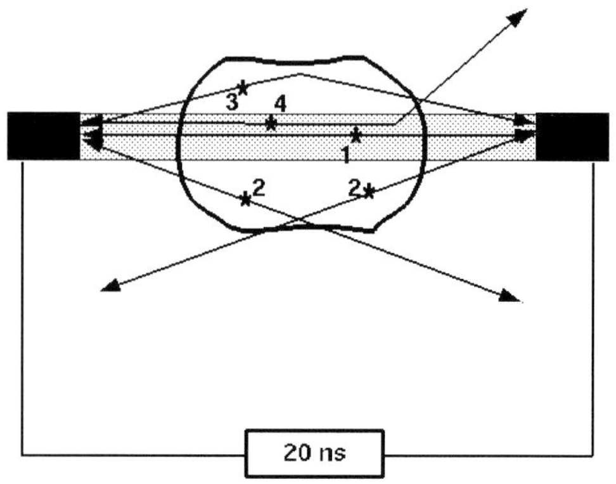

Fig. 13.5. Coincidence detector pair. True (*1*), random (*2*) and scattered (*3*) coincidence events, and attenuation (*4*). The *20 ns* is the time interval within which coincidence events occur for the 1-m distance between the detectors

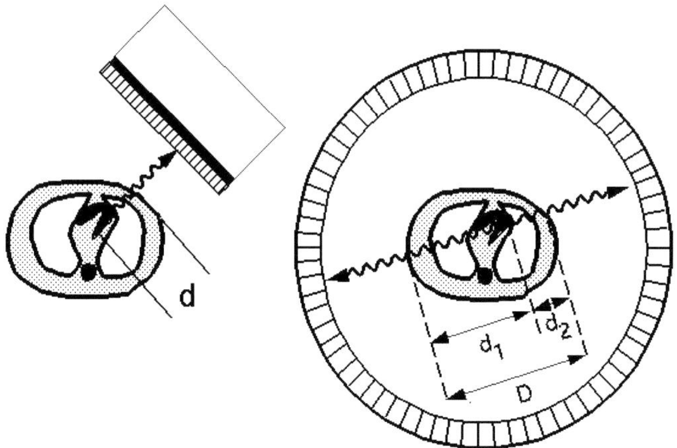

Fig. 13.6. Attenuation in SPECT (*left*) depends on the depth d of tissues in the body. In PET (*right*) one photon traverses d_1, and the other, d_2, which is the total length *D* through the body

scattered events, in which at least one of the gamma rays lost its original direction of flight through Compton scattering in the patient (Fig. 13.5). Scattering is also responsible for the loss of counts along a given line of response if one of the gamma rays is scattered so that it does not reach the detector. This effect, the attenuation of counts, is much more pronounced in PET, as compared with SPECT, since both gamma quanta have to reach the detectors (Fig. 13.6). Attenuation causes artifacts in the reconstructed images which result in distortions or inhomogeneity. Heterogeneous attenuation in the thorax especially affects myocardial scans. Hardware and software approaches have been developed for both SPECT and PET imaging (Bacharach and Buvat 1995). In contrast to SPECT, attenuation in PET can precisely be corrected because the total length through the body determines the attenuation factor along a coincidence line. By doing so, quantitative information about the tracer distribution can be obtained. Compensation for count loss through attenuation can be achieved by individually measuring the attenuation factor for 511-keV gamma rays. This is routinely done by rotating positron (^{68}Ge/^{68}Ga) rod sources. The ratio of a reference (blank) scan without object in the field-of-view and the transmission data results in correction factors for the projection data. Measured integral attenuation factors can be reconstructed into two-dimensional attenuation images. While this reconstruction step is not necessarily needed for attenuation correction in coincidence imaging, it is essential in attenuation correction methods in SPECT.

Limited count statistics in the transmission data is the reason for intensive research on optimizing measurement and processing in transmission acquisitions (BAILEY 1998).

The main difference between single photon and coincidence measurements is the necessity of lead collimators for the definition of the angle of incidence, compared with electronic collimation in the case of positron imaging. The use of collimators results in a very low detection efficiency of approximately 10^{-4} times the emitted number of gamma rays. Positron imaging by coincidence counting is much more sensitive. For example, even a triple-head SPECT system, designed to image Tc-99m-labeled tracers in the brain, is 15 times less sensitive than a positron tomograph if a 1-cm resolution is assumed in both systems (BUDINGER 1996). When imaging the body, this proportion becomes even less favorable (1:30).

The situation is even worse if annihilation quanta are detected in single photon mode by use of a ultra-high-energy collimator. The septa of such a collimator would cover more than half of the camera head. Taking into account that the efficiency of a 9.5 mm NaI(Tl) crystal is 50% lower at 511 than at 140 keV, the sensitivity for a SPECT system with 10-mm resolution would be 45 times less than a system for 140 keV and the same resolution (BUDINGER 1998). Therefore, the clinical potential of collimated detection of 511-keV single photons is found mainly in myocardial viability studies, where at the expense of spatial resolution (typically 2 cm FWHM) sensitivity is just 14 times lower than PET (VAN LINGEN et al. 1992; MACFARLANE et al. 1995; CHEN et al. 1997).

Spatial resolution in coincidence detection is defined by the size of the detectors. Crystals were read out by individual PMTs in the first tomographs. Demands for higher resolution and closely packed channels led to the invention of the block detector (CASEY and NUTT 1986). Most commercially available positron tomographs utilize this scheme. The small (4×4 cm) crystal blocks are segmented such that the light emitted from one block is distributed onto four photomultiplier tubes and Anger logic can be applied for segment identification, e.g. 64 segments. The function of a BGO block-detector therefore is very similar to a small gamma camera. The blocks are arranged in rings to cover the whole 360° around the patient and extend over 10–25 cm in the axial direction. The size of the sub-crystals in a block defines the intrinsic spatial resolution and thus is kept small.

Traditionally, PET acquisition is performed in transverse slices through the body, with inter-plane septa to reduce the scatter contribution (2D mode, Fig. 13.7a). In most of the current PET scanners, the septa can be retracted to allow three-dimensional data acquisition for enhanced sensitivity (Fig. 13.7b; BENDRIEM and TOWNSEND 1998). Although this acquisition mode has a higher scatter and random fraction than a 2D tomograph, the gain in true coincidence counts in brain scans obviates the use of smooth filters in the reconstruction process, thus image contrast is noticeably improved. Acquisitions in the abdomen or whole body in 3D mode are more affected by scattered radiation and random events originating outside the axial coincidence field of view. This measurement situation needs to be further

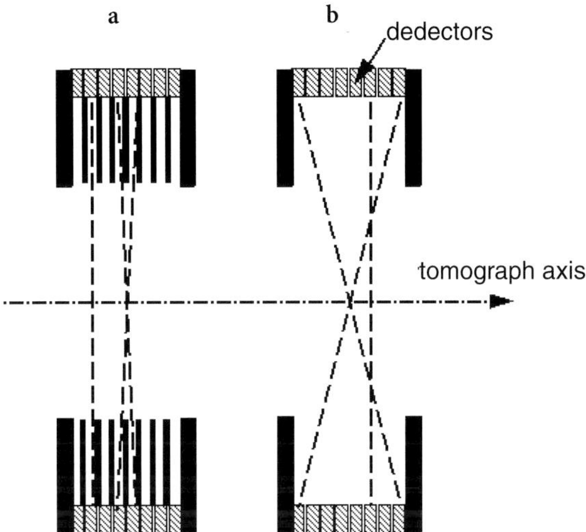

Fig. 13.7. **a** Two-dimensional PET uses inter-plane septa, restricting the events to direct slices and next neighbors. **b** In 3D PET septa are retracted, allowing all possible angles for coincidence detection

evaluated and normalization and correction methods for quantitative information have to be validated (BENDRIEM and TOWNSEND 1998). To fully utilize the advantages of 3D acquisition, methods for scatter correction and random subtraction have to be implemented along with suitable reconstruction or rebinning algorithms.

Tomographs with full rings of BGO-, and in the future LSO-, block detectors will remain the high performance PET scanners. However, clinical PET has gained much attention in the recent years, mostly triggered by the successes of using FDG in cancer diagnosis and treatment evaluation. Reducing the cost of PET instrumentation is the goal of new paths of scanner development: one being the introduction of positron tomographs with fewer or cheaper scintillation detectors, the other being hybrid dual head cameras offering SPECT as well as coincidence acquisition mode. The first category (dedicated positron imaging systems) is represented by a tomograph with large NaI(Tl) scintillation crystals arranged in a hexagon (UGM Quest, Philadelphia, Pennsylvania; ADAC C-PET, Milpitas, California). This is an intrinsically 3D system (MUEHLLEHNER and KARP 1986; KARP et al. 1990). From Table 13.1 it is clear that thicker NaI crystals are needed to improve coincidence detection efficiency. Thus, the crystals in this scanner are 25 mm thick. Since NaI(Tl) is less expensive than BGO, the price for this tomograph is lower. This tomograph has very good spatial resolution, good contrast and detection efficiency, but low count rate efficiency. Further improvements of this type of tomograph are underway, one being the use of curved crystals for better homogeneity in spatial resolution.

Another design to reduce the cost is a 3D tomograph which consists of only two sectors with BGO block detectors (Siemens CTI ECAT ART, Siemens, Erlangen, Germany), continuously rotating around the patient to cover all projection angles (TOWNSEND et al. 1993; BAILEY et al. 1997). This scanner has a good spatial resolution, and a sensitivity comparable to a full ring BGO tomograph which is operated in 2D. The most important physical performance parameters of some commercial positron imaging systems are summarized in Table 13.2.

Various realizations of hybrid cameras are available; all consist of a dual-head NaI(Tl) camera operated in either SPECT or coincidence mode (Fig. 13.8). In coincidence mode the camera is operated without collimators, and events detected in both detectors within a narrow time window (15 ns) are assigned to one coincidence event. The exact location of the coincidence line is calculated by the coordinates of gamma radiation detection on the camera heads (equivalent to 3D operation). For each angular position of the heads, therefore, coincidence events in different directions are recorded, in contrast to a parallel-hole collimator, which only records the photons that appear at right angles to the camera head.

Because a dual-head coincidence camera is meant to be operated both in the coincidence mode and in the conventional SPECT mode, compromises must be

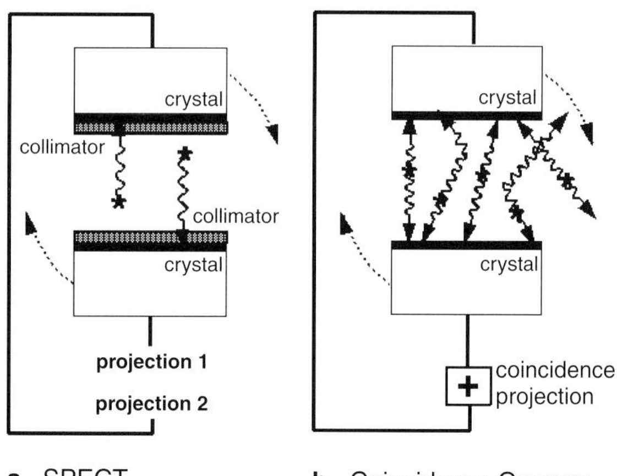

Fig. 13.8. Dual-head camera operated with collimators in **a** SPECT mode, and **b** without collimators in coincidence mode

Table 13.2. Performance parameters of dedicated ring tomographs (Siemens CTI ECAT EXACT47 and ART, Siemens, Erlangen, Germany; GE Advance and UGM Quest, General Electric Medical Systems, Milwaukee, Wis.; and a coincidence camera (ADAC Vertex MCD ADAC Laboratories, Milpitas, Calif.). *FWHM* full width at half maximum

	EXACT47		Advance		ART	Quest	MCD[c]
	2D[a]	3D[b]	2D[a]	3D[b]			
Axial field of view (cm)	16.2	16.2	15.2	15.2	16.2	25	38
Resolution in the center							
Transaxial FWHM (mm)	5.8	5.8	4.5	4.5	5.7	5.5	5.0
Axial FWHM (mm)	5.0	5.0	4.0	6.0	6.0	6.0	5.3
Sensitivity (cps/Bq per milliliter)[d]	5.8	40.5	5.7	30.4	7.5	12.2	3.2
Scatter fraction (%)[d]	17	48	10	34	37	28	32

[a] With tungsten septa
[b] Without tungsten septa
[c] Two energy windows (511 and 310 keV) 30% width, detector distance 62 cm
[d] Measured in a cylinder (20 cm diameter), homogeneously filled with ^{18}F

made in the design since some requirements are contradictory. For example, a thin scintillation crystal (generally 9.5 mm) is required for SPECT so that the best possible spatial resolution can be achieved (MUEHLLEHNER 1979). However, if high-energy annihilation photons are to be recorded efficiently, thicker crystals must be used. With a 6.4-mm-thick NaI(Tl) crystal, only 7% of the photons deposit their entire energy (511 keV) in the crystal, and with double the crystal thickness the proportion is 17% (ANGER and DAVIS 1964), resulting in a coincidence detection efficiency of 3%. Digital correction techniques are used in modern cameras; thus, despite increased crystal thickness, there is no resolution degradation in the detection of low-energy photons.

Since large-area camera heads are involved, events are also detected that have their origin outside the actual field of view of the camera and increase the singles count rate in the heads (Fig. 13.9). Similarly, the detectors are sensitive to photons that are scattered in the patient and reach the crystal. High singles count rates contribute to the background of random coincidences and, because of the open design, depend on the distribution outside the field of view, a fact that makes correction techniques more difficult or even impossible. The fraction of coincidence events is approximately 1–2% of all events, depending on crystal thickness. The singles count rates in a camera head during coincidence operation can be as high as 1 million/s. Compared with count rates of much less than 100 kcps, which normally occur in SPECT imaging, this imposes stringent demands on the camera's count rate performance. To solve the problem of a system that is less sensitive but may nevertheless be subjected to high count rates, pulse processing techniques become more important (MANKOFF et al. 1990).

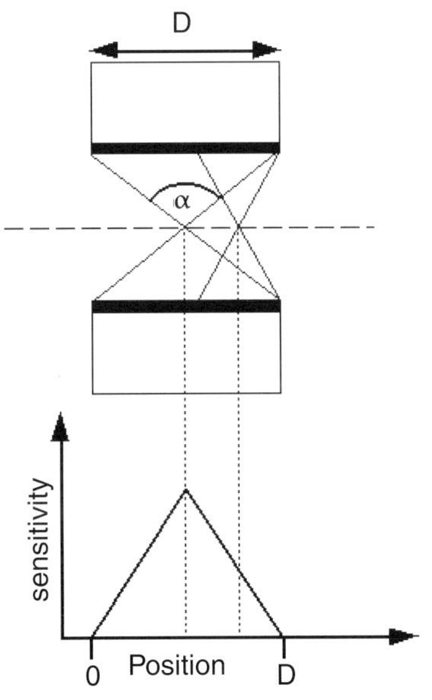

Fig. 13.9. The sensitivity profile in 3D imaging systems varies across the detector head *D*, depending on the axial acceptance angle α. The highest sensitivity is in the center

Although it provides a much higher sensitivity than a gamma camera equipped with an ultra-high-energy lead collimator, the dual-head coincidence camera is less sensitive than a full-ring PET scanner because of solid angle restrictions and lower detection efficiency at 511 keV in the NaI crystal. Therefore, a longer scan time is needed and the use of coincidence cameras is limited to the detection of ^{18}F labeled substances. Without attenuation correction, PET studies of the heart are not meaningful. Present implementations of coincidence cameras show a spatial resolution comparable to full-ring PET scanners, but with an increased scatter and random fraction (Table 13.2), causing the detectability of small lesions within background activity to be lower in coincidence cameras as compared with full-ring PET scanners (SHREVE et al. 1998). These systems are still being improved. Thus, it is very important to know where the coincidence cameras are applicable – these areas may be different from dedicated PET scanners (COLEMAN 1997).

Attenuation correction in dual-head coincidence imaging is currently being developed either by measured attenuation factors or by including attenuation into iterative reconstruction algorithms. Together with random and scatter correction techniques, this will be the basis for potential quantitative information from dual-head coincidence imaging (see chap. 14).

Obviously, a scintillator with higher detection efficiency for gamma rays of 511 keV would greatly enhance the performance of a hybrid system. Cerium activated lutetium oxy-orthosilicate, the scintillator which is most promising for coincidence measurements, unfortunately has a disadvantage in single photon detection: the natural radioactivity in the material causes non-zero count rates at background levels. In positron imaging, these events are suppressed by the coincidence window. Therefore, a new hybrid system is being developed in which the combination of two scintillation materials in a type of sandwich geometry is used. Each scintillator is specially suited for the detection either of low-energy or high-energy photons. The SPECT technique can be performed with signals from the front layer, positron imaging with coincidence counting from the back layers. For the front layer yttrium oxy-orthosilicate (YSO; DAHLBOM et al. 1997) or NaI(Tl) (SCHMAND et al.

1998a,b) were proposed in combination with a back layer made of LSO. The light decay constants of the two materials are different (Table 13.1); thus, pulse shape analysis can be used to discriminate which crystal was hit by the gamma ray. To meet the strict count rate requirements, the system consists of granulated detectors. The first cameras will merge SPECT and PET even closer.

13.2 Requirements of Imaging Systems

13.2.1 Fundamentals of Clinical Imaging Protocols and Technical Factors

The optimal use of any imaging system can only be provided if the technical parameters, such as resolution, sensitivity and scatter fraction, are evaluated in their influence on image quality.

Whereas spatial resolution is important for a realistic representation of the organ under study and quantitative information, it is not the only technical parameter determining image quality in terms of lesion detectability. Background due to septa penetration, scattered radiation or random coincidences affect contrast in the image. Thus, depending on the amount of background in the image, small lesions can get lost, even if the system resolution is the same.

For different imaging situations using gamma cameras, the most adequate collimator has to be chosen, depending on the energy of the incoming gamma ray, the size of the structures to be investigated and an acceptable scan duration for acquisition of sufficient count statistics. The highest-resolution collimator available for a given energy may be advantageous (Muehllehner 1985; Mueller et al. 1990), even if some sensitivity is lost.

In single-photon imaging, collimator resolution degrades rapidly with increasing distance from the collimator surface; therefore, the camera heads are kept as close as possible to the patient during acquisition. On the other hand, spatial resolution of coincidence detectors is almost independent of the position in-between the two detectors of a pair (Hoffman et al. 1982). However, coincidence sensitivity depends on the area of detector that is seen by each point in the object (solid angle), which is reduced with increased distance between the detector.

In camera systems utilizing lead collimators, performance is usually defined in terms of intrinsic (camera inherent properties) and extrinsic (including the collimator) system performance parameters. For patient imaging, the extrinsic values are more important since they reflect the actual clinical situation.

The system spatial resolution results from the combination of intrinsic detector resolution and resolution of the lead collimator. Measurement of the system spatial resolution is performed by imaging a ^{99m}Tc line source and using full width at half maximum (FWHM) and full width at tenth maximum (FWTM) as parameters of resolution. Whereas in most currently available gamma cameras the intrinsic spatial resolution is 4 mm FWHM, the limited resolution of the collimators degrades the system resolution to approximately 10 mm.

Intrinsic spatial resolution in camera-based systems is a result of PMT signal centroid-calculation (Fig. 13.1). Thus, it is affected by the statistical nature of scintillation light collection and random errors during conversion into electrons at the PMT cathode. Interaction of the 140-keV gamma ray, of ^{99m}Tc, produces more light in the scintillator and therefore less error in the positioning algorithm, than the 70–80 keV ray of ^{201}Tl. In order to detect a high-energy gamma ray efficiently, a thick crystal is favorable, but spread of light is more pronounced in thick crystals, causing the intrinsic spatial resolution to degrade in this situation.

It is important to eliminate image distortion by assuring spatial linearity; otherwise, images of line sources would not be straight. In modern gamma cameras, the digitized PMT signals are corrected before the event position is calculated (Muehllehner et al. 1980). Also, the event positioning in a gamma camera has to be independent of the total amount of light generated in the scintillation crystal. This is achieved by energy normalization of the centroid calculation.

One of the most important parameters is system sensitivity, describing the fraction of incoming gamma rays which are actually detected by the system. Single-photon devices suffer mainly from the low collimator efficiency needed to enhance spatial resolution. The total efficiency is also determined by the intrinsic gamma interaction probability in the crystal and the energy range selected.

The type of detection system in coincidence cameras permits 3D data acquisition with continuous sampling. The sensitivity of 3D systems strongly depends on the position within the field of view, both in axial and transaxial directions. The maximum acceptance angle for coincidence events defines the sensitivity profile. It has the shape of a pyramid or trapezoid (Fig. 13.9; CLACK et al. 1984). This fact causes lesions to be detected with different statistical accuracy, depending on their location in the field of view.

Energy resolution, determined mainly by the crystal material, measures how well gamma rays with two different energies can be distinguished. Good energy resolution also provides a means of reducing the fraction of scattered gamma rays entering into the image, because a narrow energy window can be used. For instance, a 20% energy window accepts gamma rays of up to 52° scattering angle for an incident energy of 140 keV, visible as background events distributed across the image.

13.2.2 Acquisition Parameters and Procedural Factors

13.2.2.1 Sampling Requirements

The quality of scintigraphic images is influenced by several procedural parameters. Firstly, the projection data have to be acquired in agreement with the system performance; thus, it is important to choose the pixel size of the acquisition matrix at approximately one half the size of the smallest structure to be resolved, which depends on the collimator. Gamma-camera images show variations in count density due to the limited number of photons which form the image. Therefore, detection of lesions depends on object contrast and size. Lesion contrast has to be much higher than noise levels in order to detect a lesion. A high number of counts reduces noise and smaller and/or lower-contrast lesions can be detected. For tomographic imaging the number of counts to detect a structure can be estimated, given the spatial resolution and the uncertainty with which the structure is to be imaged (BUDINGER et al. 1978).

Planar scintigraphy is performed by acquiring data with the gamma-camera viewing one direction of the patient. The data represent the projection of the tracer distribution; thus, overlapping structures result in summed signals and blurring in the image. Tomographic images, representing the activity distribution in a transaxial slice through the body, are generated from measured projections by the use of mathematical reconstruction algorithms. Full-ring dedicated positron tomographs collect all projections at once. Rotating single or multi-head gamma cameras acquire the data either during continuous motion or at a number of predefined angles (step-and-shoot). Depending on the duration of the gantry to rotate and switch between acquisition and motion, continuous rotation may be more efficient than step-and-shoot techniques. If, for instance, many angular steps with short measuring time per step are performed, continuous rotation is advantageous. In the case of larger angular steps, step-and-shoot acquisition should be preferred because of its higher angular precision and little loss in time.

To minimize resolution degradation in tomographic imaging, angular sampling should equal linear spatial sampling. Therefore, the number of angular views which are acquired in a 180° rotation (M_{180}) corresponds to the length of the arc of the selected rotation diameter (D), divided by the sampling distance Δl (Eq. 13.1; HUESMAN 1977):

$$M_{180} = \frac{\pi \cdot D}{2 \cdot \Delta l} \quad (13.1)$$

If this requirement is not met, image artifacts will show up in the reconstructed transverse slices. For a given system resolution, defined by the collimator in single-photon cameras, the pixel size in the matrix and the angular steps are defined. Patient tolerance restricts total imaging duration, limiting the count statistics. Thus, deviations from the ideal parameter set are common in clinical practice, mainly to reach a compromise between low counts in many views or high counts in fewer views, violating the sampling requirements. Since the strict requirement on count density from planar imaging does not necessarily apply to each individual projection image in a SPECT acquisition, protocols tend to favor a large number of angular steps. Resolution in the reconstructed SPECT image is not spatially invariant since the distance between detector and source organ varies between steps. Usually, SPECT resolution is worse than planar imaging. This is due in part to the fact that the camera head is farther away from the patient in SPECT. On the other hand, the limited number of events per view and the necessity to use smoothing filters in the reconstruction process further decrease the resolution. The main advantage of SPECT over planar imaging is the higher image contrast because overlapping structures are eliminated.

In PET scanners with BGO block detectors, the spatial resolution is defined by the size of the individual crystal; therefore, stationary rings cannot fulfill the sampling requirements. Although wobbling mechanisms had been developed to overcome this problem and increase sampling, these approaches have been abandoned in the recent designs, due mainly to the fact that in clinical situations the number of detected events is not high enough to fully utilize the finer sampling grid. Large-area crystals offer continuous sampling; thus, the binning process and subsequent sampling frequency have to meet the intrinsic spatial resolution (KARP et al. 1990).

13.2.2.2 Whole-Body Acquisition

A diagnostically valuable tool is the whole-body acquisition of ^{18}F labeled substances by sorting the sinogram data of a PET scanner into projection images, yielding images similar to planar body scans (GUERRERO et al. 1990; DAHLBOM et al. 1992). A stack of reconstructed transverse slices provides a volume data set which can be resliced into coronal and sagittal sections. Since most dedicated positron tomographs extend over 10 to 16 cm, numerous axial steps (or bed positions) have to be acquired in order to cover the whole body. Thus, acquisition duration per position has to be short (1–5 min), causing statistical noise in the reconstructed images. Despite the short scan time, image quality can be improved by optimized sampling schemes (DAHLBOM et al. 1992) and careful normalization of variations in detector efficiencies. Since the sensitivity of a tomograph drops at the edges of the axial field of view, adequate overlap of the neighboring bed positions needs to be applied to reduce artifacts due to variations in statistical quality of the data. Although currently not supported by commercial systems, a continuous axial motion may be advantageous in septumless, 3D PET acquisition (CHERRY et al. 1992; DAHLBOM et al. 1994). In addition to an increased scatter fraction, 3D whole-body acquisitions are specially affected by activity outside the axial field of view (SOSSI et al. 1995). Scatter correction methods based on the information from within the field of view show deviations (FERREIRA et al. 1998), causing some differences in quantitative information compared with 2D PET scanning. Numerous research groups are actively evaluating and improving this methodology.

Especially during acquisitions which involve rotating camera heads for sequential measurement of projection data (SPECT or dual-head coincidence cameras) it is important to minimize patient motion; otherwise, not only blurring but also distortions will be introduced in the reconstructed image. Therefore, it was suggested to fractionate scan times in order to reduce motion artifacts (GERMANO et al. 1994).

13.2.2.3 Attenuation Correction

Transmission measurements are frequently used as a basis for attenuation correction in nonhomogeneous objects. Whereas the projections can be pre-corrected in coincidence measurements, in SPECT imaging the measured transmission data are reconstructed and the attenuation maps are used as a basis in various correction methods, mostly applying iterative reconstruction methods (see chap. 14). Simultaneous transmission and emission scanning is most desirable so that misalignment is eliminated. This goal is achieved in SPECT imaging by using nuclides which emit gamma rays of different energy. Careful choice of transmission nuclides is important to minimize crosstalk effects and accurate determination of attenuation factors (FICARO et al. 1994). ^{153}Gd and ^{241}Am have been implemented in clinical routine. Currently, scanning line sources for single and dual-head cameras (TAN et al. 1993), or stationary line sources in combination with fan-beam collimators in triple-head systems (TUNG et al. 1992), are in use. Stationary multiple line sources are a new approach in overcoming the problem of count statistics in some areas of the body (CELLER et al. 1998).

Despite the higher energy, attenuation factors for coincidence measurements are much higher than in SPECT, since the total path for both gamma rays is longer; thus, along certain coincidence lines, attenuation factors of more than 100 can occur. The transmission data in PET are routinely acquired in coincidence using rotating rod sources made of ^{68}Ge. Spatial windowing reduces the amount of scatter in the transmission data and the contamination of emission into transmission. Contrary to SPECT scanning, simultaneous acquisition is not performed clinically, since it requires low-activity transmission sources and therefore long scan times. Generally, count-rate limitations of full-ring BGO-ring tomographs do not allow the use of intense transmission sources in coincidence mode. Due to prolonged transmission measurements, misregistration of transmission and emission may result because of patient motion. To overcome this problem, singles acquisition was proposed using high activity of either a positron emitter or of ^{137}Cs (DEKEMP and NAHMIAS 1994; KARP et al. 1995; YU and NAHMIAS 1995), which emits gamma rays with an energy of 662 keV. As in SPECT, the attenuation factors have to be scaled accordingly; however, the low-energy resolution of BGO crystals (>20%) results in high scatter fraction. NaI(Tl) systems have the advantage of intrinsically better energy resolution. The method has been implemented in a dual-head coincidence system using two collimated ^{137}Cs sources.

The clinical value of attenuation correction in whole-body PET imaging is discussed controversially (BENGEL et al. 1997; BEDIGIAN et al. 1998; IMRAN et al. 1998). Up to 40% of the total scanning time has to be dedicated to transmission measurement for optimal noise characteristics in 3D total-body PET using $^{68}Ge/^{68}Ga$ transmission sources and coincidence measurement (BEYER et al. 1997). Reduced imaging time using strong ^{137}Cs sources and singles acquisition mode may offer the possibility of applying a short interleaved emission/transmission scan protocol (KARP et al. 1995; SMITH et al. 1997). Thus, statistical quality of transmission data, which is a major obstacle in conventional transmission measurements, is improved and potential patient motion during the shorter scan is minimized. The results of ongoing investigations will show its clinical value.

13.2.3 Quality Control

Quality control of nuclear medicine instrumentation is essential to assure that the equipment functions within the known specifications and that image artifacts are avoided which could lead to misdiagnosis. There are recommendations of the manufacturers and medical physics society (NEMA 1986, 1994) on which camera parameters should be tested and how often this should be done according to a detailed protocol. The basis of quality control and action to be taken in cases of irregularities are the system performance parameters obtained during acceptance testing after the instrument has been installed in the department. These values are used as reference in the periodical checkout of the camera. Most vendors provide software tools for the routine quality control of modern digital cameras. It is important to be aware that any part in the imaging process can influence image quality, especially with automated tuning and correction processes implemented in the modern complex systems.

Besides the visual inspection of the camera, collimators and peripheral devices, certain measurements should be performed regularly. The results of these measurements have to be documented and reviewed to detect changes and obvious artifacts.

In camera-based systems, i.e. single-head planar, single- or multi-head SPECT and dual-head coincidence cameras, the basic quality control concerns the scintillation camera itself. Since the camera performance is dependent on the energy of the incident gamma ray, the implemented methods for correcting these differences have to be tested. Thus, every day before the first scan and each time a different nuclide is being used, the position and width of the energy window have to be checked. A point source in air and count rates below noticeable pileup yields the best results. This peaking of the camera is easily performed on the multi-channel display of the energy spectrum in modern systems. An evaluation of crystal, light pipe, photomultipliers, electronics and display system is achieved by the daily acquisition of a flood image. This is the most important check, yielding information on the global performance of the camera. The most convenient procedure is to measure the intrinsic uniformity. For this measurement the collimator is removed from the camera and the camera is irradiated by a point source (^{99m}Tc) which is positioned more than three times the camera diameter away. The total number of collected counts should be more than 1–3 million depending on the detector size. Comparison with the flood image taken after the last adjustment of the camera shows changes in the system, and in the case of obvious nonuniformities (e.g. defective PMT) the camera should not be used for clinical studies. Digital processing of the acquired flood images is used to quantify the nonuniformities in these images. Integral uniformity is defined as the maximum deviation of counts per pixel and differential uniformity measures the maximum change of count density over five neighboring pixels.

Nonuniformities can be produced by spatial nonlinearity, shifting events towards the center of the photomultiplier entrance window. In modern cameras this effect is reduced automatically by applying correction maps for linearity and multi-energy registration. Resolution and linearity should be checked on a weekly basis using a lead bar phantom on the camera without collimator, assessing nonlinearities and distortions in different areas of the camera. Also, the efficiency of the system can be determined weekly by calculating the ratio of counts per second in the uniformity test and the known activity in the point source which is placed at a fixed distance from the detector head. A fillable planar source (^{99m}Tc) or a ^{57}Co sheet source is needed for a monthly measurement of extrinsic uniformity, i.e. including the collimator.

Every 3 months the count rate performance and multienergy spatial registration should be checked according to the protocols used during acceptance testing. Special attention is needed for cameras used in whole-body imaging. Although they presently only need one scan covering the whole patient (older cameras with smaller fields of view needed two sweeps), alignment and electronic timing errors can severely affect the whole-body images, depending on the acquisition type. If a series of static images is acquired, misalignment between the individual images causes horizontal stripes in the image. During continuous head motion electronic timing errors will lead to areas of lower counts. A whole-body uniformity check shows these problems, which are not seen on normal flood images (O'Connor 1996).

Artefacts in planar images are propagated and even amplified in tomographic acquisitions. Linearity and uniformity are of primary importance in this context. Even small nonuniformities, not visible on the daily low-count flood images, cause artifacts in the tomographic images. Thus, quality control for SPECT systems includes some additional measurements. A weekly measurement of the extrinsic uniformity using a planar source and measurement times resulting in 10–30 million counts is incorporated in the data processing to eliminate even small nonuniformities in the camera which would cause concentric ring artifacts in the reconstructed SPECT image. Differential nonuniformity after applying the uniformity correction matrix should not exceed 1.0–2.5% to prevent ring artifacts in the tomographic image (O'Connor 1996). Especially in multi-head systems the uniformity measurement for each individual head is required. In addition, uniformity needs to be independent of the rotational position of the camera head. It is advisable to check this once per year. Careful alignment of the mechanical and electronic axis of rotation is required to prevent resolution loss or even distortion in the tomographic images. A difference of 0.5 pixel can cause serious distortions in a 128×128 image matrix. Most systems provide an automated procedure to detect deviations from the correct center of rotation (COR). In multi-head SPECT cameras, strict alignment of all axes of rotation has to be assured. Due to the improved stability of modern SPECT systems, the suggested test frequency of once per week may be prolonged. Once a month the mechanical head tilt in a SPECT system should be checked to avoid malpositioning of transaxial data. The pixel calibration, i.e. the number of pixels measured between two point sources of known distance, should be measured every month. With point sources of different energy, the multi-energy spatial registration of the camera can be checked, which not only assures the same magnification but also the applicability of COR and nonuniformity corrections for different energies.

The global performance of the SPECT system is best monitored by regularly (every 3 months) performing an acquisition with a phantom containing structures (e.g. Jaszczak phantom) representing the system resolution.

The coincidence camera can be seen as a special type of multi-head SPECT system; therefore, all the aforementioned remarks are also valid. Currently, little experience is available in terms of which additional tests should be performed in what time interval. The available cameras differ in their implementation of pulse processing, coincidence event localization and coincidence circuitry including time window widths. Imaging a positron emitting line source (long lived ^{68}Ge/^{68}Ga can routinely be used) at a fixed geometry may be useful to detect gross nonuniformities or changes in sensitivity on a daily basis without adding too much time to the quality control procedures.

Quality control in dedicated PET scanners with BGO detectors arranged in a full ring is performed by a daily measurement of the relative line-of-response efficiency (corresponds to the flood images on scintillation cameras; Spinks et al. 1989). Data are acquired similar to a transmission scan using rotating rod sources. A defective block detector or electronics bank can easily be seen as a count-depressed line in the sinogram display of the data. The counts per block in the blank scan are compared with reference data. If there is a statistically significant deviation from the expected pattern, adjustment of the system, like tuning of a gamma camera, is needed.

If quantitative PET measurements are performed, the tomograph counts are related to the injected dose and careful cross-calibration between PET scanner and dose calibrator is essential. A cylindrical phantom of known volume is filled with positron activity and imaged. Calibration factors (cps/Bq per milliliter) are calculated for each plane from the counts in the reconstructed image and the known activity concentration in the phantom. This factor should be a constant.

Currently, the recommendations apply to full ring PET scanners with BGO block detectors. Standard procedures are being evaluated for rotating BGO, large area NaI full-ring tomographs, and dual-head coincidence cameras.

Independent of the acquisition system, patient-related quality control can be summarized as reduction in motion, choice of injection site relative to target organ, time of scan after injection (biokinetics) and positioning (truncation).

13.3 Is There a Future for Dedicated Systems?

The historical division of nuclear medicine imaging into single-photon (traditionally nonquantitative) and positron imaging (quantitative) becomes more and more artificial as data processing and camera technology evolve, yielding devices capable of providing different acquisition modes and/or methodology for quantitative PET as well as SPECT. On the other hand, the imaging situation differs largely if, for example, brain or whole-body studies are performed; thus, high-performance instrumentation may have to be designed for its specific application. For instance, in single-photon detection it is indispensable to move the detector head as close as possible to the patient for optimal spatial resolution, but due to the design of the cameras this can sometimes not be accomplished. Therefore, in the past few years, investigators have concentrated on developing dedicated systems for imaging the breast or the brain.

Small, compact cameras which can be used in standard mammography systems may provide better image quality with reduced background as well as higher resolution and sensitivity than large-area conventional gamma cameras. The first feasibility studies (Levin et al. 1997; Gruber et al. 1998; Patt et al. 1998) point out that photodiode readout of luminous scintillators and the use of highly integrated electronics may be the most promising combination for this task. A prototype system showed excellent energy resolution (Patt et al. 1998) with pixelated CsI crystals and silicon photodiodes in combination with very high spatial resolution (1.5 mm). Once this technology is scaled up to a larger camera covering the whole breast, improved overall sensitivity and resolution in comparison with currently available large-area gamma cameras is expected. As important as the improvements in detector technology is the development of matched collimators for these cameras (Gruber et al. 1998).

The limitations of positron imaging in the breast are sought to be overcome with inexpensive, high-resolution dedicated systems with improved lesion detectability (Freifelder and Karp 1997). Flexible geometry will be one of the requirements for the successful clinical acceptance of these devices. The concept of just two opposing BGO detectors, mounted in an X-ray mammography gantry, is tested in two systems (Thompson et al. 1995; Weinberg et al. 1996). Owing to the position close to the breast, these systems provide much higher sensitivity than PET body scanners. Focal plane or limited-angle tomography is performed in the same geometry as X-ray imaging. Double-layer, finely pixelated BGO block detectors (Robar et al. 1997) are used in the prototype yielding a resolution of approximately 2 mm.

A high-resolution positron tomograph is being built for brain studies using LSO block detectors with two layers, providing depth-of-interaction information (Casey et al. 1997; Schmand et al. 1998a,b). This dedicated system will be the first complete tomograph utilizing this technology and is expected to yield brain images of unsurpassed quality. Cost will probably restrict the use of this tomograph type to research applications.

Clinical studies using these new dedicated imaging devices will reveal if they can improve patient care by cost-effective introduction of high-quality nuclear medical imaging.

References

Anger H (1958) Scintillation camera. Rev Sci Instr 29:27–33

Anger H, Davis D (1964) Gamma-ray detection efficiency and image resolution in sodium iodide. Rev Sci Instr 35:693–697

Bacharach SL, Buvat I (1995) Attenuation correction in cardiac positron emission tomography and single-photon emission computed tomography. J Nucl Cardiol 2:246–255

Bailey D (1998) Transmission scanning in emission tomography. Eur J Nucl Med 25:774–787

Bailey D, Young H, Bloomfield P et al. (1997) ECAT ART – a continuously rotating PET camera: performance characteristics, initial clinical studies, and installation considerations in a nuclear medicine department. Eur J Nucl Med 24:6–15

Bedigian M, Benard F, Smith R et al. (1998) Whole-body positron emission tomography for oncology imaging using singles transmission scanning with segmentation and ordered subsets-expecteation maximization (OS-EM) reconstruction. J Nucl Med 25:659–661

Bendriem B, Townsend D (1998) The theory and practice of 3D PET. Kluwer Academic, Dordrecht

Bengel F, Ziegler S, Avril N et al. (1997) Whole-body positron emission tomography in clinical oncology: comparison between attenuation-corrected and uncorrected images. Eur J Nucl Med 24:1091–1098

Beyer T, Kinahan P, Townsend D (1997) Optimization of transmission and emission scan duration in 3D whole-body PET. Trans Nucl Sci 44:2400–2407

Budinger T (1996) Single photon emission computed tomography. In: Sandler M, Patton J, Coleman R et al. (eds) Diognostic nuclear medicine, vol 1. Williams and Wilkins, Baltimore, pp 121–138

Budinger T (1998) PET Instrumentation: what are the limits? Semin Nucl Med 28:247–267

Budinger T, Derenzo S, Greenberg W et al. (1978) Quantitative potentials of dynamic emission computed tomography. J Nucl Med 19:309–315

Butler J, Lingren C, Friesenhahn S et al. (1998) CdZnTe Solid-state gamma camera. IEEE Trans Nucl Sci 45:359–363

Casey M, Nutt R (1986) Multicrystal two dimensional BGO detector system for positron emission tomography. IEEE Trans Nucl Sci 33:460–463

Casey M, Eriksson L, Schmand M et al. (1997) Investigation of LSO crystals for high resolution positron emission tomography. IEEE Trans Nucl Sci 44:1109–1113

Celler A, Sitek A, Stoub E et al. (1998) Multiple line source array for SPECT transmission scans: simulation, phantom and patient studies. J Nucl Med 39:2183–2189

Chen E, MacIntyre W, Go R et al. (1997) Myocardial viability studies using fluorine-18-FDG SPECT: a comparison with fluorine-18-FDG PET. J Nucl Med 38:582–586

Cherry S, Dahlbom M, Hoffman E (1992) High sensitivity, total body PET scanning using 3D data acquisition and reconstruction. IEEE Trans Nucl Sci 39:1088–1092

Clack R, Townsend D, Jeavons A (1984) Increased sensitivity and field of view for a rotating positron camera. Phys Med Biol 29:1421–1431

Coleman R (1997) Camera-based PET: the best is yet to come. J Nucl Med 38:1796–1797

Dahlbom M, Cutler P, Digby W et al. (1994) Characterization of sampling schemes for whole body PET imaging. IEEE Trans Nucl Sci 41:1571–1576

Dahlbom M, Hoffman E, Hoh C et al. (1992) Whole-body positron emission tomography: part I. Methods and performance characteristics. J Nucl Med 33:1191–1199

Dahlbom M, MacDonald L, Eriksson L et al. (1997) Performance of a YSO/LSO detector block for use in a PET/SPECT system. IEEE Trans Nucl Sci 44:1114–1119

deKemp RA, Nahmias C (1994) Attenuation correction in PET using single photon transmission measurement. Med Phys 21:771–778

Ferreira N, Trebossen R, Bendriem B (1998) Assessment of 3-D PET quantitation: influence of out of the field of view radioactive sources and of attenuating media. IEEE Trans Nucl Sci 45:1670–1675

Ficaro EP, Fessler JA, Rogers WL et al. (1994) Comparison of americium-241 and technetium-99 m as transmission sources for attenuation correction of thallium-201 SPECT imaging of the heart. J Nucl Med 35:652–663

Freifelder R, Karp J (1997) Dedicated PET scanners for breast imaging. Phys Med Biol 42:2463–2480

Germano G, Kavanagh P, Kiat H et al. (1994) Temporal image fractionation: rejection of motion artifacts in myocardial SPECT. J Nucl Med 35:1193–1197

Gruber G, Moses W, Derenzo S et al. (1998) A discrete scintillation camera module using silicon photodiode readout of CsI(Tl) crystals for breast cancer imaging. IEEE Nucl Instr Methods 45:1063–1068

Guerrero T, Hoffman E, Dahlbom M et al. (1990) Characterization of a whole body imaging technique for PET. IEEE Trans Nucl Sci 37:676–679

Hoffman E, Huang S, Plummer D et al. (1982) Quantitation in positron emission computed tomography: effect of nonuniform resolution. J Comput Assist Tomogr 6:987–999

Huber J, Moses W, Derenzo S et al. (1997) Characterization of a 64 channel PET detector using photodiodes for crystal identification. IEEE Trans Nucl Sci 44:1197–1201

Huesman R (1977) The effects of a finite number of projection angles and finite lateral sampling of projections on the propagation of statistical errors in transverse section reconstruction. Phys Med Biol 22:511–521

Imran M, Kubota K, Yamada S et al. (1998) Lesion-to-background ratio in nonattenuation-corrected whole-body FDG PET images. J Nucl Med 39:1219–1223

Karp J, Muehllehner G, Mankoff D et al. (1990) Continuous-slice PENN-PET: a positron tomograph with volume imaging capability. J Nucl Med 31:617–627

Karp JS, Muehllehner G, Qu H et al. (1995) Singles transmission in volume-imaging PET with a 137 Cs source. Phys Med Biol 40:929–944

Kipper M, Yeung D, Halpern S et al. (1998) Quality of planar images using a solid-state (CdZnTe) gamma camera, compared with conventional gamma scintillation cameras. J Nucl Med 39:P132

Kojima A, Matsumoto M, Takahashi M et al. (1993) Effect of energy resolution on scatter fraction in scintigraphic imaging: Monte Carlo study. Med Phys 20:1107–1113

Lecomte R, Cadorette J, Rodrigue S et al. (1996) Initial results from the Sherbrooke avalanche photodiode positron tomograph. IEEE Trans Nucl Sci 43:1952–1957

Levin C, Hoffman E, Tornai M et al. (1997) PSPMT and photodiode designs of a small scintillation camera for imaging malignant breast tumors. IEEE Trans Nucl Sci 44:1513–1520

Macfarlane D, Cotton L, Ackermann R et al. (1995) Triple-head SPECT with 2-[fluorine-18]fluoro-2-deoxy-D-glucose (FDG): initial evaluation in oncology and comparison with FDG PET. Radiology 194:425–429

Mankoff D, Muehllehner G, Miles G (1990) A local coincidence triggering system for PET tomographs composed of large-area positron-sensitive detectors. IEEE Trans Nucl Sci 37:730–736

Melcher CL, Schweitzer JS (1992) A promising new scintillator: cerium- doped lutetium oxyorthosilicate. Nucl Instr Methods 314:212–214

Muehllehner G (1979) Effect of crystal thickness on scintillation camera performance. J Nucl Med 20:992–993

Muehllehner G (1985) Effect of resolution improvement on required count density in ECT imaging: a computer simulation. Phys Med Biol 30:163–173

Muehllehner G, Karp J (1986) A positron camera using position-sensitive detectors: PENN-PET. J Nucl Med 27:90–98

Muehllehner G, Colsher J, Stoub E (1980) Correction for field nonuniformity in scintillation cameras through removal of spatial distortion. J Nucl Med 21:771–776

Mueller S, Foley Kijewski M, Moore S et al. (1990) Maximum-likelihood estimation: a mathematical model for quantitation in nuclear medicine. J Nucl Med 31:1693–1701

NEMA (1986) Performance measurements of scintillation cameras, National Electrical Manufacturers Association

NEMA (1994) Performance measurements of positron emission tomographs, National Electrical Manufacturers Association

O'Connor M (1996) Instrument- and computer-related problems and artifacts in nuclear medicine. Semin Nucl Med 26:256–277

Patt B, Iwanczyk J, Tull C et al. (1998) High resolution CsI(Tl)/Si-PIN detector development for breast imaging. IEEE Trans Nucl Sci 45:2126–2131

Robar J, Thompson C, Murthy K et al. (1997) Construction and calibration of detectors for high-resolution metabolic breast cancer imaging. Nucl Instr Methods A 392:402–406

Schmand M, Dahlbohm M, Eriksson L et al. (1998a) Performance of a LSO/NaI(Tl) phoswich detector for a combined PET/SPECT imaging system. J Nucl Med 39:9P

Schmand M, Eriksson L, Casey M et al. (1998b) Detector design of a LSO based positron emission tomograph with depth of interaction capability for high resolution brain imaging. J Nucl Med 39:133P

Schmelz C, Bradbury SM, Holl I et al. (1995) Feasibility study of an avalanche photodiode readout for high resolution PET with nsec time resolution. IEEE Trans Nucl Sci 42:1080–1084

Shreve P, Steventon R, Deters E et al. (1998) Oncologic diagnosis with 2-[fluorine-18]fluoro-2-deoxy-D-glucose imaging: dual head coincidence gamma camera versus positron emission tomographic scanner. Radiology 207:431–437

Smith R, Karp J, Muehllehner G et al. (1997) Singles transmission scans performed post-injection for quantitative whole body PET imaging. IEEE Trans Nucl Sci 44:1329–1335

Sossi V, Barney J, Harrison R (1995) Effect of scatter from radioactivity outside of the field of view in 3-D PET. IEEE Trans Nucl Sci 42:1157–1161

Spinks T, Jones T, Heather J et al. (1989) Quality control procedures in positron tomography. Eur J Nucl Med 15:736–740

Tan P, Bailey DL, Meikle SR et al. (1993) A scanning line source for simultaneous emission and transmission measurements in SPECT. J Nucl Med 34:1752–1760

Thompson C, Murthy K, Picard Y et al. (1995) Positron emission mammography (PEM): a promising technique for detecting breast cancer. IEEE Trans Nucl Sci 42:1012–1017

Townsend D, Wensveen M, Byars L et al. (1993) A rotating PET scanner using BGO block detectors: Design, performance and applications. J Nucl Med 34:1367–1376

Tung CH, Gullberg GT, Zeng GL et al. (1992) Non-uniform attenuation correction using simultaneous transmission and emission converging tomography. IEEE Trans Nucl Sci 39:1134–1143

van Lingen A, Huijgens PC, Visser FC et al. (1992) Performance characteristics of a 511-keV collimator for imaging positron emitters with a standard gamma-camera. Eur J Nucl Med 19(5):315–321

Weinberg I, Malewski S, Weisenberger A et al. (1996) Preliminary results for positron emission mammography: real-time functional breast imaging in a cenventional mammography gantry. Eur J Nucl Med 23:804–806

Yu S, Nahmias C (1995) Single-photon transmission measurements in positron emission tomography using ^{137}Cs. Phys Med Biol 40:1255–1266

14 Image Formation and Data Processing

J. Nuyts

Contents

14.1 Introduction 237
14.2 Image Formation 237
14.2.1 Filtered Backprojection 238
14.2.1.1 The Algorithm 238
14.2.1.2 Regularisation 238
14.2.2 Maximum Likelihood/ Expectation Maximisation 238
14.2.2.1 Iterative Reconstruction as a Feed-back Mechanism 238
14.2.2.2 Theoretical Considerations 239
14.2.2.3 Regularisation 239
14.2.3 Comparison of FBP and MLEM 240
14.2.3.1 Computation Time 240
14.2.4 Attenuation 241
14.2.5 Scatter 244
14.2.6 Detector Resolution 245
14.2.7 Motion Correction 245
14.3 Image Analysis 246
14.3.1 Diagnostic Value of an Image 246
14.3.2 Region of Interest Analysis 247
14.3.3 Analysing Dynamic Images 247
14.4 Future Developments 247

14.1 Introduction

For the past several years, computer speeds have tended to double every year. This is an exponential growth curve, and the cumulative gain is impressive: programs running for a day 10 years ago now require a minute. This allows algorithm designers to follow new strategies. Ingenious mathematics and clever numerical analysis now must face competition from inefficient and ugly brute-force computations, and soon will no longer be necessary. An important advantage is that problems which cannot be solved analytically can now be tackled with computation-intensive numerical procedures.

A good example of this is reconstruction from projections. Until recently, reconstruction was almost exclusively done with filtered backprojection (FBP), a relatively fast, analytical method. The current proliferation of iterative reconstruction algorithms is a direct result of the increasing computer speed. Most of the algorithms applied presently have been around for several years, waiting for the computers to become sufficiently powerful. Many iterative algorithms have been proposed (Herman 1980; Schmidlin 1972), but at least currently, the best for emission tomography seems to be the maximum likelihood/expectation maximisation (MLEM) algorithm (Rockmore and Mackovski 1976; Dempster et al. 1977; Shepp and Vardi 1982; Lange and Carson 1984), accelerated using the ordered subsets approach (Hudson and Larkin 1994). In part, this is due to the appealing theory behind it: the algorithm takes into account the statistical nature of the data, assuming that the data are Poisson distributed, which is exact or nearly exact in most cases. Convergence is guaranteed, and no tuning of mysterious parameters is required. Moreover, at least in emission tomography, it leads to a beautiful, simple mathematical expression which is very easy to program. To some extent, the success of MLEM is also due to historical reasons: it appeared at the right time, just when computers allowed application to real images in a reasonable time, and rapidly became the standard iterative method. Some other algorithms, such as weighted least squares, produce images of similar quality. In transmission tomography, where MLEM does not yield an expression of similar simplicity, weighted least-squares algorithms are more successful (Fessler et al. 1997). The high computer speed, and the availability of powerful commercial software packages, has also led to the development of sophisticated, interactive data processing techniques.

14.2 Image Formation and Reconstruction Techniques

We compare filtered backprojection and MLEM, and describe how more accurate reconstructions are ob-

J. Nuyts
Department of Nuclear Medicine, K.U. Leuven, Herestraat 49, B-3000 Leuven, Belgium

tained. In addition, some image analysis methods are discussed.

14.2.1 Filtered Backprojection

14.2.1.1 The Algorithm

The emission tomograph is unable to measure directly the tracer distribution in which we are interested; instead, it measures some complex transformation of that distribution. The mathematical model of this transformation is known by several names, including "the Radon transform", "a set of line integrals" or simply "the projection". Reconstruction from projections is thus a series of computations required to undo this undesirable transformation. The dominating reconstruction algorithm is still FBP.

Herein we focus on the two-dimensional, discrete case: a finite set of sampled projections (i.e. all images acquired by the camera over 360° around the patient) from a two-dimensional tracer distribution (i.e. a slice through the body of the patient) must be reconstructed into a discrete image.

Filtered backprojection consists of two steps: filtering and backprojection. Backprojection is *not* the inverse of projection, it is its *transpose*. Taking the transpose of an operator basically means that very similar computations must be carried out, but in reverse order. In a *projection*, pixels along projection lines in the image are summed and the resulting value is assigned to a projection pixel; thus, every pixel in the projection pixel is computed as a weighted sum of image pixels, possibly with a different weight in every image pixel. In the transpose operation, the *backprojection*, the whole computation is reversed: the image pixel is computed as a weighted sum of projection pixels, using exactly the same weights as in the projection. Therefore, image pixels that contribute little in the projection step get little back in the backprojection step.

Since backprojection is not the inverse of projection, good reconstruction by applying simple backprojection methods cannot be expected. Indeed, the resulting image is a blurred one. With some non-trivial mathematics, which are not discussed here, these images can be deblurred, such that an image of the original distribution is obtained. This is the filtering step. It does not matter whether filtering precedes or follows backprojection. In most implementations, first the projections are filtered, and then the filtered projections are backprojected. In the two-dimensional (2D) case there is no choice: the only filter that does the job is the ramp filter.

Filtered backprojection is an *exact inverse* of projection, when all possible line integrals of the two-dimensional tracer distribution are used. This implies an infinite number of angles, with an infinite number of pixel values for each angle, using a pixel size of zero. In reality, only a finite number of projection pixels for a finite number of angles is available. In addition, real single photon emission computed tomography (SPECT) or positron emission tomography (PET) measurements are not true line integrals. Real projection lines have a finite and position-dependent width, and the number of detected photons is not nicely proportional to the total activity along that "line" because of photon-electron interaction and Poisson noise. Consequently, FBP only produces an approximate image of the tracer distribution in the patient.

14.2.1.2 Regularisation

When FBP is applied to noisy projections, the noise propagates dramatically, resulting in very noisy reconstruction images. To suppress the noise, low-pass filtering (smoothing) is applied. Inevitably, smoothing also reduces the spatial resolution. For reasons of computational efficiency, a one-dimensional smoothing filter on the projections was formerly applied, which resulted in smoothing within the transverse slice. The efficiency came from the fact that the smoothing filter could be combined with the ramp filter into a single operation. However, computational speed and computer memory are no longer an issue, and it is preferable to apply a two-dimensional smoothing filter on the projections. This is equivalent to three-dimensional smoothing after FBP. The advantage of three-dimensional smoothing is that the effect of the filter is isotropic. In addition, smoothing volumes is more effective than smoothing slices, because more pixels are involved for the same kernel size.

14.2.2 Maximum Likelihood/Expectation Maximisation

14.2.2.1 Iterative Reconstruction as a Feed-back Mechanism

Iterative reconstruction algorithms start from an initial, arbitrary estimate of the unknown tracer distribution. This can be a very poor estimate, such as a completely homogeneous image. In every iteration the algorithm checks the current estimate and improves it based on that evaluation.

A key feature of iterative algorithms is that they are based on a feed-back mechanism. Feed-back mechanisms are very common in biological and man-made systems because of their robustness. The speed of a car is controlled by a feed-back path, which consists of the speedometer and the eyes and brain of the driver, who compares the measured speed with the desired one. The feed-forward path, which consists of the driver's foot and the accelerator, is there to change the speed, until the feed-back path is "satisfied". In MLEM the feed-back path is the projection of the current estimate of the tracer distribution, which is compared with the measurement. Comparison is done by computing the ratio of the measured and computed values in every projection pixel. If all these ratios are unified, then the current estimate must be excellent. If a ratio is higher than one, the measured photon count is higher than the estimated activity along the corresponding projection line; thus, the estimated activity must be increased by the feed-forward path. In MLEM the feed-forward path consists of multiplying the current estimate with the backprojection of the ratios. If all ratios are one, all backprojection pixels are also equal to one. In this case multiplication will not change anything, which is what we want because the estimate is then perfect. If ratios tend to be higher than one, multiplication with the backprojected ratios increase the estimated activity, again as desired.

The performance of a feed-back mechanism is very sensitive to its feed-back path, whereas it is less sensitive to the feed-forward path. As a result, virtually all iterative algorithms share the same feed-back path, i.e. the computation of the projection. The differences are in the feed-forward path.

Iterative reconstruction algorithms converge towards the inverse of the operation in the feed-back path. Consequently, the projector in the feed-back path should be a good model of the acquisition process. If not, artefacts can be expected. In MLEM the feed-forward path contains the transpose of the projection operator, which is the backprojection operator. As has been stated, deriving the transpose is usually not too difficult. If the projector takes into account blurring and attenuation, the backprojector should do likewise: a blurring and attenuating backprojector is required. Since projector and backprojector basically apply the same operations in a different order, the computation time of both should be similar.

14.2.2.2 Theoretical Considerations

When applied to real measurements, the algorithm is not able to make all ratios equal to one. Because the measured photon count is subject to Poisson noise, it is almost always impossible to find a tracer distribution which corresponds perfectly to the measured values. One can show that in this case, MLEM produces the most likely tracer distribution, taking into account the characteristics of the Poisson distribution. In fact, this is the main difference between MLEM and other iterative reconstruction algorithms. Because we *know* that the number of measured photons is Poisson distributed, and because nice mathematical tools are available to deal with Poisson distributions, we can *compute* the probability of measuring what we actually did measure, assuming that the current estimate really represents the true tracer distribution. It seems logical to choose the estimate that *maximises* that probability as the reconstruction of the measurement.

Note that this probability is always extremely small, though. It is so small that it is zero in clinical practice (that is why two consecutive emission scans of the same distribution are *never* identical). So we are in fact sure that the ML estimate is not the true distribution. We only select it, because all other solutions are less likely. In addition, we hope that the most likely solution is at least similar in many interesting features to the true distribution.

The MLEM algorithm maximises the likelihood function (ML). It does so by applying an iterative strategy, which belongs to a particular class of algorithms, named expectation maximisation (EM). The good thing about EM is that convergence is guaranteed; no step size or other parameter has to be tuned.

14.2.2.3 Regularisation

Many authors have reported noise deterioration in MLEM reconstruction from noisy projections. Noise levels do increase with increasing iteration numbers. At very high iteration numbers, i.e. close to the actual MLEM solution, the noise is often so high that the image is useless for clinical purposes. The MLEM algorithm "knows" that the measurement is subject to Poisson noise, but it does not know whether a particular measured count rate is too high or too low due to that noise. The best guess is that it is correct, implying that as much noise as possible should be included in the reconstruction. The noise must be suppressed, or in mathematical language, regularisation is needed. Several effective approaches are available.

In MLEM low spatial frequencies converge faster than high spatial frequencies. This means that image detail and noise only show up at higher iterations. So one can use the iteration number in much the same way as the cut-off frequency of the low-pass filter in FBP. This technique is often applied in clinical practice: it combines two advantages: the noise level remains acceptable and the computation time is minimised. The resulting so-called MLEM images are not really ML reconstructions. They are just "HL" (high likelihood) images.

Stopping early is fine, but stopping too early is dangerous: convergence may be insufficient, resulting in large errors, both in absolute and relative quantification. The images do not warn against this: intermediate images from MLEM nearly always look good, even at early iterations. Several authors have investigated stopping rules (Coakley and Llacer 1991; Falcon et al. 1998; Veklerov and Llacer 1987; Llacer and Veklerov 1989; Liow and Strother 1993).

The very noisy ML image is not as useless as it seems. When filtered with a low-pass filter, an image with good visual and quantitative characteristics appears. An important advantage of this approach is that the risk of insufficient convergence is low (Beekman et al. 1998; Hutton and Lau 1998).

In standard MLEM any reconstruction pixel is treated as an independent variable; thus, it may end up with a value very different from that of the neighbours. Some authors propose to use overlapping bell-shaped functions instead of non-overlapping pixel values. Since noisy images with overlapping blobs cannot be made, this leads to very effective noise suppression (Lewitt 1992; Snyder and Miller 1985). Unfortunately, it also leads to some artefacts, usually called "edge artefacts" or "Gibbs overshoot" (Snyder et al. 1987). This artefact appears as soon as one tries to produce sharp edges without using high spatial frequencies. The MLEM algorithm can be extended to a maximum-a-posteriori (MAP) algorithm by including a-priori knowledge. (The posterior is the product of the likelihood and the prior.) This means that the program is not only needed to look at the data (by maximising the likelihood function), but also to judge the reconstruction (by maximising the prior). By using a prior function that is high for smooth images and low for noisy ones, we can encourage the program to look for smooth solutions. In these algorithms there is almost always a parameter present, assigning a weight to the prior. With a low weight the algorithm reduces to regular MLEM. With a high weight only very smooth images are considered as a solution. The parameter must usually be tuned manually by a skilled observer in order to obtain a good compromise between smoothness and adherence to the measured projections. To encourage local smoothness, one often regards the image as a Markov random field and uses Gibbs distributions as a prior. The mathematics of Markov random fields have been studied extensively, because they are used in physics. This framework allows a wide variety of priors, including priors with edge-preserving characteristics (Mumcuoglu et al. 1996; Lalush and Tsui 1993). An alternative is to use a smoothed version of the current reconstruction estimate as a prior (Alenius and Ruotsolainen 1997). The MAP algorithm seems to be effective in improving diagnostic quality of the images (Chan et al. 1997).

If the patient has undergone an anatomical study, such as MR imaging or CT, one can attempt to include also the anatomical information as a-priori knowledge. In most implementations the anatomy is used to define edges over which smoothing is forbidden in the functional image (Ardekani et al. 1996; Bowsher et al. 1996). Of course, this approach is most effective in those cases were anatomical and functional boundaries tend to coincide, and it requires good alignment between the anatomical and the functional image.

14.2.3 Comparison of FBP and MLEM

14.2.3.1 Computation Time

Since backprojection is the dominating operation in FBP, and because backprojection and projection are of similar complexity, computing a single MLEM iteration takes about twice as long as computing the FBP reconstruction.

Typically at least several tens of iterations are required, and many researchers have studied techniques to accelerate MLEM (Kaufman 1987; Tanaka 1987). Currently, the most successful one is the use of ordered subsets (Hudson and Larkin 1994). A single MLEM iteration is computed using only a subset of the projections. For every iteration a different subset is used, so all projections still contribute to the final image. Acceleration factors of 10 or higher can be obtained, depending on the number of projections, the noise in the projections, the stopping rule, etc. However, the noise in the reconstruction tends to increase with increasing number of subsets. If that is to be avoided, one can use a scheme with a gradually decreasing number of subsets. The MLEM algorithm accelerated with ordered subsets is often called OSEM.

Filtered backprojection is a linear algorithm, MLEM is not. Consequently, FBP can be characterised by its point spread function, or equivalently, by its modulation transfer function. There is a direct relation between resolution and recovery. Recovery is the ratio of the reconstructed tracer uptake to the real one. If we know the size of an object, the resolution of the scanner and the low-pass filter used in FBP reconstruction, we can predict the recovery coefficient for that object.

For MLEM all this is impossible. The MLEM reconstructions do not have a point-spread function, and prediction of recovery is more of an art than a science.

Filtered backprojection is designed under the assumption that both the projections and the tracer distribution are defined in continuous space. This means that FBP can only be applied to reconstruction problems where the number of projections and the number of pixels per projection is sufficiently large. In contrast, MLEM is designed for digital data.

The difference in behaviour between the two algorithms can be shown with a few very simple simulations. In the first example only two projections from a point source are available (at 0 and 90°). Figure 14.1 shows the true distribution, and the FBP and MLEM reconstructed images. Filtered backprojection produces positive and negative streaks. The streaks cross near the point source, but the reconstruction is of poor quality. Filtered backprojection fails because the number of projections is too low. The MLEM image is exact. Indeed, two projections are sufficient to find a point source, provided that negative tracer uptakes are impossible.

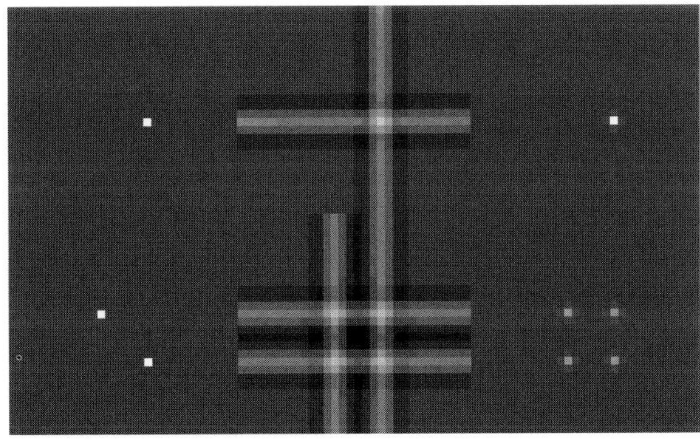

Fig. 14.1. True image (*left*), filtered backprojection (FBP; *centre*) and maximum likelihood/expectation maximisation (MLEM; *right*) reconstruction from two simulated perpendicular projections. *Top:* one point source; *bottom:* two point sources

In the bottom row of Fig. 14.1, the experiment was repeated, but now there were two point sources. Filtered backprojection projection simply produces the cross-pattern twice. This was expected: FBP is linear, so we should see the point-spread function (i.e. the response to a single point source) twice. In contrast, MLEM now shows four points, not two, clearly illustrating that MLEM is non-linear. This image is not the exact reconstruction, but it is one that produces exactly the same two perpendicular projections. Because the number of projections is too low, there are multiple solutions.

Figure 14.2 shows images from a software phantom with two homogeneous regions and two identical point sources. The MLEM images at iterations 40 and 200 are displayed. This figure also shows a horizontal profile intersecting the two point sources. It is clear that the isolated source converges much faster than the one surrounded by activity. In addition, there is no simple relationship between the width of the response in each point and the recovery of that point. To further illustrate this, the right panel of the figure plots the full width at half maximum as a function of the maximum for subsequent iterations. For comparison, a similar plot for FBP was produced, by using different cut-off frequencies. The two MLEM curves converge to the same, exact reconstruction, but following different trajectories. The FBP curve shows a third relation between recovery and resolution, and does not reach the exact solution because of some residual blurring.

If position-independent resolution is required, one could iterate until convergence is sufficient, and then smooth with a linear filter. Resolution will then be dominated by the filter, so the effective point-spread function of the image would be the point spread function of the filter. (Note that in these examples the resolution of the projections was ideal. In reality, the resolution of the reconstruction images is directly affected by the finite resolution of the measured projections.)

14.2.4 Attenuation

Filtered backprojection is the inverse of the projection operator. In practice, this operator is a poor model of the true radio-activity acquisition. Due to

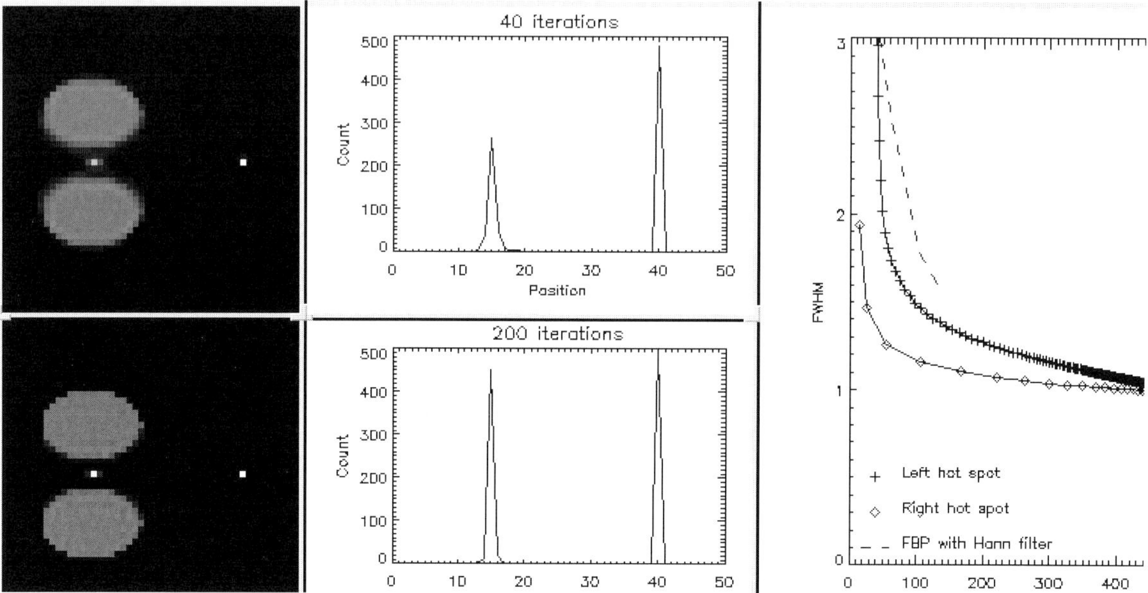

Fig. 14.2. *Left:* MLEM reconstruction after 40 and 200 iterations. *Centre:* the horizontal profile intersecting the two points. *Right:* the full width at half maximum as a function of the maximum pixel value for the two point sources. Each point corresponds to an iteration. The same relation is also shown for FBP (same curve for both point sources), by varying the cut-off frequency of the Hann low-pass filter

photon-electron interactions, many photons are lost, an effect usually called attenuation. Between 0.1 and 0.5 MeV, Compton scatter is the main cause of attenuation in tissue. Consequently, we need the inverse of the attenuated projection operator. In PET the effect of attenuation can be separated from the projection, because all photon pairs contributing to the same projection pixel have undergone the same attenuation. Consequently, the acquisition can be modelled as the successive application of two independent operators: first projection, and then attenuation. The inverse operator is then easily obtained: attenuation compensation (a single correction factor in every projection pixel), followed by FBP.

In SPECT this separation is not possible: photons contributing to the same projection pixels have undergone different attenuation. Consequently, for reconstruction we need the inverse of the attenuated projector, where the attenuation is position dependent.

In the case of an homogeneously attenuating object, this inverse can be computed analytically, leading to an adapted version of FBP (Bellini et al. 1979). For non-homogeneous attenuation, iterative algorithms are required (King et al. 1996). Extension of MLEM to attenuated projection is straightforward. In the feed-back path the projector is replaced with the attenuated projector. In the feed-forward path, the transpose operator must be inserted, which is attenuated backprojection.

Attenuation is supposed to be known. In some cases it can be easily derived from the emission projections (Michel et al. 1989), and in other cases a transmission measurement is needed. In PET the raw transmission data can be used directly. In SPECT they can be used to reconstruct an attenuation map with FBP, which is then inspected by the projector/backprojector pair of the MLEM algorithm to compute the effect of attenuation. However, both in PET and in SPECT, it may be useful to compute an ML or MAP reconstruction of the transmission scan (Lange and Carson 1984; Mumcuoglu et al. 1996; Fessler et al. 1997), which may reduce the contribution of the transmission noise to the final image.

Figure 14.3 shows the FBP, the ML and a MAP reconstructed attenuation map from the same 1-min PET transmission sinogram, and the corresponding reconstruction of the emission ^{18}F-fluorodeoxyglucose image. Transmission reconstructions were done with a gradient-ascent algorithm (Nuyts et al. 1998). It is clear that short transmission scans may contribute significantly to the noise in the final attenuation-corrected image, and that this contribution also depends on the attenuation-correction method. The MAP reconstruction can be regarded as a combination of reconstruction and segmentation. Segmenta-

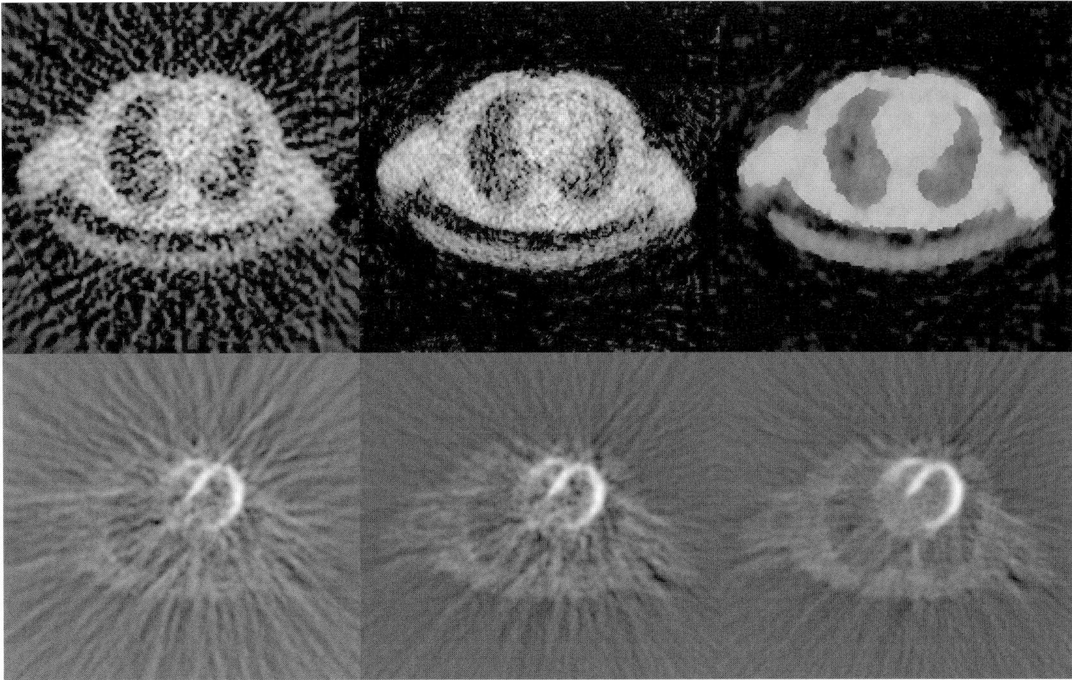

Fig. 14.3. *Top:* reconstruction of the attenuation map from a short transmission scan with FBP (*left*), a gradient ascent ML algorithm (*centre*) and a gradient ascent maximum-a-posteriori (MAP) algorithm (*right*). *Bottom:* the corresponding attenuation-corrected PET-FDG images produced with FBP

tion is the classification of pixels with the attenuation correction factor, according to tissue type, i.e. a regrouping of measured or calculated factors in a certain number of tissue classes (lung, bone, soft tissue). Several authors have obtained significant noise reduction with the consecutive application of these operations: first reconstruction with FBP, then segmentation to reduce the noise (Meikle et al. 1993; Tai et al. 1996; Xu et al. 1996).

Some authors have investigated the alignment requirements of the transmission map with the emission reconstruction for SPECT (Matsunari et al. 1998) and PET (Chatziioannou and Dahlbom 1996; McCord et al. 1992). In SPECT deviations of more than 1 cm can cause significant artefacts. In PET appropriate alignment is even more delicate.

In Fig. 14.4 we simulated projections of an object with a small air bubble (zero activity, zero attenuation). They were reconstructed based on a transmission map in which this region was labelled as tissue. Scatter and resolution effects were not simulated. As shown in Fig. 14.4, the SPECT reconstruction shows low activity in the region. The PET reconstruction, however, shows a marked hot spot in that region. The reconstructions were done with MLEM, but FBP shows the same artefacts. Consequently, air bubbles in the colon can cause artefactual hot spots in PET.

For many years non-attenuation-corrected images have been used in SPECT. As a result, physicians are used to those images, and they have developed powerful mental attenuation-correction skills. It is easy to show that attenuation correction dramatically improves quantification of tracer concentration and eliminates artefacts (Nuyts et al. 1995), but this does not prove that diagnostic value has improved as well. Attenuation correction eliminates severe artefacts but introduces or amplifies some others, such as overcorrection due to contribution of scattered photons or the position-dependent effect of collimator blurring. Because physicians are not used to these new artefacts, the diagnostic value of the "superior" corrected images may actually be lower than that of the familiar "poor" images. In a receiver operating characteristics (ROC) study, Jang et al. (1998) found that a group of physicists performed similar on attenuation-corrected and attenuation-uncorrected myocardial SPECT images, whereas a group of experienced physicians performed significantly worse on attenuation-corrected images. Similarly, Gilland et al. (1992) found in an ROC analysis based on simulated cardiac studies that attenuation correction had an adverse effect, and that MLEM was not statistically better than FBP. In contrast, in an ROC study involving PET brain

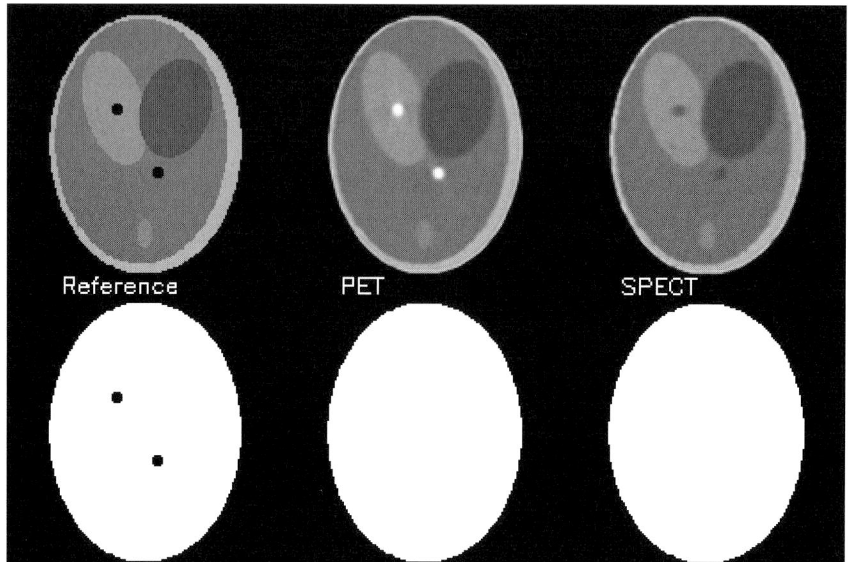

Fig. 14.4. Reconstruction artefact due to a region of zero attenuation and activity, which was missed in the transmission map. *Top:* reference image, reconstruction from PET and single photon emission computed tomography (SPECT) projections. *Bottom:* the true attenuation map, and the maps used for attenuation correction in PET and SPECT reconstruction (aligned respective to their upper counterparts)

studies, LLACER et al. (1993) found MLEM to be superior to FBP.

When new techniques are introduced, a learning phase should be implemented in which both the old and new method are used in parallel.

In SPECT, transmission measurements are often carried out with convergent beam configurations; thus, the influence of image truncation has been studied as well (MANGLOS et al. 1993; CASE et al. 1995). There seems to be agreement that, at least in SPECT, attenuation correction should be combined with scatter correction to obtain good results (IIDA et al. 1998). When collimator blurring is significant, such as in 180° acquisition or with a high-sensitivity collimator, blurring must be corrected for as well.

14.2.5 Scatter

Compton scatter not only prevents photons from being detected, it also deflects into the detector some photons that should not have been detected. This undesirable contribution to the projections is usually called scatter. Compton scatter can be well modelled as an elastic collision between two particles of different mass, an electron and a photon. It follows that photons lose energy in the process. Fortunately, we know the energy of unscattered photons, and we can measure the energy of detected photons with the tomograph, so we can distinguish between scattered and unscattered photons. Unfortunately, the resolution of the energy measurement is limited, so the separation of photons based on measured energy is not very reliable. Consequently, many scattered photons pass the energy test, and further correction is required.

Many algorithms have been proposed, both in SPECT and in PET. Because acquisition at different energy windows is valuable in SPECT (different isotopes emit photons with different energies), this approach has also been applied for scatter estimation. Acquisition at energy levels just below and/or above the photopeak are used to estimated to number of scattered photons that are accepted by the photopeak window (JASZCZAK et al. 1984; GAGNON et al. 1989; BUVAT et al. 1995; KING et al. 1997). Alternatively, the scatter can be estimated using a model. This can be a simple stationary convolution (AXELSSON et al. 1984), a transmission-scan-dependent convolution model (NARITA et al. 1997), or an attenuation-map-dependent model based on measurements (BEEKMAN et al. 1996; HUTTON et al. 1996; NUYTS et al. 1993) or on the Klein-Nishina equation for Compton scatter (WALRAND et al. 1994; WELLS et al. 1997).

For PET, energy-based methods are less obvious, because PET systems were originally designed for 511 keV only, and because the energy resolution of most current PET systems is relatively poor. There-

Herman GT (1980) Image reconstruction from projections, the fundamentals of computerized tomography. Academic, New York

Huang SC, Phelps ME (1986) In: Phelps ME, Mazziotta JC, Schelbert HR (eds) Positron emission tomgoraphy and autoradiography. Raven, New York, pp 287–346

Hudson HM, Larkin RS (1994) Accelerated image reconstruction using ordered subsets of projection data. IEEE Trans Med Imaging 13:601–609

Huesman RH (1984) A new fast algorithm for the evaluation of regions of interest and statistical uncertainty in computed tomography. Phys Med Biol 29:543–552

Hutton BF, Lau YH (1998) Application of distance-dependent resolution compensation and post-reconstruction filtering for myocardial SPECT. Phys Med Biol 43:1679–1693

Hutton BF, Osiecki A, Meikle SR (1996) Transmission-based scatter correction of 180 degrees myocardial single-photon emission tomographic studies. Eur J Nucl Med 23:1300–1308

Iida H, Narita Y, Kado H et al. (1998) Effects of scatter and attenuation correction on quantitative assessment of regional cerebral blood flow with SPECT. J Nucl Med 39:181–189

Jang S, Jaszczak RJ, Tsui BMW et al. (1998) ROC evaluation of SPECT myocardial lesion detectability with and without single iteration non-uniform Chang attenuation compensation using an anthropomorphic female phantom. IEEE Trans Nucl Sci 45:2080–2088

Jaszczak RJ, Greer KL, Floyd CE et al. (1984) Improved SPECT quantification using compensation for scattered photons. J Nucl Med:25:893–900

Karp JS, Becker AJ, Matej S et al. (1998) Data processing and image reconstruction methods for the HEAD PENN-PET scanner. Phys Med Biol 45:1144–1151

Kaufman L (1987) Implementing and accelerating the EM algorithm for positron emission tomography. IEEE Trans Med Imaging MI-6:37–51

King MA, Schwinger RB, Penney BC et al. (1986) Digital restoration of indium-111 and iodine-123 SPECT images with optimized Metz filters. J Nucl Med 27:1327–1336

King MA, Tsui BMW, Pan TS et al. (1996) Attenuation compensation for cardiac single-photon emission computed tomographic imaging: 2. Attenuation compensation algorithms. J Nucl Cardiol 3:55–64

King MA, de Vries DJ, Pan TS et al. (1997) An investigation of the filtering of TEW scatter estimates used to compensate for scatter with ordered subset reconstructions. IEEE Trans Nucl Sci 44:1140–1145

Kohli V, King MA, Glick SJ et al. (1998) Comparison of frequency-distance relationship and Gaussian-diffusion-based methods of compensation for distance-dependent spatial resolution in SPECT imaging. Phys Med Biol 43:1025–1037

Lalush DS, Tsui BM (1993) A generalized Gibbs prior for maximum a posteriori reconstruction in SPECT. Phys Med Biol 38:729–741

Lange K, Carson R (1984) EM reconstruction algorithms for emission and transmission tomography. J Comp Assist Tomogr 8:306–316

Lewitt RM (1992) Alternatives to voxels for image representation in iterative reconstruction algorithms. Phys Med Biol 37:705–716

Li J, Jaszczak RJ, Wang H et al. (1995) A filtered backprojection algorithm for fan beam SPECT which corrects for patient motion. Phys Med Biol 40:283–294

Liow JS; Strother SC (1993) The convergence of object dependent resolution in maximum likelihood based tomographic image reconstruction. Phys Med Biol 38:55–70

Llacer J, Veklerov E (1989) Feasible images and practical stopping rules for iterative algorithms in emission tomography. IEEE Trans Med Imaging 8:186–193

Llacer J, Veklerov E, Baxter LR et al. (1993) Results of a clinical receiver operating characteristic study comparing filtered backprojection and maximum likelihood estimator images in FDG PET studies J Nucl Med 34:1198–1203

Manglos SH, Gagne GM, Bassano DA (1993) Quantitative analysis of image truncation in focal-beam CT. Phys Med Biol 38:1443–1457

Matsunari I, Boning G, Ziegler SI et al. (1998) Effects of misalignment between transmission and emission scans on attenuation-corrected cardiac SPECT. J Nucl Med 39:411–416

McCord ME, Bacharach SL, Bonow RO et al. (1992) Misalignment between PET transmission and emission scans: its effect on myocardial imaging. J Nucl Med 33:1209–1214

Meikle SR, Dahlbom M, Cherry SR (1993) Attenuation correction using count-limited transmission data in positron emission tomography. J Nucl Med 34:143–144

Meikle SR, Matthews JC, Cunningham VJ et al. (1998) Parametric image reconstruction using spectral analysis of PET projection data. Phys Med Biol 43:651–666

Michel C, Bol A, De Volder AG, Goffinet AM (1989) Online brain attenuation correction in PET: towards a fully automated data handling in a clinical environment. Eur J Nucl Med 15:712–718

Mumcuoglu EU, Leahy RM, Cherry SR (1996) Bayesian reconstruction of PET images: methodology and performance analysis. Phys Med Biol 41:1777–1807

Narita Y, Iida H, Eberl S et al. (1997) Monte Carlo evaluation of accuracy and noise properties of two scatter correction methods for Tl-201 cardiac SPECT. IEEE Trans Nucl Sci 44:2465–2472

Nuyts J, Bosmans H, Suetens P (1993) An analytical model for scatter in a homogeneously attenuating medium. IEEE Trans. Med. Imaging 12:421–429

Nuyts J, Dupont P, Van den Maegdenbergh V et al. (1995) A study of the liver-heart artifact in emission tomography. J Nucl Med 36:133–139

Nuyts J, Maes A, Vrolix M et al. (1996) Three-dimensional correction for spill-over and recovery of myocardial PET images. J Nucl Med 37:767–774

Nuyts J, De Man B, Dupont P et al. (1998) Iterative reconstruction for helical CT: a simulation study. Phys Med Biol 4:729–737

Ollinger JM (1996) Model-based scatter correction for fully 3D PET. Phys Med Biol 41:153–176

Raylman RR, Hutchins GD, Beanlands RSB et al. (1994) Modeling of carbon-11-acetate kinetics by simultaneously fitting data from multiple ROIs coupled by common parameters. J Nucl Med 35:1286–1291

Rockmore AJ, Macovski A (1976) A maximum likelihood approach to emission image reconstruction from projections. IEEE Trans Nucl Sci NS-23:1428–1432

Schiepers C, Nuyts J, Wu C et al. (1997) PET with F-18 fluoride: effects of iterative versus filtered backprojection reconstruction on kinetic modeling. IEEE Trans Nucl Sci 44:1591–1593

Schmidlin P (1972) Iterative separation of sections in tomographic scintigrams. Nuklearmedizin 11:1–16

Shepp LA, Vardi Y (1982) Maximum likelihood reconstruction for emission tomography. IEEE Trans Med Imaging MI-1:113–122

Snyder DL, Miller MI (1985) The use of sieves to stabilize images produced with the EM algorithm for emission tomography. IEEE Trans Nucl Sci NS-32:3864–3872

Snyder DL, Miller MI, Thomas LJ et al. (1987) Noise and edge artifacts in maximum likelihood reconstructions for emission tomography. IEEE Trans Med Imaging MI-6:228–238

Tai YC, Lin KP, Dahlbom M, Hoffman EJ (1996) A hybrid attenuation correction technique to compensate for lung density in 3D total body PET. IEEE Trans Nucl Sci 43:323–330

Tanaka E (1987) A fast reconstruction algorithm for stationary positron emission tomography based on a modified EM algorithm. IEEE Trans Med Imaging MI-6:98–105

Veklerov E, Llacer J (1987) Stopping rule for the MLE algorithm based on statistical hypothesis testing. IEEE Trans Med Imaging MI-6:313–319

Walrand SHM, van Elmbt LR, Pauwels S (1994) Quantitation in SPECT using an effective model of the scattering. Phys Med Biol 39:719–734

Welch A, Gullberg GT (1997) Implementation of model-based nonuniform scatter correction scheme for SPECT. IEEE Trans Med Imaging 16:717–726

Wells RG, Celler A, Harrop R (1997) Experimental validation of an analytical method of calculating SPECT projection data. IEEE Trans Nucl Sci 44:1283–1290

Wilson DW, Tsui BMW, Barrett HH (1994) Noise properties of the EM algorithm: II. Monte Carlo simulations. Phys Med Biol 39:833–846

Wu HM, Huang SC, Allada et al. (1996) Derivation of input function from FDG-PET studies in small hearts. J Nucl Med 37:1717–1722

Xia W, Lewitt RM, Edholm PR (1995) Fourier correction for spatially variant collimator blurring in SPECT. IEEE Trans Med Imaging 14:100–115

Xu M, Cutler PD, Luk WK (1996) Adaptive, segmented attenuation correction for whole-body PET imaging. IEEE Trans Nucl Sci 43:331–336

Yang JT, Yamamoto K, Sadato N et al. (1997) Clinical value of triple-energy window scatter correction in simultaneous dual-isotope single-photon emission tomography with I-123-BMIPP and Tl-201. Eur J Nucl Med 24:1099–1106

Zhou Y, Cloughesy T, Hoh CK et al. (1997) A modeling-based factor extraction method for determining spatial heterogeneity of Ga-68 EDTA kinetics in brain tumors. IEEE Trans Nucl Sci 44:2522–2527

Outlook

15 Imaging Gene Expression: Concepts and Future Outlook

S. S. Gambhir

Contents

15.1 Introduction 253
15.2 Fundamentals of Gene Expression 254
15.2.1 Gene Promoters/Enhancers 254
15.3 Imaging Technology for Monitoring Gene Expression in Animals 254
15.4 Targets for Imaging Gene Expression 255
15.4.1 Conventional Probes Targeted for Proteins 255
15.4.2 Antibody and Antibody Fragments Targeted for Proteins 255
15.4.3 Oligodeoxynucletoide Antisense Probes Targeted for mRNA 255
15.4.4 Oligodeoxynucleotide (Aptamer) Probes Targeted for Proteins 259
15.5 Gene Delivery 259
15.5.1 Transgenics 260
15.5.2 Non-Viral Vectors 260
15.5.3 Adenoviral Vectors 260
15.5.4 Retroviral Vectors 261
15.5.5 Adeno-Associated Viral Vectors 261
15.5.6 Lentiviral Vectors 261
15.6 Reporter Gene Imaging 261
15.6.1 Fundamental Principles of Reporter Genes 261
15.6.2 Properties of the Ideal Reporter Genes for Imaging 262
15.6.3 Cytosine Deaminase Reporter Gene 263
15.6.4 Herpes-Simplex Virus Type-1 Thymidine Kinase Reporter Gene 263
15.6.5 Dopamine 2 Receptor Reporter Gene 265
15.6.6 Reporter Genes for use with Magnetic Resonance Imaging 266
15.7 Signal Amplification for Imaging Gene Expression 266
15.8 Imaging Endogenous Gene Expression 266
15.8.1 Imaging Endogenous Gene Expression with Antisense Probes 266
15.8.2 Imaging Endogenous Gene Expression with a Reporter Gene 266
15.9 Human Gene Therapy Imaging 267
15.9.1 Suicide Gene Therapy and Imaging 267
15.9.2 Therapeutic Gene Therapy and Imaging 267
15.10 Future Outlook 268

S. S. Gambhir
Crump Institute for Biological Imaging, Department of Molecular & Medical Pharmacology, Laboratory of Structural Biology & Molecular Medicine (DOE), UCLA School of Medicine, 700 Westwood Plaza, Los Angeles, CA, USA

15.1 Introduction

Advances in molecular biology are making it possible to develop assays for imaging specific molecular processes, including those directly related to gene expression. Imaging gene expression entails determining the location(s) of those cells expressing a particular gene of interest, as well as monitoring the magnitude and persistence of gene expression. The gene of interest may be an endogenous gene or it may be an "exogenous" gene introduced into the organism/tissue(s) of interest. Imaging gene expression with generalized approaches applicable to any gene of interest have recently been reported. Conventional nuclear imaging techniques can be used to image gene expression if a radiolabeled substrate can be developed to interact with the protein of the gene of interest. However, more general methods are emerging to image gene expression without the need for developing new radiolabeled substrates for each new gene of interest.

In this chapter two general approaches for imaging gene expression are reviewed. The first approach uses an antisense oligodeoxynucleotide targeted towards the messenger ribonucleic acid (mRNA) of a gene of choice. The second approach uses a reporter gene to track the expression of an endogenous or exogenous gene. Methods to introduce genes into target tissue(s) are presented. Principles and applications of assays for imaging gene expression in animals and in human clinical gene therapy trials are also presented and discussed.

15.2 Fundamentals of Gene Expression

The process of gene expression (Fig. 15.1) and the components of gene regulation are only partially understood and are reviewed in detail elsewhere (Lewin, 1994). Not all genes are expressed in all cells, leading to a wide variety of cellular functions or phenotypes. Many phenomena, including cellular development, maturation, proliferation, and oncogenesis can be attributed to the differential expression of genes. As advances in molecular and cell biology lead to a better understanding of the mechanisms leading to altered cellular functions, imaging assays may be able to allow imaging of these alterations in living animals and humans.

15.2.1 Gene Promoters/Enhancers

Specific sequence motifs, about 100 nucleotide bases from the transcription initiation start site, are referred to as the promoter region of the gene. The promoter is directly involved in RNA polymerase (a RNA synthesizing enzyme) binding and the initiation of transcription. Eukaryotic promoters do not always function alone, but can be influenced by enhancers. The position of the enhancer can be quite variable and can be upstream or downstream from the location of the promoter, and sometimes the enhancer is located within the transcription unit itself. The enhancer can increase the efficiency of initiation or be involved in specific regulation of a given gene. A complex of proteins and RNA polymerase are involved in the transcription process, which begins by interactions with the promoter. For the purposes of imaging gene expression, two main types of promoters need to be described. Constitutive promoters can be used to produce continuous transcription of a gene, and inducible promoters can be used to provide external control for varying the levels of transcription. Constitutive promoters can be those of exogenous genes (e.g., cytomegalovirus (CMV)) or those of endogenous genes (e.g., GAPDH, a protein made in all cells). Inducible promoters can also be those of exogenous genes (e.g., tetracycline regulable) or those of endogenous genes (e.g., c-jun).

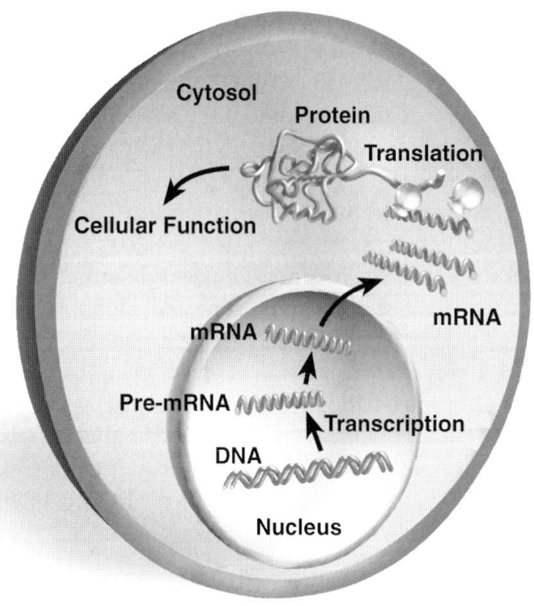

Fig. 15.1. Gene expression. Transcription of DNA in the nucleus leads to the synthesis of pre-messenger RNA (pre-mRNA), which is then processed into mRNA, transported into the cytoplasm, and translated into protein. The final protein product may serve as an enzyme, cell surface receptor, structural component, etc. Conventional targets for *in vivo* nuclear imaging have been aimed at the protein level. Newer targets for gene expression include mRNA through the use of small modified antisense oligodeoxynucleotides.

15.3 Imaging Technology for Monitoring Gene Expression in Animals

The mouse has long been used by molecular biologists to study fundamental cellular events *in vivo*. The relatively small size of the mouse makes it difficult to image using conventional imaging technology. Noninvasive imaging of mice/rats *in vivo* is now possible using microPET technology recently developed at the Crump Institute for Biological Imaging (Cherry et al., 1997). This new PET scanner design facilitates imaging of small animals with a volumetric resolution of 2^3 mm^3 (a significant advantage over current systems with a resolution of $(4\text{-}6)^3$ mm^3). The microPET system and others like it should significantly improve over the next several years, facilitating even better resolution and dynamic imaging capabilities. The next generation of microPET technology has a goal of improving volumetric resolution by another factor of ~10. Anatomical based imaging with MRI and combined PET and MRI imaging with joint PET/MRI systems (Shao et al., 1997), and animal SPECT systems (Kastis et al., 1998) should also further facilitate the development of various imaging assays.

15.4 Targets for Imaging Gene Expression

In order to image gene expression, one could attempt to image (i) if transcription has occurred, or (ii) if transcription and translation have occurred. Potential targets for imaging gene expression include proteins on the cell surface, intracellular proteins, RNA (pre-mRNA, mRNA, other RNA) and least likely DNA (by targeting open transcription complexes). For both, an endogenous gene or an administered (exogenous) gene, the same types of probes can be used to image gene expression. Targeting DNA is particularly difficult because of the limited number of copies present within a cell, as well as limited accessibility to the target DNA sequence. Targeting of RNA and proteins is possible and will be discussed in detail in upcoming sections.

15.4.1 Conventional Probes Targeted for Proteins

Conventional radiotracer imaging methods have focused primarily on the final products of gene expression by utilizing radiolabeled substrates that interact with the proteins originating from specific genes. These interactions are based on either receptor-radioligand binding (e.g., binding of the dopamine 2 receptor to 3-(2'-^{18}F-fluoroethyl)spiperone (^{18}F-FESP)) or enzyme mediated trapping of a radiolabeled substrate (e.g., ^{18}F-2-fluoro-2-deoxyglucose (^{18}F-FDG) phosphorylation by hexokinase). The fundamental limitation of a majority of these conventional approaches is that new substrates must be discovered and radiolabeled for each new protein to be targeted. Due to the difficulty of radiolabeling new substrates, and characterizing all their interactions *in vivo*, alternate methods are needed in order to develop new assays that can categorically image gene expression of any gene of interest.

15.4.2 Antibody and Antibody Fragments Targeted for Proteins

For imaging gene expression, one could potentially develop an antibody targeted against the protein product of the gene. The antibody could then be radiolabeled non-specifically using the same methodology, regardless of the antibody type. The antibody approach, however, is predominantly limited to genes whose products are proteins that have a component on the cell surface. Most genes lead to protein products that remain in the intracellular space, and would therefore be difficult to target with an antibody based approach. In addition, high background signal due to the slow clearance of antibodies from the blood pool, and an immune response to them, limits their overall utility (Goldenberg, 1997). Newer *molecularly engineered* antibody fragments that are smaller in size, with rapid targeting and fast blood clearance, may help resolve existing problems with conventional antibody approaches. These antibody fragments can be constructed by retaining the active binding site of the antibody (e.g., Fab and F(ab')^2), and removing the Fc region leading to lower immunogenicity. A very small antibody fragment (e.g., a "minibody") has also been developed. An example of this category is an antibody fragment targeted against carcinoembryonic antigen (CEA) with useful *in vivo* properties of rapid targeting and fast blood clearance (Hu, et al.. 1996). If general labeling strategies can be applied to the various antibody fragments, then these engineered antibodies may be useful for imaging gene expression for those genes leading to protein products that have a component at the cell surface.

15.4.3 Oligodeoxynucleotide Antisense Probes Targeted for mRNA

In order to image transcription directly, one has to develop tracers that can interact with pre-mRNA or mRNA. Assays for imaging mRNA levels are currently being investigated through the use of small (11-30 nucleobases long) modified radiolabeled antisense oligodeoxynucleotide (RASON) probes targeted toward a specific mRNA (Fig. 15.2). This RASON "antisense" probe is complementary to a small segment of target mRNA. RASON probes have the potential for imaging gene expression specifically at the transcription level. The RASON must be stable against degradation from nucleases, be able to enter and efflux from cells, and be of sufficient specific activity to detect relatively low levels of mRNA. The antisense method is a general approach, because the RASON probe sequence could easily be modified (by changing the sequence of bases) in order to target many mRNAs of interest.

The pharmaceutical industry has been investigating both DNA and mRNA as targets for antisense drugs for over a decade (Agrawal and Iyer, 1997; Crooke, 1997; Crooke and Lebleu, 1993). DNA is an ideal target for a drug, because by binding of an antisense drug to a specific gene (via Hoogsteen base pairing in the major groove) one could theoretically prevent the production of mRNA, and therefore stop protein production. For diseases in which stopping

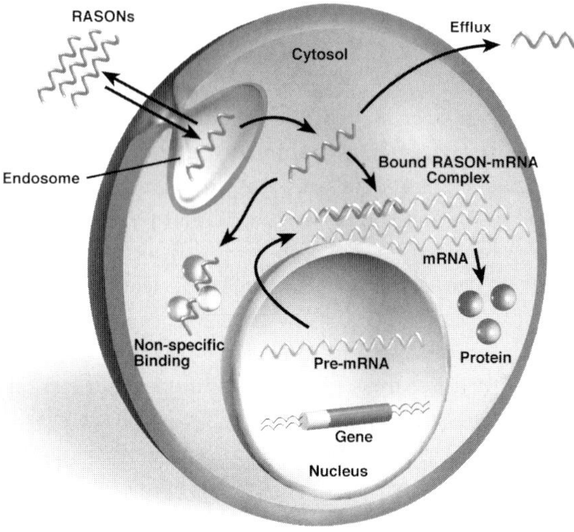

Fig. 15.2. Radioactive antisense oligodeoxynucleotides (RASONs) as probes for imaging gene expression. RASON probes can be designed to target a specific mRNA of a gene of interest. The RASON must be able to enter cells, hybridize to target mRNA. Intracellular RASONs are likely to be in endosomes, and must be able to leave the endosome prior to interaction with target mRNA. Non-specific interactions with proteins as well as efflux out of the cell are key processes which must be considered for developing RASONs as effective probes for imaging gene expression. The target mRNA may be that of an endogenous gene or an administered gene.

the production of an aberrant protein is beneficial, this approach holds significant promise. Companies that focus specifically on the development and testing of antisense drugs (e.g., Isis Pharmaceuticals, Carlsbad, CA) targeted towards various mRNAs are now testing third-generation antisense drugs. However to date, clinical trials using antisense drugs have met with limited success (Wagner and Flanagan, 1997). Much of what may be possible with imaging applications utilizing RASON probes is dependent on the significant progress on antisense pharmaceuticals made by the pharmaceutical industry over the last decade.

Messenger RNA concentrations are typically in the range of 1–1000 pM (Hargrove et al., 1990). Messenger RNA molecules are ideal targets due to their ability to very specifically pair with antisense oligonucleotides through hydrogen bonds. The binding affinity of antisense drugs for mRNA is very high, but a single mismatch can drop the affinity by as much as 300-fold (Crooke and Lebleu, 1993). It has been mathematically shown that a minimum of only 11–15 bases need to be targeted in order to hybridize *uniquely* to any mRNA in the human genome (Helene and Toulme, 1989). This calculation is based on assuming that 0.5% of the human genome is expressed as mRNA. The two numbers correspond to the extreme cases where the oligonucleotide contains only C and G (n=11) or only A and T (n=15). Therefore, an antisense probe of relatively short length can be used to target a given mRNA (Fig. 15.3).

Messenger RNA molecules are typically several hundred to thousands of base pairs long, but not all of these bases are accessible to an antisense probe due to the secondary and tertiary structure of the mRNA molecule. Intracellular mRNA is invariably protein bound, and only a few sites are probably available for base pairing. The location of the best targets for the antisense mRNA approach has been pursued in detail (Goodchild, 1989). The main findings are that in general, the best mRNA locations are the 5' cap or initiation codon (AUG) regions. There are, however, exceptions to this rule, and the tertiary structure of the mRNA must be considered in order to predict potential binding sites. It is important not to generalize mRNA regions that are useful for targeting; instead for each mRNA careful studies must be performed in order to identify good target sites.

Since mRNA-antisense probe interaction is stoichiometric, and therefore equivalent to a receptor-

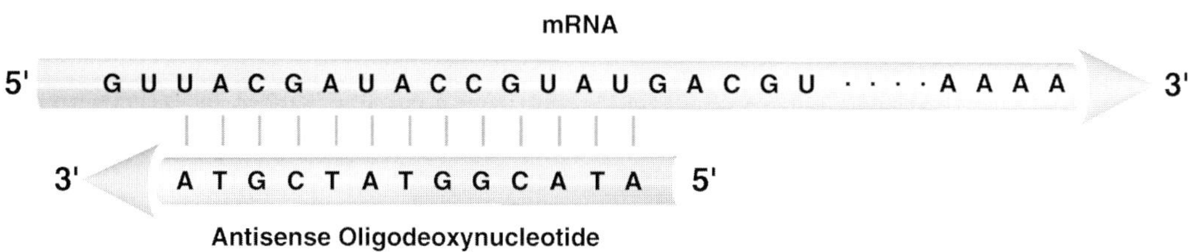

Fig. 15.3. Hybridization of an antisense oligodeoxynucleotide probe with a target mRNA. The antisense probe has a very high specificity for a target mRNA sequence. Although the mRNA can contain hundreds to thousands of bases, an antisense probe of small length (11–15 bases) can uniquely target any mRNA. A: adenine, T: thymidine, G: Guanine, C: cysteine

ligand interaction, one can attempt to answer questions about the minimal levels of mRNA that can be detected by a given antisense probe. Variables such as the concentration of target mRNA, binding affinities of receptor and ligand, antisense probe specific activity, free intracellular antisense tracer concentration, sensitivity of detection (typically only 0.5–2% of annihilation events are detected by PET), and target to background levels all play key roles. Based on these parameters it has been estimated that mRNA concentrations as low as 1 pM tissue can probably be imaged with PET, using RASON probes with specific activities of ~1,000–10,000 Ci/mmole (Pan et al., 1998).

Oligonucleotides are readily cleaved by nucleases *in vivo* (Wickstrom, 1986). A non-hydrolyzable analogue of an oligonucleotide is therefore required so that sufficient amounts can reach the target in effective concentrations. Oligodeoxynucleotides are more stable *in vivo* when compared with oligoribonucleotides (Wickstrom, 1986), and are therefore the probes of choice. Various investigators have investigated modified oligodeoxynucleotides (e.g., phosphorothioates) for greater stability against degradation (Agrawal and Iyer, 1997; Matsukura et al., 1978; Murakami et al., 1985) (Fig. 15.4). Additional modifications that confer stability are alpha oligodeoxynucleotides, as well as 2' modified moieties (Crooke, 1997). Modifications at the 3' end may be particularly useful because they can hinder exonuclease based degradation. Polypeptide nucleic acids (PNAs) (Good and Nielsen, 1997), in which nucleobases are attached to a pseudopeptide, have also been explored as potential drugs, but they may suffer from little to no cellular uptake. PNAs do however have improved stability against nucleases, and may even have enhanced sequence selectivity for target mRNA.

Uptake of oligodeoxynucleotides by cells appears to occur via several mechanisms. The surprising and essential feature is that oligodeoxynucleotides are readily taken up by many different cells. This uptake is critical to insure that a probe can be delivered to the intracellular target mRNA by injection into the venous plasma space. Most oligodeoxynucleotides (except methylphosphonates) are polyanionic and do not passively diffuse across cell membranes. Trans-

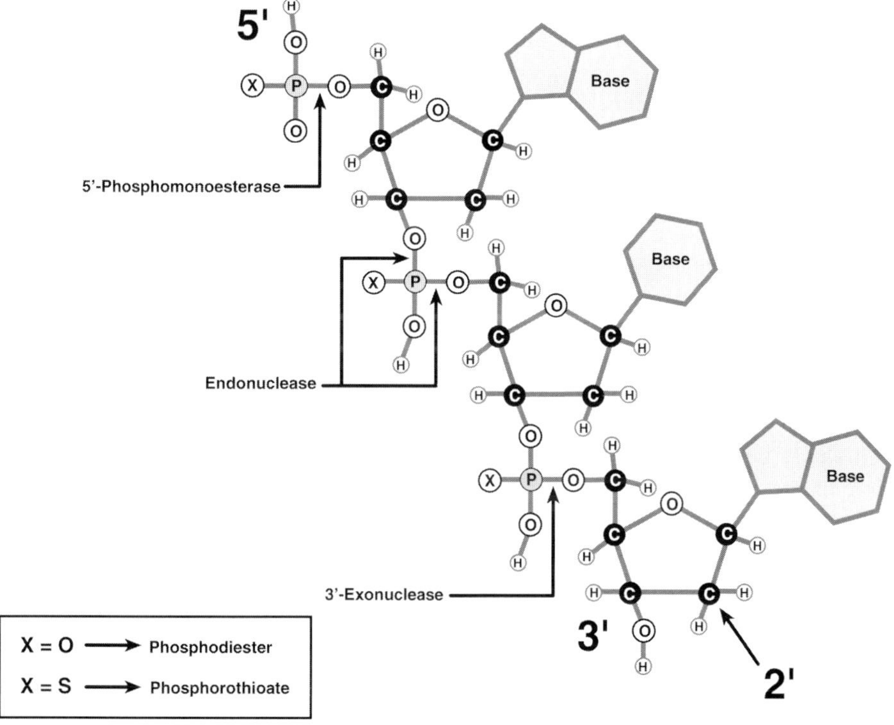

Fig. 15.4. Structure of an oligodeoxynucleotide. Shown is a three-mer. The ribose sugars are interlinked through a backbone composed of phosphodiester bonds. The backbone can be modified in order to achieve greater stability against degradation from nucleases. Phosphorothioates have significant increased stability as compared to phosphodiesters. 2′ modification of the ribose can also lead to more stable oligodeoxynucleotides. Degradation sites are as indicated.

port mechanisms include receptor mediated endocytosis, adsorptive endocytosis, as well as fluid-phase pinocytosis (Cotten et al., 1993; Loke et al., 1989; Wu-Pong et al., 1992; Wu-Pong et al., 1994). There is a fast component as well as a slow component of uptake. An approximately 80-kD protein has also been isolated from several cell types that seems to be responsible for oligodeoxynucleotide binding and possible internalization (Cotten et al., 1993; Loke et al., 1989). The exact transport mechanism seems to be different for various cell types. There have been some preliminary attempts to model oligonucleotide cell transport (Wu-Pong et al., 1992), but no mathematical model is currently available. It is likely that non-diffusible oligodexoynucleotides end up in cellular endosomes, but it is not clear how they leave the endosomes or the efflux rate from endosomes. Several groups have shown that exogenously administered oligonucleotides appear to localize readily in the nucleus, mitochondria or both (Wu-Pong et al., 1992).

The oligonucleotide, once inside the cell, must be able to bind to the target mRNA, and excess unhybridized oligonucleotide must also be able to leave cells during the time in which the oligonucleotide and target mRNA complex is stable. Charged oligonucleotides can nonspecifically interact with intracellular proteins. This may lead to nonspecific binding, and the potential inhibition of oligonucleotide internalization (Loke et al., 1989). To obtain sufficient specificity of the image signal, the rates of exocytosis and mRNA binding must exceed the rate of nonspecific binding. Exocytosis follows a multi-compartmental model, with a rapid phase (half-life of 10 minutes) as well as a slower phase (half-life of 30 minutes) in some cases, but varies depending on the cell type and the type of oligodeoxynucleotide. Both truncated fragments as well as chain extension products efflux from cells. Some studies have reported desired pharmacologic effects of a decrease in protein production with *non-antisense* oligodeoxynucleotides; this may be due to interaction of the drug with proteins. It is important that a true antisense mechanism be demonstrated by using controls with sequentially increasing number of nucleobase mismatches, before proceeding with *in vivo* studies. As the number of mismatches in bases increases, the binding to target mRNA should decrease. Without these appropriate controls, it is possible that nonspecific binding of oligodeoxynucleotide to protein(s) is leading to a desired effect (e.g., reduction in protein production).

Numerous investigators have explored the use of antisense oligonucleotides, both *in vitro* and *in vivo*, as therapeutic agents for decreasing protein production (Stein and Cheng, 1993). These include targeting the 35S RNA of the Rous sarcoma virus (Zamecnik and Stephenson, 1978), various mRNAs for use against HIV (Zamecnik et al., 1986), as well as many oncogene mRNA's including c-myc. Most of this work has shown that antisense oligodeoxynucleotides can work effectively in suppressing mRNA translation. After binding of oligodeoxynucleotide to target mRNA, the mRNA can be digested by ribonuclease H. Direct translation inhibition can also occur. In either case, the net result is a direct decrease in translation of mRNA and production of protein product.

Biodistribution of oligodeoxynucleotides in normal animals has been reported (Crooke, 1995). Phosphorothioate oligonucleotides, for example, bind to serum proteins (~400 μM dissociation constant for albumin). The plasma disappearance is extremely rapid, and is well described by a two-compartment model. A large volume of distribution (~20 ml with a dose of 3.6 mg/kg) is observed for phosphorothioates demonstrating a very wide-spread distribution to many tissues *in vivo*. Peaks of blood activity occur within 2–4 hours after bolus injection. The kidneys and liver have the greatest concentrations, with no significant penetration across the blood-brain-barrier. Natural phosphodiester oligonucleotides are very rapidly degraded to monomers in vivo, and would probably have limited use for targeting gene expression. Animal whole-body autoradiography has also been used to assess the biodistribution of various radiolabeled oligodeoxynucleotides (Phillips et al., 1997).

Although much can be learned from the development and use of antisense oligodeoxynucleotides as drugs, several distinctions must be kept in mind for using them as imaging probes. First, any isotope labeling modification to the oligodeoxynucleotide must not significantly decrease its stability as well as its cellular influx, efflux, specific interaction, or hybridization ability. Second, the relative rate of hybridization to target mRNA must exceed the net effect of the non-specific interactions and efflux rates. Also, the efflux rate must dominate if no target mRNA is present, so as to lead to minimal background signal. The isotope half-life, biological half-life, and specific activity of the RASON are also important parameters to consider when attempting to target a specific mRNA *in vivo*.

The first RASON probe to be developed specifically for nuclear imaging was an indium-labeled oligodeoxynucleotide targeted against the amplified c-myc oncogene (Dewanjee et al., 1994). A 15-mer oligonucleotide sequence was synthesized, amino linked (sense and antisense phosphodiester and monothioester) and bound with diethylenetriamine pentaacetate (DTPA) containing ^{111}In. Subsequently, oligodeoxynucleotides labeled with ^{99m}Tc (HNATOWICH et al., 1995) and ^{125}Iodine (CAMMILLERI et al., 1996) have been reported. More recently fluorine labeled oligodeoxynucleotides for use with PET (PAN et al., 1998; TAVITIAN et al., 1998) have been synthesized. As described earlier, it is essential that high specific-activity probes be developed for targeting the lowest possible levels of mRNA. ^{18}F labeling may achieve high specific activities of 1,000–10,000 Ci/mmole, but has the disadvantage of a relatively short isotope half-life of 110 minutes.

15.4.4 Oligodeoxynucleotide (Aptamer) Probes Targeted for Proteins

Small oligodeoxynucleotide probes can also be used to target *proteins* in addition to targeting RNA. In vitro selection, or systematic evolution of ligands by exponential enrichment (SELEX), has been used both to characterize the interaction of natural nucleic acids with proteins and to generate novel nucleic acid-binding species, or aptamers (CONRAD et al., 1995). Large libraries of potential aptamers can be screened in order to arrive at a high affinity probe targeted towards a specific protein of interest. Since many aptamers can probably be transported into the cell, the products of many genes could potentially be targeted. A single application of the use of an aptamer targeted towards neutrophil elastase (a surface protein) for *in vivo* inflammation imaging with a gamma camera has been reported (CHARLTON et al., 1997). A rat reverse passive Arthus reaction model for inflammation was utilized. The aptamer achieved a peak target-to-background ratio of approximately 4 in two hours, with fast blood clearance of the aptamer. More research in this important arena may lead to other imaging applications in which proteins can be targeted with aptamers. This could allow for imaging gene expression, by developing aptamers targeted towards the protein of the gene of interest.

15.5 Gene Delivery

For some applications a gene has to be introduced into the organism of interest. Prior to the introduction of any gene, a decision must be made as to what promoter to couple to the gene to drive its transcription. As described in section 15.2.1, the choices include constitutive or inducible promoters based on the intended application.

Ex vivo gene delivery in which target cells are first removed from the host, transfected with a specific gene, and then re-delivered to the host are one possible mechanism for some gene delivery applications. Alternatively, gene delivery can be preformed *in vivo* by using one of several vectors to deliver the gene into some specific tissue(s) of interest.

Introduction of genes into *animals* can be accomplished by one of two general methods. Transgenic animals can be made in which every cell in the animal carries the gene of interest (HAIDER et al., 1998). The transgene can be driven by a constitutive or inducible promoter. Only certain tissues can be made to express this gene, depending on the type of promoter used. Alternatively, a wide variety of non-viral (ROLLAND, 1998) and viral vectors (MILLER and VILE, 1995) can be used to introduce a gene of interest into target somatic tissue.

Delivery of genes into *humans* continues to remain a challenge for a wide variety of investigations, and is reviewed in detail elsewhere (SMITH, 1995). Although not sufficient, a necessary condition for the success of gene therapy in humans will be efficient delivery of the gene(s) of interest into the appropriate target tissue(s). The use of a plasmid (an autonomously replicating DNA molecule) *in vivo* has been investigated, but is limited by a poor efficiency of transfer into cells. Plasmid vectors can also be delivered by the use of cationic liposomes, which enhance transfer of genetic material into the cell. The use of adenoviral vectors, retroviral vectors, adeno-associated vectors, and most recently lentiviral vectors are all being pursued and are discussed in upcoming sections.

When two genes need to be introduced into the same tissue (e.g., a therapeutic gene and a reporter gene for monitoring human gene therapy), it is preferable to have a system in which a fixed relationship holds between the expression of both genes. Such fixed expression of two genes is possible through the use of an internal ribosomal entry site (IRES) (GALLARDO et al., 1997; LEVENSON et al., 1998). In this case transcription of both genes (driven by a common promoter of choice) leads to a *single* mRNA, and translation produces both protein products from the same transcript because of the IRES (Fig. 15.5). A validation of this approach for imaging bicistronic gene expression in animals with microPET has been published (YU et al., in press)

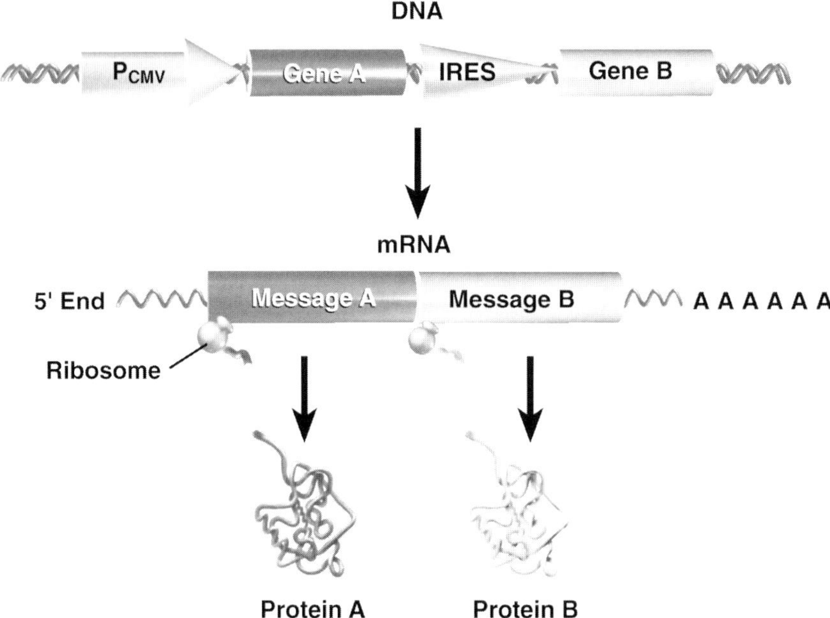

Fig. 15.5. A bicistronic vector with an internal ribosomal entry site (IRES). In applications in which two genes (A and B) need to be jointly expressed through a common promoter, an IRES can be used. A single mRNA (containing both genes) is transcribed, but translation of this single transcript leads to two distinct proteins. Ribosomes can enter at the IRES leading to only translation of message B, and production of protein B.

15.5.1 Transgenics

Animals in which a specific new or altered gene (driven by a promoter of choice) has been introduced into every cell of the entire organism are referred to as transgenics. The recombinant gene (transgene) is introduced into the fertilized ovum of an animal at the two-cell stage of development. The fertilized ovum is reimplanted into a surrogate female (a pseudo-pregnant mouse primed for implantation), and animals that are born which contain the transgene can be identified. The mouse model has been the most frequently used, but other animal models are also possible.

15.5.2 Non-Viral Vectors

A gene and its promoter could be injected directly into the blood stream, but as discussed in section 15.4.3, breakdown by nucleases, and poor delivery across cell membranes limit this approach. The use of a plasmid (an autonomously replicating DNA molecule) *in vivo* has been investigated, but limited by a poor efficiency of transfer into cells. Plasmid vectors can also be delivered by the use of cationic liposomes, which enhance transfer of genetic material into the cell. These vectors also lead to only transient expression of the delivered gene, which may limit their utility for many applications.

15.5.3 Adenoviral Vectors

Adenoviral vectors are relatively large (38 Kb) DNA viral vectors. The wild-type adenovirus can be modified by deleting one or more early genes (e.g., E1a, E2, and E3) which are responsible for activation of other genes. Through deletion of one or more of these genes, one can incorporate a segment of DNA that can then be delivered into cells capable of being infected by the adenovirus. The E1a gene is needed for viral replication, but the E2 and E3 genes are not. Additional genes can also be deleted to increase the packaging capacity if needed.

Since the adenoviral vector with the E1a gene deleted can not replicate, the isolation of high titers of adenovirus requires cells which express the E1a gene. 293 human kidney cell lines which constitutively express the E1a protein can be used to grow an adenovirus in which the E1a gene is replaced by a gene of interest. Standard purification techniques can be used to isolate relatively high titers (10^{11} pfu/ml) of the desired adenoviral vector.

Adenoviral vectors like the wild-type adenovirus are capable of transducing both replicating and non-dividing cells. These vectors can transfect a wide variety of cells, with respiratory airway epithelium being particularly susceptible. The adenoviral vectors do not integrate their DNA into host DNA, but do lead to an immune response. The immune response can be particularly worsened by repeated administration of the viral vector. Adenoviral vectors lead to a transient level of gene expression, primarily due to host response to viral proteins in transduced cells. Future research may lead to adenoviral vectors with a decreased immune response, and improved specificity for the tissue(s) of choice.

15.5.4 Retroviral Vectors

Retroviruses have a RNA genome, which is converted into DNA in the infected cell followed by its integration into host DNA. Entry of the retrovirus into target cells is critically dependent on appropriate receptors on the cell surface. Packaging cell lines which are capable of generating retroviruses of a variety of host ranges have been used to combat this problem. Also, mitosis of the target cells is necessary for proviral integration to occur. The retroviral genome is composed of three genes termed gag, pol, and env, which are flanked by long terminal repeats (LTRs), and a packaging sequence (Ψ) which allows viral RNA to be distinguished from other RNAs in the cell. The LTRs serve to control expression of the viral genes, and also define the beginning and end of the viral genome. Viral genes can be replaced with a gene of interest (transgene) to deliver this gene into host cells. The transgene can be under the control of the LTRs or a promoter which is a part of the transgene. Packaging cells can be used that allow production of high titers of replication-deficient recombinant virus. Retroviruses are primarily limited by their ability to integrate only into replicating cells, and their relative lability as compared to other viruses.

15.5.5 Adeno-Associated Viral Vectors

Adeno-associated virus (AAV) is a single-stranded DNA virus that is capable of infecting non-replicating cells. It can integrate into host genome at a specific site on chromosome 19. AAV is a small virus which is relatively difficult to propagate *in vitro* and can only be purified in low titers. AAV vectors have low packaging ability (4 Kb) because of their small size, but have the advantage of a decreased host immune response because of their structural simplicity.

15.5.6 Lentiviral Vectors

Lentiviruses belong to the retrovirus family and are capable of infecting both dividing and non-dividing cells. The human immunodeficiency virus (HIV) is an example of a lentavirus. A disabled HIV virus has been developed and could be used for *in vivo* gene delivery. A portion of the viral genome which encodes for accessory proteins can be deleted without affecting production of the vector and efficiency of infection. The lentiviral vectors have been produced in small scale (>10^9 virus particles per ml). Lentiviral delivery into various rodent tissues shows sustained expression of the transgene of up to six months. Furthermore, there seems to be little or no immune response with these vectors. These lentiviral vectors hold significant promise for *in vivo* gene delivery.

15.6 Reporter Gene Imaging

15.6.1 Fundamental Principles of Reporter Genes

Molecular biologists have used reporter genes both *in vitro* and *in vivo* for over a decade to monitor gene expression. Reporter genes are used to study promoter/enhancer elements involved in gene expression, inducible promoters to look at the induction of gene expression, and endogenous gene expression through the use of transgenes containing endogenous promoters fused to the reporter gene. In all of these cases transcription of the reporter gene can be tracked and therefore gene expression can be studied.

Specific examples of reporter genes include the bacterial gene chloramphenicol acetyl transferase (CAT), and the lacZ gene which codes for β-galactosidase. Autoradiography of a chromatogram (when using CAT) or enzyme assay (when using lacZ) can then be used to assay cell extracts for the product of the reporter gene (Lewin, 1994). For tissue specimens, the same reporter genes can also be used, with the use of immunohistochemistry or histochemical staining. In studies of reporter gene expression, the introduction of a chimeric fusion gene (a gene coupled to some endogenous or exogenous promoter) into the target tissue has to be accomplished. A reporter gene (e.g., alkaline phosphatase) which can lead to a protein product secreted into the blood stream can also be used, thereby allowing monitoring in living animals (Fig.15.6). However, the location(s) of the reporter gene are not able to be determined in this case, because only the blood can easily be sampled.

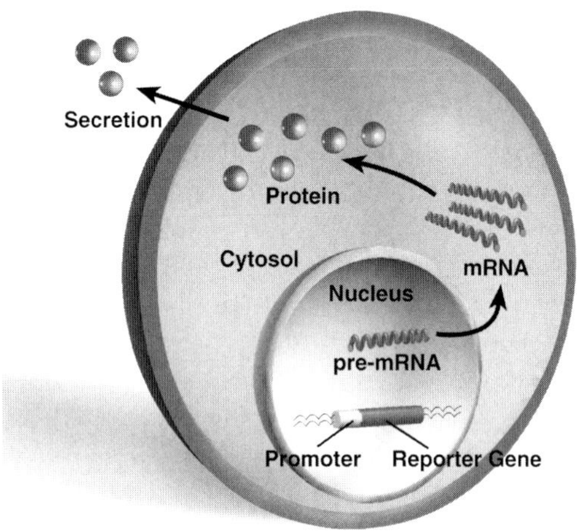

Fig. 15.6. The reporter gene concept for *in vivo* applications. A reporter gene driven by a promoter of choice must first be introduced into the cell(s) of interest. If the reporter gene is transcribed, a protein product is eventually made which can be secreted into the blood and therefore detected. Sampling the blood will not reveal the location(s) where the reporter gene is active, but it will reveal that it is being transcribed and translated. Changes in magnitude of protein product may also allow for the determination of the degree to which the promoter is actively driving the gene of interest.

Conventional reporter gene methods are limited by their inability to determine the *location(s)* of gene expression in *living* animals. Approaches using green fluorescent protein (GFP) (Chalfie et al., 1994; Misteli and Spector, 1997) and luciferase (Jacobs et al., 1993) as reporter genes whose products directly interact with light, allow for localization in some living animals. Animals that are transparent to light can be imaged with simple video cameras because of the ability of these reporter genes to produce products that interact with visible light. However, these imaging techniques are very limited because of their lack of generalizability (e.g., GFP would not work with humans) and detailed tomographic resolution. Radionuclide imaging techniques offer the possibility of monitoring the location, magnitude, and persistence of reporter gene expression (with potentially a very high sensitivity) for *in vivo* use in animals and humans. Shown in Figures 15.7 and 15.8 are approaches in which a reporter gene which encodes for an enzyme and receptor respectively can lead to trapping of an imaging probe, thereby allowing the imaging of reporter gene expression.

15.6.2 Properties of the Ideal Reporter Genes for Imaging

The ideal reporter gene/reporter probe imaging system would have the following characteristics: (a) The reporter gene should be present in mammalian cells, but not expressed (this will prevent an immune response). (b) When expressed, the reporter gene protein should produce specific reporter probe accumulation only in those cells in which it is expressed. (c) When the reporter gene is not expressed, there should be no significant accumulation of reporter probe in cells. (d) There should be no significant immune reaction to the reporter gene product. (e) The reporter probe should be stable *in vivo* and not be converted to *peripheral* metabolites that complicate the development of a quantitative assay. (f) The reporter probe should be rapidly cleared from the

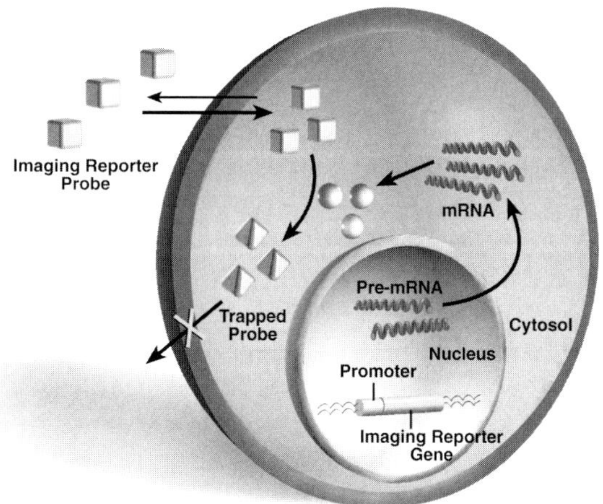

Fig. 15.7. An imaging reporter gene with enzyme mediated trapping of the imaging reporter probe. An imaging reporter gene driven by a promoter of choice must first be introduced into the cell(s) of interest. If the reporter gene is transcribed, a enzyme product (spheres) is eventually made which can lead to the trapping (tetrahedrons) of the imaging reporter probe (cubes). The imaging reporter probe must be able to enter cells. Signal amplification by accumulation of trapped imaging reporter probe leads to the ability to determine the location(s), magnitude, and persistence of reporter gene expression.

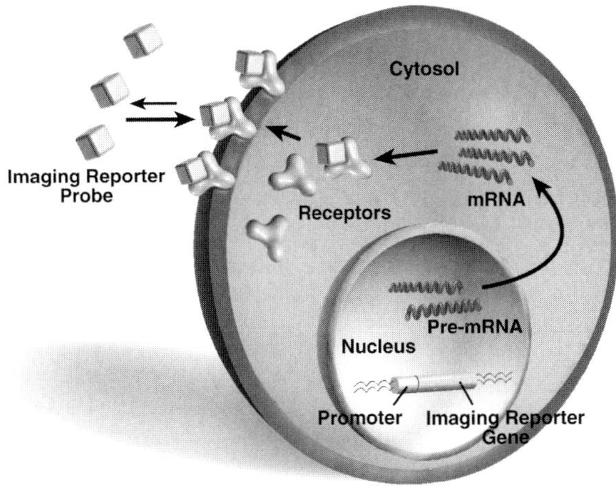

Fig. 15.8. An imaging reporter gene with receptor mediated trapping of the imaging reporter probe (a ligand). An imaging reporter gene driven by a promoter of choice must first be introduced into the cell(s) of interest. If the reporter gene is transcribed, a receptor protein (Y) is eventually made which leads to binding of the imaging reporter probe (cubes). Signal amplification by receptor-ligand interaction leads to the ability to determine the location(s), magnitude, and persistence of reporter gene expression. The receptor protein can be intracellular and/or at the cell surface. If the receptor protein is only intracellular, than the imaging reporter probe must be able to enter cells.

blood and non-specific sites in tissues, and preferably have an elimination route that does not interfere with the detection of specific signal. (g) The reporter probe should be conveniently radiolabeled with a variety of radionuclides without significant change in its properties, and should be labeled with an appropriate specific activity. (h) The reporter probe or its metabolites should not be cytotoxic at the concentrations used. This is likely to be the case for most tracer applications, which are based on very low concentrations of tracer. (i) The size of the reporter gene and the promoter driving it should be small enough to fit in the delivery vehicle (e.g., for a conventional adenoviral vector the upper limit is ~ 7 Kb). This requirement can be relaxed for animal applications such as transgenics in which a delivery vehicle is usually not needed. (j) The reporter probe must be able to reach the area(s) of interest without transport across membranes being a significant limitation. (k) The reporter probe image signal should correlate well (over the range of concentration relevant to the study paradigm) with levels of reporter gene mRNA and protein *in vivo.* (l) The reporter gene assay should correlate well with levels of endogenous gene expression, if the reporter gene is being used to monitor endogenous gene expression.

No single reporter gene/reporter probe system currently meets all these criteria. It is likely that each reporter gene /reporter probe system will only meet some of the above criteria, and therefore different reporter systems will have to be chosen based on the intended application. The development of multiple reporter gene/reporter probe systems will help to provide a choice, based on their application of interest, for future investigators. Furthermore, by having multiple reporter gene assays, it should be possible to monitor the expression of more than one reporter gene in the same living animal or human.

15.6.3 Cytosine Deaminase Reporter Gene

Cytosine deaminase (CD) was one of the first reporter genes to be studied for imaging reporter gene expression. CD is found primarily in yeasts and bacteria and its expression is responsible for the deamination of cytosine to form uracil. Mammalian cells lack CD and therefore can not convert cytosine to uracil. In those cells expressing CD, 5-fluorocytosine is converted to 5-fluorouracil which is cytotoxic. CD has been used in animal (Nishiyama et al., 1985) and human (Wallace et al., 1994) cancer therapy models with 5-fluorocytosine. The reporter probe 6-^{3}H-5-fluorocytosine has been studied in human glioblastoma cells stably transfected with the Escherichia coli CD reporter gene, because of its ability to be converted to 6-^{3}H-5-fluorouracil only in cells expressing CD (Haberkorn et al., 1996). Rapid cellular efflux of 6-^{3}H-5-fluorouracil limits the utility of this reporter probe and further exploration of the CD reporter gene with 5-^{18}F-fluorocytosine and PET. Furthermore, very slow uptake of ^{3}H-5-fluorocytosine, in part attributable to different transporters between prokaryotes and eukaryotes, is also a problem. Times of up to 48 hours are needed to see differences in radioactivity accumulation between cells expressing CD and control cells. Alternative substrates for CD, which are rapidly transported, deaminated, and trapped intracellularly, may eventually allow the use of CD to develop an assay for imaging reporter gene expression.

15.6.4 Herpes-Simplex Virus Type-1 Thymidine Kinase Reporter Gene

There are two known *mammalian* thymidine kinases: a mitochondrial and a cytosolic enzyme (Arner and ERIKSSON, 1995). These kinases are responsible for catalyzing the transfer of the γ-phosphate from ATP to the 5'-terminus of deoxythymidine to form deoxythymidine monophosphate (dTMP). When cells are infected with the Herpes simplex virus (HSV), the *viral* thymidine kinase is expressed. The viral thymidine kinase (tk) has relaxed substrate specificity as compared to the mammalian thymidine kinases, and is capable of phosphorylating pyrimidine and purine nucleoside derivatives (DE CLERCQ, 1993), as well as deoxythymidine. These compounds, when phosphorylated, are trapped intracellularly.

The discovery that acyclovir (9-(2-hydroxyethoxymethyl)guanine) is specifically phosphorylated by the viral thymidine kinase resulted in one of the most successful approaches to the treatment of Herpes simplex virus infection (ELION, 1993). Subsequent phosphorylation of acyclovir monophosphate by guanylate kinase to form acyclovir diphosphate, followed by phosphorylation by various cellular enzymes leads to the formation of acyclovir triphosphate. Acyclovir triphosphate leads to chain termination when it is incorporated into DNA, and acts as a more potent inhibitor of the viral DNA polymerases than of cellular polymerases. The DNA polymerases of HSV1 and HSV2 also use acyclovir triphosphate as a substrate and incorporate it into the DNA primer-template to a much greater extent than do the cellular enzymes. The viral DNA polymerase binds strongly to the acyclovir triphosphate-terminated template, and is thereby inactivated (ELION, 1993). Multiple substrates for HSV1-TK* including ganciclovir (9-[[2-hydroxy-1-(hydroxymethyl)ethoxy]methyl]guanine) and penciclovir (9-(4-hydroxy-3-hydroxymethylbutyl)guanine) have subsequently been synthesized and reported in the literature as antiviral agents (ALRABIAH and SACKS, 1996).

Two main categories of substrates; uracil nucleoside derivatives (e.g., 5-iodo-2'-fluoro-2'-deoxy-1-β-D-arabinofuranosyl-5-iodouracil (FIAU)) and acycloguanosine derivatives (e.g., 8-^{18}F-fluoroganciclovir (^{18}F-FGCV)) have recently been investigated as reporter probes for imaging HSV1-tk reporter gene expression. These reporter probes are transported into cells, and trapped as a result of phosphorylation by HSV1-TK. The details of various reporter probes for imaging HSV1-tk reporter gene expression are reviewed elsewhere (GAMBHIR et al., 1999a,b). Two distinct *in vivo* imaging applications of the HSV1-tk reporter gene have been published and are discussed next.

* *Note that HSV1-tk denotes the gene and HSV1-TK denotes the enzyme.*

TJUVAJEV et. al. (1995) used a recombinant replication-deficient STK retrovirus containing HSV1-tk to transduce RG2 glioma cells *in vitro* and *in vivo*. HSV1-tk gene expression was then imaged using quantitative autoradiography of 2-^{14}C-FIAU in an intracerebral tumor model in rats. Transduction of the RG2 tumor cells with the HSV1-tk gene *in vivo* resulted in tumors which accumulated 2-^{14}C-FIAU and produced good autoradiographic images of gene expression. Imaging relatively late, at 24 hours after the injection of 2-^{14}C-FIAU, reduced the effects of background radioactivity by taking advantage of a long washout time. These authors also explored 8-^{3}H-ganciclovir *in vitro*, but it was not explored *in vivo* because it showed less accumulation in cell culture when compared to 2-^{14}C-FIAU. In a subsequent study, TJUVAJEV et. al. (1996) used ^{131}I-FIAU and scintigraphy. In this study, using rats, tumors were transduced *in vitro* with the HSV1-tk gene, and also *in vivo* using direct intratumoral injection of retroviral vector-producer cells. Animals were imaged with a planar and tomographic scintigraphy 24–48 hours after injection of ^{131}I-FIAU. The authors concluded that "clinically relevant" levels of HSV1-tk gene expression can be imaged with ^{131}I-FIAU and scintigraphy. Studies with ^{124}I-FIAU and PET have also recently been reported (TJUVAJEV et al., 1998) and demonstrate that tumors with various levels of HSV1-tk expression can be distinguished by PET imaging at 30 hours after injection of ^{124}I-FIAU. Good correlations between sensitivity of the transduced tumors to ganciclovir (IC_{50}) and the ^{124}I-FIAU %ID/g, as well as the incorporation constant (Ki) were shown.

The UCLA Gene Imaging Consortium (GAMBHIR et al., 1998) has used an adenoviral-directed delivery mechanism in which a replication-deficient adenovirus carrying the HSV1-tk reporter gene driven by the cytomegalovirus promoter is used to deliver the HSV1-tk reporter gene primarily to the murine liver (Fig.15.9). Peripheral intravenous injection of adenovirus causes a predominant infection of the mouse liver (HERZ and GERARD, 1993; STRATFORD-PERRICAUDET et al., 1990). Forty-eight hours after tail-vein injection of either control virus or virus carrying HSV1-tk to the mice, the animals were injected with 8-^{14}C-ganciclovir and imaged one hour later. Digital whole-body autoradiography was used to evaluate the specificity and sensitivity of this assay. Correlations *in vivo* between relative levels of HSV1-TK enzyme, HSV1-tk mRNA, and %ID/g, show the feasibility of quantitatively relating the *in vivo* imaging signal from the liver to the level of reporter gene

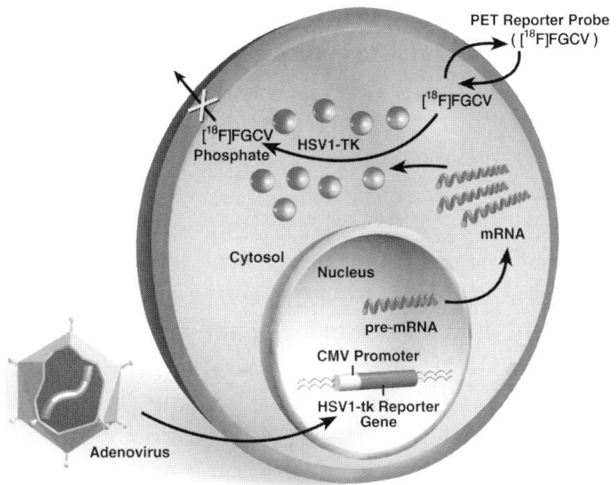

Fig. 15.9. Adenoviral mediated delivery of the Herpes Simple Type 1 virus thymidine kinase (HSV1-tk) reporter gene followed by subsequent 8-[^{18}F]-fluoroganciclovir ([^{18}F]FGCV) PET reporter probe trapping. An adenovirus carrying the HSV1-tk reporter gene has been used to deliver the HSV1-tk reporter gene (driven by a constitutive cytomegalovirus (CMV) promoter). Transcription and translation of HSV1-tk lead to production of HSV1-TK enzyme which can phosphorylate and trap [^{18}F]FGCV. PET imaging can thereby detect the location(s), magnitude, and persistence of HSV1-tk reporter gene expression.

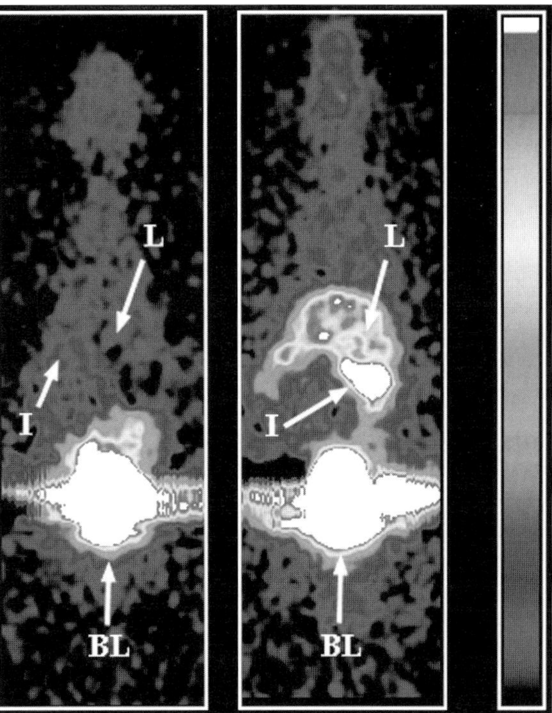

Fig. 15.10. Coronal microPET images from a mouse injected with control adenovirus (left) and adenovirus carrying the HSV1-tk gene (right). Each viral vector was injected 48 hours prior to imaging. The images were obtained one hour after the injection of 150 μCi of [^{18}F-]FGCV using 8 bed positions and 8 minutes/bed. Each image is normalized to a common global maximum with thresholding and represents approximately 1 mm depth and an in-plane resolution of approximately 3 mm. The color white representing maximum counts. (L)-liver; (I)-intestine; (BL)-bladder. Reproduced with permission (from Gambhir et al, 1998).

expression. MicroPET (Cherry et al., 1997) studies using the same murine model and ^{18}F-FGCV also show encouraging results (Fig. 15.10) (Gambhir et al., 1998 and 1999). ^{18}F-FGCV shows some decreased affinity for HSV1-tk as compared to ganciclovir, leading to a decreased accumulation in HSV1-TK positive tissue(s) per unit level of HSV1-tk gene expression (Gambhir et al., 1999). 9-(3-^{18}F-Fluoro-1-hydroxy-2-propoxy)methyl]guanine ^{18}F-FHPG has also been preliminarily studied in primates in order to demonstrate the absence of catabolism and relative uptake into transduced cells (Alauddin et al., 1997; Bading et al., 1997).

15.6.5 Dopamine-2 Receptor Reporter Gene

The dopamine-2 receptor (D2R) is primarily expressed in the brain striatum and in the pituitary gland. The D2R is a 415 amino acid protein with a seven transmembrane domain topology (Bunzow et al., 1988). Ligand-activated D2R interacts with G proteins to inhibit adenylate cyclase (Strange, 1990). Several PET D2R ligands (labeled with either ^{11}C or ^{18}F) for the D2R reporter gene have been well validated in animal and human applications (Ehrin et al., 1985; Wagner et al., 1983). 3-(2'-^{18}F-Fluoroethyl)spiperone (^{18}F-FESP), a D2R antagonist is one of these ligands (Barrio et al., 1989). ^{123}I-Iodobenzamine is also potentially useful for imaging D2R expression with SPECT (Kessler et al., 1991).

A PET reporter gene/PET reporter probe assay based on D2R/^{18}F-FESP has been developed by the UCLA Gene Imaging Consortium and investigated in nude mice using both an adenoviral-directed hepatic gene delivery system, and in tumors transfected with D2R *ex vivo,* then implanted in nude mice (MacLaren et al., 1999). The D2R reporter gene when expressed, leads to accumulation of ^{18}F-FESP by direct binding to D2R (cell membrane and intracellular). Good correlations ($r^2 > 0.88$) with PET image signal *in vivo,* and with GAPDH normalized levels of D2R mRNA and receptor concentrations, as quantified from tissue extracts *in vitro* were demonstrated.

15.6.6
Reporter Genes for Use with Magnetic Resonance Imaging

In order to be useful with MRI, a reporter gene would have to lead to a change in relaxivity in cells in which the reporter gene is expressed. Intrinsically, MRI has a sensitivity of $\sim 10^{-4} - 10^{-5}$ M, and does not compete well with PET where the sensitivity is $\sim 10^{-10}$ M. Therefore a PET based approach would need much less accumulation of a reporter probe than would an MRI based approach for a given level of gene expression. However, an MRI based approach might have an advantage of improved spatial and temporal resolution which in part is based on signal strength. Reporter genes for use with MRI have preliminarily been studied in cell culture (ENOCHS et al., 1997; WEISSLEDER et al., 1997) and are reviewed in detail elsewhere (BOGDANOV and WEISSLEDER, 1998). An example of this approach is the use of the β-Galactosidase reporter gene which when expressed can lead to the hydrolysis of a compound complexed with gadolinium. Free gadolinium would increase proton relaxation times with subsequent changes in MRI signal (BOGDANOV and WEISSLEDER, 1998). Other approaches use the tyrosinase reporter gene leading to greater production of melanin, and subsequent trapping of heavy metals by melanin binding thereby changing cell relaxivity (WEISSLEDER et al., 1997). Future *in vivo* studies will be needed to better define the potential role of these and other approaches for imaging reporter gene expression with MRI.

15.7
Signal Amplification for Imaging Gene Expression

Signal amplification is a key issue in imaging gene expression. Higher levels of imaging signal per unit level of gene expression lead to a higher sensitivity for any particular gene imaging assay. The antisense approach has the lowest concentration of the target (mRNA), and is the most challenging of the methods discussed in this respect. The receptor based reporter gene approach is better because one mRNA leads to many receptor proteins. The enzyme based reporter gene approach has the greatest signal amplification, because one mRNA leads to many enzyme molecules, and each enzyme molecule can lead to the trapping of a large number of reporter probe molecules. These differences must be kept in mind based on the imaging application desired prior to selecting an optimal approach.

15.8
Imaging Endogenous Gene Expression

15.8.1
Imaging Endogenous Gene Expression with Antisense Probes

In vivo imaging applications with antisense probes have been limited to date. DEWANJEE et al., (1994) were the first to demonstrate the targeting of endogenous gene expression with ^{111}In-labeled antisense probes and gamma camera imaging using a tumor bearing model in mice. This study demonstrated rapid targeting to a tumor expressing the c-myc oncogene as compared to a control tumor with imaging performed at two hours after injection. Control probes were used, but sequential mismatch probes were not studied. No subsequent applications have been reported, and no other laboratories have reported verification of these preliminary, but encouraging results. Most recently TAVITIAN et. al. (1998) reported the biodistribution of antisense probes in baboons *in vivo,* using PET. 18-mer oligodeoxynucleotides labeled at the 3' end with fluorine-18 (specific activity 1000-2000 Ci/mmole) were studied. Phosphodiester, phosphorothioate, and 2'-O-methyl oligodeoxynucleotides were each studied. The 18-mer sequence chosen was complementary to a murine virus with computer database verified lack of matches to any mammalian mRNA target. This study demonstrated that each of the three types of ^{18}F labeled oligodeoxynucleotides studied behaved very differently *in vivo* (as expected), that the 3' labeling with ^{18}F did not affect the biodistribution of each probe, and that PET could be used to quantitate the biodistribution of oligodeoxynucleotides. This study focused on the *in vivo* pharmacokinetics of the RASONs, and did not attempt to target any particular mRNA, as would be needed for eventual application of imaging gene expression. All antisense imaging applications to date have been preliminary, but with further validation and continued exploration should lead to reproducible assays for imaging gene expression.

15.8.2
Imaging Endogenous Gene Expression with a Reporter Gene

In imaging applications to date, reporter genes driven by a constitutive promoter such as the CMV promoter have been used (GAMBHIR et al., 1998). This allows for continued transcription of the reporter gene (up to the cellular life-time of the reporter gene), but does not allow for tracking of *endogenous* gene expression. Through the creation of a chimeric fusion gene, in which the promoter of an endogenous gene is coupled to the reporter gene, endogenous gene expression can be monitored (Fig. 15.11).

A reporter gene assay to *specifically* monitor *endogenous* gene expression in living animals through the use of a radiotracer imaging technique has not yet been reported. However, because methods to image a reporter gene with a constitutive promoter have been demonstrated (see sections 15.6.4–15.6.5), it should soon be possible to image endogenous gene expression while utilizing a reporter gene. This should allow for many new questions to be asked and answered in which repeated, noninvasive, imaging of endogenous gene expression is needed to monitor the location, magnitude, and persistence of endogenous gene expression. In order to use reporter methods for monitoring endogenous gene expression, levels of endogenous mRNA and reporter mRNA should be *independently* assayed in order to verify that reporter gene expression correlates with endogenous gene expression. There need not be a linear relationship between levels of reporter and endogenous gene mRNA if a reporter gene approach is used. This potential lack of linearity must be kept in mind, as one seeks to interpret and *quantify* assays for measuring endogenous gene expression.

15.9 Human Gene Therapy Imaging

No specific applications of imaging gene expression in humans using either the reporter gene or antisense approach have been published to date. In human gene therapy trials physicians deliver either a therapeutic or a suicide gene (a gene which can inhibit tumor cell growth). To date no imaging of the expression of either therapeutic or suicide genes has been reported.

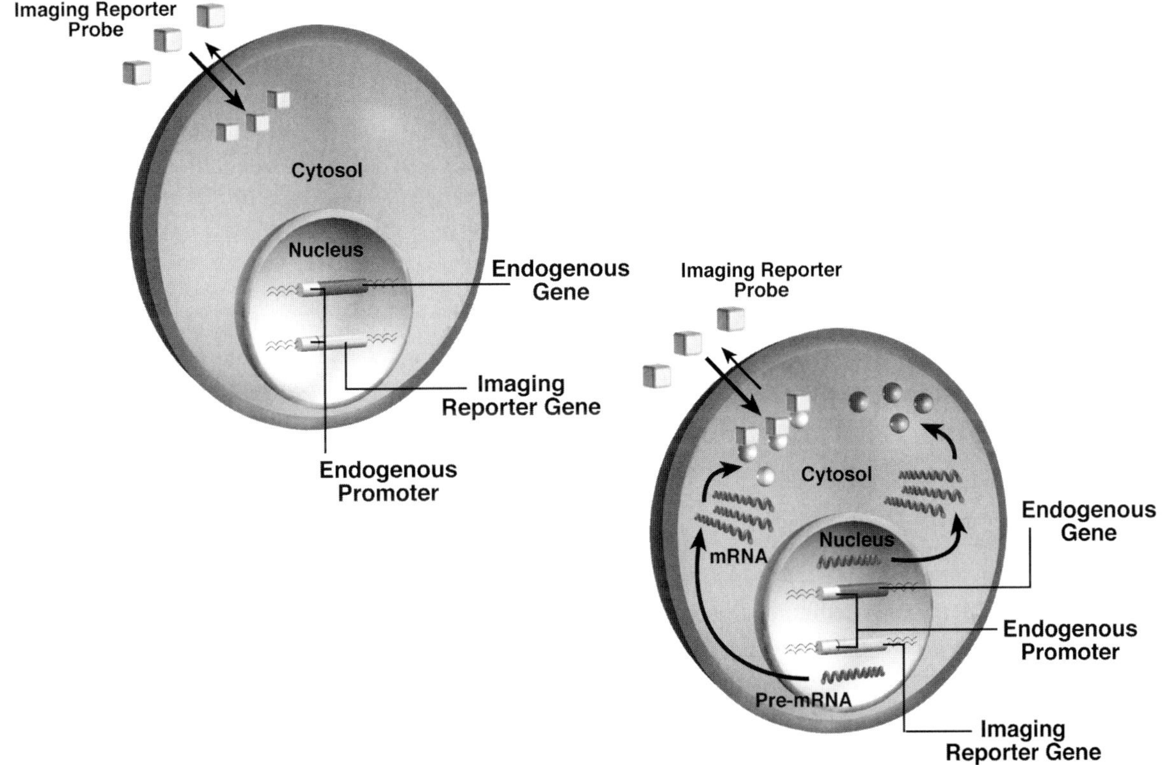

Fig. 15.11. Monitoring of endogenous gene expression through the use of a reporter gene. The endogenous gene and the reporter gene share the *same* promoter. If the endogenous gene is not transcribed, then the reporter gene is not transcribed, and there is no accumulation of the imaging reporter probe (cubes) (upper left panel). If the endogenous gene is transcribed, leading to transcription of the imaging reporter gene, then imaging reporter probe (cubes) is accumulated (lower right panel). The interaction of reporter gene protein and imaging reporter probe can be enzyme based or receptor-ligand based. Accumulation of imaging reporter probe allows for the potential indirect monitoring of the *endogenous* gene expression *in vivo.*

15.9.1 Suicide Gene Therapy and Imaging

A suicide gene is a gene that when delivered to cells, renders the cell susceptible to an administered pro-drug. Moolten first demonstrated the transfer of the HSV1-tk suicide gene into neoplasms in 1986 (Moolten, 1986). Subsequent systemic treatment with the pro-drug ganciclovir resulted in neoplasm reduction. The mechanism of ganciclovir trapping was described in section 15.6.4. Cancer cells are unable to replicate leading to a decrease in tumor burden and tumor cell death. Multiple clinical trials in which the HSV1-tk suicide gene is being used are underway. Retroviral vector producer cells or adenoviral vectors are both being used. Most gene therapy trials using the suicide gene approach have employed the HSV1-tk gene; therefore imaging the expression of this gene with PET to determine the successful delivery and optimal start time for ganciclovir therapy should soon be possible. During treatment with ganciclovir, the use of a reporter gene distinct from HSV1-tk would be useful because of the potential pharmacologic competition of ganciclovir with the PET reporter probe. It should be possible to use a construct in which both HSV1-tk (as a suicide gene) and a second gene (e.g., the D2R gene) serving as a reporter gene (through the use of an IRES) for imaging suicide gene expression. Furthermore, concurrent PET imaging of tumor metabolism with FDG may also be useful. Issues related to delivery across the blood-brain-barrier (BBB) (for brain tumors) will need to be investigated further because many substrates for HSV1-tk do not cross the BBB, and therefore may only be able to reach target sites where the BBB has broken down.

15.9.2 Therapeutic Gene Therapy and Imaging

Currently, therapeutic gene therapy is being aimed only at somatic (non-reproductive) cells (Knoell and Yiu, 1998). Specifically, hematopoetic stem cells are potentially an optimal target because transduction and transplantation of these cells would hopefully lead to continuous expression of the transgene during the life-time of the patient. The β-globin gene for β-thalassemia and sickle cell anemia has been used for stem cell transduction with limited results. Therapeutic genes such as the low density lipoprotein receptor (LDL-R) targeted for expression in hepatocytes, and the cystic fibrosis transmembrane conductance regulator (CFTR) have also been investigated (Rosenfeld et al., 1992). In the case of human gene therapy with therapeutic genes (e.g., for treating cystic fibrosis), the use of a bicistronic vector with an IRES should make possible the monitoring of the therapeutic gene through the use of an imaging reporter gene. Monitoring of the delivery of the therapeutic gene and the magnitude of its expression over time should help to determine the reasons for the success or failure of gene therapy. It should also be possible to directly target the therapeutic gene mRNA through the use of antisense probes (see section 15.4.3), thereby circumventing the need to introduce a reporter gene.

15.10 Future Outlook

Significant progress has been made in the last few years in developing preliminary assays for imaging gene expression *in vivo*. Much more work remains to be done in the development of practical, highly sensitive, and specific quantitative assays for *in vivo* applications. For the antisense based approach many key issues including those related to stability of probes, minimization of non-specific interaction, and sufficient efflux of probes for minimizing the background will need to be resolved. It is likely that the antisense based approaches will lag behind the reporter gene approach because of the numerous issues that have yet to be resolved. However, when successful (both for the pharmaceutical industry and for imaging applications) the antisense approach will provide a more general method to imaging gene expression, as well as to be able to identify the early changes in gene expression signaling the transformation of normal cellular function to that of an altered state of disease. Reporter approaches have already proven themselves in preliminary animal applications. Studies with transgenic animals, *in vivo* inducible expression, bicistronic vectors, and the monitoring of endogenous gene expression with a reporter gene, are all areas of active research. Human applications of reporter gene technology will likely be reported within the next year, and will probably involve imaging the delivery of the HSV1-tk suicide gene, prior to ganciclovir therapy for treating tumors.

References

Agrawal S and Iyer RP (1997) Perspectives in antisense therapeutics. Pharmacology and Therapeutics 76:151-60.

Alauddin MM, Raman RK, Kundun R, *et al.* (1997) Evaluation of F-18 9[(3-[^{18}F]fluoro-1-hydroxy-2-propoxy)methyl]guanine (F-18 FHPG) in HT-29 cells. Journal of Nuclear Medicine 38:176P.

Alrabiah FA and Sacks SL (1996) New Anti-herpes virus agents: their targets and therapeutic potential. Drugs 52:17-32.

Arner ES and Eriksson S (1995) Mammalian deoxyribonucleoside kinases. Pharmacology and Therapeutics 67:155-186.

Bading JR, Alauddin MM, Fissekis JD, *et al.* (1997) Pharmacokinetics of F-18 fluorohydroxy-propoxymethylguanine (FHGP). Journal of Nuclear Medicine 38:43P.

Barrio JB, Satyamurthy N, Huang SC, *et al.* (1989) 3-(2'-[^{18}F]fluoroethyl)spiperone: In vivo biochemical and kinetic characterization in rodents, nonhuman primates, and humans. Journal of Cerebral Blood Flow and Metabolism 9:830-839.

Bogdanov A and Weissleder R (1998) The development of in vivo imaging systems to study gene expression. Trends in biotechnology 16:5-10.

Bunzow JR, Van Tol HH, Grandy DK, *et al.* (1988) Cloning and expression of a rat D2 dopamine receptor cDNA. Nature 367:783-787.

Cammilleri S, Sangrajrang S, Perderau B, *et al.* (1996) Biodistribution of iodine-125 dyramine transforming growth factor alpha antisense oligonucleotide in athymic mice with a human mammary tumor xenograft following intratumoral injection. European Journal of Nuclear Medicine 23:448-452.

Chalfie M, Tu Y, Euskirchen W, *et al.* (1994) Green fluorescent protein as a marker for gene expression. Science 263:802-805.

Charlton J, Sennello J and Smith D (1997) In vivo imaging of inflammation using an aptamer inhibitor of human neutrophil elastase. Chemistry and Biology 4:809-816.

Cherry SR, Shao Y, Silverman RW, *et al.* (1997) MicroPET: A high resolution PET scanner for imaging small animals. IEEE Transactions on Nuclear Science 44:1161-1166.

Conrad RC, Baskerville S and Ellington AD (1995) In vitro selection methodologies to probe RNA function and structure. Molecular Diversity 1:69-78.

Cotten M, Wagner E and Birnstiel M (1993) Receptor-mediated transport of DNA into eukaryotic cells. Methods in Enzymology 217:618-644.

Crooke S (1997) Progress in antisense therapeutics discovery and development. CIBA Foundation Symposium 209:158-168.

Crooke ST (1995) Progress in antisense therapeutics. Hematologic Pathology 9:59-72.

Crooke ST and Lebleu B (1993) Antisense Research and Applications. CRC Press, Inc., Ann Arbor, pp 579.

De Clercq E (1993) Antivirals for the treatment of herpes virus infections. J. Antimicrob. Chemother. 32:121-132.

Dewanjee MK, Ghafouripour AK, Kapadvanjwala M, *et al.* (1994) Noninvasive imaging of c-myc oncogene messenger RNA with indium-111-antisense probes in a mammary tumor-bearing mouse model. J. of Nucl. Med. 35:1054-1063.

Ehrin E, Farde L, de Paulis T, *et al.* (1985) Preparation of 11C-labelled raclopride, a new potent dopamine receptor antagonist: preliminary PET studies of cerebral dopamine receptors in the monkey. International Journal of Applied Radiation and Isotopes 36:269-273.

Elion GB (1993) Acyclovir: discovery, mechanism of action, and selectivity. Journal of Medical Virology 2-6.

Enochs WS, Petherick P, Bogdanova A, *et al.* (1997) Paramagnetic metal scavenging by melanin: MR imaging. Radiology 204:417-423.

Gallardo HF, Tan C and Sadelain M (1997) The internal ribosomal entry site of the encephalomyocarditis virus enables reliable coexpression of two transgenes in human primary T lymphyocytes. Gene Therapy 4:1115-1119.

Gambhir SS, Barrio J, Wu L, *et al.* (1998) Imaging of Adenoviral Directed Herpes Simplex Virus Type 1 Thymidine Kinase Gene Expression in Mice with Ganciclovir. Journal of Nuclear Medicine 39:2003-2011.

Gambhir SS, Barrio JR, Phelps ME, Iyer M, Namavari M, Satyamurthy N, Wu L, Green LA, Bauer E, MacLaren DC, Nguyen K, Berk AJ, Cherry SR, Herschman HR (1999a) Imaging Adenoviral-Directed Reporter Gene Expression in Living Animals with Positron Emission Tomography. Proc Natl Acad Sci (USA), 96(5):2333-2338.

Gambhir SS, Barrio JR, Herschman HR, Phelps ME (1999b) Assays for Non-Invasive Imaging of Reporter Gene Expression. Nuclear Medicine and Biology, 26:481-490

Goldenberg DM (1997) Perspectives on oncologic imaging with radiolabeled antibodies. Cancer 80:2431-2435.

Good L and Nielsen PE (1997) Progress in developing PNA as a gene-targeted drug. Antisense and Nucleic Acid Drug Development 7:431-437.

Goodchild J (1989) Oligodeoxynucleotides: Antisense inhibitors of gene expression. Macmillan, London.

Haberkorn U, Oberdorfer F, Gebert J, *et al.* (1996) Monitoring of gene therapy with cytosine deaminase: in vitro studies using 3H-5-fluorocytosine. Journal of Nuclear Medicine 37:87-94.

Haider N, Iyer RR and Narula J (1998) Topics in Molecular Biology: Techniques and Methods. Journal of Nuclear Cardiology 5:343-354.

Hargrove JL, Hulsey MG, Schmidt FH, *et al.* (1990) A computer program for modeling kinetics of gene expression. BioTechniques 8:654-660.

Helene C and Toulme JJ (1989) Oligodeoxynucleotides: Antisense Inhibitors of Gene Expression. In Cohen JS (ed). Macmillan, London, pp 137-172.

Herz J and Gerard RD (1993) Adenovirus-mediated transfer of low density lipoprotein receptor gene acutely accelerates cholesterol in normal mice. Proceedings of the National Academy of Sciences USA 90:2812-2816.

Hnatowich DJ, Winnard Pj, Virzi F, *et al.* (1995) Technetium-99m labeling of DNA oligonucleotides. J. Nucl. Med. 36:2306-2314.

Hu S, Shively L, Raubitschek A, *et al.* (1996) A novel engineered anti-carcinoembryonic antigen antibody fragment (single-chain Fv-CH3) which exhibits rapid, high-level targeting of xenografts. Cancer Research 56:3055-3061.

Jacobs WR, Barletta RG, Udani R, *et al.* (1993) Rapid assessment of drug susceptibilities of mycobacterium tuberculosis by means of luciferase reporter phages. Science 260:819-822.

Kastis GK, Barber HB, Barrett HH, *et al.* (1998) High resolution SPECT imager for three-dimensional imaging of small animals (abstract). Journal of Nuclear Medicine 39:9P.

Kessler RM, Ansari MS, de Paulis T, *et al.* (1991) High affinity dopamine D2 receptor radioligands. 1. Regional rat brain distribution of iodinated benzamines. Journal of Nuclear Medicine 32:1593-1600.

Knoell DL and Yiu IM (1998) Human gene therapy for hereditary diseases. American Journal of Health-System Pharmacy 55:899-904.

Levenson VV, Transue ED and Roninson IB (1998) Internal ribosomal entry site-containing retroviral vectors with green fluorescent protein and drug resistance markers. Human Gene Therapy 9:1233-1236.

Lewin B (1994) Genes V. Oxford University Press, New York.

Loke SL, Stein CA, Zhang XH, *et al.* (1989) Characterization of oligonucleotide transport into living cells. Proceedings of the National Academy of Sciences USA 86:7595-7599.

MacLaren DC, Gambhir SS, Satyamurthy N, Barrio JR, Sharfstein S, Toyokuni T, Wu L, Berk AJ, Cherry SR, Phelps ME, Herschman H (1999) Repetitive, Non-invasive Imaging of the Dopamine D2 Receptor as a Reporter Gene in Living Animals. Gene Therapy, 6:785-791

Matsukura M, Shinozuka K, Zon G, *et al.* (1978) Phosphorothioate analogs of oligodeoxynucleotides: novel inhibitors of replication and cytopathic effects of human immunodeficiency virus (HIV). Proceedings of the National Academy of Sciences USA 84:7706-7710.

Miller N and Vile R (1995) Targeted vectors for gene therapy. FASEB Journal 9:190-199.

Misteli T and Spector D (1997) Applications of the green fluorescent protein in cell biology and biotechnology. Nature Biotechnology 15:961-964.

Moolten FL (1986) Tumor chemosensitivity conferred by inserted herpes thymidine kinase genes: paradigm for prospective cancer control strategy. Cancer Res. 46:5276-5281.

Murakami A, Blake K and Miller PS (1985) Characterization of sequence-specific oligodeoxynucleoside methylphosphonates and their interaction with rabbit globin mRNA. Biochemistry 24:.

Nishiyama T, Kawamura Y and Kawamoto Kea (1985) Antineoplastic effects of 5-fluorocytosine in combination with cytosine deaminase capsules. Cancer Res. 45:1753-1761.

Pan D, Gambhir SS, Toyokuni T, *et al.* (1998) Rapid synthesis of a 5'-Fluorinated Oligodeoxynucletoide: A model antisense probe for use in imaging with Positron Emission Tomography (PET). Bioorganic & Medicinal Chemistry Letters 8:1317-1320.

Phillips JA, Craig SJ, Bayley D, *et al.* (1997) Pharmacokinetics, metabolism, and elimination of a 20-mer phosphorothioate oligodeoxynucleotide (CGP 69846A) after intravenous and subcutaneous administration. Biochemical Pharmacology 54:657-668.

Rolland AP (1998) From genes to gene medicines: recent advances in nonviral gene delivery. Critical Reviews in Therapeutic Drug Carrier Systems 15:143-198.

Rosenfeld MA, Yoshimura K, Trapnell BC, *et al.* (1992) In vivo transfer of the human cystic fibrosis transmembrane conductance regulator gene to the airway epithelium. Cell 68:143-155.

Shao Y, Cherry SR, Member, IEEE, Farahani K, *et al.* (1997) Development of a PET Detector System Compatible with MRI/NMR Systems. IEEE Transactions on Nuclear Science 44:1167-1171.

Smith AE (1995) Viral vectors in gene therapy. Annual Review of Microbiology 49:807-838.

Stein CA and Cheng YC (1993) Antisense oligonucleotides as therapeutic agents-is the bullet really magical. Science 261:1004-1011.

Strange PG (1990) Aspects of the structure of the D2 dopamine receptor. Trends in Neurosciences 13:373-378.

Stratford-Perricaudet LD, Levrero M, Chasse J-F, *et al.* (1990) Evaluation of the transfer and expression in mice of an enzyme-encoding gene using a human adenovirus vector. Human Gene Therapy 1:241-256.

Tavitian B, Terrazzino S, Kühnast B, *et al.* (1998) In vivo imaging of oligonucleotides with positron emission tomography. Nature Medicine 4:467-471.

Tjuvajev JG, Avril N, Oku T, *et al.* (1998) Imaging herpes virus thymidine kinase gene transfer and expression by positron emission tomography. Cancer Research 58:4333-4341.

Tjuvajev JG, Finn R, Watanabe K, *et al.* (1996) Noninvasive imaging of herpes virus thymidine kinase gene transfer and expression: A potential method for monitoring clinical gene therapy. Cancer Research 56:4087-4095.

Tjuvajev JG, Stockhammer G, Desai R, *et al.* (1995) Imaging the expression of transfected genes in vivo. Cancer Research 55:6126-6132.

Wagner HNJ, Burns HD, Dannals RF, *et al.* (1983) Imaging dopamine receptors in the human brain by positron tomography. Science. 221:1264-1266.

Wagner RW and Flanagan WM (1997) Antisense technology and prospects for therapy of viral infections and cancer. Molecular Medicine Today 3:31-38.

Wallace PM, MacMaster JF, Smith VF, *et al.* (1994) Intratumoral generation of 5-fluorouracil mediated by an antibody-cytosine deaminase conjugate in combination with 5-fluorocytosine. Cancer Res. 54:2719-2723.

Weissleder R, Simonova M, Bogdanova A, *et al.* (1997) MR imaging and scintigraphy of gene expression through melanin induction. Radiology 204:425-429.

Wickstrom E (1986) Oligodeoxynucleotide stability in subcellular extracts and culture media. J. Biochem. Biophys. Methods. 13:97-102.

Wu-Pong S, Weiss TL and Hunt AC (1992) Antisense c-myc oligodeoxyribonucleotide cellular uptake. Pharmaceutical Research 9:1010-1017.

Wu-Pong S, Weiss TL and Hunt AC (1994) Antisense c-myc oligonucleotide cellular uptake and activity. Antisense Research and Development 4:155-163.

Yu Y, Annala AJ, Barrio JR, Toyokuni T, Satyamurthy N, Namavari M, Cherry SR, Phelps ME, Herschman, HR, Gambhir SS. Quantitation of Target Gene Expression by Imaging Reporter Gene Expression in Living Animals. Nature Medicine (in press)

Zamecnik PC, Goodchild J, Yaguchi Y, *et al.* (1986) Inhibition of replication of expression of human T-cell lymphotropic virus type III in cultured cells by exogenous synthetic oligonucleotides complementary to viral RNA. Proceedings of the National Academy of Sciences USA 83:4143-4146.

Zamecnik PC and Stephenson M (1978) Inhibition of Rous sarcoma virus replication and cell transformation by a specific oligodeoxynucleotide. Proceedings of the National Academy of Sciences USA 75:280-284.

Acknowledgements

I would like to thank my mentors Drs. Barrio, Herschman, and Phelps who have helped me to rapidly move forward in this new and exciting arena of biomedical imaging. I would like to thank the growing body of undergraduate and graduate students, post-doctoral fellows, research scientists, and faculty who have joined the UCLA Gene Imaging Consortium in bringing together different disciplines to form a new science of biological imaging targeted towards specific cellular events. I sincerely thank K. Akhoon, Ph.D., E. Bauer, M.S., A. Berk, Ph.D., A. Borghei, B.S., A. Chatziioannou, Ph.D., S. Cherry, Ph.D., R. Goldman, B.S., S. Golish, B.S., L.A. Green, M.S., M. Iyer, Ph.D., Q. Liang, Ph.D., D. MacLaren Ph.D., M. Namavari, Ph.D., K. Nguyen, B.S., D. Pan, Ph.D., N. Satyamurthy, Ph.D., P. Shah, B.S., S. Sharafstein, Ph.D., X. Sun, Ph.D., T. Toyokuni, Ph.D., A. Wu, Ph.D., L. Wu, Ph.D., S. Yahgoubi, B.S., Y. Yu, Ph.D. for all their efforts in helping to evolve imaging gene expression *in vivo.* I also thank T. Sama, P. Zaslav, and G. Lacson for assistance with preparing this chapter.

16 Imaging Gene Expression in Cancer: Functional Identification of Multidrug Resistance P-glycoprotein In Vivo

D. Piwnica-Worms, G. D. Luker, K. E. Luker, V. V. Rao, V. Sharma

Contents

16.1 Introduction 273
16.2 Biochemical Properties of the Multidrug Resistance P-glycoprotein 273
16.3 Radiopharmaceuticals for Functional Assessment of Pgp Transport Activity 275
16.4 Clinical Applications: General Principles 277
16.4.1 Imaging MDR in Breast Cancer 277
16.4.2 Imaging MDR in Lung Cancer 279
16.4.3 Imaging MDR Reversal In Vivo 279
16.5 Conclusion 280

16.1 Introduction

Resistance of malignant tumors to chemotherapeutic agents is a major cause of treatment failure in cancer patients (Gottesman and Pastan 1993; Bosch and Croop 1996). One resistance phenotype, known as multidrug resistance (MDR), is characterized by the failure to respond to a variety of structurally and functionally diverse drugs, despite initial treatment with only a single drug. Classically, this refractory behavior to multiple chemotherapeutic agents was observed to occur in recurring tumors; however, recent clinical data have indicated that tumors, even at presentation, also may exhibit a MDR phenotype. Molecular mechanisms of MDR were first analyzed in studies with tumor cell lines in culture, which had been selected for resistance by growth survival in the presence of high concentrations of cytotoxic drugs. Several different mechanisms involving overlapping, but distinct, patterns of multidrug resistance have been identified; these include changes in topoisomerases, superoxide dismutases, glutathione transferases, and expression of transport proteins such as the multidrug resistance P-glycoprotein (*MDR1* Pgp) and the multidrug resistance-associated protein (MRP; Cole et al. 1992; Morrow et al. 1992; Gottesman and Pastan 1993; Tuccari et al. 1993; Schneider et al. 1994; Zyad et al. 1994). These different forms of multidrug resistance in tumors may occur independently or in combination, and their relationship to other types of therapeutic resistance (due to mutations or deletions of p53, regulation of bcl2, and modulation of the programmed cell death cascade) remain active areas of research. Of the mechanisms of MDR, overexpression of *MDR1* Pgp is one of the best characterized and clinically validated mediators of the multidrug resistance phenotype (Bosch and Croop 1996). This chapter provides a brief overview of the biochemical mechanisms of transporter-mediated multidrug resistance, and then focuses on the clinical studies and potential for functional scintigraphic imaging of the multidrug resistance phenotype attributed to expression of *MDR1* Pgp in tumors.

16.2 Biochemical Properties of the Multidrug Resistance P-glycoprotein

Multidrug resistance in cancer mediated by the *MDR1* Pgp, a 140- to 180-kDa plasma membrane protein (Gros et al. 1986; Bosch and Croop 1996), is thought to render chemotherapeutic treatment ineffective by "pumping" a variety of natural product cytotoxic agents and xenobiotic compounds out of cancer cells (Gottesman and Pastan 1993; Stein 1997). The *MDR1* gene is often amplified, and consequently overexpressed, in malignant tissues (Pastan and Gottesman 1987; Bosch and Croop 1996; Trock et al. 1997) and transfection (see 15.5) of a full-length cDNA of 4.5 kilobase pairs into drug-sensitive cells in culture is sufficient to cause multidrug resistance in experimental systems (Gros et al. 1986). Two family members have been identified in humans (*MDR1* and *MDR3*), whereas three family members are present in rodents (mdr1a, mdr1b and mdr2).

D. Piwnica-Worms, G. D. Luker, K. E. Luker, V. V. Rao, V. Sharma
Mallinckrodt Institute of Radiology, 510 S. Kingshighway Blvd., Saint Louis, MO 63310, USA

Only human *MDR1* and rodent mdr1a/mdr1b confer multidrug resistance. The key characteristic aspect of multidrug resistance is the apparent capacity of Pgp to recognize a large group of cytotoxic compounds sharing little or no structural or functional similarities. Doxorubicin, etoposide, paclitaxel, and the *Vinca* alkaloids, such as vinblastine, are among the clinically important compounds which are substrates for transport by *MDR1* Pgp (Ford and Hait 1990; Gottesman and Pastan 1993). While there exists a large number of compounds transported by Pgp, most drugs recognized by Pgp are relatively small, hydrophobic, cationic, and biplanar (Ford and Hait 1990), and are usually thought to enter cells by passive diffusion across the lipid bilayer (Ford and Hait 1990). Whereas *MDR1* Pgp has been conventionally thought to function as an ATP-dependent efflux transporter of these compounds, alternative mechanisms for diminished drug accumulation have been proposed. Cells transfected with *MDR1* Pgp have a more alkaline intracellular pH and reduced membrane potential compared with non-transfected cells (Hoffman and Roepe 1997). The MDR cells also may have intracellular organelles which are more acidic than in non-MDR cells (Hurwitz et al. 1997; Altan et al. 1998). These changes in pH and membrane potential could decrease the distribution of chemotherapeutic drugs into cells and/or sequester drugs from their targets within cells. In addition, *MDR1* Pgp has been reported to modulate pathways of programmed cell death (Robinson et al. 1997; Smyth et al. 1998), thus protecting cells from chemotherapeutic drugs as well as other classes of agents. Overall, by mechanisms which result in decreased net intracellular concentration of drugs, *MDR1* Pgp renders tumors resistant to chemotherapy.

In addition to its expression in multidrug resistant tumors, *MDR1* Pgp is normally located in several tissues, including the brush border of proximal tubule cells in the kidney, on the biliary surface of hepatocytes, and on the apical surface of mucosal cells in the small intestine and colon (Thiebaut et al. 1987). *MDR1* is also highly expressed on luminal surfaces of endothelial cells lining capillaries in the brain and testis (Cordon-Cardo et al. 1989) and on the apical surface of choroid plexus epithelial cells (Rao et al. 1998). Despite its widely disseminated expression, the function of *MDR1* Pgp in normal physiology has not been clearly defined. For example, based on its function as an ATP-dependent efflux pump for cytotoxic agents, some researchers have proposed that *MDR1* Pgp functions to protect humans against ingested xenobiotics (Schinkel et al. 1994; Leveille-Webster and Arias 1995). The tissue distribution would be consistent with a role for *MDR1* Pgp in active excretion of xenobiotics into the urine, bile, or bowel lumen, whereas sensitive organs, such as the brain, would be protected from entry of potentially toxic compounds. Furthermore, recent data also suggest a role as a phospholipase, transporting compounds such as short-chain phosphatidylcholine from the inner leaflet to the outer leaflet of the plasma membrane (van Helvoort et al. 1996; Bosch et al. 1997). However, the exact relationship of this activity to drug transport is unknown.

High levels of Pgp expression have been reported in tumors derived from tissues that normally express Pgp, including tumors of the adrenal gland, colon, kidney, pancreas, and acute myelogenous leukemia (for a review see Bosch and Croop 1996). Systematic evaluation of many other tumor types has also shown high levels of Pgp expression in subgroups of sarcomas, breast cancer, lymphomas, neuroblastomas, acute lymphocytic leukemia, and chronic myelogenous leukemia (Bosch and Croop 1996). Expression of *MDR1* Pgp and related transporters, e.g., MRP (Cole et al. 1992), are independent prognostic indicators of poor outcomes in patients with cancer, and increased levels of *MDR1* Pgp and MRP are often detected in tumor biopsies from relapsing cancer patients (Goldstein et al. 1990; Yoshimura et al. 1990; Chan et al. 1991; Baldini et al. 1995; Norris et al. 1996).

Because studies have shown the clinical relevance associated with *MDR1* Pgp expression in tumors, reversal of multidrug resistance by nontoxic agents that block the transport activity of *MDR1* Pgp has been an important target for pharmaceutical development (Ford and Hait 1990). When co-administered with a cytotoxic agent, these nontoxic compounds, known as MDR modulators or reversal agents, enhance net accumulation of cytotoxic drugs within the tumor cells. Many compounds known to have other pharmacological sites of action initially were used to reverse MDR in cancer cells grown in culture (Ford and Hait 1990). These compounds included verapamil, cyclosporin A, quinidine, trifluperazine and derivatives thereof (Ford and Hait 1990). However, these agents have limited clinical utility because of their toxicity at levels needed to modulate *MDR1* Pgp. New second-generation modulators (dexverapamil, BASF Pharma, Basel, Switzerland; and PSC 833, Novartis, Basel, Switzerland) and third-generation modulators (GF120918, Glaxo-Welcome, Research Triangle Park, N.C.; LY335979, Eli Lilly, Indianapolis, Ind.;

and VX710, Vertex, Cambridge, Mass.) have been subsequently developed, and phase-I/II clinical trials are currently in progress with these new, more specific compounds (GAVERIAUX et al. 1991; HYAFIL et al. 1993; DANTZIG et al. 1996; GERMANN et al. 1997). Thus, there exists considerable promise that the MDR phenotype may be therapeutically modulated in patients with these more selective reversal agents.

In the practice of clinical oncology, a priori identification of the presence of the molecular target of a therapeutic agent is becoming increasingly common to select patients most likely to benefit from the therapy. For optimal application of modulators in chemotherapeutic protocols, identification of *MDR1* Pgp at the time of presentation would provide important information which could guide the choice of chemotherapeutic agents and the intensity of therapy in patients. However, expression of *MDR1* Pgp, as detected at the level of messenger RNA or protein, is not always directly correlated with functional transport activity. Because Pgp transport activity is affected by specific mutations as well as the phosphorylation state of the protein (GERMANN et al. 1990; GOTTESMAN and PASTAN 1993), altered or less active forms of Pgp may be detected by polymerase chain reaction (PCR) or immunohistochemistry which do not accurately reflect the tumor cell resistance status. Thus, methods to functionally interrogate Pgp transport activity have been sought (HOMOLYA et al. 1993). Imaging with a radiopharmaceutical that is transported by *MDR1* Pgp may be one promising method to identify those tumors in which the transporter is expressed and functional. Non-invasive detection of successful inhibition of *MDR1* Pgp-mediated transport in tumors is also required to evaluate the likelihood of success of therapy with modulators. Conversely, detection of inhibition of Pgp in normal tissues may allow oncologists to anticipate toxicity from chemotherapeutic drugs in the MDR phenotype, allowing adjustments in dosing schedules. All of these applications potentially may improve the success of chemotherapy in patients with cancer.

16.3 Radiopharmaceuticals for Functional Assessment of Pgp Transport Activity

To meet the need for non-invasive detection of Pgp, gamma-emitting compounds have been discovered and characterized as substrates for *MDR1* Pgp, and new ^{99m}Tc-labeled radiopharmaceuticals specifically targeted to Pgp have been developed (Fig. 16.1; PIWNICA-WORMS et al. 1993; CRANKSHAW et al. 1998). Additionally, substrates of *MDR1* Pgp suitable for positron emission tomography (PET) imaging are under development for possible applications in oncologic imaging (MEHTA et al. 1994; ELSINGA et al. 1996; SHARMA et al. 1996). However, because several of the ^{99m}Tc-based agents are already approved for other clinical uses, these single-photon agents are more likely to contribute significantly to clinical diagnosis and treatment of multidrug resistant tumors in the near future.

^{99m}Tc-sestamibi, ^{99m}Tc-tetrofosmin, and ^{99m}Tc-furifosmin ("Tc-Q12"-complex) are lipophilic cationic radiotracers commercially available for imaging myocardial perfusion (WACKERS et al. 1989; HIGLEY et al. 1993; ROSSETTI et al. 1994). Each compound is a nonmetabolizable radiopharmaceutical with a delocalized monocationic charge (ABRAMS et al. 1983; KRONAUGE et al. 1990; HIGLEY et al. 1993; ROSSETTI et al. 1994; PLATTS et al. 1995). The mechanisms of uptake and retention of ^{99m}Tc-sestamibi and analogous ^{99m}Tc-based agents have been extensively studied in a variety of cellular and subcellular preparations in vitro. For example, biophysical analysis has shown that ^{99m}Tc-sestamibi is a high-fidelity probe of transmembrane potential (PIWNICA-WORMS et al. 1990; CHERNOFF et al. 1993), with passive inward movement of this lipophilic cation being driven (in the absence of *MDR1* Pgp) by the transmembrane potentials generated in living cells (DELMON-MOINGEON et al. 1990; PIWNICA-WORMS et al. 1990). Biochemical analysis and direct localization in situ by electron probe X-ray microanalysis have determined that the intracellular target for ^{99m}Tc-sestamibi in living tissues is the mitochondrial inner matrix (BACKUS et al. 1993). The complex is reversibly sequestered within this organelle by the serial thermodynamic driving forces of the negative plasma membrane and mitochondrial inner membrane potentials. These data confirm fractionation data suggesting localization of the radioprobe to mitochondrial fractions in vivo (CARVALHO et al. 1992). Similarly, ^{99m}Tc-tetrofosmin has been shown to respond to membrane potential in an analogous manner (PLATTS et al. 1995; YOUNES 1995), whereas ^{99m}Tc-furifosmin responds to a lesser extent (CRANKSHAW et al. 1998). Thus, whereas these ^{99m}Tc-based lipophilic cations can rapidly permeate lipid bilayers, they primarily reside in the steady state within intracellular compartments. In humans, this likely accounts for the initial distribution of these agents into mitochondria-rich tissues such as heart, kidney, liver, and many tumors in vivo.

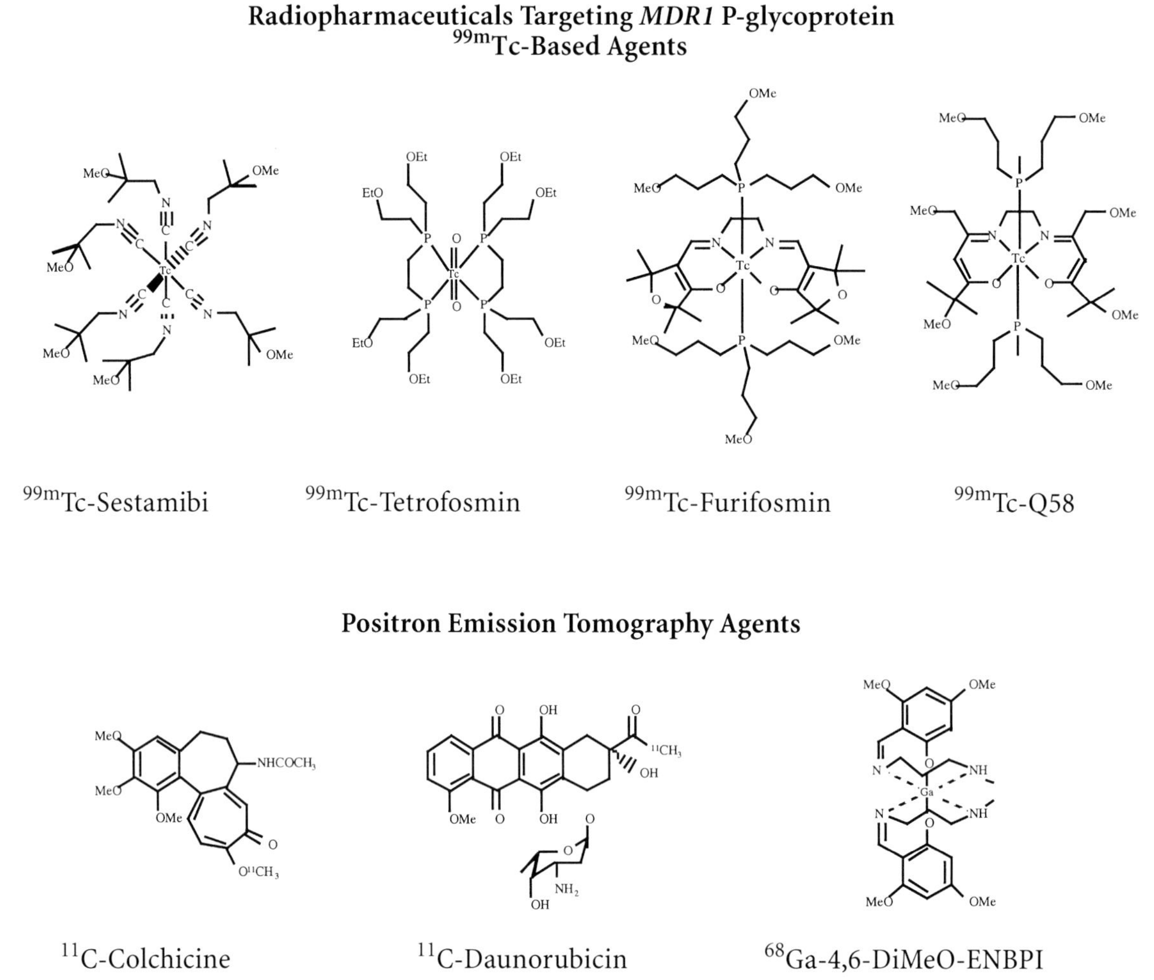

Radiopharmaceuticals Targeting *MDR1* P-glycoprotein
^{99m}Tc-Based Agents

^{99m}Tc-Sestamibi ^{99m}Tc-Tetrofosmin ^{99m}Tc-Furifosmin ^{99m}Tc-Q58

Positron Emission Tomography Agents

^{11}C-Colchicine ^{11}C-Daunorubicin ^{68}Ga-4,6-DiMeO-ENBPI

Fig. 16.1. Structures of single photon emission computed tomography (SPECT) and positron emission tomography (PET) radiopharmaceuticals recognized as transport substrates by multidrug resistance type I P-glycoprotein (*MDR1* Pgp)

^{99m}Tc-sestamibi and several of these other Tc-based cationic radiopharmaceuticals also are substrates recognized by rodent and human *MDR1* Pgp (Piwnica-Worms et al. 1993; Rao et al. 1994; Ballinger et al. 1995a). Baculoviral expression of recombinant human *MDR1* in insect cells confers decreased accumulation of ^{99m}Tc-sestamibi (Rao et al. 1994), and, in addition, MDR cells expressing Pgp accumulate ^{99m}Tc-sestamibi in inverse proportion to the amount of immunodetectable transporter (Piwnica-Worms et al. 1993, 1995). ^{99m}Tc-tetrofosmin and ^{99m}Tc-furifosmin also have been validated as transport substrates for Pgp in a variety of multidrug-resistant human and rodent cells (Ballinger et al. 1995a,b, 1996; Crankshaw et al. 1995, 1998; Cordobes et al. 1996). Net cellular accumulation of these tracers is inversely proportional to the level of Pgp expression, and enhancement of radiotracer content is observed upon administration of MDR modulators such as verapamil, cyclosporin A, or the new high-potency agents such as GF120918 or PSC 833 (Luker et al. 1997). Optimization of the *MDR1* Pgp recognition properties of the "Tc-Q" series of non-reducible Tc(III) cations (Jurisson et al. 1984; Rossetti et al. 1994) has resulted in the discovery of ^{99m}Tc-Q58 and ^{99m}Tc-Q63 (Luker et al. 1997; Crankshaw et al. 1998); each has properties that are essentially equivalent to ^{99m}Tc-Sestamibi and ^{99m}Tc-tetrofosmin as *MDR1* Pgp transport substrates in vitro (Crankshaw et al. 1998).

Net cell content of these ^{99m}Tc-based agents generally is a function of both passive potential-dependent influx and *MDR1* Pgp-mediated extrusion (Fig. 16.2). Addition of an MDR modulator blocks the function of Pgp and thus enables the tracer to accumulate within

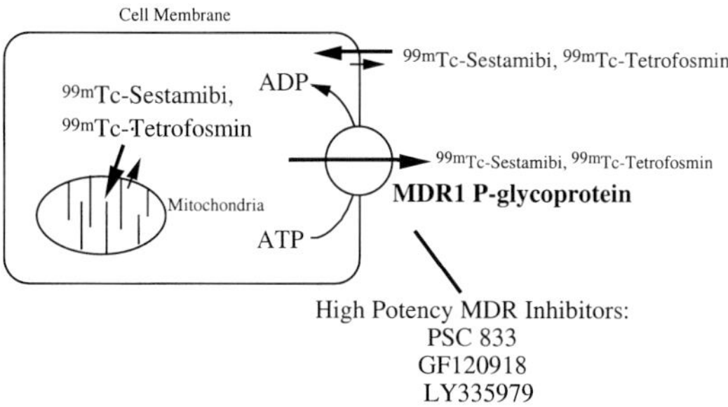

Fig. 16.2. Model of cellular influx and efflux pathways for ^{99m}Tc-based lipophilic cations such as ^{99m}Tc-sestamibi and ^{99m}Tc-tetrofosmin. Cellular accumulation of the agents into drug-sensitive tumor cells will be high in response to the inwardly directed driving forces of the inside-negative plasma membrane and mitochondrial potentials. This will translate into a hot spot on scintigraphic imaging or a slow washout rate from a tumor focus. Conversely, expression of the *MDR1* Pgp (or the MRP) transporter on the cell surface will outwardly transport the tracers, thereby resulting in reduced net accumulation. This will be detected either as a photopenic tumor or as a rapid washout rate from a tumor focus. A two-step "rest-pharmacological stress" protocol for imaging MDR reversal is proposed: After baseline imaging (rest), administration of a potent modulating agent (inhibitor), such as Glaxo-Wellcome GF120918 (Glaxo-Wellcome, Research Triangle Park, N.C.), Novartis PSC 833 (Novartis, Basel, Switzerland), or Eli Lilly LY335979 (Eli Lilly, Indianapolis, Ind.), and reinjection of the ^{99m}Tc tracer (stress), would be performed. After administration of the modulator, those tumors showing higher accumulation of the tracer within the tumor and/or reduced washout rates would specifically indicate expression of *MDR1* Pgp

the cell. This forms the basis for a functional approach to assessment of *MDR1* Pgp in patients. However, several issues remain as these concepts begin to be translated into the clinic. For example, the relationship of homologous ATP-binding-cassette (ABC) transporters, such the *MDR3* Pgp (Van der Bliek et al. 1987) and the multidrug resistance-associated protein (MRP) (Cole et al. 1992), to extrusion of these ^{99m}Tc-based agents is under evaluation (Crankshaw and Piwnica-Worms 1996; Kabasakal et al. 1996; Luker et al. 1997; Hendrikse et al. 1998; Moretti et al. 1998).

16.4 Clinical Applications: General Principles

All of the radiopharmaceuticals developed for potential clinical use in imaging of *MDR1* Pgp are substrates for transport by this protein. Based primarily on data from in vitro studies, net accumulation of radiotracer in tumor or normal tissue is expected to be inverse to expression of functional Pgp, and rates of efflux of radiopharmaceutical from tissues should increase with greater expression of this transporter. Assuming adequate perfusion, tumors with functional *MDR1* Pgp will have low (or undetectable) uptake of radiopharmaceutical, and washout of activity from tumors with *MDR1* Pgp will be faster because of active extrusion by this protein. Following successful therapy with a modulator of *MDR1* Pgp, net uptake of radiopharmaceutical should increase and the rate of efflux should decrease in tumors which express Pgp, due to inhibition of the transport function of this protein. Although these principles for functional imaging of *MDR1* Pgp with scintigraphy have been supported by several clinical studies, the optimal protocol(s) and agent(s) for scintigraphic detection of Pgp in vivo remain to be determined. Based on published studies to date, scintigraphy of *MDR1* Pgp-mediated transport has been used for two clinical applications: (a) detection and quantification of functional Pgp in various tumors at the time of diagnosis; and (b) identification of successful inhibition of transport function following therapy with a modulator. While many case reports and anecdotal clinical studies correlating imaging results with patient outcomes have appeared in the context of MDR, these often fail to independently validate the presence or absence of Pgp in the tumor specimens. At this early stage in the clinical development of MDR imaging, such validation is important to enhance the rigor of each study.

In the remainder of this chapter, we survey results from many of the most robust of the validated clinical studies published to date.

16.4.1 Imaging MDR in Breast Cancer

Recently, Pgp has been studied extensively in breast tumors because of the observation that breast tumors frequently express clinically relevant Pgp, and that Pgp expression in breast tumors may be closely associated with treatment failure. Expression of Pgp could result in treatment failure for breast cancer, because several drugs which are widely used in treatment of this tumor, such as doxorubicin, vincristine, and paclitaxel, are transported by Pgp in vitro. A meta-analysis (Trock et al. 1997) of 31 published studies examining *MDR1* Pgp expression in breast cancer revealed that 41.2% of breast tumors expressed Pgp according to the various detection methods used in the studies, and that patients with tumors expressing Pgp were three times more likely to fail chemotherapy than those with tumors that were Pgp-negative; thus, imaging studies designed to functionally detect *MDR1* Pgp in breast tumors have received considerable attention.

DEL VECCHIO et al. (1997a) determined rates of efflux of ^{99m}Tc-sestamibi in 30 patients with untreated breast cancer. Dynamic imaging of tumor was performed for 15 min, followed by static planar images at 0.5, 1, 2, and 4 h after injection of 20 mCi of ^{99m}Tc-sestamibi. Tumor specimens were obtained 24 h after scintigraphy, and quantitative autoradiography of Pgp in each tumor was performed for correlation with the calculated rate of efflux (Fig. 16.3). Rates of efflux of ^{99m}Tc-sestamibi were 2.7-fold greater in tumors expressing increased *MDR1* Pgp compared with tumors that expressed Pgp at a level comparable to benign breast lesions. Estimates of sensitivity and specificity for in vivo detection of *MDR1* Pgp using ^{99m}Tc-sestamibi were 80 and 95%, respectively. From these data, the authors concluded that efflux rate constants of ^{99m}Tc-sestamibi may be used for non-invasive identification of *MDR1* Pgp. The overall correlation of tumor efflux rate constants and expression of Pgp was 0.62 which the authors inferred may be too low to be used for quantification of Pgp on follow-up examinations, but this remains to be tested. Of note, the expression of *MDR1* Pgp in untreated breast cancers also suggests that drug-resistant cells are present at the time of diagnosis and are selected by subsequent chemotherapy rather than being induced by therapy.

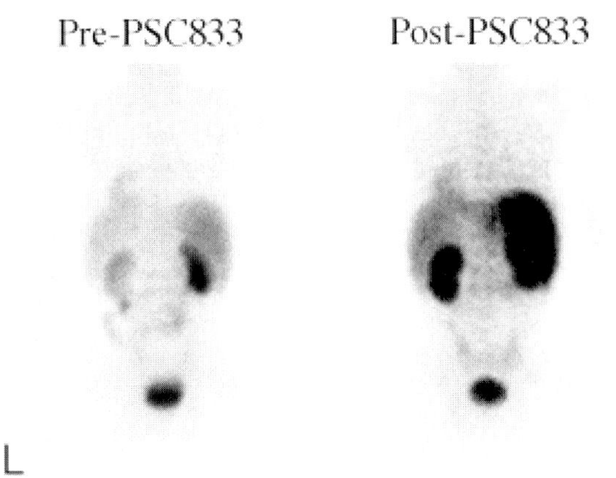

Fig. 16.3. Effect of PSC 833 on the pharmacokinetics of ^{99m}Tc-Sestamibi. *Left panel:* Pre-treatment PSC 833. Posterior planar image obtained at 120 min after injection of ^{99m}Tc-sestamibi shows significant clearance of radiotracer from liver and kidneys, a result of prompt Pgp-mediated clearance. Note enlarged spleen. *Right panel:* Following 24 h of oral split-dose treatment with PSC 833 (5 mg/kg times four doses). Image obtained 120 min after re-injection of ^{99m}Tc-Sestamibi now depicts significantly enhanced retention of activity in liver and kidneys, especially in comparison with myocardial uptake. The heart, a Pgp negative tissue which serves as an internal control, shows little difference in retention of activity

To explore the potential merit of a simplified, more practical approach to scintigraphic assessment of *MDR1* Pgp in breast cancer, fractional retention values of ^{99m}Tc-sestamibi in breast cancers were evaluated (DEL VECCHIO et al. 1997b). Twenty-seven patients with histologically proven breast carcinoma were injected with ^{99m}Tc-sestamibi and static planar images of the breast obtained at 10, 60, and 240 min. Fractional retention of ^{99m}Tc-sestamibi in the tumors was calculated from ratios of regions of interest drawn over the tumor images between 60 and 10 min (R60/10) and between 240 and 10 min (R240/10). Subsequently, Pgp expression of excised tumors was determined by quantitative autoradiography using the mAb MRK16 and correlated with tracer retention. Fractional retentions, in particular the R240/10 values, were significantly higher in the low Pgp expressing group compared with the high Pgp expressing group (r=–0.74). Depending on the cutoff value chosen, sensitivity for detection of high Pgp expression by analysis of fractional retention was 78–100% with an associated specificity of 95 to 83%. The investigators conclude that this practical protocol has the potential to identify non-invasively tumors with a high probability of expressing *MDR1* Pgp.

The prospective value of high tumor clearance rates of ^{99m}Tc-sestamibi to predict poor therapeutic outcomes is being evaluated in locally advanced breast cancer. In a study by CIARMIELLO and colleagues (1998), 39 patients with stage-III disease were enrolled in a prospective clinical trial to receive pretreatment mammoscintigraphy with ^{99m}Tc-sestamibi before neoadjuvant chemotherapy. Breast tumor clearance of ^{99m}Tc-sestamibi was determined out to 4 h post-injection and half-times calculated from the image sets using monoexponential curve fitting. Patients were subsequently treated with standard chemotherapy (epirubicin) for 6 weeks and then underwent surgery within 3 weeks of completion of chemotherapy. Tumor burden was assessed by pathologic examination of the mastectomy specimens. Of the 39 patients, 17 showed a tumor clearance half-time of $<$204 min, a value previously shown by this group to correspond to the mean tracer clearance rate minus one standard deviation in tumors with high Pgp content. Of these rapidly effluxing tumors, 15 of 17 showed a highly cellular residual tumor indicating lack of response to neoadjuvant chemotherapy. Conversely, 22 patients showed prolonged tumor clearance (half-time of >204 min) and of these, only 8 showed highly cellular residual tumor at the time of surgery. As pointed out by the investigators, the lack of slow clearance rates to be highly predictive of a good response is consistent with mechanisms of drug resistance other than Pgp at play in breast cancer patients. Interestingly, no patient with a half-time of <164 min, which was approximately two standard deviations faster than the mean half-time of high Pgp expressing breast tumors, showed evidence of pathologic response to neoadjuvant chemotherapy (DEL VECCHIO et al. 1997b). Thus, pre-treatment scintigraphy of advanced breast tumor was highly predictive of subsequent response to neoadjuvant chemotherapy. Especially noteworthy was the ability of dynamic mammoscintigraphy to identify that subset of patients with very rapid clearance rates who all failed chemotherapy.

Similar data were reported by KOSTAKOGLU et al. (1994) in a prospective study of 48 patients with either breast (30 patients) or lung (18 patients) cancer at the time of presentation (37 patients) or after therapy (11 patients). Scintigraphy was done with whole-body planar images and single photon emission computed tomography (SPECT) beginning 30 min after injection of 20 mCi of ^{99m}Tc-sestamibi. Tumor-to-background ratios of radioactivity from regions of interest were correlated with immunohistochemistry of specimens obtained 3–5 days after imaging. Overall, tumor-to-background ratios of ^{99m}Tc-sestamibi were significantly inversely correlated with expression of *MDR1* Pgp, although five exceptions were noted. The authors also noted that strong but focal expression of *MDR1* Pgp in a specimen did not alter ratios for uptake of ^{99m}Tc-sestamibi. In this study, the effects of perfusion to tumor and necrosis on uptake ratios of ^{99m}Tc-sestamibi were not addressed, potentially accounting for the five patients in whom uptake of ^{99m}Tc-sestamibi and expression of *MDR1* Pgp were not inversely correlated.

16.4.2
Imaging MDR in Lung Cancer

Several studies have begun to examine the correlation of ^{99m}Tc-sestamibi pharmacokinetics with Pgp expression in other tumor types. For example, in a prospective study of 46 lung cancer patients, KOSTAKOGLU and colleagues (1998) calculated washout rates and the degree of ^{99m}Tc-sestamibi accumulation in the lung tumors by analysis of early (30 min) and delayed (180 min) SPECT and planar images of the thorax. These were correlated with Pgp expression as determined by immunohistochemical analysis of tumor sections with the mAb JSB-1. A strong inverse correlation was again observed between tumor-to-background ratios at 30 min and levels of Pgp expression (p=0.001). However, no appreciable correlation between tumor washout rates of ^{99m}Tc-sestamibi and Pgp expression in lung cancer was found. The investigators correctly pointed out that the MRP gene may be more relevant than *MDR1* Pgp in mechanistically determining the MDR phenotype of lung cancer (GIACCONE et al. 1996), thus accounting for the low numbers of strongly positive Pgp expressing tumors in their study. Given that MRP may also transport ^{99m}Tc-sestamibi (CRANKSHAW and PIWNICA-WORMS 1996; HENDRIKSE et al. 1998; MORETTI et al. 1998), this could potentially contribute to the lack of correlation of washout rates in lung cancer with Pgp expression alone.

16.4.3
Imaging MDR Reversal In Vivo

In clinical trials with novel potent modulators of *MDR1* Pgp, validation of successful inhibition of the transporter is necessary to assess the effects of these drugs on patient outcome. Initial experience with ^{99m}Tc-sestamibi suggests that this radiopharmaceutical can be used to detect inhibition of Pgp function in patients. LUKER et al. (1997) reported the results of scintigraphy in three patients with relapsed cancer who were imaged before and after treatment with PSC 833, a potent second generation modulator of *MDR1* Pgp, during a phase-I clinical trial. Planar images were obtained 15–30 and 60–90 min after injection of approximately 20 mCi ^{99m}Tc-sestamibi. Compared with images obtained 24 h earlier in the absence of PSC 833, delayed clearance of ^{99m}Tc-sestamibi from the liver and kidneys was seen in all patients following treatment with the modulator at a dose known to inhibit *MDR1* Pgp (Fig. 16.3). These findings were consistent with inhibition by PSC 833 of *MDR1* Pgp expressed normally in these organs, markedly reducing Pgp-mediated transport of ^{99m}Tc-sestamibi into bile and urine. Uptake of radiotracer in tumors of two patients did not change after treatment with PSC 833, suggesting absence of functional Pgp; however, expression of *MDR1* Pgp in tumors was not independently verified. In one patient, a tumor in the abdomen was obscured by background activity in the intestine due to biliary excretion of ^{99m}Tc-sestamibi. Although routine use of SPECT and changes in imaging protocols may improve visualization of known tumors in the abdomen and pelvis, results from this patient demonstrated a potential limitation of abdominal imaging of *MDR1* Pgp with ^{99m}Tc-sestamibi.

Further support for the usefulness of scintigraphy in detection of *MDR1* Pgp function and modulation in patients is provided by a study of ten patients with metastatic cancer (nine with renal cell carcinoma and one with adrenal cortical carcinoma) by CHEN et al. (1997). Expression of *MDR1* Pgp in these tumors was verified by PCR. Scintigraphic studies were performed at baseline, 1 day following treatment with vinblastine (a drug transported by Pgp), and during therapy with PSC 833 (a potent inhibitor). Sequential 1-min images were obtained for 30 min, followed by 5-min planar images at 1, 2, 3, and 5 h after injection of 20 mCi of ^{99m}Tc-sestamibi. In all patients, vinblastine had no effect, whereas visualization of tumor was enhanced on images obtained during treatment with PSC 833, and in two patients, tumor was seen only following therapy with the modulator. Delayed clearance of ^{99m}Tc-sestamibi from liver but not other organs was also apparent after treatment with PSC 833. Scintigraphic images were used to generate time-activity curves for tumor, liver, heart, lung, and muscle. Area-under-the-curve analysis of radiotracer activity in each site over 3 h was performed, using a ratio of organ or tumor activity to heart (an organ which does not express *MDR1* Pgp in humans). Quantitatively, time to peak uptake of ^{99m}Tc-sestamibi in liver was 12 min on baseline scintigraphy and significantly delayed (30 to >200 min) after treatment with the modulator. By area-under-the-curve analysis, uptake of ^{99m}Tc-sestamibi increased 20 and 79% in tumor and liver, respectively, after inhibition of Pgp by PSC 833. PSC 833 did not affect time to peak uptake or ^{99m}Tc-sestamibi uptake by area-under-the-curve analysis in any other organ. Washout rates of ^{99m}Tc-sestamibi from tumor or normal organs were not always detectably affected by PSC 833 over the time course of the 30-min dynamic scan, although this may have been too short an interval to resolve this parameter (DEL VECCHIO et al. 1997b). Rate constants could not be determined for liver because of the delay to peak uptake of radiopharmaceutical. Both liver and tumor expressed similar levels of *MDR1* Pgp as determined by PCR, so differences in pharmacokinetics of ^{99m}Tc-sestamibi in these tissues were not due to differences in relative expression of MDR1 Pgp. The authors proposed that the greater effect of PSC 833 on uptake of ^{99m}Tc-sestamibi in liver vs tumor could relate to relatively decreased perfusion of the tumor, overlap of tumor with adjacent normal tissues which do not express Pgp, or to alternative mechanisms for elimination of ^{99m}Tc-sestamibi in liver which are blocked by PSC 833 but are not present in tumor.

Although it is possible to demonstrate increased accumulation of ^{99m}Tc-sestamibi in tumors and tissues expressing Pgp in the presence of reversal agents (CHEN et al. 1997; LUKER et al. 1997), the utility of this information for predicting response to chemotherapy remains to be clinically validated. However, a pilot study in patients with small cell lung cancer has provided provocative data regarding the combined use of ^{99m}Tc-sestamibi and the MDR reversal agent dipyridamole for prediction of chemotherapeutic response (BOM et al. 1997). In 27 patients undergoing pre-treatment scintigraphy, all 5 patients with no subsequent clinical response showed enhanced 1-h tumor-to-normal-lung ratios when imaged after administration of dipyridamole (0.84 mg/kg) compared with pre-modulator imaging, whereas the 3 patients with a complete response showed diminished dipyridamole-induced ratios. Although independent assessment of *MDR1* Pgp status was not performed, this functional scintigraphic approach with an MDR modulator provides guidance for further rigorous evaluation of the method.

16.5 Conclusion

Overall, these studies support the use of validated radiopharmaceuticals, such as ^{99m}Tc-sestamibi and ^{99m}Tc-tetrofosmin, and others in the future, for detection of function and modulation of *MDR1* Pgp in vivo. We envision that functional imaging of *MDR1* Pgp will be performed as a two-part study, with scintigraphy performed before and after treatment with a MDR modulator. More data are needed to determine the optimum imaging protocol for detecting and quantifying function and modulation of *MDR1* Pgp in tumors and normal tissues. Such a protocol likely will require both initial dynamic imaging and delayed static images to acquire data for time-activity curves and calculations of rate constants of washout and/or area-under-the-curve analyses. Eventually, imaging of transport mediated by *MDR1* Pgp may provide prognostic information at the time of diagnosis, guide the type of chemotherapy and timing of administration of drugs in combination with a modulator, and possibly predict side effects, such as neurotoxicity, of combined treatment with chemotherapeutic agents and MDR modulators.

References

Abrams MA, Davison A, Jones AG, Costello CE, Pang H (1983) Synthesis and characterization hexakis(alkyl isocyanide) and hexakis(arylisocyanide) complexes of technetium(I). Inorg Chem 22:2798–2800

Altan N, Chen Y, Schindler M, Simon S (1998) Defective acidification in human breast tumor cells and implications for chemotherapy. J Exp Med 187:1583–1598

Backus M, Piwnica-Worms D, Hockett D, Kronauge J, Lieberman M, Ingram P et al. (1993) Microprobe analysis of Tc-MIBI in heart cells: calculation of mitochondrial potential. Am J Physiol Cell 265:C178–C187

Baldini N, Scotlandi K, Barbanti-Brodano G, Manara M, Maurici D, Bacci G et al. (1995) Expression of P-glycoprotein in high-grade osteosarcomas in relation to clinical outcome. N Eng J Med 333:1380–1385

Ballinger J, Hua H, Berry B, Firby P, Boxen I (1995a) ^{99m}Tc-Sestamibi as an agent for imaging P-glycoprotein-mediated multi-drug resistance: in vitro and in vivo studies in a rat breast tumour cell line and its doxorubicin-resistant variant. Nucl Med Comm 16:253–257

Ballinger JR, Sheldon KM, Boxen I, Erlichman C, Ling V (1995b) Differences between accumulation of Tc-99m-MIBI and Tl-201-thallous chloride in tumor cells: role of P-glycoprotein. Q J Nucl Med 39:122–128

Ballinger JR, Bannerman J, Boxen I, Firby P, Hartman NG, Moore MJ (1996) Technetium-99m-tetrofosmin as a substrate for P-glycoprotein: in vitro studies in multidrug-resistant breast tumor cells. J Nucl Med 37:1578–1582

Bom H, Kim Y, Lim S, Park K (1997) Dipyridamole modulated Tc-99m-sestamibi (mibi) scintigraphy: a predictor of response to chemotherapy in patients with small cell lung cancer. J Nucl Med 38:240P

Bosch I, Croop J (1996) P-glycoprotein multidrug resistance and cancer. Biochim Biophys Acta 1288:F37–F54

Bosch I, Dunussi-Joannopoulos K, Wu R-L, Furlong S, Croop J (1997) Phosphatidylcholine and phosphatidylethanolamine behave as substrates of the human MDR1 P-glycoprotein. Biochemistry 36:5685–5694

Carvalho PA, Chiu ML, Kronauge JF, Kawamura M, Jones AG, Holman BL et al. (1992) Subcellular distribution and analysis of technetium-99m-MIBI in isolated perfused rat heart. J Nucl Med 33:1516–1521

Chan HSL, Haddad G, Thorner PS, DeBoer G, Lin YP, Ondrusek N et al. (1991) P-glycoprotein expression as a predictor of the outcome of therapy for neuroblastoma. N Engl J Med 325:1608–1614

Chen C, Meadows B, Regis J, Kalafsky G, Fojo T, Carrasquillo J et al. (1997) Detection of in vivo P-glycoprotein inhibition by PSC 833 using Tc-99m-Sestamibi. Clin Cancer Res 3:545–552

Chernoff DM, Strichartz GR, Piwnica-Worms D (1993) Membrane potential determination in large unilamellar vesicles with hexakis(2-methoxyisobutyl isonitrile) technetium(I). Biochim Biophys Acta 1147:262–266

Ciarmiello A, Del Vecchio S, Silvestro P, Potena MI, Carriero MV, Thomas R et al. (1998) Tumor clearance of technetium-99m-Sestamibi as a predictor of response to neoadjuvant chemotherapy for locally advanced breast cancer. J Clin Oncol 16:1677–1683

Cole SPC, Bhardwaj G, Gerlach JH, Mackie JE, Grant CE, Almquist KC et al. (1992) Overexpression of a transporter gene in a multidrug-resistant human lung cancer cell line. Science 258:1650–1654

Cordobes M, Starzec A, Delmon-Moingeon L, Blanchot C, Kouyoumdjian J-C, Prevost G et al. (1996) Technetium-99m-Sestamibi uptake by human benign and malignant breast tumor cells: correlation with *mdr* gene expression. J Nucl Med 37:286–289

Cordon-Cardo C, O'Brien JP, Casals D, Rittman GL, Biedler JL, Melamed MR et al. (1989) Multidrug-resistance gene (P-glycoprotein) is expressed by endothelial cells at blood-brain barrier sites. Proc Natl Acad Sci USA 86(2):695–698

Crankshaw C, Piwnica-Worms D (1996) Tc-99m-Sestamibi may be a transport substrate of the human multidrug resistance-associated protein (MRP). J Nucl Med 37:247P

Crankshaw CL, Marmion M, Burleigh BD, Deutsch E, Piwnica-Worms D (1995) Non-reducible mixed ligand Tc(III) cations (Q complexes) are recognized as transport substrates by the human multidrug-resistance (MDR) P-glycoprotein. J Nucl Med 36:130P

Crankshaw C, Marmion M, Luker G, Rao V, Dahlheimer J, Burleigh B et al. (1998) Novel Tc(III)-Q-complexes for functional imaging of the multidrug resistance (*MDR1*) P-glycoprotein. J Nucl Med 39:77–86

Dantzig A, Shepard R, Cao J, Law K, Ehlhardt W, Baughman T et al. (1996) Reversal of P-glycoprotein-mediated multidrug resistance by a potent cyclopropyldibenzosuberane modulator, LY335979. Cancer Res 56:4171–4179

Del Vecchio S, Ciarmiello A, Potena MI, Carriero MV, Mainolfi C, Botti G et al. (1997a) In vivo detection of multidrug resistance (MDR1) phenotype by technetium-99m-sestamibi scan in untreated breast cancer patients. Eur J Nucl Med 24:150–159

Del Vecchio S, Ciarmiello A, Pace L, Potena M, Carriero M, Mainolfi C et al. (1997b) Fractional retention of technetium-99m-sestamibi as an index of P-glycoprotein expression in untreated breast cancer patients. J Nucl Med 38:1348–1351

Delmon-Moingeon LI, Piwnica-Worms D, Van den Abbeele AD, Holman BL, Davison A, Jones AG (1990) Uptake of the cation hexakis (2-methoxy isobutylisonitrile) technetium-99m by human carcinoma cell lines in vitro. Cancer Res 50:2198–2202

Elsinga PH, Franssen JF, Hendrikse NH, Fluks L, Weemaes A-MA, van der Graaf WTA et al. (1996) Carbon-11-labeled daunorubicin and verapamil for probing P-glycoprotein in tumors with PET. J Nucl Med 37:1571–1575

Ford JM, Hait WN (1990) Pharmacology of drugs that alter multidrug resistance in cancer. Pharmacol Rev 42(3):155–199

Gaveriaux C, Boesch D, Jachez B (1991) PSC 833 a non-immunosuppressive cyclosporin analog is a very potent multidrug-resistance modifier. J Cell Pharmacol 2:225–234

Germann UA, Willingham MC, Pastan I, Gottesman MM (1990) Expression of the human multidrug transporter in insect cells by a recombinant baculovirus. Biochemistry 29:2295–2303

Germann U, Ford P, Schlakhter D, Mason V, Harding M (1997) Chemosensitization and drug accumulation effects of VX-710, verapamil, cyclosporin A, MS-209, and GF120918 in multidrug resistant HL60/ADR cells expressing the multidrug resistance-associated protein MRP. Anticancer Drugs 8(2):141–155

Giaccone G, van Ark-Otte J, Rubio G, Gazdar A, Broxterman H, Dingemans A et al. (1996) MRP is frequently expressed in human lung cancer cell lines, in non-small cell lung cancer and in normal lungs. Int J Cancer 66:760–767

Goldstein LJ, Fojo AT, Ueda K, Crist W, Green A, Brodeur G et al. (1990) Expression of the multidrug resistance, MDR1, gene in neuroblastomas. J Clin Oncol 8(1):128–136

Gottesman MM, Pastan I (1993) Biochemistry of multidrug resistance mediated by the multidrug transporter. Annu Rev Biochem 62:385–427

Gros P, Ben Neriah Y, Croop JM, Housman DE (1986) Isolation and expression of a complementary DNA that confers multidrug resistance. Nature 323(6090):728–731

Hendrikse N, Franssen E, van der Graaf W, Meijer C, Piers D, Vaalburg W et al. (1998) ^{99m}Tc-sestamibi is a substrate for P-glycoprotein and the multidrug resistance-associated protein. Br J Cancer 77:353–358

Higley B, Smith FW, Smith T, Gemmell HG, Gupta PD, Gvozdanovic DV et al. (1993) Technetium-99m-1,2-bis[bis(2-ethoxyethyl)phosphino]ethane: human biodistribution, dosimetry and safety of a new myocardial perfusion imaging agent. J Nucl Med 34:30–38

Hoffman M, Roepe P (1997) Analysis of ion transport perturbations caused by hu MDR1 protein overexpression. Biochemistry 36:11153–11168

Homolya L, Hollo Z, Germann UA, Pastan I, Gottesman MM, Sarkadi B (1993) Fluorescent cellular indicators are extruded by the multidrug resistance protein. J Biol Chem 268(29):21493–21496

Hurwitz S, Terashima M, Mizunuma N, Slapak C (1997) Vesicular anthracycline accumulation in doxorubicin-selected U-937 cells: participation of lysosomes. Blood 89:3745–3754

Hyafil F, Vergely C, Du Vignaud P, Grand-Perret T (1993) In vitro and in vivo reversal of multidrug resistance by GF120918, an acridonecarboxamide derivative. Cancer Res 53(19):4595–4602

Jurisson SS, Dancey K, McPartlin M, Tasker PA, Deutsch E (1984) Synthesis, characterization, and electrochemical properties of technetium complexes containing both tetradentate Schiff base and monodentate tertiary phosphine ligands: single-crystal structure of trans-(N,N'-ethylenebis(acetylacetone iminato))bis(triphenylphosphine)technetium(III) hexafluorophosphate. Inorg Chem 23:4743–4749

Kabasakal L, Ozker K, Hayward M, Akansel G, Griffith O, Isitman A et al. (1996) Technetium-99m sestamibi uptake in human breast carcinoma cell lines displaying glutathione-associated drug-resistance. Eur J Nucl Med 23:568–570

Kostakoglu L, Elahi N, Kirarli P, Ruacan S, Sayek S, Baltali E et al. (1994) Clinical validation of the influence of P-glycoprotein on technetium-99m-Sestamibi uptake in malignant tumors. J Nucl Med 38:1003–1008

Kostakoglu L, Kirath P, Ruacan S, Hayran M, Emri S, Ergun E et al. (1998) Association of tumor washout rates and accumulation of technetium-99m-MIBI with expression of P-glycoprotein in lung cancer. J Nucl Med 39:228–234

Kronauge JF, Kawamura M, Lepisto E, Holman BL, Davison A, Jones AG et al (1990) Metabolic studies of the myocardial perfusion agent Tc-(MIBI). In: Nicolini M, Bandoli G, Mazzi U (eds) Technetium and rhenium in chemistry and nuclear medicine. Cortina International, , pp 677–682

Leveille-Webster, C. and Arias, I (1995) The biology of the P-glycoproteins. J Membr Biol 143:89–102

Luker G, Rao V, Crankshaw C, Dahlheimer J, Piwnica-Worms D (1997a) Characterization of phosphine complexes of technetium (III) as transport substrates of the multidrug resistance (MDR1) P-glycoprotein and functional markers of P-glycoprotein at the blood-brain barrier. Biochemistry 36:14218–14227

Luker GD, Fracasso PM, Dobkin J, Piwnica-Worms D (1997b) Modulation of the multidrug resistance P-glycoprotein: detection with Tc-99m-Sestamibi in vivo. J Nucl Med 38:369–372

Mehta B, Rosa E, Biedler J, Larson S (1994) In vivo uptake of carbon-14-colchicine for identification of tumor multidrug resistance. J Nucl Med 35:1179–1184

Moretti J-L, Cordobes M, Starzec A, de Beco V, Vergote J, Benazzouz F et al. (1998) Involvement of glutathione in loss of technetium-99m-MIBI accumulation related to membrane MDR protein expression in tumor cells. J Nucl Med 39:1214–1218

Morrow C, Chiu J, Cowan K (1992) Posttranscriptional control of glutathione S-transferase pi gene expression in human breast cancer cells. J Biol Chem 267:10544–10550

Norris M, Bordow S, Marshall G, Haber P, Cohn S, Haber M (1996) Expression of the gene for multidrug-resistance-associated protein and outcome in patients with neuroblastoma. N Engl J Med 334:231–238

Pastan I, Gottesman M (1987) Multiple-drug resistance in human cancer. N Engl J Med 316:1388–1393

Piwnica-Worms D, Kronauge JF, Chiu ML (1990) Uptake and retention of hexakis (2-methoxy isobutyl isonitrile) technetium(I) in cultured chick myocardial cells: mitochondrial and plasma membrane potential dependence. Circulation 82:1826–1838

Piwnica-Worms D, Chiu ML, Budding M, Kronauge JF, Kramer RA, Croop JM (1993) Functional imaging of multidrug-resistant P-glycoprotein with an organotechnetium complex. Cancer Res 53:977–984

Piwnica-Worms D, Rao V, Kronauge J, Croop J (1995) Characterization of multidrug-resistance P-glycoprotein transport function with an organotechnetium cation. Biochemistry 34:12210–12220

Platts E, North T, Pickett R, Kelly J (1995) Mechanism of uptake of Tc-tetrofosmin I: uptake into isolated rat venticular myocytes and subcellular localization. J Nucl Cardiol 2:317–326

Rao VV, Chiu ML, Kronauge JF, Piwnica-Worms D (1994) Expression of recombinant human multidrug resistance P-glycoprotein in insect cells confers decreased accumulation of technetium-99m-SESTAMIBI. J Nucl Med 35:510–515

Rao V, Dahlheimer J, Bardgett M, Snyder A, Piwnica-Worms D (1998) MDR1 Pgp mediates the blood-cerebrospinal fluid permeability barrier in choroid plexus epithelium. Proc Am Assoc Cancer Res 38:76

Robinson L, Roberts W, Ling T, Lamming D, Sternberg S, Roepe P (1997) Human MDR1 protein overexpression delays the apoptotic cascade in Chinese hamster ovary fibroblasts. Biochemistry 36:11169–11178

Rossetti C, Vanoli G, Paganelli G, Kwiatkowski M, Zito F, Colombo F et al. (1994) Human biodistribution, dosimetry and clinical use of technetium(III)-99m-Q12. J Nucl Med 35:1571–1580

Schinkel A, Smit J, van Tellingen O, Beijnen J, Wagenaar E, van Deemter L et al. (1994) Disruption of the mouse mdr1a P-glycoprotein gene leads to a deficiency in the blood-brain barrier and to increased sensitivity to drugs. Cell 77:491–502

Schneider E, Horton J, Yang C, Nakagawa M, Cowan K (1994) Multidrug resistance-associated protein gene overexpression and reduced drug sensitivity of topoisomerase II in a hman breast carcinoma MCF7 cell line selected for etoposide resistance. Cancer Res 54:152–158

Sharma V, Wey SP, Bass L, Crankshaw CL, Green MA, Welch MJ et al. (1996) Monocationic N_4O_2 Schiff-Base phenolate complexes of gallium(III): novel PET imaging agents of the human multidrug resistance (*MDR1*) P-glycoprotein. J Nucl Med 37:51P

Smyth MJ, Krasovskis E, Sutton VR, Johnstone RW (1998) The drug efflux protein P-glycoprotein additionally protects drug-resistant tumor cells from multiple forms of caspase-dependent apoptosis. Proc Natl Acad Sci USA 95:7024–7029

Stein W (1997) Kinetics of the multidrug transporter (P-glycoprotein) and its reversal. Physiol Rev 77:545–590

Thiebaut F, Tsuruo T, Hamada H, Gottesman MM, Pastan I, Willingham MC (1987) Cellular localization of the multidrug-resistance gene product P-glycoprotein in normal human tissues. Proc Natl Acad Sci USA 84(21):7735–7738

Trock B, Leonessa F, Clarke R (1997) Multidrug resistance in breast cancer: a meta-analysis of MDR1/gp170 expression and its possible functional significance. J Natl Cancer Inst 89:917–931

Tuccari G, Rizzo A, Giuffre G, Barresi G (1993) Immunocytochemical detection of DNA topoisomerase type II in primary breast carcinomas: correlation with clinico-pathological features. Virchows Arch A Pathol Anat Histopathol 423:51–55

Van der Bliek AM, Baas F, Ten Houte de Lange T, Kooiman PM, Van der Velde Koerts T, Borst P (1987) The human mdr3 gene encodes a novel P-glycoprotein homologue and gives rise to alternatively spliced mRNAs in liver. EMBO J 6(11):3325–3331

van Helvoort A, Smith AJ, Sprong H, Fritzsche I, Schinkel AH, Borst P et al. (1996) MDR1 P-glycoprotein is a lipid translocase of broad specificity, while MDR3 P-glycoprotein specifically translocates phosphatidylcholine. Cell 87:507–517

Wackers FJ, Berman D, Maddahi J, Beller G, Straus H, Boucher C et al. (1989) Tc-99m-hexakis 2-methoxy isobutylisonitrile: human biodistribution, dosimetry, safety and preliminary comparison to thallium-201 for myocardial perfusion imaging. J Nucl Med 30:301–309

Yoshimura A, Shudo N, Ikeda SI, Ichikawa M, Sumizawa T, Akiyama SI (1990) Novel screening method for agents that overcome classical multidrug resistance in a human cell line. Cancer Lett 50(1):45–51

Younes A (1995) Mechanism of uptake of Tc-tetrofosmin II: uptake into isolated adult rat heart mitochondria. J Nucl Cardiol 2:327–333

Zyad A, Benard J, Tursz T, Clarke R, Chouaib S (1994) Resistance to TNF-alpha and adriamycin in the human breast cancer MCF-7 cell line: relationship to MDR1, MnSOD, and TNF gene expression. Cancer Res 54:825–831

17 Quo Vadis?

C. Schiepers

In the foregoing chapters, an update was given on the progress in the 1990s. Promising developments in receptor and metabolic imaging support the notion that they are here to stay.

For the classical NM studies, image quality improved due to better cameras and faster computers. Newer, mostly ^{99m}Tc-based radiopharmaceuticals were manufactured, taking advantage of the optimization of the equipment to the radionuclide ^{99m}Tc. Adaptation of existing tests and imaging protocols, mainly by adding pharmacological interventions, also improved the efficiency and efficacy of many studies.

Metabolic imaging appeared as the "new kid on the block" and propelled the field of diagnostic imaging in oncology. FDG soon became the workhorse of positron emission tomography (PET) and in the US a network was set up for distribution of FDG over the densely populated areas. Dedicated PET instruments are still expensive and not widely available, so the development of hybrid gamma camera systems was accelerated and appears to have a bright future. Another development was the introduction of mobile PET systems, to spread this relatively expensive technology over wider geographic areas.

How will NM look in the next century? Various opinions have been expressed encompassing the whole spectrum from negative to positive, as has been clearly put forward by Henry N. Wagner Jr. The key word of the 1960s civil rights movement, "integration", is currently the catchword of business management (Kotz 1999). "Merger" and "fusion" not only have been frequently used and heard words, but actually have happened in hospitals, telecommunication industries, media networks and other businesses. Several academic disciplines are now doing the same.

C. Schiepers
Department of Molecular and Medical Pharmacology, UCLA School of Medicine, 10833 Le Conte Avenue, AR-144 CHS, Los Angeles, CA 90095-6942, USA

Nuclear medicine as a relatively small specialty will have to follow suit. In the clinical section of this book, the progress in certain fields is obvious, and the integration in immunology and oncology applications is evident (see Chaps. 9, 10). The field of oncology is a perfect example for the integration movement: tumor boards consisting of surgical, medical and radiation oncologists, imaging specialists (radiology and NM) and pathologists, in joint discussion, decide which therapy is best for the individual cancer patient. This approach appears to be effective and provides the patient with the optimal treatment plan available for a particular institution.

An interesting approach is the fusion of imaging modalities. This effort is driven by the desire to merge anatomical and biological information into one device, procedure and image, so that perfect alignment for fusion is obtained. The PET/CT (Townsend 1998) and PET/MR (Shao 1997) combinations are being investigated.

At our institution, UCLA, the integration of NM with medical and molecular pharmacology is another example of bringing together basic science with clinical science. All this is done with the intention to develop new assays for diagnostic imaging, manufacture new radiopharmaceuticals and design equipment. Instruments such as micro-PET scanner, combined CT/PET and MR/PET scanners, and dedicated breast PET imaging device, are being developed for future applications. These innovations will keep NM in the forefront of the imaging field and will result in new diagnostic strategies for work-up of patients with disease.

In this book the cost-effectiveness of diagnostic tests and combination of imaging modalities to yield optimal results, i.e. arrive at the diagnosis in the shortest amount of time with an adequate balance between tests performed and costs spent, is mentioned sporadically. In the present environment of managed care, at least in the US, or budget constraints elsewhere, there is a need for objective assessment and evaluation of imaging strategies for certain clinical problems. At UCLA, Gambhir and coworkers have developed a method based on decision-tree analysis to furnish these results. Models have been designed for staging of lung cancer (Gambhir 1996; Scott 1998) and management of solitary pulmonary nodules (Gambhir 1998). At the annual meeting of the Society of Nuclear Medicine a combined model for detection and staging of lung lesions was proposed (Shepherd 1999).

Nuclear medicine as a biological imaging modality will evolve and keep expanding in the next century, a technology which is meant to stay despite the "doom and gloom" of some opponents. This tendency will not come for free and will mandate continuous input from scientists and clinicians. In addition, new ways of interdisciplinary collaboration need to be explored to assemble the best team of experts that will arrive at the diagnosis in the shortest amount of time, without prohibitive costs of health care to society. In this way the patient will benefit by being provided with optimum care.

References

Kotz D (1999) Nuclear medicine in the 21st century: integration with other specialties. J Nucl Med 40: 13N-15N

Gambhir SS, Hoh CK, Phelps ME, Madar I, Maddahi J(1996) Decision tree sensitivity analysis for cost-effectiveness of FDG-PET in the staging and management of non-small-cell lung carcinoma. J Nucl Med 37:1428–1436

Gambhir SS, Shepherd JE, Shah BD, Hart E, Hoh CK, Valk PE, Emi T, Phelps ME (1998) Analytical decision model for the cost-effective management of solitary pulmonary nodules. J Clin Oncol 16: 2113–2123

Scott WJ, Shepherd J, Gambhir SS (1998) Cost effectiveness of FDG-PET for staging non-small cell lung cancer: a decision analysis. Ann Thorac Surg 66: 1876–1885

Shao Y, Cherry S, Farahani K, et al (1997) Development of a PET detector system compatible with MRI/NMR systems. IEEE Trans Nucl Sci 44: 1167–1171

Shepherd JE, Phelps ME, Czernin J, Gambhir SS (1999) Cost effectiveness analysis for the role of FDG-PET in lung carcinoma. J Nucl Med 40: 56P

Townsend DW, Beyer T, Kinahan PE, et al. The SMART scanner: a combined PET/CT tomograph for clinical oncology. IEEE Medical Imaging Conference Record, Toronto, Canada, 1998

Glossary

Accuracy	probability that a test will yield the correct diagnosis
ACEI	angiotensin-converting enzyme inhibitors
AD	Alzheimer's dementia
ADHD	attention deficit hyperactivity disorder
Anion	electro negative ion, element or molecule
Antisense	in molecular genetics: strand of DNA having set of nucleotides complementary to the sense strand
Apoptosis	programmed cell death, suicidal pathway of cell stored in the genes
Aptamer	novel nucleic acid-binding species
BGO	bismuth germanate
Cation	electro positive ion, element or molecule
Chelate	chemical compound that sequesters and firmly binds a metallic ion into a ring, thus shielding the chemical effects of the metal
Chemotaxis	orientation of a cell along a chemical gradient, or movement in the direction of the gradient
Compartmental analysis	method of analyzing the data, in which the organ or system under study is represented as a set of compartments, e.g. intra-vascular, extra-cellular fluid (ECF), intra-cellular, and excretion compartments.
DAS	dynamic antral scintigraphy
Deconvolution analysis	mathematical technique to reconstruct a function at time T from measurements at a later time.
DLBD	diffuse Lewy body disease
Dose, absorbed	radiation energy absorbed in the body, expressed in mSv (milli Sievert); 1 Sievert = 1 Gray · Q (Q is quality factor, which equals 1 for gamma and beta radiation); 1 Gray = 1 Joule/kilogram
Dose, administered	amount of radioactivity, e.g. mCi – (milli Curie), or Bq (Becquerel; 1 Bq is 1 disintegration per second); the prefix indicates the power of 10, e.g. M is mega for 10^6 and T is for tera or 10^{12}; 1 mCi = $3.7 \cdot 10^7$ Bq
Dose, exposed	amount of radiation emitted to the organ or system or body under study, expressed in Coulombs/kilogram in the current SI system, or mR (milli Roentgen) in the old system: 1 Roentgen = $2.58 \cdot 10^{-4}$ Coulombs/kilogram
Eluate	product of elution, i.e. separation by washing, such as freeing an enzyme from its absorbent
EOB	end of bombardment, i.e. of the target in a cyclotron
Epitope	antigenic determinant
ER	estrogen receptor (in breast cancer)
ETT	esophageal transit time, (in gastro-enterology); or exercise treadmill test (in cardiology)

FBP	filtered back-projection; reconstruction algorithm for tomography
FNA	fine- needle aspiration
FWHM	full width at half maximum
FWTM	full width at one tenth of the maximum
Genome	the full set of genes of an individual
GFR	glomerular filtration rate
Glucose clamp	method to keep serum glucose within a specific range by infusing insulin and glucose simultaneously: originally developed for arterial glucose levels (invasive), but in most PET centers applied to keep venous glucose levels constant in myocardial metabolism studies
GLUT	glucose transporter: subtypes are indicated with an Arabic numeral
Glycolysis	breaking down of sugars into simpler compounds; specifically, the metabolic degradation path of glucose
Glycoprotein	conjugated protein, having protein(s) with a carbohydrate group
HAMA	human anti-mouse antibody
HPLC	high- pressure liquid chromatography
hSSTR	human somatostatin receptor
hVIPR	human vasoactive intestinal peptide receptor
Hydrophilic	having affinity for water
Hygroscopic	material that attract water or water vapors
IBD	inflammatory bowel disease
ICAM	intercellular adhesion molecule
K_a	association constant of a chemical reaction, e.g. binding of an agonist or antibody to its receptor on the cell membrane
K_d	dissociation constant of a chemical reaction
keV	kilo electron Volt: energy an electron accumulates after acceleration over 1000 Volts
Ligand	molecule or compound active in biological processes, usually a small molecule that binds specifically to a larger one, e.g. antibody binding to an antigen, hormone or neurotransmitter binding to a receptor, substrate binding to an enzyme
Lipophilic	having affinity for fat
LSO	cerium- activated lutetium oxy-orthosilicate; high energy scintillator
LVEF	left ventricular ejection fraction
MDR	multidrug resistance
Micturition	voiding of bladder
MIRD	medical internal radiation dose
MLEM	maximum-likelihood expectation -maximization
MoAB, MAB	monoclonal antibody
MSA	multi-system atrophy
Normoxic	having normal oxygen tension
NPV	negative predictive value, likelihood that a negative test result indicates absence of disease
NSCLC	non-small- cell lung cancer
OCD	obsessive compulsive disorder
Oncogene	gene with properties for inducing cancer

Oncogenesis	the formation of cancer cells
OSEM	ordered subsets maximum-likelihood expectation -maximization; iterative reconstruction algorithm
PCR	polymerase chain reaction
PET	positron emission tomography: the term ET for emission tomography, combining both SPECT and PET, has not been generally accepted
Pgp	P-glycoprotein
PIOPED	Prospective Investigation of Pulmonary Embolism Diagnosis (study)
Plasmid	an autonomously replicating DNA molecule
PMT	photomultiplier tube
PNA	polypeptide nucleic acid
PPV	positive predictive value; likelihood that a positive test result indicates presence of disease
PR	progesterone receptor (of tumors)
PTCA	percutaneous transluminal coronary angioplasty
Radiolysis	decomposition of a radio-labeled compound by the radiation emitted by its own radioactive nuclide
Radionuclide	radio-active element:, formerly isotope
Radiopharmaceutical	biological compound or pharmaceutical labeled with a radioactive element to trace its pathway; used for diagnostic or therapeutic purposes
RASON	radiolabeled antisense oligodeoxynucleotide
RBF	renal blood flow
rCBF	regional cerebral blood flow
rCMR-Xx	regional cerebral metabolic rate of substance Xx
Rebinning	regrouping of data, for faster processing by computer algorithms
ROI	region of interest
Scintillator	substance that emits light after interaction with high- energy photons
Sensitivity	probability that a test will detect presence of disease
Specificity	probability that a test will determine absence of disease
SPECT (or SPET in Europe)	single photon emission computed tomography
SPM	statistical parametric mapping
SPN	solitary pulmonary nodule
SUV	standardized uptake value: ratio of measured activity in a certain area to the expected activity if the radioactivity were homogeneously distributed through the body
TCA cycle	tricarboxylic acid cycle
TER	tubular extraction rate
Transduction	transfer of DNA via a bacteriophage to another cell, thereby changing the constitution of the second organism, also called genetic recombination
Transfection	artificial infection of cells by nucleic acid isolated from virus or bacteriophage, resulting in production of mature virus or phage particles
Transgenic animal	animal in which every cell carries a specific new or altered gene of interest
TTNA	trans-thoracic needle aspiration
USP	United States Pharmacopoeia
YSO	yttrium oxy-orthosilicate; high- energy scintillator

Subject Index

Abscess and FDG 114
Achalasia 124
Acute tubular necrosis (ATN) 83
Alzheimer's disease (AD) 15
Ambulatory renal monitor (ARM) 82
Angiotensin converting enzyme (ACE) 82
Annihilation 224
Antibodies,
 Anti-granulocytes 110
 Approach 255
 Monoclonal 27
Anticoagulation 58
Attention deficit hyperactivity disorder (ADHD) 188
Attenuation 161, 230, 242
Autism 190

Bayes' theorem 74
Brain,
 AIDS 27
 Energy metabolism 8
 Lymphoma 27
 Tumors 25, 163
 Death 187
Brain development 184
Binding potential (BP) brain receptors 12
Blood-brain-barrier (BBB) 9
Blood flow / Metabolism mismatch 46, 48

Cancer,
 Breast 146, 165, 277
 Colorectal 140, 167
 Lung 144, 164, 279
  Non-small cell lung cancer 145, 165
  Solitary Pulmonary Nodule (SPN) 145, 164
 Ovarian 170
 Pancreatic 142, 168
 Prostate 169
 Renal cell 170
 Testicular 170
 Thyroid 151
Captopril test 84
Cerebral blood flow (CBF) 12
Cerebral glucose metabolism 15, 26, 185
Cerebral palsy 186
Cerebro-vascular disease (CVD) 19
Cerebro-vascular reserve 186
Cholecystitis 131-133
Cholescintigraphy,
 Cholecystokinin (CCK) augmented 131
 Morphine augmented 131
Coincidence events 227
Collimator 223
Compartments 10
Compression ultrasound 69
Compton scattering 224, 244
Condensed image (GI-scintigraphy) 124
Connective tissue disorders 125
Constipation 128
Crohn's disease (CD) 179, 182
CT-angiography 70

D-dimer test 69
Deep venous thrombosis 69, 210
Diabetic gastroparesis 127
Diaschisis 20
Diffuse Lewy body disease (DLBD) 15
Diuresis renography 87
DNA 255
Duodenal ulcer 179
Dysfunctional myocardium 50
Dyspepsia 127

Effective renal plasma flow (ERPF) 79
Efflux (rate) 278
Epilepsy 21
 Temporal lobe 186

Factor Analysis 247
Fever of unknown origin 110, 115
Filtered backprojection 238

Gallbladder dyskinesia 133
Gastrointestinal (GI)-bleeding 129
Gene,
 Delivery,
  In vivo 259
  Ex vivo 259
 Multi drug resistance 200, 273
 Signal amplification 266
 Suicide 268
 Therapy 267
Genome 1
Glomerular filtration rate (GFR) 79
Grading of tumors 163

Head injury 188
Helicobacter pylori 178
Hexokinase enzyme 160
Hibernating myocardium 37
High pressure liquid chromatography (HPLC) 198
Hybrid camera 226
Hydronephrosis 87, 89

Immunology 1
Immunoscintigraphy 112
Imaging,
 Biological 1, 286
 Clinical service 162
 Correlative 98
 Gene expression 253
 Metabolic 163, 204, 285
 MDR reversal 279
 NM (nuclear medicine) 160
 Peptide 137
 Positron 96
 Receptor 13
 Reporter genes 262
 Single photon 96
 Three phase bone 97
Inflammatory bowel disease (IBD) 109, 110, 179, 181
Interleukin 104
IRES – internal ribosomal entry site 260

Kinetic model 10

Lag phase 126
Landau-Kleffner syndrome 187
Legg-Calve-Perthes disease 100
Likelihood ratio 73
Luxury perfusion 20
Lymphoma 152, 170

MAP – maximum a posteriori reconstruction 240
Mammography (MX) 165
Match and Mismatch patterns,
 Heart 46
 Lung 65
Meckel scan 180
Medical decision making 59, 72
Melanoma 151, 171
MicroPET 254
MLEM – maximum likelihood expectation maximization 239
Modulators, MDR 275, 279
Molecular biology 253
Motion artifacts 230, 245
Multidrug resistance (MDR) gene 200, 274

NaI(Tl) thallium activated sodium iodide crystal 221
Neuro-psychiatric disorders, childhood 188
Neurotransmission 8, 9
Neurotransmitter 11
Neuroreceptor 11
Northern blotting 152

Obsessive-compulsive disorder (OCD) 189
Obstructive uropathy 87
OSEM – ordered subset expectation maximization 241
Osteomyelitis 99, 109
Osteonecrosis 101
Osteoporosis 98

P-glycoprotein 200, 274
Paget's disease 98
Pancreatitis 169
Parkinson's disease (PD) 17
Phenotype 254
Pick's disease 15
PIOPED 64
Platelet activating factor 104
Probability notation 72
Probes,
- Antibody 255
- Antisense 255, 266
- Aptamer 259
- Protein 255

Prosthesis
- Infection 100
- Loosening 100

Pulmonary embolism 57

Quality control 231

Radiation necrosis 163
Radiation safety, pediatric 177
Radiation risks 178
Radiopharmaceuticals,
- Acetate 44
- Aerosols 63
- Ammonia 45
- BMIPP 44
- DISIDA 131
- DMSA 89
- EC 80
- ECD 184, 201
- Fluoride 95
- Fluoro-deoxy-glucose (FDG) 1, 114, 160
- F- DOPA 12
- FESP 13
- Flumazenil 21, 211
- Furofosmin 276
- Gallium 105
- Hippuran 79
- HMPAO 105, 184, 201
- Iomazenil 21, 211
- IMP 20, 184
- IBZM 13, 19
- IPPA 43
- Krypton 63, 203
- Labeled WBC 105, 108, 181, 215
- Labeled RBC 214
- MAA 63
- MAG3 80
- MIBI 27, 42
- Methyl-Tyrosine 27
- Octreotide 137, 207
- Oxine 108
- Polyphosphonates (MDP, HDP) 95
- Sestamibi 42, 276
- Sulfur colloid 123
- Technegas 203
- Tetrosfosmin 42, 276
- Thallium 26, 38, 198
- VIP 137, 208
- Water 45
- Xenon 20, 63, 184, 203

Receiver-operating characteristic (ROC) 73
Receptors,
- Affinity (K_D) 12
- Density (B_{max}) ^{123}I-VIP 12
- Types,
  - Benzodiazepine 17, 21, 25, 210
  - Cholinergic 14
  - Dopaminergic 13, 213
  - Estrogen 147
  - Muscarinic 14
  - Nicotinic 13,
  - Opioid 13, 25
  - Peptide 210
  - Progesteron 147
  - Serotonergic 13, 211
  - Somatostatin 138, 207,

Reconstruction,
- Filtered backprojection 238
- Iterative 238

Reflex Sympathetic Dystrophy (RSD) 101
Renal blood flow (RBF) 81
Renal artery stenosis (RAS) 84
Renovascular hypertension (RVH) 84
Repetitive stunning 38
Reporter gene 261, 262
Resolution,
- Angular 229
- Energy 229
- Extrinsic 228
- Intrinsic 228, 245
- Spatial 225, 228

Rett's syndrome 190
Reversibility 41
RNA 255
ROI – region of interest analysis 246

Sarcoidosis 107, 116
Scintillator 221
Sedation, pediatric 177
Seizures 21, 24
Solitary Pulmonary Nodules 145
Staging,
- Tumors 162
- Initial 162
- Nodal 164
- Axillary 166

Standardized uptake value (SUV) 161
Statistical Parametric Mapping (SPM) 11
Stress fracture 99
Sports injury 99
Stroke 20
Stunned myocardium 37
Substance P 104
System sensitivity 228

Thymidine kinase 264
Time activity curve (TAC) 247
Tourette syndrome 190
Transient ischemic attacks (TIA) 20
Tracers,
- Amino acids 204
- Brain perfusion 201
- Glucose metabolism 203
- Hypoxia agents 205
- Lung ventilation 203
- Myocardial perfusion 198
- Positron emitters 197
- Renal function 203

Transporters,
- Dopamine (DAT) 18,
- Glucose (GLUT) 160
- Vesicular acetyl choline (VAChT) 16

Tuberculosis 116
Tumors,
- also, see Cancer
- Carcinoid 149
- Insulinoma 150
- Lymphoma 152, 170
- Melanoma 151, 171
- Neuroendocrine 148
- Teratoma 170
- VIPoma 150

Ulcerative colitis (UC) 180
Urea breath test 179,180
Urinary tract infection (UTI) 89

Vectors 260, 261
Vesico-ureteric reflux (VUR) 90
Viability,
- Brain 20
- Bone graft 98
- Myocardium 38

List of Contributors

W. Becker
Department of Nuclear Medicine
University of Göttingen
Robert-Koch-Strasse 40
37075 Göttingen
Germany

R. Campisi
Department of Molecular and Medical Pharmacology
UCLA School of Medicine
10833 Le Conte Avenue
Los Angeles, CA 90095-1735
USA

J. J. Frost
Johns Hopkins Hospital
600 N. Wolfe Street
Nelson Tower Bl-130
Baltimore, MD 21205
USA

S. S. Gambhir
Crump Institute for Biological Imaging
Department of Molecular & Medical Pharmacology
Laboratory of Structural Biology & Molecular Medicine (DOE)
UCLA School of Medicine
700 Westwood Plaza
Los Angeles, CA 90095-1770
USA

D. A. Hillier
Division of Nuclear Medicine
Mallinckrodt Institute of Radiology
510 S. Kingshighway Blvd.
Saint Louis, MO 63110
USA

C. K. Hoh
Department of Molecular and Medical Pharmacology
UCLA School of Medicine
10833 Le Conte Avenue, AR-144 CHS
Los Angeles, CA 90095-6942
USA

F. Jamar
Center of Nuclear Medicine
University of Louvain Medical School UCL 54.30
Avenue Hippocrate 54
1200 Brussels
Belgium

C. Johnson
Department of Diagnostic Imaging
Temple University Hospital
3401 North Broad Street
Philadelphia, PA 19140
USA

F. Y. J. Keng
Department of Molecular and Medical Pharmacology
UCLA School of Medicine
10833 Le Conte Avenue
Los Angeles, CA 90095-1735
USA

G. Lucignani
Department of Nuclear Medicine
University of Milan H.S. Raffaele
Via Olgettina 60
20132 Milan
Italy

G. D. Luker
Mallinckrodt Institute of Radiology
510 S. Kingshighway Blvd.
Saint Louis, MO 63310
USA

K. E. Luker
Mallinckrodt Institute of Radiology
510 S. Kingshighway Blvd.
Saint Louis, MO 63310
USA

H. R. Nadel
Department of Nuclear Medicine
B.C. Children's Hospital
4480 Oak Street
Vancouver, B.C. V6H 3V4
Canada

J. Nuyts
Department of Nuclear Medicine,K.U. Leuven
Herestraat 49
3000 Leuven
Belgium

D. Piwnica-Worms
Mallinckrodt Institute of Radiology
510 S. Kingshighway Blvd.
Saint Louis, MO 63310
USA

V. V. Rao
Mallinckrodt Institute of Radiology
510 S. Kingshighway Blvd.
Saint Louis, MO 63310
USA

H. D. Royal
Division of Nuclear Medicine
Mallinckrodt Institute of Radiology
510 S. Kingshighway Blvd.
Saint Louis, MO 63110
USA

H. R. Schelbert
Department of Molecular and Medical Pharmacology
UCLA School of Medicine
10833 Le Conte Avenue
Los Angeles, CA 90095-1735
USA

C. Schiepers
Department of Molecular and Medical Pharmacology
UCLA School of Medicine
10833 Le Conte Avenue, AR-144 CHS
Los Angeles, CA 90095-6942
USA

V. Sharma
Mallinckrodt Institute of Radiology
510 S. Kingshighway Blvd.
Saint Louis, MO 63310
USA

M. E. Stilwell
Department of Nuclear Medicine
B.C. Children's Hospital
4480 Oak Street
Vancouver, B.C. V6H 3V4
Canada

J. L. C. Urbain
Department of Diagnostic Imaging
Temple University Hospital
3401 North Broad Street
Philadelphia, PA 19140
USA

M. C. Vekemans
CHGH
Route de Mons 63
7301 Hornu
Belgium

K. Verbeke
Department of Radiopharmacy
UZ Gasthuisberg
Herestraat 49
3000 Leuven
Belgium

A. Verbruggen
Department of Radiopharmacy
UZ Gasthuisberg
Herestraat 49
3000 Leuven
Belgium

I. Virgolini
Department of Internal Medicine
University of Vienna
Währinger Gürtel 18–20
1030 Vienna
Austria

S. I. Ziegler
Nuklearmedizinische Klinik und Poliklinik
Klinikum rechts der Isar der TU München
Ismaninger Strasse 22
81675 Munich
Germany

Medical Radiology

Diagnostic Imaging and Radiation Oncology

Titles in the series already published

Diagnostic Imaging

Innovations in Diagnostic Imaging
Edited by J.H. Anderson

Radiology of the Upper Urinary Tract
Edited by E.K. Lang

The Thymus - Diagnostic Imaging, Functions, and Pathologic Anatomy
Edited by E. Walter, E. Willich, and W.R. Webb

Interventional Neuroradiology
Edited by A. Valavanis

Radiology of the Pancreas
Edited by A.L. Baert, co-edited by G. Delorme

Radiology of the Lower Urinary Tract
Edited by E.K. Lang

Magnetic Resonance Angiography
Edited by I.P. Arlart, G.M. Bongartz, and G. Marchal

Contrast-Enhanced MRI of the Breast
S. Heywang-Köbrunner and R. Beck

Spiral CT of the Chest
Edited by M. Rémy-Jardin and J. Rémy

Radiological Diagnosis of Breast Diseases
Edited by M. Friedrich and E.A. Sickles

Radiology of the Trauma
Edited by M. Heller and A. Fink

Biliary Tract Radiology
Edited by P. Rossi

Radiological Imaging of Sports Injuries
Edited by C. Masciocchi

Modern Imaging of the Alimentary Tube
Edited by A. R. Margulis

Diagnosis and Therapy of Spinal Tumors
Edited by P. R. Algra, J. Valk, and J. J. Heimans

Interventional Magnetic Resonance Imaging
Edited by J. F. Debatin and G. Adam

Abdominal and Pelvic MRI
Edited by A. Heuck and M. Reiser

Orthopedic Imaging
Techniques and Applications
Edited by A.M. Davies and H. Pettersson

Radiology of the Female Pelvic Organs
Edited by E.K.Lang

Magnetic Resonance of the Heart and Great Vessels
Clinical Applications
Edited by J. Bogaert, A. J. Duerinckx, and F. E. Rademakers

Modern Head and Neck Imaging
Edited by S. K. Mukherji and J. A. Castelijns

Radiological Imaging of Endocrine Diseases
Edited by J. N. Bruneton in collaboration with B. Padovani and M.-Y. Mourou

Trends in Contrast Media
Edited by H. S. Thomsen, R. N. Muller, and R. F. Mattrey

Functional MRI
Edited by C. T. W. Moonen and P. A. Bandettini

Radiology of the Pancreas
2nd Revised Edition
Edited by A. L. Baert
Co-edited by G. Delorme and L. Van Hoe

Radiology of Peripheral Vascular Diseases
Edited by E. Zeitler

Emergency Pediatric Radiology
Edited by H. Carty

Spiral CT of the Abdomen
Edited by F. Terrier, M. Grossholz, and C. Becker

Liver Malignancies
Diagnostic and Interventional Radiology
Edited by C. Bartolozzi and R. Lencioni

Medical Imaging of the Spleen
Edited by A. M. De Schepper and F. Vanhoenacker

Diagnostic Nuclear Medicine
Edited by C. Schiepers

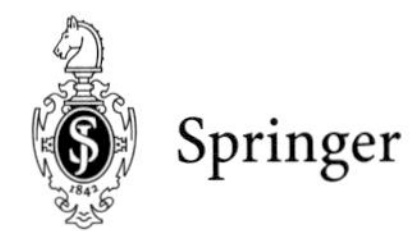

Medical Radiology
Diagnostic Imaging and Radiation Oncology

Titles in the series already published

Radiation Oncology

Lung Cancer
Edited by C.W. Scarantino

Innovations in Radiation Oncology
Edited by H.R. Withers
and L.J. Peters

Radiation Therapy of Head and Neck Cancer
Edited by G.E. Laramore

Gastrointestinal Cancer – Radiation Therapy
Edited by R.R. Dobelbower, Jr.

Radiation Exposure and Occupational Risks
Edited by E. Scherer, C. Streffer,
and K.-R. Trott

Radiation Therapy of Benign Diseases - A Clinical Guide
S.E. Order and S.S. Donaldson

Interventional Radiation Therapy Techniques - Brachytherapy
Edited by R. Sauer

Radiopathology of Organs and Tissues
Edited by E. Scherer,
C. Streffer, and K.-R. Trott

Concomitant Continuous Infusion Chemotherapy and Radiation
Edited by M. Rotman
and C.J. Rosenthal

Intraoperative Radiotherapy – Clinical Experiences and Results
Edited by F.A. Calvo,
M. Santos, and L.W. Brady

Radiotherapy of Intraocular and Orbital Tumors
Edited by W.E. Alberti
and R.H. Sagerman

Interstitial and Intracavitary Thermoradiotherapy
Edited by M.H. Seegenschmiedt
and R. Sauer

Non-Disseminated Breast Cancer
Controversial Issues
in Management
Edited by G.H. Fletcher
and S.H. Levitt

Current Topics in Clinical Radiobiology of Tumors
Edited by H.-P. Beck-Bornholdt

Practical Approaches to Cancer Invasion and Metastases
A Compendium of Radiation Oncologists' Responses to 40 Histories
Edited by A.R. Kagan with the
Assistance of R.J. Steckel

Radiation Therapy in Pediatric Oncology
Edited by J.R. Cassady

Radiation Therapy Physics
Edited by A.R. Smith

Late Sequelae in Oncology
Edited by J. Dunst and R. Sauer

Mediastinal Tumors. Update 1995
Edited by D.E. Wood
and C.R. Thomas, Jr.

Thermoradiotherapy and Thermochemotherapy

Volume 1:
Biology, Physiology, and Physics

Volume 2:
Clinical Applications
Edited by M.H. Seegenschmiedt,
P. Fessenden, and C.C. Vernon

Carcinoma of the Prostate
Innovations in Management
Edited by Z. Petrovich,
L. Baert, and L.W. Brady

Radiation Oncology of Gynecological Cancers
Edited by H.W. Vahrson

Carcinoma of the Bladder
Innovations in Management
Edited by Z. Petrovich,
L. Baert, and L.W. Brady

Blood Perfusion and Microenvironment of Human Tumors
Implications for Clinical Radiooncology
Edited by M. Molls and P. Vaupel

Radiation Therapy of Benign Diseases. A Clinical Guide
2nd Revised Edition
S.E. Order and S.S. Donaldson

Carcinoma of the Kidney and Testis, and Rare Urologic Malignancies
Innovations in Management
Edited by Z. Petrovich,
L. Baert, and L.W. Brady

Progress and Perspectives in the Treatment of Lung Cancer
Edited by P. Van Houtte, J. Klastersky,
and P. Rocmans

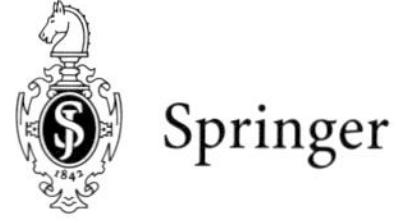

Springer

Printing and Binding: Stürtz AG, Würzburg